Video Atlas of Advanced Minimally Invasive Surgery

Video Atlas of Advanced Minimally Invasive Surgery

Constantine T. Frantzides, MD, PhD, FACS
Director
Advanced Laparoscopic and Bariatric Fellowship Program
Resurrection Health Care
St. Francis Hospital
Evanston, Illinois
Director
Chicago Institute of Minimally Invasive Surgery
Chicago, Illinois

Mark A. Carlson, MD, FACS
Professor
Department of Surgery
Department of Genetics, Cell Biology, and Anatomy
University of Nebraska Medical Center
VA Nebraska Western-Iowa Health Care System
Omaha, Nebraska

Illustrations by
DNA Illustrations, Inc.
Asheville, North Carolina

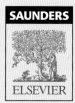

SAUNDERS

ELSEVIER

1600 John F. Kennedy Blvd.
Ste 1800
Philadelphia, PA 19103-2899

VIDEO ATLAS OF ADVANCED MINIMALLY INVASIVE SURGERY   ISBN: 978-1-4377-2723-4

Notices

Knowledge and best practice in this field are constantly changing. As new research and experience broaden our understanding, changes in research methods, professional practices, or medical treatment may become necessary.

   Practitioners and researchers must always rely on their own experience and knowledge in evaluating and using any information, methods, compounds, or experiments described herein. In using such information or methods they should be mindful of their own safety and the safety of others, including parties for whom they have a professional responsibility.

   With respect to any drug or pharmaceutical products identified, readers are advised to check the most current information provided (i) on procedures featured or (ii) by the manufacturer of each product to be administered, to verify the recommended dose or formula, the method and duration of administration, and contraindications. It is the responsibility of practitioners, relying on their own experience and knowledge of their patients, to make diagnoses, to determine dosages and the best treatment for each individual patient, and to take all appropriate safety precautions.

   To the fullest extent of the law, neither the Publisher nor the authors, contributors, or editors assume any liability for any injury and/or damage to persons or property as a matter of products liability, negligence or otherwise, or from any use or operation of any methods, products, instructions, or ideas contained in the material herein.

Library of Congress Cataloging-in-Publication Data

Video atlas of advanced minimally invasive surgery / [edited by] Constantine T. Frantzides, Mark A. Carlson.
      p. ; cm.
   Advanced minimally invasive surgery
   Companion vol. to: Atlas of minimally invasive surgery / [edited by] Constantine T. Frantzides, Mark A. Carlson. c2009.
   Includes bibliographical references and index.
   ISBN 978–1–4377–2723–4 (hardcover : alk. paper)
   I. Frantzides, Constantine T.   II. Carlson, Mark A.   III. Atlas of minimally invasive surgery.
IV. Title: Advanced minimally invasive surgery.
   [DNLM: 1. Surgical Procedures, Minimally Invasive—methods—Atlases.   2. Laparoscopy—methods—Atlases.   WO 517]
   LC classification not assigned
   617.5′507545—dc23   2012017972

Content Strategists: Judith Fletcher/Michael Houston
Content Development Specialist: Roxanne Halpine Ward
Publishing Services Manager: Patricia Tannian
Project Manager: Linda Van Pelt
Design Direction: Louis Forgione
Marketing Manager: Abigail Swartz

Printed in China

Last digit is the print number: 9   8   7   6   5   4   3   2   1

Dedication

To my wife, Lena, and my children, Marlena and Alexander

—**CF**

To my wife, Sarah; to my children, Kirsten, Ty, Trent, Blake, and Weston; and to my father and mother, Ken and Mary Jane Carlson

—**MC**

Contributors

Shahab F. Abdessalam, MD
Associate Professor of Surgery
Department of General Surgery
University of Nebraska Medical Center
Staff Surgeon
Department of Pediatric Surgery
Children's Hospital and Medical Center
Omaha, Nebraska

Nora Alghothani, MD
Fellow
The Ohio State University
Columbus, Ohio

Carlo Enrico Ambrosini, MD, PhD
Department of Surgery
University of Pisa
Pisa, Italy

Basil J. Ammori, FRCS, MD
Professor
Hepatobiliary and Bariatric Surgery
The University of Manchester
Consultant Laparoscopic and Bariatric Surgeon
Salford Royal Hospital
Consultant Hepatobiliary Surgeon
North Manchester General Hospital
Director
International Bariatric Centre of Excellence
Manchester, United Kingdom

Stavros A. Antoniou, MD
Surgical Fellow
Department of Visceral, Thoracic, and Vascular Surgery
Phillipps University Marburg
Surgical Fellow
Department of General and Visceral Surgery
Center of Minimally Invasive Surgery
Hospital Neuwerk
Mönchengladbach
Marburg, Germany

Georgios D. Ayiomamitis, MD, MSc, PhD
Consultant General Surgeon
Laparoscopic Surgeon
Second Surgical Department
Tzanio General Hospital
Piraeus, Attica, Greece
Member
Department of Advanced Minimally Invasive and Bariatric Surgery
Chicago Institute of Minimallly Invasive Surgery
Skokie, Illinois

Kenneth S. Azarow, MC, FACS, FAAP
Alton S. K. Wong Distinguished Professor of Surgery
Department of Surgery
University of Nebraska Medical Center
College of Medicine
Omaha, Nebraska

Paul R. Balash, MD
Resident
General Surgery
Rush University Medical Center
Chicago, Illinois

Jonathan W. Berlin, MD, MBA
Clinical Associate Professor of Radiology
The University of Chicago Pritzker School of Medicine
Chicago
Department of Diagnostic Radiology
NorthShore University HealthSystem
Evanston, Illinois

Jeffrey A. Blatnik, MD
Resident
General Surgery
University Hospitals Case Medical Center
Cleveland, Ohio

Robert E. S. Bowen, BA
Student Researcher
Center for Advanced Surgical Technology
University of Nebraska Medical Center
Omaha, Nebraska

Russell E. Brown, MD
Surgical Oncologist
Cancer Surgery of Mobile
Mobile Infirmary Medical Center
Mobile, Alabama

Mark A. Carlson, MD, FACS
Professor
Department of Surgery
Department of Genetics, Cell Biology, and Anatomy
University of Nebraska Medical Center
VA Nebraska Western-Iowa Health Care System
Omaha, Nebraska

Marco Casaccia, MD
Assistant Professor of Surgery
Department of General and Transplant Surgery
University of Genoa
San Martino Hospital
Genoa, Italy

Jovenel Cherenfant, MD
Endocrine Surgery Fellow
Department of Surgery
NorthShore University HealthSystem
Evanston, Illinois

Lawrence Crist, MD
Assistant Professor of Surgery
Department of Cardiothoracic Surgery
Division of Thoracic Surgery
University of Pittsburgh Medical Center
Pittsburgh, Pennsylvania

Robert A. Cusick, MD, FACS, FAAP
Associate Professor of Surgery
Division of Pediatric Surgery
University of Nebraska Medical Center
Division of Pediatric Surgery
Children's Hospital and Medical Center
Omaha, Nebraska

Celia M. Divino, MD, FACS
Professor
Department of Surgery
Mount Sinai School of Medicine
Chief
Division of General Surgery
Mount Sinai Hospital
New York, New York

Natalie Donn, MS
Research Assistant
Center for Outpatient Research Excellence
Tampa General Hospital
Tampa, Florida

George S. Ferzli, MD, FACS
Professor of Surgery
State University of New York Downstate Medical Center
College of Medicine
Chairman
Department of Surgery
Lutheran Medical Center
Brooklyn, New York

Alexander T. Frantzides
Member
Chicago Institute of Minimally Invasive Surgery
Skokie, Illinois

Constantine T. Frantzides, MD, PhD, FACS
Director
Advanced Laparoscopic and Bariatric Fellowship Program
Resurrection Health Care
St. Francis Hospital
Evanston, Illinois
Director
Chicago Institute of Minimally Invasive Surgery
Chicago, Illinois

Richard M. Gore, MD
Professor of Radiology
Department of Radiology
The University of Chicago Pritzker School of Medicine
Chicago, Illinois
Chief of Radiology
Department of Radiology
NorthShore University HealthSystem
Evanston, Illinois

Adam S. Gorra, MD
Pediatric Surgeon
Division of Pediatric Surgery
Children's Hospital Central California
Madera, California

Frank A. Granderath, MD
Medical Director
Department of General, Visceral and Minimally Invasive Surgery
Neuwerk Hospital
Moenchengladbach, Germany

Andrew A. Gumbs, MD, FACS
Director of Minimally Invasive Hepatic-Pancreatic-Biliary Surgery Program
Summit Medical Group
Department of Surgical Oncology
Berkeley Heights, New Jersey

Woong Kyu Han, MD, PhD
Assistant Professor
Urology
Yonsei University Health System
Urological Sciences Institute
Seoul, Republic of Korea

Oz Harmanli, MD
Associate Professor of Obstetrics and Gynecology
Director of Urogynecology and Pelvic Surgery
Department of Obstetrics and Gynecology
Tufts University School of Medicine
Baystate Medical Center
Springfield, Massachusetts

Eric S. Hungness, MD, FACS
Assistant Professor of Surgery
Department of Surgery
Feinberg School of Medicine
Northwestern University
Chicago, Illinois

Kris Jardon, MD
Associate Professor
Department of Obstetrics and Gynecology
Division of Gynecologic Oncology
McGill University Health Centre
Montreal, Quebec, Canada

Boris Kirshtein, MD
Senior Lecturer
Faculty of Health Sciences
Ben Gurion University of the Negev
Deputy Chief
Department of Surgery A
Soroka University Medical Center
Beer Sheva, Israel

Seigo Kitano, MD, PhD
President
Oita University
Yufu City, Oita, Japan

Yohei Kono, MD
Department of Gastroenterological Surgery
Oita University Faculty of Medicine
Yufu City, Oita, Japan

David M. Krpata, MD
Resident
General Surgery
University Hospitals Case Medical Center
Cleveland, Ohio

Rudy P. Lackner, MD, FACS
Professor
Department of Surgery
Division of Surgical Oncology
Chief
Section of Thoracic Surgery
University of Nebraska Medical Center
Omaha, Nebraska

Chad A. LaGrange, MD
Assistant Professor
Director of Minimally Invasive Urology
Division of Urology
University of Nebraska Medical Center
Omaha, Nebraska

Eric C. H. Lai, MBChB, MRCS(ed), FRACS
Clinical Assistant Professor (Honorary)
Surgery
The Chinese University of Hong Kong
Associate Consultant
Surgery
Pamela Youde Nethersole Eastern Hospital
Hong Kong SAR
Honorary Associate Professor
Eastern Hepatobiliary Surgery Hospital
Second Military Medical University
Shanghai, China

Stephanie Hiu Yan Lau, MBChB, MRCS(Ed)
Resident
Department of Surgery
Queen Elizabeth Hospital
Hong Kong, China

Wan Yee Lau, MD, FRACS(Hon)
Professor of Surgery
Faculty of Medicine
The Chinese University of Hong Kong
Master
Lee Woo Sing College
The Chinese University of Hong Kong
Shatin, New Territories
Hong Kong SAR

Bernard Lelong, MD
Department of Surgical and Digestive Oncology
Paoli Calmettes Institute
Comprehensive Anticancer Center
Marseilles, France

Marc S. Levine, MD
Professor of Radiology and Advisory Dean
Perelman School of Medicine at the University of Pennsylvania
Chief
Gastrointestinal Radiology Section
Department of Radiology
Hospital of the University of Pennsylvania
Philadelphia, Pennsylvania

Alessandro Loddo, MD
Dipartimento Chirugico, Materno Infantile e di Scienze delle immagini
Clinica Ginecologica, Ostetrica e di Fisiopatologia della Riproduzione Umana
University of Cagliari
Cagliari, Italy

Kenneth Luberice, BS
Clinical Research Data Coordinator
Center for Outpatient Research Excellence
Tampa General Hospital
Tampa, Florida

James D. Luketich, MD
Chairman and Henry T. Bahnson Professor of Cardiothoracic Surgery
Department of Cardiothoracic Surgery
University of Pittsburgh School of Medicine
Pittsburgh, Pennsylvania

Gauri Luthra, MD
Resident
Department of Obstetrics and Gynecology
Baystate Medical Center and Tufts University School of Medicine
Springfield, Massachusetts

Minh B. Luu, MD
Assistant Professor of Surgery
General Surgery
Rush University Medical Center
Chicago, Illinois

Robert C. G. Martin II, MD, PhD, FACS
Professor of Surgery
Academic Advisory Dean
Sam and Lolita Weakley Endowed Chair in Surgical Oncology
Director
Division of Surgical Oncology
Director
Upper GI and HPB Multi-Disciplinary Clinic
University of Louisville School of Medicine
Louisville, Kentucky

Gabriele Materazzi, MD
Researcher
Department of Surgery
University of Pisa
Pisa, Italy

Uday K. Mehta, MD
Associate Professor of Radiology
The University of Chicago Pritzker School of Medicine
NorthShore University HealthSystem
Chicago, Illinois

Paolo Miccoli, MD
Professor of Surgery
Head
Department of Surgery
University of Pisa
Pisa, Italy

Tricia Moo-Young, MD
Staff Surgeon
Department of Surgery
NorthShore University HealthSystem
Evanston, Illinois

Geraldine M. Newmark, MD
Clinical Assistant Professor of Radiology
Department of Radiology
NorthShore University HealthSystem
Evanston, Illinois

Scott Q. Nguyen, MD, FACS
Assistant Professor
Department of Surgery
Mount Sinai School of Medicine
New York, New York

Dmitry Oleynikov, MD, FACS
Professor of Surgery
General Surgery/Minimally Invasive Surgery
University of Nebraska Medical Center
Omaha, Nebraska

Pavlos Papavasiliou, MD
Department of Surgical Oncology
Fox Chase Cancer Center
Philadelphia, Pennsylvania

Sejal Dharia Patel, MD
Associate Professor
Department of Obstetrics and Gynecology
University of Central Florida College of Medicine
Partner
Center for Reproductive Medicine
Orlando, Florida

Harold Paul, MS
Clinical Research Data Coordinator
Center for Outpatient Research Excellence
Tampa General Hospital
Tampa, Florida

Rudolph Pointner, MD
Head
Department of General Surgery
General Public Hospital Zell am See
Zell am See, Austria

Andrew M. Popoff, MD
Resident
Department of Surgery
Rush University Medical Center
Chicago, Illinois

Richard A. Prinz, MD
Clinical Professor of Surgery
Department of Surgery
The University of Chicago Pritzker School of Medicine
Chicago, Illinois
Attending Physician
Vice Chairman
Department of Surgery
NorthShore University HealthSystem
Evanston, Illinois

Denis Querleu, MD
Professor and Chairman
Department of Obstetrics and Gynecology
McGill University
Montreal, Quebec, Canada
Professor and Head
Department of Surgery
Institut Claudius Regaud
Toulouse, France

Stephen C. Raynor, MD
Professor
Department of Surgery
University of Nebraska College of Medicine
Clinical Service Chief
Department of Pediatric Surgery
Children's Hospital and Medical Center
Omaha, Nebraska

Sean Rim, MD
Attending Surgeon
Department of Bariatric and Minimally Invasive Surgery
Lutheran Medical Center
Brooklyn, New York

Jacob E. Roberts, DO
Surgeon
Advanced Laparoscopic Surgical Associates
St. Mary Mercy Hospital
Livonia, Michigan

Alexander Rosemurgy, MD, FACS
Chief of General Surgery
Tampa General Medical Group
Tampa General Hospital
Tampa, Florida

Michael J. Rosen, MD, FACS
Associate Professor of Surgery
Department of Surgery
Case Western Reserve University School of Medicine
Chief
Division of Gastrointestinal and General Surgery
University Hospitals Case Medical Center
Cleveland, Ohio

Sharona Ross, MD, FACS
Assistant Professor of Surgery
Division of General Surgery
University of South Florida College of Medicine
General Surgeon
Tampa General Hospital
Tampa, Florida

Alfonso Rossetti, MD
Gynecological Endoscopic Division
Nuova Villa Claudia Hospital
Rome, Italy

Timothy M. Ruff, MD
Member
Advanced Minimally Invasive and Bariatric Surgery
Chicago Institute of Minimally Invasive Surgery
Skokie, Illinois

Jesse D. Sammon, DO
Vattikuti Urology Institute
Henry Ford Hospital
Detroit, Michigan

Elizabeth M. Schmidt, MD
General Surgeon
Union Associated Physicians Clinic
Terre Haute, Indiana

Norio Shiraishi, MD, PhD
Professor
Surgical Division
Center for Community Medicine
Oita University Faculty of Medicine
Yufu City, Oita, Japan

Veeraiah Siripurapu, MD
Department of Surgical Oncology
Fox Chase Cancer Center
Philadelphia, Pennsylvania

Ornella Sizzi, MD
Gynecological Endoscopic Division
Nuova Villa Claudia Hospital
Rome, Italy

Nathaniel J. Soper, MD
Loyal and Edith Davis Professor of Surgery
Chair
Department of Surgery
Northwestern University Feinberg School of Medicine
Surgeon-in-Chief
Northwestern Memorial Hospital
Chicago, Illinois

Charles R. St. Hill, MD
Fellow
Division of Surgical Oncology
Department of Surgery
University of Louisville
Louisville, Kentucky

Stephen E. Strup, MD
James F. Glenn Professor and Chief of Urology
Department of Surgery
University of Kentucky
Lexington, Kentucky

Kiran H. Thakrar, MD
Clinical Assistant Professor
Radiology
NorthShore University HealthSystem
Evanston, Illinois

Michael F. Timoney, MD
Associate Director of Surgery
Lutheran Medical Center
Brooklyn, New York

Quoc-Dien Trinh, MD, FRCSC
Co-Director
Cancer Prognostics and Health Outcomes Unity
University of Montreal Health Centre
Montreal, Quebec, Canada
Senior Fellow
Vattikuti Urology Institute
Henry Ford Health System
Detroit, Michigan

Tzu-Jung Tsai, MD
Koo Foundation Sun Yat-Sen Cancer Center
Department of Surgical Oncology
Taipei, Taiwan

Olga A. Tusheva, BS
Medical Student
University of Central Florida College of Medicine
Orlando, Florida

Michelle Vice, BS
Research Assistant
Center for Outpatient Research Excellence
Tampa General Hospital
Tampa, Florida

Benny Weksler, MD, FACS
Associate Professor of Cardiothoracic Surgery
Department of Cardiothoracic Surgery
University of Pittsburgh Medical Center
Pittsburgh, Pennsylvania

Scott N. Welle, DO, FACOS
Assistant Professor
School of Osteopathic Medicine in Arizona
A.T. Still University
Mesa, Arizona
Private Practice
Tucson Bariatrics
Tucson, Arizona
Member
Chicago Institute of Minimally Invasive Surgery
Chicago, Illinois

Dennis C. T. Wong, MBBS(Lond), MRSC(Ed), FRACS, FCSHK, FHKAM
Hon. Clinical Assistant Professor
Surgery
University of Hong Kong
Associate Consultant
Surgery
Pamela Youde Nethersole Eastern Hospital
Hong Kong, China

Shannon L. Wyszomierski, PhD
Scientific Grant Writer
Department of Cardiothoracic Surgery
University of Pittsburgh
Pittsburgh, Pennsylvania

Seung Choul Yang, MD, PhD
Professor
Department of Urology
Urological Science Institute
Yonsei University Health System
Seoul, Republic of Korea

Tallal M. Zeni, MD
Director
Minimally Invasive and Bariatric Surgery
Department of Surgery
St. Mary Mercy Hospital
Livonia, Michigan

Linda P. Zhang, MD
General Surgery Resident
Department of Surgery
Mount Sinai School of Medicine
New York, New York

John G. Zografakis, MD, FACS
Associate Professor of Surgery
Northeast Ohio Medical University
Rootstown, Ohio
Director
Bariatric Care Center
Director
Advanced Laparoscopic Surgical Services
Department of Surgery
Summa Akron City Hospital
Summa Health System
Division Chief
General Surgery
Department of Surgery
Summa Western Reserve Hospital
Akron, Ohio

Kevin C. Zorn, MDCM, FACS, FRCSC
Director of Robotic and Laparoscopic Surgery
Department of Surgery
Section of Urology
University of Montreal Hospital Centre
Montreal, Quebec, Canada

Preface

In the past 20 years, laparoscopy has invaded and conquered all bastions of open surgery. It is the first time in the history of surgery that such drastic and sweeping changes have occurred in such a short period of time. It is now inconceivable for any discipline of surgery not to offer the patient a minimally invasive approach. Furthermore, laparoscopic surgery has become a major component of the teaching of surgical residents. The era when surgeons and residents had to learn basic and advanced laparoscopic techniques through a weekend course is in the past. It is now expected that surgeons in training will be exposed to laparoscopy through their residency or specialized fellowship programs.

The metamorphosis of surgical techniques has prompted a change in the surgical treatise. Instead of the simple description of techniques by means of drawings, the addition of high-definition digital videography enabled by laparoscopy has created a combined instructional format. The 2009 *Atlas of Minimally Invasive Surgery* was the first multimedia surgical textbook to be published; this video/text *Atlas* contains all the commonly performed laparoscopic procedures in one presentation. The success of the 2009 *Atlas* prompted this 2013 *Video Atlas of Advanced Minimally Invasive Surgery*, which includes more complex and technically demanding procedures. Some of these procedures, such as laparoscopic esophagectomy, laparoscopic pancreatoduodenectomy, laparoscopic bariatric revisional surgery, and thoracoscopic pneumonectomy, are rare or performed only in specialized centers. Indeed, these procedures are expected to be performed by very experienced laparoscopic surgeons. However, a multitude of different techniques and procedures described in this *Video Atlas* can be employed by most surgeons. Such examples include cholecystectomy in the presence of cholecystitis, management of perforated peptic ulcer, small bowel resection, and repair of scrotal or parastomal hernias. Unlike the previous 2009 *Atlas*, which focused on general surgery, the present text includes other disciplines such as thoracic, gynecologic, urologic, and pediatric surgery. In addition, new approaches to minimally invasive surgery, such as single port, natural orifice transluminal endoscopic, robotic, and microrobotic surgery, are described. This *Video Atlas* combines the traditional illustrated textbook with edited and narrated videos of 62 procedures, available on DVD as well as on the book website at ExpertConsult.com.

We have made every effort to include world-renowned authorities on each subject covered in the *Video Atlas*. It is our hope that we managed to cover each topic in a concise yet informative format to contribute to the teaching of medical students, surgical residents, and surgeons.

Constantine T. Frantzides, MD, PhD, FACS
Mark A. Carlson, MD, FACS

Acknowledgments

The authors would like to acknowledge Teresa Wojtusiak for her indispensable editorial assistance and Dr. Timothy M. Ruff for the narration of the video portion of this atlas.

Contents

Video Contents

Thyroid Gland

PAOLO MICCOLI, CARLO ENRICO AMBROSINI, AND GABRIELE MATERAZZI

Minimally Invasive Video-Assisted Thyroidectomy

1

The videos associated with this chapter are listed in the Video Contents and can be found on the accompanying DVDs and *on Expertconsult.com.*

Video-assisted parathyroidectomy was the first minimally invasive procedure in the neck. Parathyroid adenomas are ideal for minimal access surgery because these tumors usually are benign and of small size. Various minimally invasive approaches soon thereafter were proved suitable for removing small thyroid nodules. In 1998, we began performing minimally invasive video-assisted thyroidectomy (MIVAT), which uses external retraction to create operative space in the neck. This approach to the thyroid resection has been used in our Department of Surgery on more than 3000 patients with results that rival those of traditional open resection. The main limitation to MIVAT is that only 10% to 30% of patients who need a thyroid resection fulfill the inclusion criteria for this procedure.

OPERATIVE INDICATIONS

The inclusion criteria and the main contraindications for MIVAT are summarized in Table 1-1. The main limiting factor is the size of both the nodule and the thyroid gland, as measured by preoperative ultrasonography. In geographic areas with endemic goiter, the gland volume can vary considerably compared with the nodule volume. Thus, if the gland was not adequately imaged before attempting MIVAT, there is increased risk for conversion to open thyroidectomy. Ultrasonography also may be useful to exclude thyroiditis, which can increase the difficulty of the dissection. If thyroiditis is suspected by ultrasonography, then serum autoantibodies should be determined. In general, thyroiditis by itself should not be an indication for MIVAT.

One of the most controversial operative indications for MIVAT is malignancy. Although low-risk papillary carcinoma (characterized by female sex, age <30 years, absence of distant metastasis, no extrathyroidal extension, and tumor dimension <2 cm) generally has been thought to be amenable to MIVAT, a careful evaluation for possible lymph node involvement in the neck has to be done in the thyroid cancer patient who is considered for this procedure. Great caution should be taken with disease metastatic to lymph nodes or with extracapsular invasion. In these cases, MIVAT may not allow for complete lymphadenectomy or for adequate excision of a mass infiltrating into the trachea or esophagus and therefore is not advisable. Accurate preoperative ultrasonography is paramount for the proper selection of a patient with thyroid cancer who may undergo MIVAT.

PREOPERATIVE EVALUATION, TESTING, AND PREPARATION

All patients should be rendered euthyroid before the procedure. Preoperative preparation of the patient with thyrotoxicosis is critical to avoid perioperative thyroid storm. During the informed consent process, the possibility of conversion to open surgery should be explained to the patient, particularly if the diagnosis is cancer. It is our opinion that in addition to neck ultrasonography, preoperative laryngoscopy should be performed in all patients undergoing thyroid surgery to identify asymptomatic vocal cord hypokinesia or palsy.

PATIENT POSITIONING

The operation is performed with the patient under general anesthesia; alternatively, a deep bilateral cervical block may be used. The patient is placed supine without neck hyperextension (Fig. 1-1). After aseptic preparation, the skin is protected with a transparent adhesive film (e.g., Tegaderm, 3M, St. Paul, Minn.) and then draped. The surgeon stands on the patient's right, the first assistant is opposite the surgeon on the left, the second assistant is at the head of the table, the camera operator is on the patient's left and caudal to the first assistant, and the scrub technician is on the right and caudal to the surgeon (Fig. 1-2). Two monitors, one facing the surgeon and the other facing the first assistant, are optimum. The basic instrumentation used for MIVAT is shown in Figure 1-3. Other helpful instruments include a suction dissector, thin ear forceps, vascular clip applier, and straight scissors.

OPERATIVE TECHNIQUE

Preparation of the Operative Space

A 1.5-cm horizontal skin incision is performed 2 cm above the sternal notch. Subcutaneous fat and platysma are carefully dissected to minimize bleeding. During this step of the procedure, the use of the insulated electrocautery blade (see Fig. 1-3) is preferred to avoid damage to the skin and the superficial planes. Two small retractors are used to expose the deep cervical fascia, which is incised in the vertical midline in a bloodless plane for 2 to 3 cm (Fig. 1-4). The thyroid lobe is then bluntly dissected from

Table 1-1 Indications and Contraindications for MIVAT

Indications	Contraindications
Benign disease*	Recurrent disease
Low risk papillary carcinoma	Locally advanced and/or metastatic carcinoma
Graves disease	Short neck in an obese patient

*Thyroid volume less than 25 mL and nodule diameter less than 3 cm.

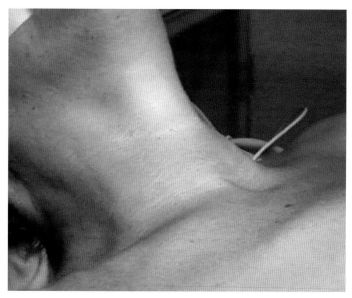

FIGURE 1-1 Patient positioning on the operating table for MIVAT. The neck is not extended.

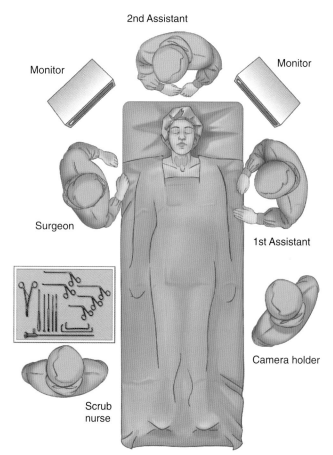

FIGURE 1-2 Operating team setup for MIVAT.

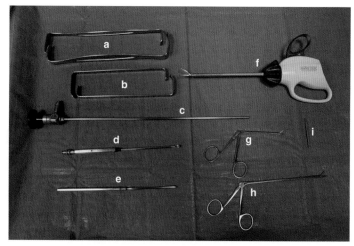

FIGURE 1-3 Basic instrument tray for MIVAT, including large double-ended retractor, Army-Navy-type (a); small double-ended retractor (length 12 cm) (b); forward-oblique endoscope, 30-degree viewing angle, diameter 5 mm, length 30 cm (c); aspirating spatula (d); dissecting spatula (e); ultrasonic scalpel (f); endoscopic scissors (g); endoscopic forceps (h); and insulated monopolar electrocautery tip (i).

the strap muscles using small spatulas (see Fig. 1-3) and gentle retraction. When the thyroid lobe is almost completely dissected from the strap muscles, larger double-ended retractors (Army-Navy type; see Fig. 1-3) can be inserted to maintain the operative space during the endoscopic portion of the procedure (Fig. 1-5). A 30-degree, 5-mm (or 7-mm) endoscope is then introduced through the skin incision to commence the endoscopic portion of the procedure (Fig. 1-6).

Ligation of the Main Thyroid Vessels

The thyrotracheal groove should be dissected under endoscopic vision with small (2-mm diameter) instruments, such as spatulas, forceps, spatula suckers, or scissors. Avoiding electrocautery is important at this point because both laryngeal nerves have not yet been identified. The ultrasonic scalpel may be used for almost all the vascular structures. If a vessel runs close to the inferior laryngeal nerve, then small vascular clips may be placed. The first major vessel to be ligated is the middle thyroid vein, if present (Fig. 1-7A); otherwise, the small veins running between the jugular vein and the lateral thyroid capsule are ligated first. During this step, the 30-degree endoscope is introduced from the lateral direction and is rotated to allow a posterior view. The middle thyroid vein is exposed with medial retraction of the thyroid lobe and lateral retraction of the jugular vein and strap muscles (Fig. 1-7B). This step permits subsequent dissection of the thyrotracheal groove, where the recurrent laryngeal nerve should reside. The inferior thyroid artery may be identified at this point (see Fig. 1-7B), but not yet ligated.

To visualize the upper pedicle, the 30-degree endoscope approaches inferiorly and parallel to the trachea and is rotated to provide an upward view. The upper pedicle is exposed with downward and medial retraction on the thyroid lobe, using the medial retractor and a spatula (Fig. 1-8). The lateral retractor is used to displace the strap muscles. A second spatula can be used to pull the vessels laterally, which should allow the external branch of the superior laryngeal nerve to be identified (see Fig. 1-8). Thermal injury to this nerve branch can be avoided by keeping the inactive blade of the ultrasonic scalpel posterior. The

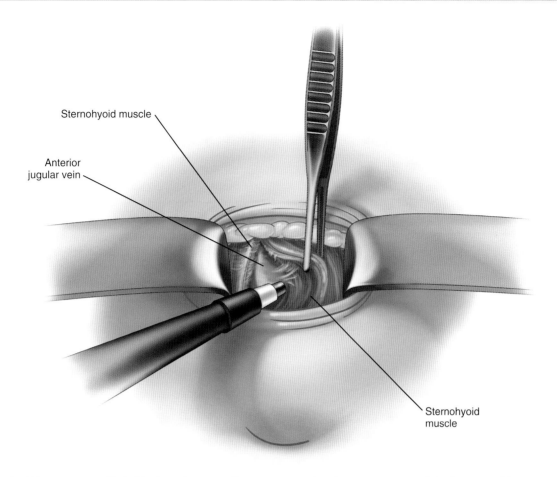

Sternohyoid muscle

Anterior jugular vein

Sternohyoid muscle

FIGURE 1-4 After the 1.5-cm transverse skin incision is made, two small retractors open the subcutaneous space, and the deep cervical fascia is opened vertically in the midline with electrocautery.

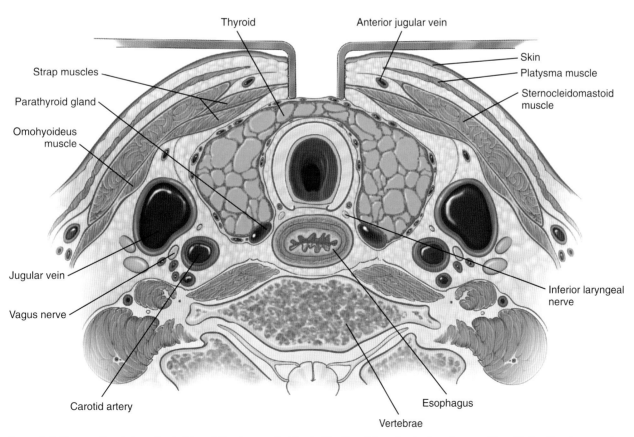

Thyroid

Anterior jugular vein

Strap muscles

Parathyroid gland

Omohyoideus muscle

Skin

Platysma muscle

Sternocleidomastoid muscle

Jugular vein

Vagus nerve

Inferior laryngeal nerve

Carotid artery

Esophagus

Vertebrae

FIGURE 1-5 Cross-sectional view after incision of the deep cervical fascia. The tips of the retractor have been positioned below the strap muscles.

upper pedicle vessels may be ligated individually or en masse with the ultrasonic scalpel (Fig. 1-9).

Identification of Recurrent Laryngeal Nerve and Parathyroid Glands

For this portion of the procedure, the 30-degree endoscope should approach from the lateral direction and look downward. The thyroid lobe is retracted medially and anteriorly. Using gentle blunt dissection, the recurrent laryngeal nerve may be identified in the thyrotracheal groove posterior to the Zuckerkandl tuberculum (Fig. 1-10). The latter is a posterior projection of the thyroid that, because it is present in most patients, may serve as a landmark to locate the recurrent laryngeal nerve. The nerve

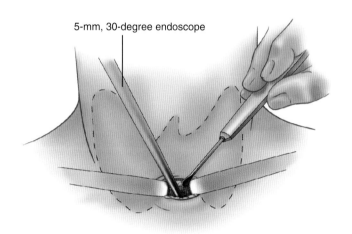

FIGURE 1-6 Insertion of the 30-degree, 5-mm endoscope through the cervical incision to visualize the MIVAT.

should be mobilized away from the thyroid capsule; however, dissection of the nerve from its mediastinal exit to its laryngeal entrance typically is not necessary.

The inferior and superior parathyroid glands also are identified and preserved at this time. The inferior gland has a variable location; inspection for this gland usually starts on the inferior posterolateral thyroid lobe. The color of the parathyroid glad is reddish brown or yellowish brown, distinguishing it from the surrounding fat. Once identified, the parathyroid gland is gently swept off the thyroid lobe, taking care to preserve the former's blood supply. If the inferior parathyroid gland is not found on the inferior posterolateral thyroid lobe, then the next most common location is inferior, along the thyrothymic ligament. The superior parathyroid gland has a more constant location, 1 to 2 cm superior to where the inferior thyroid artery enters the lobe. This gland also should be swept away gently from the thyroid lobe to preserve the gland's vasculature. Most of the blood supply to both parathyroid glands is from the inferior thyroid artery. The latter should be clipped and transected distal to the parathyroid branches.

Extraction of the Lobe

The endoscope and retractors are removed, and the upper portion of the gland is rotated and pulled out of the incision, using conventional forceps and gentle traction. After exteriorization of the lobe, the operation is completed under direct vision. The lobe is separated from the trachea by ligating small vessels and transecting the ligament of Berry. The integrity of the recurrent laryngeal nerve is rechecked at this time. The thyroid isthmus is dissected from the trachea and divided, and the specimen is removed. Drainage is not necessary. The deep cervical fascia is approximated with a single stitch. The platysma is approximated with a

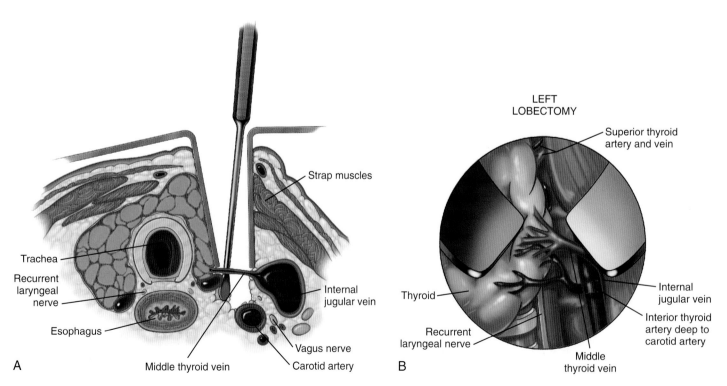

FIGURE 1-7 **A,** Cross-sectional view after the thyroid lobe has been dissected from the strap muscles (inferior perspective). The Army-Navy retractors have been positioned to expose the middle thyroid vein. **B,** Endoscopic view of the exposure of the middle thyroid vein (left side), which courses from the internal jugular vein to the thyroid lobe. The latter has been retracted medially and anteriorly. The inferior thyroid artery (originating from the thyrocervical trunk) can be seen emerging from underneath the carotid artery.

RIGHT
LOBECTOMY

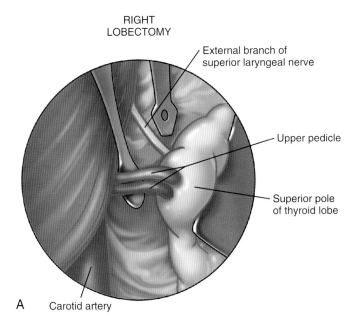

A   Carotid artery

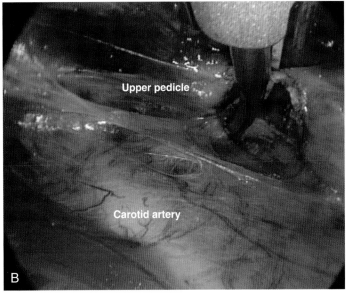

B

FIGURE 1-8 **A**, Endoscopic view of the upper pedicle dissection (right side) during MIVAT. The upper pedicle is exposed by retracting the thyroid lobe downward and medially with the retractor and spatula. The medial retractor is on the superior pole of the thyroid, and the lateral retractor (not shown) is on the strap muscles. Dissection here should reveal the external branch of the superior laryngeal nerve running superior and posterior to the upper pole vessels. **B**, Intraoperative photo of same.

subcuticular suture, and the skin is closed with cyanoacrylate sealant. If total thyroidectomy is the planned operation, the same procedure is then performed on the contralateral side.

POSTOPERATIVE CARE

Patients undergoing MIVAT require close observation during the first 5 to 10 hours after the procedure for dysphonia, airway obstruction, and neck swelling, particularly if neck drains are not used. The risk for postoperative bleeding is very low and decreases after 5 hours; therefore, we have our patients stay in bed for at least 5 to 6 hours. Oral feeding should be avoided during this observation period to decrease the risk for postoperative nausea and vomiting. If the procedure was done in the morning, then the patient may be fed in the evening. Serum calcium determination is followed for 1 to 2 days, particularly in the patient who

LEFT
LOBECTOMY

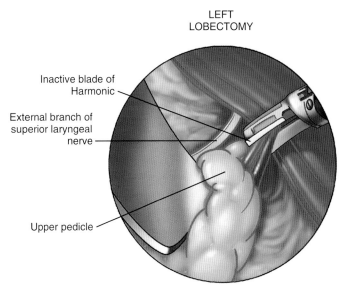

FIGURE 1-9 Endoscopic view of ligation of upper pole vessels (left side) with the ultrasonic scalpel during MIVAT. The inactive blade of the scalpel is directed posterior so as to minimize heat transmission to the external branch of the superior laryngeal nerve.

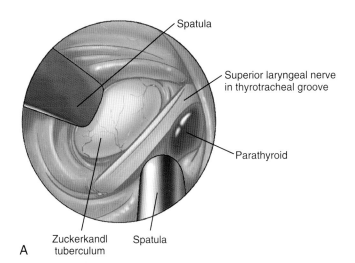

A

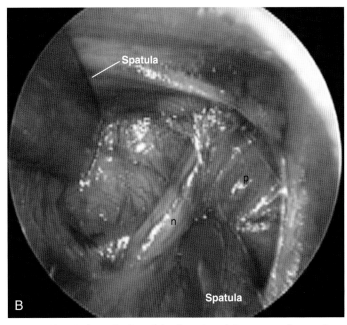

B

FIGURE 1-10 **A**, Endoscopic view of the dissection of the recurrent laryngeal nerve, occupying the thyrotracheal groove. **B**, Intraoperative photo of same. n, Nerve; p, pedicle.

Table 1-2 Management of Postoperative Hypocalcemia*

Acute symptomatic	Calcium gluconate IV
Asymptomatic, calcium ≤7.5† mg/dL	Elemental calcium‡ (3 g) + vitamin D (0.5 µg) PO daily
Asymptomatic, calcium 7.5-7.9 mg/dL	Elemental calcium (1.5 g) PO daily

*Management of hypocalcemia after thyroidectomy on the first postoperative day.
†Normal range, 8-10 mg/dL.
‡500 mg calcium carbonate = 200 mg elemental calcium.

has undergone a total thyroidectomy. Patients are discharged on the first postoperative day after the procedure and are allowed to return to normal activities. Replacement levothyroxine therapy may begin on discharge, especially in the case of total thyroidectomy. No wound care is required for the glue-sealed wound. Oral anti-inflammatory drugs may be prescribed in the postoperative period for pharyngodynia and cervical pain.

MANAGEMENT OF PROCEDURE-SPECIFIC COMPLICATIONS

If compressive symptoms and airway obstruction are present from a postoperative hematoma, then immediate hematoma evacuation is required. If the patient develops hypocalcemia from hypoparathyroidism, then treatment is instituted as described in Table 1-2. Voice impairments and subjective or objective dysphonia require an immediate postoperative vocal cord check by an otolaryngologist. For most patients with an unremarkable postoperative course, a vocal cord check usually is performed at 3 months.

RESULTS AND OUTCOME

Since developing our technique of MIVAT in June 1998, we have performed more than 3000 procedures. The mean patient age was 40.2 ± standard deviation 12.3 (range 8 to 85) years; the female-to-male ratio was 4:1. The ratio of total thyroidectomy to hemithyroidectomy was 3:1. Mean operative time was 31.1 (range 20 to 120) minutes for hemithyroidectomy and 41.1 (range 30 to 130) minutes for total thyroidectomy. Preoperative

diagnoses included follicular lesion, papillary carcinoma (low risk), toxic multinodular goiter, Graves disease, and familiar medullary carcinoma (a prophylactic operation for carriers of the RET mutation). Conversion from MIVAT to conventional technique was necessary in 2.5% of cases; causes of conversion included intraoperative bleeding, difficult dissection because of thyroiditis, and unexpected tracheal or esophageal invasion by carcinoma.

After 10 years of experience, the authors' complication rate for laryngeal nerve injury, hypoparathyroidism, and postoperative bleeding has been similar to that of conventional open thyroidectomy. Recent prospective randomized studies involving low-risk papillary carcinoma have demonstrated that MIVAT allows the same clearance at the thyroid bed level and the same outcome as the open technique. The main advantages of this minimally invasive technique over open thyroidectomy include less postoperative pain, faster postoperative recovery, and excellent cosmetic outcome.

Suggested Readings

Barczyński M, Konturek A, Cichoń S: Minimally invasive video-assisted thyroidectomy (MIVAT) with and without use of Harmonic scalpel—a randomized study, *Langenbecks Arch Surg* 393:647–654, 2008.

Del Rio P, Berti M, Sommaruga L, et al: Pain after minimally invasive videoassisted and after minimally invasive open thyroidectomy: Results of a prospective outcome study, *Langenbecks Arch Surg* 393:271–273, 2008.

Lombardi CP, Raffaelli M, D'alatri L, et al: Video-assisted thyroidectomy significantly reduces the risk of early postthyroidectomy voice and swallowing symptoms, *World J Surg* 32:693–700, 2008.

Miccoli P, Berti P, Ambrosini CE: Perspectives and lessons learned after a decade of minimally invasive video-assisted thyroidectomy, *ORL J Otorhinolaryngol Relat Spec* 70:282–286, 2008.

Miccoli P, Elisei R, Materazzi G, et al: Minimally invasive video assisted thyroidectomy for papillary carcinoma: A prospective study about its completeness, *Surgery* 132:1070–1074, 2002.

Miccoli P, Materazzi G: Minimally invasive video assisted thyroidectomy (MIVAT), *Surg Clin North Am* 84:735–741, 2004.

Miccoli P, Minuto MN, Ugolini C, et al: Minimally invasive video-assisted thyroidectomy for benign thyroid disease: An evidence-based review, *World J Surg* 32:1333–1340, 2008.

Miccoli P, Pinchera A, Materazzi G, et al: Surgical treatment of low- and intermediate-risk papillary thyroid cancer with minimally invasive video-assisted thyroidectomy, *J Clin Endocrinol Metab* 94:1618–1622, 2009.

Terris DJ, Angelos P, Steward DL, Simental AA: Minimally invasive video-assisted thyroidectomy: A multi-institutional North American experience, *Arch Otolaryngol Head Neck Surg* 134:81–84, 2008.

Thorax

Rudy P. Lackner

Thoracoscopic Lung Resections

2

The videos associated with this chapter are listed in the Video Contents and can be found on the accompanying DVDs and on Expertconsult.com.

Minimally invasive thoracic surgery was introduced almost 100 years ago, when Jacobeus first inserted a cystoscope into the pleural space. Indications for thoracoscopy at that time consisted of drainage of pleural effusion or tuberculous empyema. Another 80 years were to pass, however, before thoracic surgeons embraced video-assisted thoracic surgery (VATS) as their standard approach to intrathoracic disorders. Increasing numbers of pulmonary, esophageal, and mediastinal resections are performed by VATS, and most experts would consider this the optimal approach to the pleural space. As in general surgery, many procedures in thoracic surgery are labeled "minimally invasive" but in actuality are done through incisions larger than the typical trocar, using retractors to access the chest cavity. For the purposes of this chapter, a VATS lobectomy will be defined as one having no chest retractors placed and including individual ligation of the hilar structures.

OPERATIVE INDICATIONS

In patients undergoing thoracic surgical intervention, lung cancer is the most common indication for lobectomy. Other options for surgical resection include bilobectomy, pneumonectomy, and sleeve lobectomies. With the increased use of low-dose computed tomography (CT) scans for lung cancer screening, more subcentimeter lung cancers are being detected. This has stimulated discussion regarding the option of performing an anatomic segmentectomy to conserve lung function, while still achieving an acceptable oncologic resection. A nonanatomic wedge resection can be performed in high-risk patients with severely limited pulmonary function but generally is deemed a suboptimal cancer operation.

It is imperative that all cases of lung tumors be discussed at a multidisciplinary thoracic oncology conference to determine which treatment options are applicable for a given patient. Although surgery remains the best treatment option for patients with early-stage lung cancer, not all patients choose surgery or will be deemed suitable surgical candidates. In these patient groups, radiation therapy with or without chemotherapy will be the main alternative therapy offered. Radiofrequency ablation (RFA) is a newer modality available to treat pulmonary tumors. This modality is more applicable to patients with peripheral tumors and no associated adenopathy. This is due in part to a few case reports of fatal massive hemoptysis occurring a few days after RFA of more centrally located tumors.

Other, less common indications for lobectomy include carcinoids, mucoepidermoid tumors, adenoid cystic tumors, and sarcomas. Lobectomy also may be necessary to resect pulmonary metastases from other primary sites; however, if resectable, pulmonary metastases usually are treated with wedge resections. A lobectomy may be required to manage benign lung diseases that result from an underlying inflammatory or infectious etiology, such as an aspergilloma. These patients often are immunosuppressed and require resection due to the development of massive hemoptysis, bronchopleural and other fistulas, and empyema. Because of the presence of severe comorbidities, however, lobectomy for infectious etiology may be associated with high morbidity and mortality. In these situations, the use of antibiotics and antifungals, coupled with the use of percutaneously placed catheters or stents, may be used to temporize the patient until definitive surgical intervention can be accomplished with lower risk.

PREOPERATIVE EVALUATION, TESTING, AND PREPARATION

Patients scheduled to undergo a lobectomy should undergo a complete preoperative evaluation. Essential information regarding the patient's physiologic ability to safely undergo lobectomy will help risk-stratify the potential operative candidate. Pulmonary function testing should include a forced expiratory volume in 1 second (FEV_1), diffusion capacity of carbon monoxide (D_{LCO}), and arterial blood gas measurement. Patients determined to be marginal candidates based on the postoperative predicted values (e.g., FEV_1 <800 to 1000 cc and/or D_{LCO} <40% predicted) also may benefit from information provided by a quantitative perfusion scan or a cardiopulmonary exercise stress test, or both. Those patients still deemed at high risk after obtaining these tests may be better served by a sublobar resection or nonoperative therapy. Because cardiovascular disease may coexist in this patient population, additional cardiac evaluation also may be obtained, as indicated by the history and physical examination.

Staging

At a minimum, all patients in whom an anatomic lung resection is planned need to have a dedicated CT scan of the chest that includes the liver and adrenal glands. When available, a positron emission tomography (PET) scan will assist with the staging of patients undergoing lobectomy for cancer. The patient with no evidence of enlarged mediastinal lymph nodes on a CT scan and a PET scan typically does not require further evaluation. A patient with enlarged nodes or positive nodes on a PET scan requires invasive staging of the mediastinum before the planned resection. Staging of the mediastinum can be done by endobronchial ultrasound (EBUS), esophageal ultrasound (EUS), cervical mediastinoscopy, a Chamberlain procedure, or VATS. Those found to have mediastinal lymph involvement often require a multimodality approach to treat their cancer. Based on careful history and physical examination, a CT scan, brain magnetic resonance imaging (MRI), or a bone scan also may be helpful in staging the patient.

PATIENT POSITIONING IN THE OPERATING SUITE

A multitude of options are available for performing minimally invasive thoracic surgery. Although most complex procedures are performed using general anesthesia and a double-lumen endotracheal tube to achieve single-lung ventilation, simple diagnostic procedures can be performed using local anesthetics, with the patient awake and spontaneously breathing. Most of these will be done through a single port site, but additional instruments can be added if required.

Depending on the surgeon's preference, patients undergoing a VATS lobectomy may have a thoracic epidural placed by the anesthesia pain service to manage postoperative pain. Other options include the use of local anesthesia, administered by injection or an indwelling catheter. This is usually combined with some type of patient-controlled analgesia. Once adequate general anesthesia is obtained, a double-lumen endotracheal tube or a bronchial blocker is placed to obtain selective single-lung ventilation. In some cases, mainstem bronchial placement of a single-lumen endotracheal tube can be used, but this typically is not ideal management of the airway. Bronchoscopy should be performed routinely in all patients before an anatomic lung resection, both to assess for endobronchial disease and to confirm placement of the tube. This can be done through a single-lumen tube before the placement of the double-lumen tube.

Monitoring devices are placed at the discretion of the anesthesiologist but usually include an arterial line and one or two peripheral large-bore intravenous catheters. Central venous catheters are not mandatory in all patients undergoing lobectomy but may be helpful in selected higher-risk patients. In patients deemed to be at a higher cardiac risk, transesophageal echocardiography also can be used for real-time cardiac monitoring. An indwelling bladder catheter should be placed after the induction of anesthesia and usually will remain in place as long as the epidural is present, but it can be removed earlier in patients with other pain management strategies. Because many lobectomy patients are operated on for cancer or have multiple comorbidities, deep venous thrombosis prophylaxis (e.g., heparin or lower extremity sequential compression devices) should be used.

A VATS lobectomy most commonly is performed with the patient in the lateral decubitus position. The position can be maintained with the use of a surgical bean bag or blankets. Placement of an axillary roll is mandatory. The head should be supported so that the cervical spine is in a neutral position. The upper arm may be supported with blankets or an arm holder. The

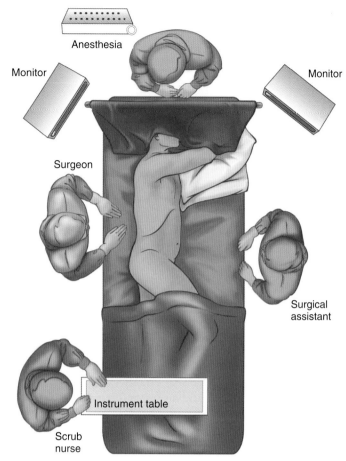

FIGURE 2-1 Patient and operating team positioning for a VATS lobectomy (right-sided procedure shown).

lower arm and both legs need to be carefully cushioned to prevent peripheral nerve injury. Once the patient is securely positioned, a body warming device should be placed.

POSITIONING AND PLACEMENT OF TROCARS

With the patient in the lateral decubitus position (Fig. 2-1), the initial port site is in the seventh or eighth intercostal space at the midaxillary line (Fig. 2-2). This port will be used for the camera in most cases; ideally, the port will be just above the level of the diaphragm. This corresponds to point A in Figure 2-2. In general, the greater the body mass index (BMI) of the patient, the higher the level of the diaphragm; this requires cephalad movement of the camera site so that the diaphragm does not impair thoracoscopic visualization. The diaphragmatic position can be determined by reviewing the preoperative chest radiograph. This port site should be created under direct visualization to avoid passing through the intercostal space and diaphragm simultaneously, which would result in intra-abdominal camera placement.

Before placing the camera port, digital examination of the pleural space should be performed to assess for the presence of adhesions or even pleural tumor implants. Many of these adhesions can be cleared by digital sweeping, but denser adhesions may need sharp dissection. Once there is an adequate space to insert the thoracoscope, the pleural space can undergo further evaluation. Because there is no need for insufflation, a simple reusable port typically is sufficient. A 30-degree scope provides excellent visualization of the upper mediastinum, the subcarinal area, the diaphragm, and the pericardium. Two additional port

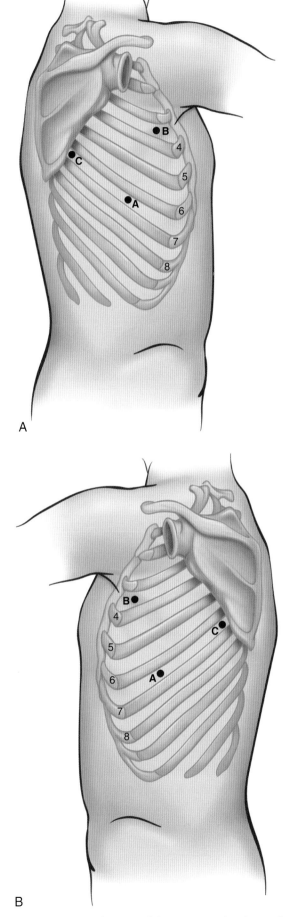

FIGURE 2-2 Port positions for a VATS lobectomy. **A,** Right side. **B,** Left side.

sites are placed under direct vision. The anterior port site (point B in Fig. 2-2) is placed in the fourth intercostal space when an upper lobectomy is planned, whereas the fifth intercostal space is used for a middle or lower lobectomy. The third (posterior) port is placed in the seventh intercostal space, anterior to the scapular edge (point C in Fig. 2-2). Unsuspected pleural metastases can be resected for biopsy if they are identified, and any adhesions are lysed at this time.

OPERATIVE TECHNIQUE

Right Upper Lobectomy

After placement of the ports, the lung is retracted anteriorly. The pleura along the posterior aspect of the hilum is opened with the electrocautery device. With gentle blunt dissection, the confluence of the right upper lobe bronchus and the bronchus intermedius is identified (Fig. 2-3). There usually is a lymph node located at this bifurcation. Clearing this area at the beginning of the operation will expedite completion of the fissure later in the procedure. The lung then is retracted posteriorly. The pleura on the anterior aspect of the hilum is opened with the cautery. The location of the phrenic nerve needs to be monitored at all times during the dissection of the anterior hilum. Clearing this portion of the pleura will identify the trunks of the superior pulmonary vein, which drain the right upper and right middle lobes. This dissection also will demarcate the fissure between the right upper lobe and right middle lobe. In some patients, a branch of the right middle lobe vein crosses the fissure and drains into the posterior segment vein. Whenever possible, this crossing branch should be spared, taking the upper lobe vein proximal to this branch.

The upper lobe vein is isolated by a combination of blunt and sharp dissection (Fig. 2-4). A large, blunt right-angle clamp can be used to clear the soft tissue behind the vein. This must be done carefully because the pulmonary artery is located immediately behind the vein. The vein then is divided with the vascular stapler. One option for positioning the stapler is to place a red rubber catheter on the stapling device to guide the blade behind the vein. Placement of the stapler blade behind the vein also can be facilitated with the use of a large right-angle clamp.

Division of the vein exposes the right pulmonary artery (Fig. 2-5). There usually is a single large arterial branch that supplies the upper lobe, although occasionally there will be two to three smaller branches. The right upper lobe pulmonary artery branch, once cleared, is divided with the stapling device. At this point there usually are two remaining structures to be divided: (1) the branch of the pulmonary artery supplying the posterior segment of the right upper lobe, and (2) the bronchus. It often is easier to clear the bronchus and divide this structure before stapling the posterior segment branch of the pulmonary artery (Fig. 2-6). Alternatively, depending on how complete the fissure is between the right upper and lower lobes, the remaining arterial branch can be divided first, followed by the bronchus. It is imperative to ensure correct placement of the stapler across the upper lobe bronchus by ventilating the middle and lower lobes before firing the stapler. After division of all hilar structures, the fissures can be completed with a laparoscopic stapler-cutter (e.g., Endo GIA, Covidien, Norwalk, Conn).

An alternative approach to right upper lobectomy is to approach the hilum from the posterior aspect. In this case, the right upper lobe bronchus is the first structure to be divided. Care must be taken when dissecting around the bronchus because the

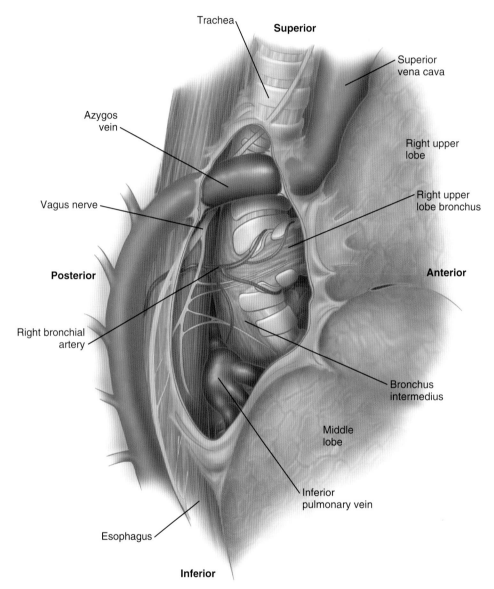

Trachea

Superior

Superior
vena cava

Azygos
vein

Right upper
lobe

Right upper
lobe bronchus

Vagus nerve

Posterior

Anterior

Right bronchial
artery

Bronchus
intermedius

Middle
lobe

Inferior
pulmonary vein

Esophagus

Inferior

FIGURE 2-3 Exposure of posterior hilum during a VATS right upper lobectomy.

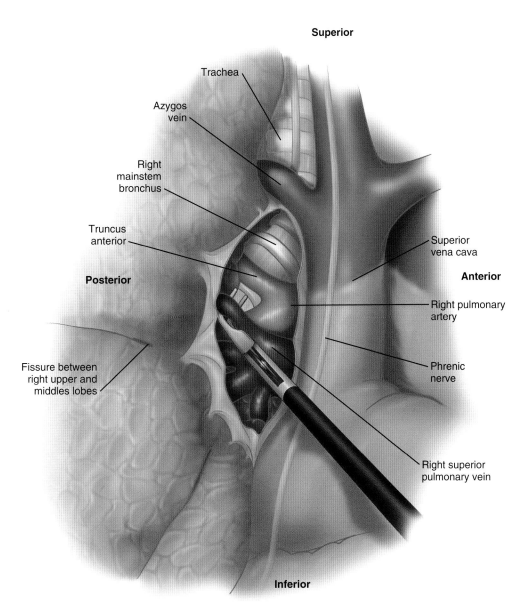

Superior

Trachea

Azygos vein

Right mainstem bronchus

Truncus anterior

Posterior

Superior vena cava

Anterior

Right pulmonary artery

Fissure between right upper and middles lobes

Phrenic nerve

Right superior pulmonary vein

Inferior

FIGURE 2-4 Exposure of the anterior hilum, with dissection of the right superior pulmonary vein (VATS RUL).

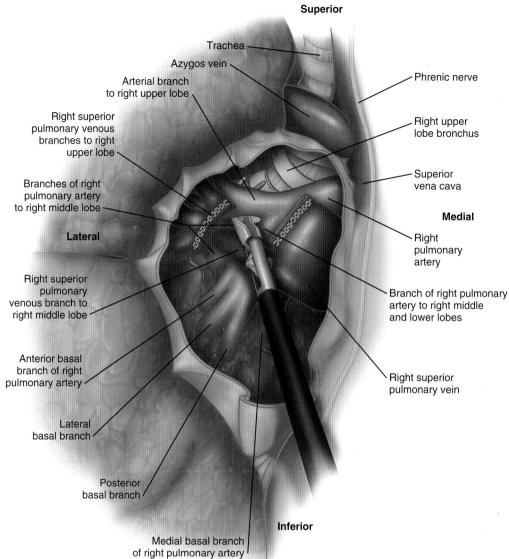

Superior

Trachea

Azygos vein

Arterial branch
to right upper lobe

Phrenic nerve

Right superior
pulmonary venous
branches to right
upper lobe

Right upper
lobe bronchus

Superior
vena cava

Branches of right
pulmonary artery
to right middle lobe

Medial

Lateral

Right
pulmonary
artery

Right superior
pulmonary
venous branch to
right middle lobe

Branch of right pulmonary
artery to right middle
and lower lobes

Right superior
pulmonary vein

Anterior basal
branch of right
pulmonary artery

Lateral
basal branch

Posterior
basal branch

Inferior

Medial basal branch
of right pulmonary artery

FIGURE 2-5 Dissection of pulmonary artery branch to the right upper lobe (VATS RUL).

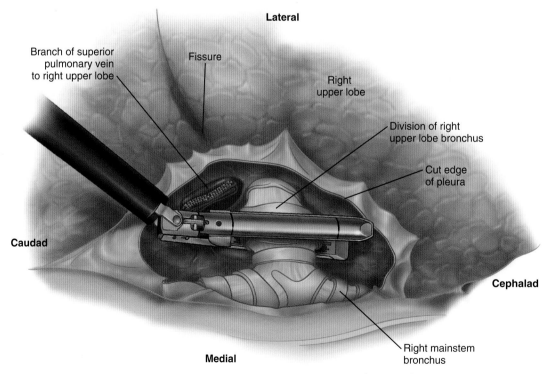

Lateral

Branch of superior
pulmonary vein
to right upper lobe

Fissure

Right
upper lobe

Division of right
upper lobe bronchus

Cut edge
of pleura

Caudad

Cephalad

Medial

Right mainstem
bronchus

FIGURE 2-6 Division of the right upper lobe bronchus (VATS RUL).

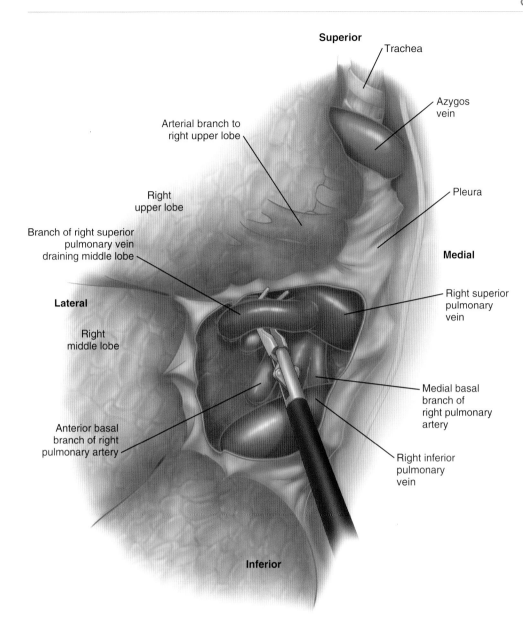

Superior

Trachea

Azygos vein

Arterial branch to right upper lobe

Pleura

Right upper lobe

Medial

Branch of right superior pulmonary vein draining middle lobe

Right superior pulmonary vein

Lateral

Right middle lobe

Medial basal branch of right pulmonary artery

Anterior basal branch of right pulmonary artery

Right inferior pulmonary vein

Inferior

FIGURE 2-7 Exposure of the anterior hilum, with dissection of the pulmonary vein branch to the right middle lobe (VATS right middle lobectomy).

pulmonary artery branch to the upper lobe may not be visible from this approach. Division of the bronchus will expose the posterior segment branch of the artery, which can be divided, and then followed by division of the larger, proximal branch. The right upper lobe vein branch is divided last.

In most patients, the fissure between the right upper and middle lobes is incomplete. In contrast, the fissure between the middle and lower lobes is relatively complete. Once the right upper lobe is removed, the middle lobe can twist on its pedicle. To prevent the disastrous complication of right middle lobe torsion, we routinely staple the middle lobe to the lower lobe after inflation.

Right Middle Lobectomy

The dissection is begun in the anterior hilum. The pleura is opened to identify the pulmonary vein branch draining the middle lobe (Fig. 2-7). Typically, this joins with the upper lobe vein to become the superior pulmonary vein. Less commonly, it drains directly into the left atrium or becomes part of the inferior pulmonary vein. Once isolated, the middle lobar vein is stapled to expose the bronchus (Fig. 2-8). At this point, the dissection can follow one of two paths. Dissection can proceed around the

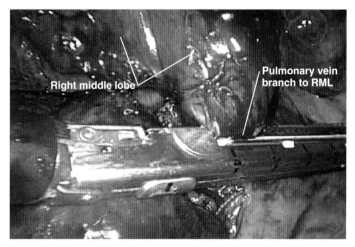

Right middle lobe

Pulmonary vein branch to RML

FIGURE 2-8 Division of the pulmonary vein branch to the right middle lobe (VATS RML).

right middle bronchus, taking care to avoid the pulmonary artery branches supplying the middle lobe. If the bronchus is taken first, then the middle lobe pulmonary artery branches will be immediately visible. Depending on the exposure, the arterial branches can be taken first (Fig. 2-9), and then the fissure between the

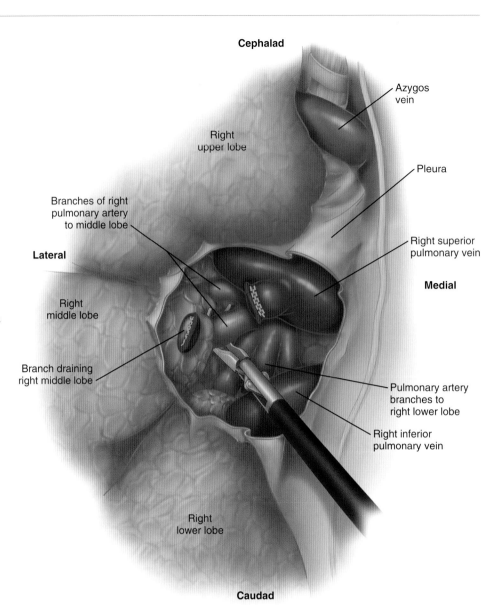

Cephalad

Azygos vein

Right upper lobe

Pleura

Branches of right pulmonary artery to middle lobe

Lateral

Right superior pulmonary vein

Medial

Right middle lobe

Branch draining right middle lobe

Pulmonary artery branches to right lower lobe

Right inferior pulmonary vein

Right lower lobe

Caudad

FIGURE 2-9 Dissection of pulmonary artery branches to the right middle lobe (VATS RML).

upper and middle lobes can be completed. This avoids undue traction on the pulmonary artery and minimizes the risk for avulsing the branches off the main pulmonary artery trunk.

Alternatively, the pulmonary artery may be traced proximally after dividing the vein, which allows identification of single or dual segmental branches supplying the right middle lobe. Depending on the anatomy, the branches can be divided simultaneously or sequentially. The right middle lobe bronchus then will be the last hilar structure divided (Figs. 2-10 and 2-11), and completion of the fissure will follow the bronchus division. Again, correct placement of the stapling device is ensured by ventilation of the upper and lower lobes before firing the stapler.

Right Lower Lobectomy

Retracting the lung superiorly allows division of the pulmonary ligament up to the level of the inferior pulmonary vein (Fig. 2-12). This pleural dissection is continued posteriorly to the takeoff of the right upper lobe bronchus; this maneuver facilitates completion of the fissure later in the procedure. The lung then is shifted posteriorly, allowing exposure of the anterior aspect of the inferior pulmonary vein. As described previously, the fissure then can be completed between the middle and lower lobes, allowing

for identification of the lower lobe pulmonary artery branches. The superior segment and basilar segment arterial branches can be isolated and divided individually or together. The camera is moved to the anterior port site, and the vascular stapling device is introduced from the inferior port to give the best angle of attack for division of the arterial branches (Figs. 2-13 and 2-14).

After the arterial divisions, the lung is retracted toward the head, allowing for isolation of the inferior pulmonary vein (Fig. 2-15). The stapling device is introduced from the anterior port site, and the inferior pulmonary vein is divided (Fig. 2-16). The lower lobe bronchus then is cleared up to the level of the right middle lobe bronchus. After confirming ventilation to the middle and upper lobes, the bronchus is stapled (Fig. 2-17), completing the dissection.

Left Upper Lobectomy

The arterial anatomy of the left upper lobe is the most variable of the pulmonary lobes, having from three to seven separate branches. The dissection begins anteriorly to identify the confluence of the superior and inferior branches of pulmonary vein. The superior pulmonary vein branch can be isolated and divided at this time (Figs. 2-18 and 2-19). With the vein out of the way,

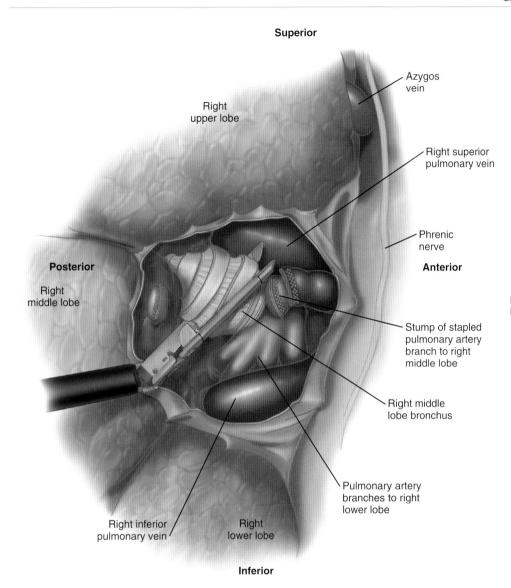

Superior

Azygos
vein

Right
upper lobe

Right superior
pulmonary vein

Phrenic
nerve

Posterior

Anterior

Right
middle lobe

Stump of stapled
pulmonary artery
branch to right
middle lobe

FIGURE 2-10 Division of the right middle lobe
bronchus (VATS RML).

Right middle
lobe bronchus

Pulmonary artery
branches to right
lower lobe

Right inferior
pulmonary vein

Right
lower lobe

Inferior

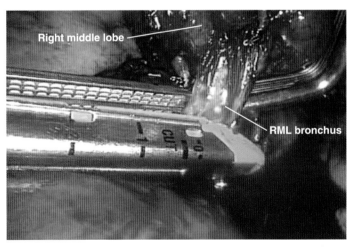

Right middle lobe

RML bronchus

FIGURE 2-11 Use of a right-angle clamp to guide the stapler across the right middle lobe bronchus (VATS RML).

the fissure can be completed with either gentle blunt dissection or electrocautery. The lingular branches of the pulmonary artery will be the first branches of this artery to be identified, followed by the upper lobe branches. Once the superior segment branch to the lower lobe is identified, an incomplete fissure can be completed with the use of the stapling device. While the fissure is

incomplete, however, the lung can be retracted anteriorly to open the pleura along the posterior aspect of the hilum. This helps identify the pulmonary artery branch to the superior segment of the lower lobe. Using this anatomic landmark, an opening above the artery can be created to place the stapler safely and complete the fissure. This should be done by retracting the lung posteriorly and working with the artery in direct view.

With the fissure completed, all of the arterial branches are sequentially divided, working from the more distal lingular branches to the more proximal upper lobe branches (Fig. 2-20). Unlike the right upper lobe arterial branch, which is anterior to the bronchus, the first upper lobe branch of the left pulmonary artery lies directly superior to the bronchus, which often limits the view of this arterial branch. If this is the only remaining arterial branch to the left upper lobe, then division of the bronchus before the division of this last arterial branch may enhance access for stapler placement (Figs. 2-21 and 2-22). Care should be exercised during dissection between the superior aspect of the left upper bronchus and the associated arterial branch. For this dissection, the camera can be moved from the inferior port to the anterior port, allowing better visualization of the superior aspect of the hilum. The stapling device then can be introduced from the inferior port, approaching the artery from the anterior aspect of the hilum.

Text continued on page 24.

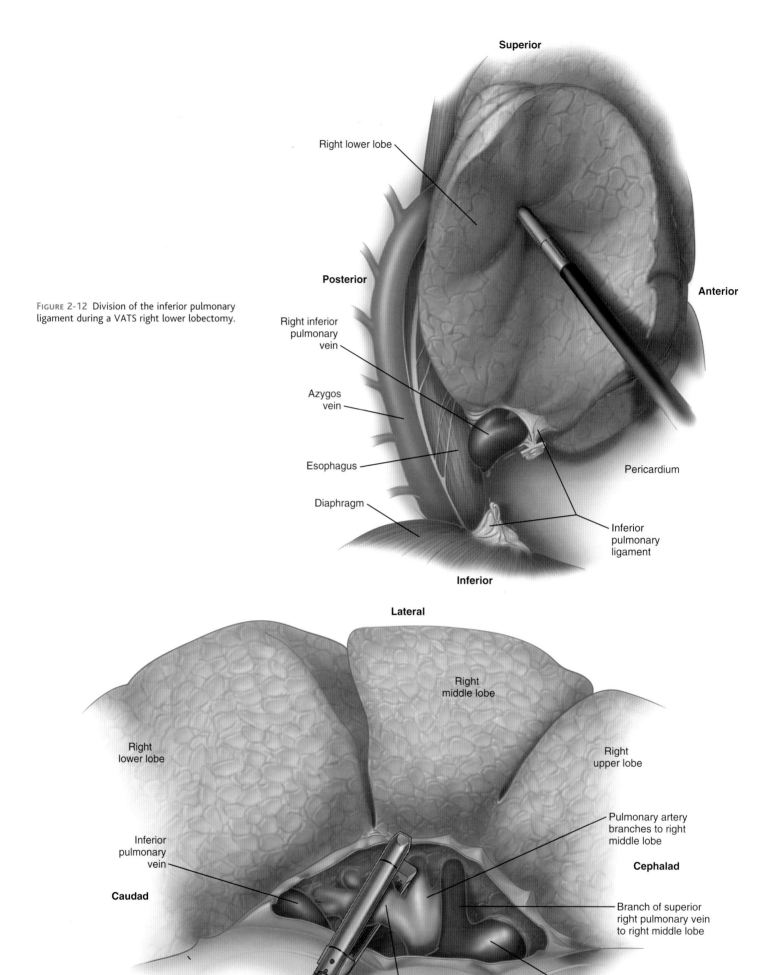

Superior

Right lower lobe

Posterior

Anterior

FIGURE 2-12 Division of the inferior pulmonary ligament during a VATS right lower lobectomy.

Right inferior pulmonary vein

Azygos vein

Esophagus

Diaphragm

Pericardium

Inferior pulmonary ligament

Inferior

Lateral

Right middle lobe

Right lower lobe

Right upper lobe

Pulmonary artery branches to right middle lobe

Inferior pulmonary vein

Cephalad

Caudad

Branch of superior right pulmonary vein to right middle lobe

Superior pulmonary vein

Pulmonary artery branch to right lower lobe

Medial

FIGURE 2-13 Exposure of the anterior hilum, with division of pulmonary artery branches to the right lower lobe (VATS RLL).

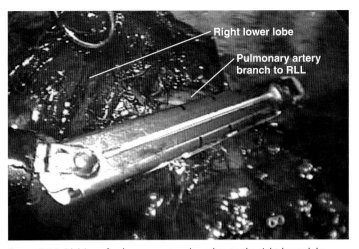

FIGURE 2-14 Division of pulmonary artery branches to the right lower lobe (VATS RLL).

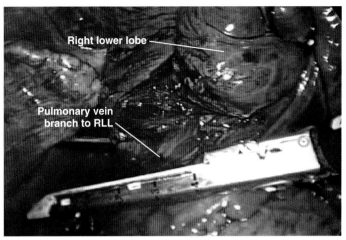

FIGURE 2-16 Division of the pulmonary vein branch to the right lower lobe (VATS RLL).

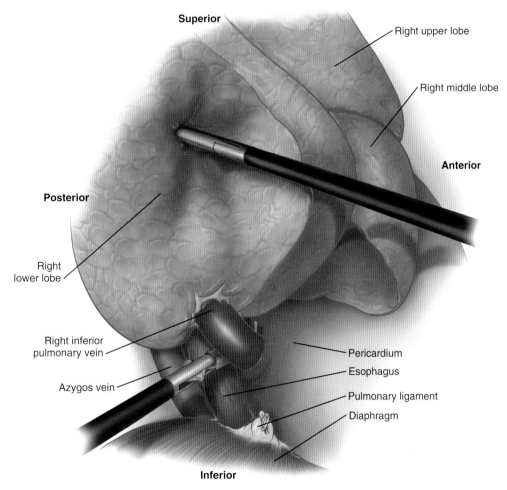

FIGURE 2-15 Dissection of the pulmonary vein branch to the right lower lobe (VATS RLL).

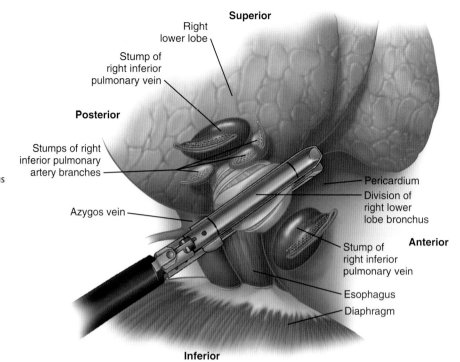

FIGURE 2-17 Division of the right lower lobe bronchus (VAT RLL).

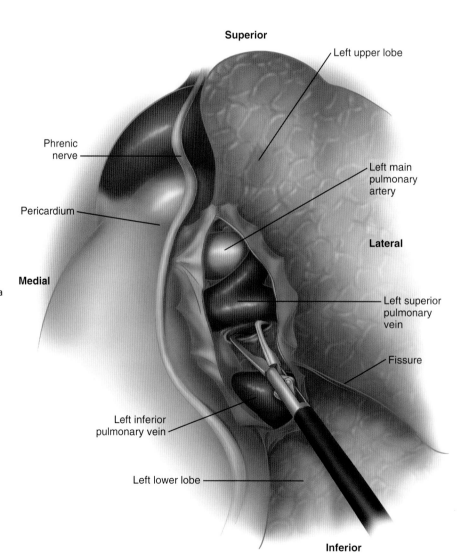

FIGURE 2-18 Exposure of the anterior hilum, with dissection of the left superior pulmonary vein during a VATS left upper lobectomy.

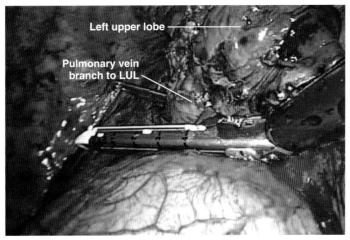

FIGURE 2-19 Division of left superior pulmonary vein during a left upper lobectomy (VATS LUL).

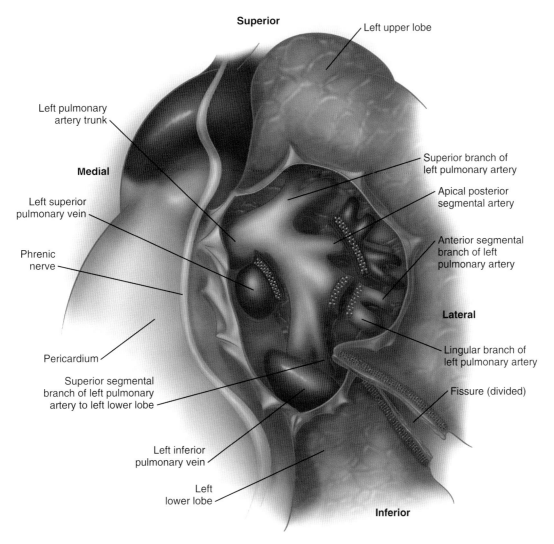

FIGURE 2-20 Division of the pulmonary artery branches to the left upper lobe (VATS LUL).

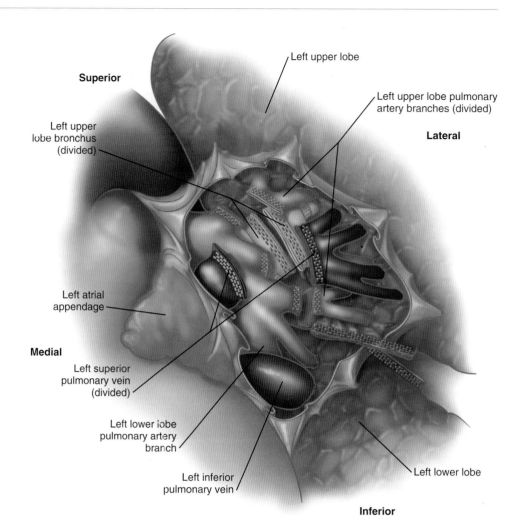

FIGURE 2-21 Division of the left upper lobe bronchus (VATS LUL).

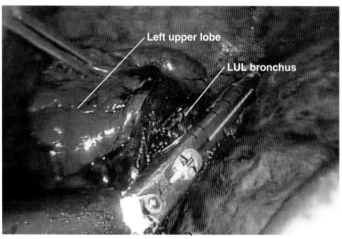

FIGURE 2-22 Division of the left upper lobe bronchus (VATS LUL).

Left Lower Lobectomy

Similar to a right lower lobectomy, the pulmonary ligament is divided up to the inferior pulmonary vein (Fig. 2-23), and the dissection is continued along the anterior and posterior aspects of the hilum. Coming across the fissure from the anterior aspect allows isolation of the two left lower lobe pulmonary arterial branches (Fig. 2-24). Division of these branches may be accomplished simultaneously or sequentially. With the arterial branches

transected, an incomplete fissure can be completed with the stapling device. Retracting the lower lobe toward the head allows for exposure of the left inferior pulmonary vein (Figs. 2-25 and 2-26). For both lower lobes, the stapler typically is introduced from the anterior port. With all of the vascular structures divided, the soft tissue around the bronchus is cleared to the level of the left upper bronchus, and the left lower bronchus then is divided with the stapler (Figs. 2-27 and 2-28).

Specimen Removal

After completion of the lobectomy, the skin incision of the anterior port site is slightly enlarged, and the underlying intercostal muscle is opened to a greater extent. A 15-mm specimen retrieval bag then is used to extract the lobe. This may require a fair amount of circumferential maneuvering to extricate the lobe. Grasping an edge of the lobe inside the bag with a sponge stick can establish a leading point, facilitating specimen removal.

Mediastinal Lymph Node Dissection

Preferably, a formal mediastinal node dissection is performed in all patients undergoing a lobectomy for cancer. Alternatively, a systematic nodal sampling may be performed. At a minimum, lymph node stations 2R, 4R, 7, 9, and 10R should be evaluated on the right side, and levels 5, 6, 7, 9, and 10L should be evaluated on the left side (see Fig. 2-29 for a map of lymph node stations).

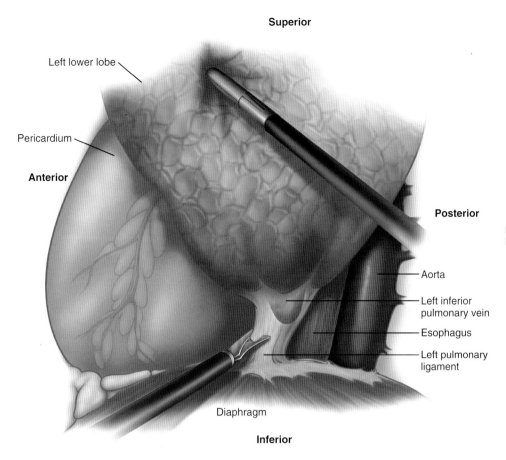

Superior

Left lower lobe

Pericardium

Anterior

Posterior

FIGURE 2-23 Division of the inferior pulmonary ligament during a VATS left lower lobectomy.

Aorta

Left inferior pulmonary vein

Esophagus

Left pulmonary ligament

Diaphragm

Inferior

After a right lobectomy, the lung is retracted anteriorly. Starting at the level of the pulmonary ligament and working up to the carina, all of the lymphatic tissue is cleared along the esophagus and bronchus. This dissection can be performed using a combination of sharp and blunt dissection. The L-hook cautery may be used, taking care to stay off the bronchus so that airway injury is avoided. The upper aspect of the dissection is started by retracting the upper lobe toward the diaphragm. The pleura overlying the azygos vein is opened, and dissection is continued along the superior vena cava toward the thoracic inlet. The vagus nerve at this level is preserved by gentle posterior retraction. All of the lymphatic tissue below the azygos vein and between the trachea and superior vena cava should be removed.

On the left side, the lymphatic tissue in the aortopulmonary window and anterior mediastinum should be included. The phrenic and left recurrent laryngeal nerves are in the immediate area and should be avoided. Posteriorly, the pleura already will have been opened during the lobectomy. The lymphatic tissue superior to the pulmonary ligament and adjacent to the esophagus are removed, in the space between the hilum and the descending aorta. The esophagus is retracted posteriorly to allow access to the level 7 lymph nodes because these are generally deeper in the mediastinum compared with the right side.

After completion of the lobectomy and lymph node dissection, the chest is copiously irrigated with saline. The chest cavity then is filled with saline, and the lung is inflated to a pressure of 30 cm H_2O to check the bronchial stump closure. Assessment and repair of other air leaks can be accomplished at this time. In patients with complete fissures and minimal adhesions, a single chest tube is placed through the inferior port site. For those needing a greater pneumonolysis or having incomplete fissures, a second tube can be placed in the anterior port site. In patients

without an epidural catheter, intercostal nerve blocks can be injected or an indwelling pleural catheter positioned for postoperative analgesia. In almost all cases, the patient should be extubated in the operating room and taken to the postanesthesia care unit. A chest radiograph is obtained before transfer to the patient's room.

POSTOPERATIVE CARE

Most patients undergoing VATS lobectomy can be transferred safely to a monitored floor bed and do not necessarily require placement in an intensive care unit. Postoperative chest physiotherapy should commence immediately. The patient who has undergone a VAT lobectomy early in the day can be expected to be out of bed to a chair (if not ambulating with assistance) later that same day. During the course of the next few days, the chest tubes, which typically are on wall suction, can be switched to water seal as air leaks resolve. While on wall suction, a patient may be disconnected to ambulate. Lower extremity sequential compression devices, anticoagulation, or both should be maintained throughout the hospital stay. After the air leaks have resolved and chest tube output reaches the threshold for removal (generally <250 cc per 24 hours), the tube can be removed.

The epidural catheter can remain in place for 5 days, although it usually is removed with the bladder catheter after the chest tube has been removed. The patient then is transitioned to oral analgesics. Many studies have suggested a decreased need for postoperative pain medications after VATS lobectomy compared with the open procedure. Oxygen therapy is weaned during the postoperative period. If the patient continues to have low saturation levels, then oxygen therapy can be continued at home. Patients with dyspnea on exertion can have a 6-minute walk test

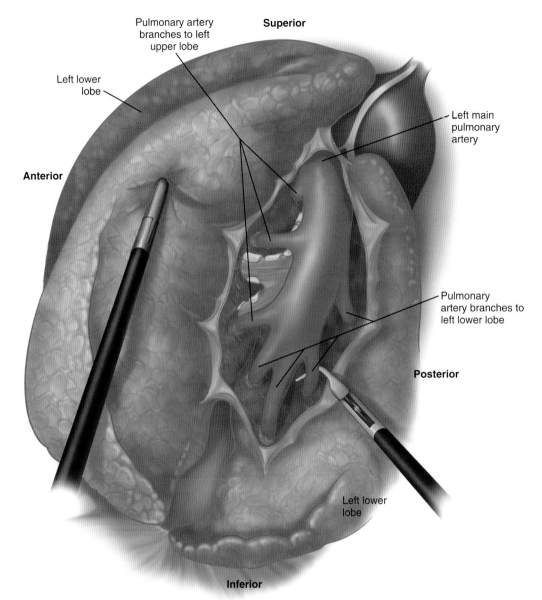

FIGURE 2-24 Dissection of the pulmonary artery branches to the left lower lobe from an anterior approach, within the fissure (VATS LLL).

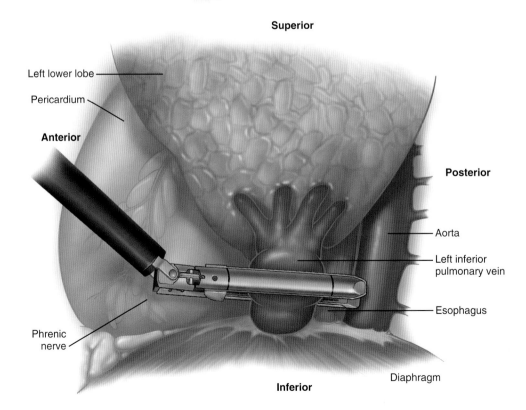

FIGURE 2-25 Exposure of the posterior hilum, with division of the pulmonary vein branch to the left lower lobe (VATS LLL).

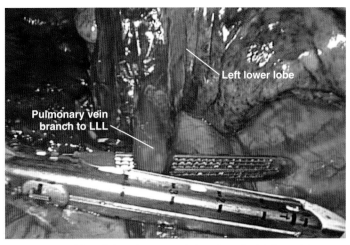

FIGURE 2-26 Division of the pulmonary vein branch to the left lower lobe (VATS LLL).

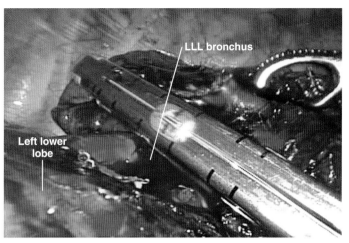

FIGURE 2-28 Division of left lower lobe bronchus (VATS LLL).

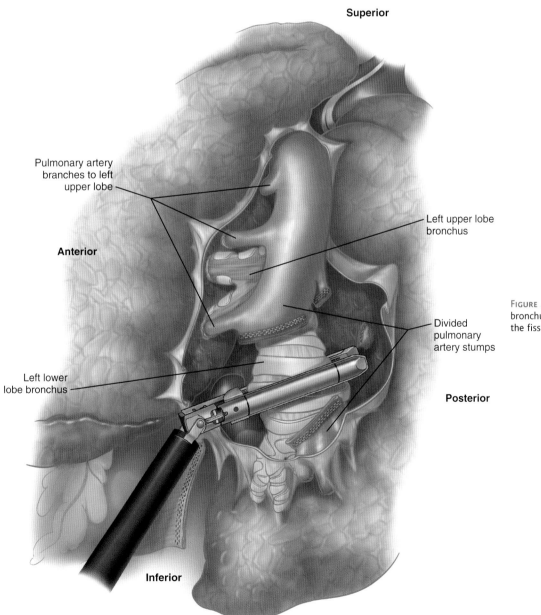

FIGURE 2-27 Division of left lower lobe bronchus from an anterior approach, within the fissure (VATS LLL).

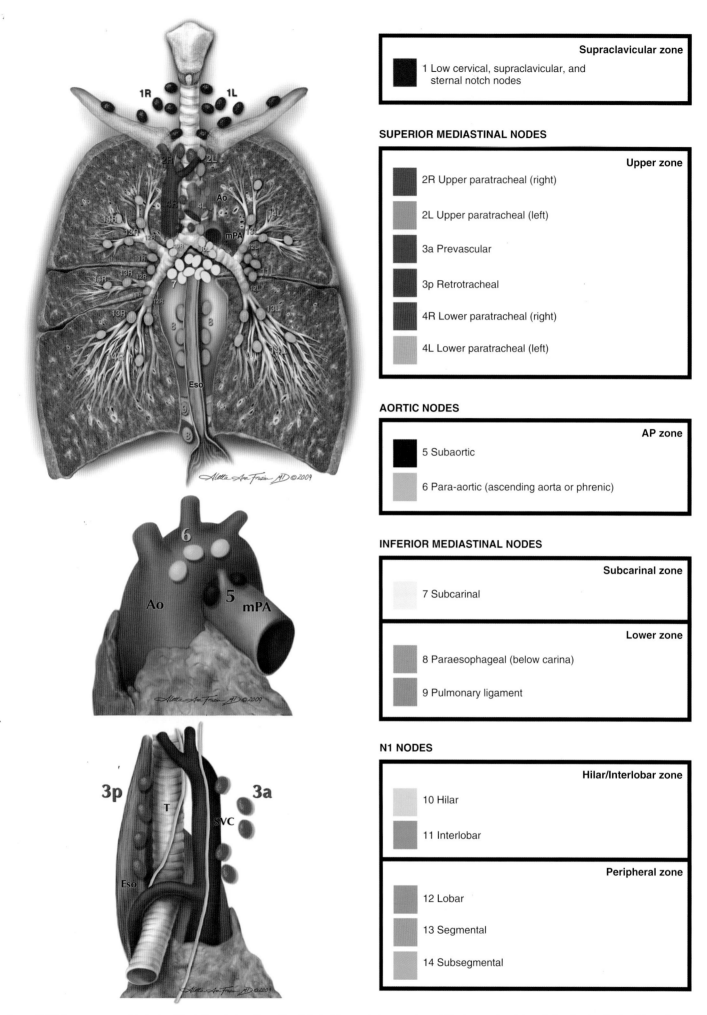

FIGURE 2-29 Lung cancer nodal chart, with station designations. (Reprinted with permission courtesy of the International Association for the Study of Lung Cancer. Copyright © 2008 Aletta Ann Frazier, MD.)

to determine need for home oxygen. Participation in some type of postoperative pulmonary rehabilitation is strongly encouraged for most patients.

MANAGEMENT OF PROCEDURE-SPECIFIC COMPLICATIONS

Even after performance of a minimally invasive lobectomy, postoperative pain control is of paramount importance. Inability to cough will increase the risk for postoperative pulmonary complications, the two most common being atelectasis and pneumonia. Moreover, this risk is greatly increased in those who continue to abuse tobacco products up until the time of surgery. Cessation of smoking for 8 weeks before surgery decreases the risk for postoperative pulmonary complications; unfortunately, few patients can comply with this abstinence.

An aggressive approach should be taken with postoperative chest physiotherapy to avoid these complications. In those with inadequate pain control and radiographic signs of increasing atelectasis, bronchoscopy should be performed earlier rather than later. In the patient with marginal pulmonary function, the development of pneumonia may progress to respiratory failure and mechanical ventilation. Noninvasive positive-pressure ventilation can be used but may increase or prolong a postoperative air leak.

Atrial fibrillation often is associated with the development of atelectasis on the second or third postoperative day. This is more common in patients older than 70 years but also can occur in patients with intrinsic cardiac disease or severe underlying lung disease. Atrial fibrillation usually responds to pharmacologic management and, depending on the patient, may not require specific medication after discharge. Because of an increased risk for postoperative bleeding, routine anticoagulation has not been used. The risk for stroke in this population generally has been very low.

Patients undergoing VATS lobectomy often have a shorter length of stay than those managed with an open lobectomy. This is attributed to a more rapid resolution of air leaks and earlier chest tube removal. This observation may be secondary to a patient selection effect because a lobectomy patient is more likely to have success with a VATS approach when there are fewer adhesions and more complete fissures. A prolonged air leak exists when it has not resolved by the fifth to seventh postoperative day (the exact definition depends on the quoted authority). Some patients with a prolonged air leak can be discharged home with the tube in place using a one-way valve device; the tube subsequently is removed in the clinic. Gentle handling of the lung and the use of sharp dissection can help minimize postoperative air leaks. The use of buttressed staple loads has been advocated by some to further reduce the risk for air leak. A number of pneumostatic agents are available that, when applied to the staple lines and raw visceral pleural areas, may reduce the risk for postoperative air leak. All of these techniques in combination may be helpful in reducing air leaks, thus shortening length of stay.

The decrease in chest tube output required before a chest tube should be removed varies by authority. Some use a cutoff of less than 250 cc of drainage in 24 hours, whereas others remove the chest tube with higher outputs. Removal of tubes with such a higher output has not resulted in an increase in pleural space complications. Maneuvers to decrease chest tube output include excellent intraoperative hemostasis; areas of lymphatic dissection should be closely examined, and any lymphatic branches secured with clips. Application of biologic sealants (e.g., fibrin glue) to these areas also may decrease chest tube drainage.

Other complications that can follow a VATS lobectomy include bleeding, chylothorax, deep venous thrombosis, pulmonary emboli, prolonged ileus, pulmonary torsion, phrenic or recurrent laryngeal nerve injuries, Horner syndrome, bronchopleural fistula, empyema, acute renal failure, and wound infection. Although most of these complications are relatively uncommon as a single occurrence following a routine VATS lobectomy, about 20% to 40% of patients undergoing this procedure experience at least one postoperative complication. Most patients can anticipate a return to most normal activities within 7 to 10 days following discharge, with a return to their preoperative sense of well-being by 4 weeks after the procedure.

RESULTS AND OUTCOME

Currently, it is estimated that only 10% of lobectomies are performed with the VATS approach. This increases to 32% if the procedure is performed by thoracic surgeons, as reported to the General Thoracic Surgery database. There presently are few prospective, randomized studies comparing VATS and open lobectomy. Based on existing nonrandomized data, lobectomies performed at experienced centers have an overall morbidity rate of 32% to 37% and an operative mortality rate of 1% to 2%. This compares with a 15% to 20% morbidity rate for VATS lobectomy, with a similar mortality rate. This trend of decreased morbidity with the VATS approach may be even greater in an elderly population, with one center reporting a complication rate of 18% and a mortality rate of 1.8% in a group of octogenarians.

A few studies have looked at the biologic advantages of VATS lobectomy compared with the open procedure. These studies have shown a reduced inflammatory response, with lower interleukin and C-reactive protein levels in VATS patients. Other reports have demonstrated less reduction in CD4 and natural killer cells, as well as less impairment in cellular cytotoxicity with the VATS procedure. Available data suggest equivalent long-term survival in patients undergoing open versus VATS lobectomy for primary lung cancer. Some data have even suggested improved survival in VATS lobectomy subjects, but these may represent a selection bias. Patients selected for VATS lobectomy generally have smaller, more peripheral tumors, which usually have less lymph node involvement. Unfortunately, it generally is believed that a prospective, randomized study comparing the two operative techniques is not feasible and is unlikely to be performed.

The number of VATS lobectomies being performed is slowly increasing. As more experience has been obtained, procedures of increasing complexity have been performed by VATS, including bilobectomy, pneumonectomy, lobectomy with chest wall resection, and sleeve lobectomy. It is likely that the VATS approach for these and other thoracic procedures will continue to increase as the use of VATS becomes more common.

Suggested Readings

Allen MS, Darling GE, Pechet TT, et al: Morbidity and mortality of major pulmonary resections in patients with early-stage lung cancer: Initial results of the randomized, prospective ACOSOG Z0030 trial, *Ann Thorac Surg* 81:1013–1019, 2006.

Gharagozloo F, Temesta B, Margolis M, et al: Video-assisted thoracic surgery lobectomy for stage I lung cancer, *Ann Thorac Surg* 76:1009–1014, 2003.

Kirby TJ, Mack MJ, Landreneau RJ, et al: Lobectomy: Video assisted thoracic surgery versus muscle-sparring thoracotomy. A randomized trial, *J Thorac Cardiovasc Surg* 109:997–1001, 1995.

McKenna RJ Jr: Lobectomy by video-assisted thoracic surgery with mediastinal lymph node dissection for lung cancer, *J Thorac Cardiovasc Surg* 107:879–881, 1994.

McKenna RJ, Jr, Houck W, Fuller CB: Video-assisted thoracic surgery lobectomy: Experience with one thousand one hundred cases, *Ann Thorac Surg* 81:421–425, 2006.

Roviaro G, Varoli F, Vergani C. et al: Long-term survival after videothoracoscopic lobectomy for stage I lung cancer, *Chest* 126:725–732, 2004.

Solaina L, Prusciano F, Bagioni P, et al: Video-assisted thoracic surgery (VATS) of the lung: Analysis of intraoperative and postoperative complications over 15 years and review of the literature, *Surg Endosc* 22:298–310, 2003.

Sugi K, Kaneda Y, Esato K: Video-assisted thoracoscopic lobectomy achieves a satisfactory long-term prognosis in patients with clinical stage IA lung cancer, *World J Surg* 24:27–30, 2000.

Swanson SJ, Herndon JE, D'Amico TA, et al: Video-assisted thoracic surgery lobectomy: Report of CALGB 39802—a prospective multi-institutional feasibility study, *J Clin Oncol* 25:4993–4997, 2007.

Villamizar NR, Darrabie MD, Burfeind WR, et al: Thoracoscopic lobectomy is associated with lower morbidity compared with thoracotomy, *J Thorac Cardiovasc Surg* 138:419–425, 2009.

Walker WS, Codispoti M, Soon SY, et al: Long-term outcomes following VATS lobectomy for non-small cell bronchogenic carcinoma, *Eur J Cardiothorac Surg* 23:397–402, 2003.

Whitson BA, Groth SS, Duval SJ, et al: Surgery for early-stage non-small cell lung cancer: A systematic review of video-assisted thoracoscopic surgery versus thoracotomy approaches to lobectomy, *Ann Thorac Surg* 86:2008–2016, 2008.

BASIL J. AMMORI AND GEORGIOS D. AYIOMAMITIS

Bilateral Thoracoscopic Splanchnotomy for Intractable Upper Abdominal Pain

3

The videos associated with this chapter are listed in the Video Contents and can be found on the accompanying DVDs and on Expertconsult.com.

Thoracoscopic splanchnotomy is a minimally invasive procedure that involves the division of the greater and lesser splanchnic sympathetic nerve afferents. The alternative terminology "thoracoscopic splanchnicectomy" that often is applied in the literature is a misnomer because no excision of the splanchnic nerves typically is performed. This procedure has been used to treat chronic severe abdominal pain, mostly from pancreatic disease.

The three splanchnic nerves of the thoracic sympathetic trunk arise from the lower eight ganglia (Figs. 3-1 and 3-2). Branches of the T5-T9 sympathetic ganglia form the greater splanchnic nerve, the T10-T11 ganglia form the lesser splanchnic nerve, and the T12 ganglion forms the least splanchnic nerve. These splanchnic nerves predominantly contain visceral efferent fibers but also carry afferent sympathetic "pain" signals from the upper abdominal viscera, including the pancreas, to the brain. At thoracoscopy, these nerves can be seen running superficial to the intercostal vessels along the vertebral spine (Figs. 3-3 and 3-4), where they can readily be divided.

OPERATIVE INDICATIONS

Chronic pancreatitis represents the most common indication for splanchnotomy. Relief of abdominal pain in patients with chronic pancreatitis poses a challenge to surgeons, gastroenterologists, and pain specialists. As the disease progresses, painful attacks become more frequent with shorter pain-free intervals, culminating in constant and often intractable abdominal pain. The management options include both nonoperative and operative approaches, such as pancreatic enzyme supplementation, nonopioid or opioid analgesia, celiac plexus block with ethanol, thoracoscopic splanchnotomy, decompression of the pancreatic duct, or pancreatic resection. Nonoperative methods may not be effective in achieving pain control in 20% to 50% of patients with chronic pancreatitis; on the other hand, pancreatic surgery carries the potential for long-term morbidity and a small risk for operative mortality. The wide variety of methods available to treat pain associated with chronic pancreatitis reflects the multifactorial nature of this condition, with no single method producing superior results. When selecting these patients for splanchnotomy, it is essential to consider the following:

- *Exclude alternative causes for pain.* Chronic duodenal ulceration is not an uncommon coexisting disorder in chronic pancreatitis patients. It also is essential to exclude pain of drug seekers and those with psychogenic disease.

- *Reserve splanchnotomy for patients who have visceral rather than somatic pain of chronic pancreatitis.* Progression of pancreatitis adds a somatic component to the pain that responds poorly to splanchnotomy. Visceral pain often is described as upper abdominal, whereas back or lower abdominal pain suggests somatic pain. Bradley and colleagues described differential epidural analgesia as a potentially useful method in selecting patients with small duct chronic pancreatitis for thoracoscopic splanchnotomy; patients who responded to sympathetic block were the best candidates for splanchnotomy. Strickland and associates suggested that a favorable response to preoperative paravertebral sympathetic (splanchnic) nerve block with local anesthetic predicted a good response to splanchnotomy.

- *Exclude disorders that require direct pancreatic surgery.* These include pancreatic pseudocyst (internal drainage or distal pancreatectomy might bring symptomatic relief), inflammatory mass in the head of the pancreas (a Beger or Whipple procedure might be necessary), and pancreatic duct dilation with or without stones (which might require a Puestow, Frey, or Beger procedure). Splanchnotomy is reserved for patients with small duct chronic pancreatitis.

- *Assess severity of the pain.* There is no clearly defined threshold for the selection of patients for thoracoscopic splanchnotomy. It is reasonable to reserve this procedure for patients in whom nonoperative measures have been explored and in whom pain severity has required escalating doses of opiates. Thoracoscopic splanchnotomy should not necessarily be the treatment of last resort, however, because its outcome is worst in patients with advanced chronic pancreatitis and previous pancreatic surgery. Although many of these patients may previously have received one or more celiac plexus blocks to relieve the pain with short-lived partial response, failure to achieve any response from such a block might predict poor outcome for thoracoscopic splanchnotomy.

- *Ensure abstinence from drinking, which is an absolute requirement in patients with alcoholic chronic pancreatitis.* Continued alcohol abuse predicts a poor response to thoracoscopic splanchnotomy.

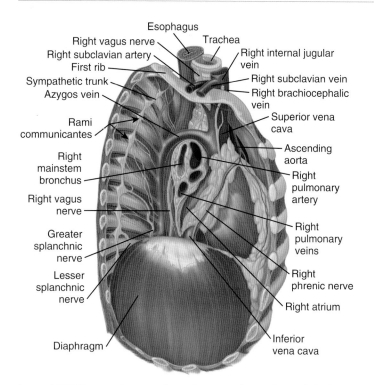

Esophagus
Right vagus nerve
Right subclavian artery
First rib
Sympathetic trunk
Azygos vein
Rami communicantes
Right mainstem bronchus
Right vagus nerve
Greater splanchnic nerve
Lesser splanchnic nerve
Diaphragm

Trachea
Right internal jugular vein
Right subclavian vein
Right brachiocephalic vein
Superior vena cava
Ascending aorta
Right pulmonary artery
Right pulmonary veins
Right phrenic nerve
Right atrium
Inferior vena cava

FIGURE 3-1 Right thoracic cavity, viewed from lateral to medial, with the lateral chest wall cut away.

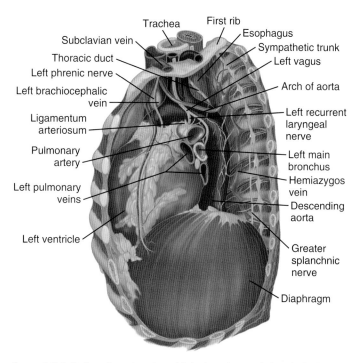

Trachea
First rib
Subclavian vein
Esophagus
Thoracic duct
Sympathetic trunk
Left phrenic nerve
Left vagus
Left brachiocephalic vein
Arch of aorta
Ligamentum arteriosum
Left recurrent laryngeal nerve
Pulmonary artery
Left main bronchus
Left pulmonary veins
Hemiazygos vein
Descending aorta
Left ventricle
Greater splanchnic nerve
Diaphragm

FIGURE 3-2 Left thoracic cavity, viewed from lateral to medial, with the lateral chest wall cut away.

The patient with advanced upper abdominal cancer (e.g., pancreatic, hepatobiliary, or gastric) causing severe abdominal pain may be a candidate for thoracoscopic splanchnotomy. The following points should be considered for this operative indication:

- The offer of thoracoscopic splanchnotomy should be timely and not delayed if optimal quality of life is to be achieved. Patients should be selected through a multidisciplinary team discussion that involves Pain and Palliative Care disciplines and should take into account the patient's life expectancy and fitness for a general anesthesia.

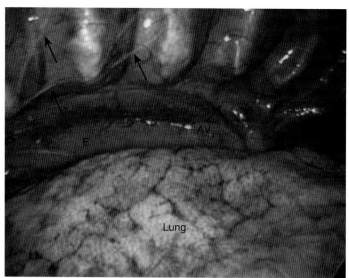

FIGURE 3-3 Thoracoscopic view of right chest, viewing in the posterior direction. *Arrows* indicate splanchnic nerves. AV, azygos vein; E, esophagus.

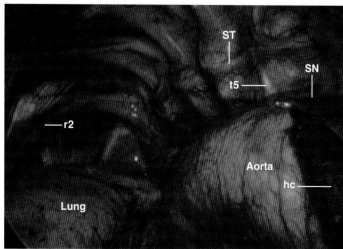

FIGURE 3-4 Thoracoscopic view of left chest, viewing in the superoposterior direction. hc, Hook electrocautery; r2, second rib; SN, greater splanchnic nerve; ST, sympathetic trunk; t5, thoracic level 5 root of greater splanchnic nerve.

- Although thoracoscopic splanchnotomy is useful for visceral cancer pain, it is ill advised if pain is considered to be predominantly secondary to peritoneal disease, subacute small bowel obstruction, or infiltration of the abdominal wall.

Contraindications to thoracoscopic splanchnotomy might include the following:

- Events or factors that might have obliterated the pleural space, such as previous thoracic surgery, recurrent severe pneumonia, empyema or need for drainage of pleural effusion, and significant pulmonary metastases. Consideration could be given to contralateral splanchnotomy in patients with unilateral thoracic surgery.

- Mediastinal radiotherapy, because this would produce thickening of the pleura, making identification of the splanchnic nerves quite difficult and hazardous.

- Severe chronic pulmonary disease, which would increase the risk for capnothorax and partial lung collapse that is induced during thoracoscopic splanchnotomy.

PREOPERATIVE TESTING, EVALUATION, AND PREPARATION

Radiologic assessment of the abdomen is required to demonstrate the state of pancreatic structural and ductal pathologic findings in chronic pancreatitis and to give an up-to-date assessment of the regional and metastatic extent of cancer. The potential role of differential epidural analgesia or paravertebral splanchnic nerve block in selecting patients for thoracoscopic splanchnotomy was discussed earlier but should not be overstated. A radiologic assessment of the chest and evaluation of any pulmonary disease might be necessary.

OPERATIVE TECHNIQUE

Thoracoscopic splanchnotomy is performed under general anesthesia. Single endotracheal tube intubation is sufficient. Parenteral prophylactic antibiotics are not required. The authors prefer a posterior thoracic approach; the patient is placed in the prone position with the arms abducted and the elbows flexed, placing the hands over the patient's head (Fig. 3-5). This allows the lungs to fall away from the posterior chest wall, facilitating bilateral thoracoscopic splanchnotomy while eliminating the disadvantages associated with double-lumen tube intubation. Insufflation of the pleural space is performed after entry with a blunt 5-mm trocar port in the intercostal space (ICS) immediately below the inferior angle of the scapula (usually the fifth ICS; see Fig. 3-5). The capnothorax is maintained at 6 to 8 mm Hg CO_2. We

routinely perform the procedure bilaterally and treat the right side first. Another 5-mm port is inserted under direct vision in the next or second-next lower ICS (usually the seventh ICS) and slightly medial to the first port. A 5-mm 30-degree endoscope is used through the upper port.

Adhesions between the lung and the parietal pleura (if present) are divided with an electrosurgical hook or scissors. The main sympathetic trunk can be seen readily in the upper chest running craniocaudad across the necks of the ribs, and the roots of the splanchnic nerves can be observed to descend obliquely and superficial to the intercostal vessels from the fifth rib downward (see Figs. 3-1 and 3-2). The uppermost rib that can be seen at thoracoscopy is the second. The greater splanchnic nerve has one to eight roots, with four being the most common; this nerve runs lateral to the main azygos vein on the right and lateral to the hemiazygos vein on the left (see Figs. 3-1 and 3-2). Division starts with the uppermost root of the greater splanchnic nerve. With electrocautery set to "cut" rather than "coagulate," the hook is used to make a small incision in the parietal pleura on both sides of the nerves or their roots, away from the sympathetic chain (Fig. 3-6). The nerve is then lifted up with the hook (Fig. 3-7) and transected so that its cut ends are seen to retract apart. Alternative techniques of nerve disruption include excision of a 1- to 2-cm nerve segment (splanchnicectomy), or division with an ultrasonic scalpel. Care should be taken during the dissection of the right lesser splanchnic nerve to avoid an injury to the thoracic duct, which runs immediately medial to the nerve (Fig. 3-8). The sympathetic trunk itself is not transected to minimize the risk for extensive visceral denervation. The division of splanchnic nerve roots is extended to the costophrenic recess, but it is unusual to find the least splanchnic nerve. The number of splanchnic nerves that must be cut to achieve pain relief is not known; there is no obvious correlation between the number of cut nerves and the postoperative results.

At completion of the procedure, the capnothorax is evacuated. The anesthesiologist is asked to manually hyperinflate the lungs to expel CO_2 from the pleural space, and the surgeon views the lung expansion through the endoscope. When the lung is fully expanded, the ports are withdrawn. A chest drain is not routinely applied. A postoperative chest radiograph is unnecessary unless clinically indicated. The right-sided procedure, which usually

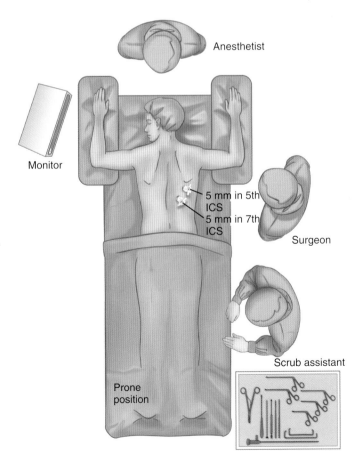

FIGURE 3-5 Patient positioning and port placement for thoracoscopic splanchnotomy. ICS, intercostal space.

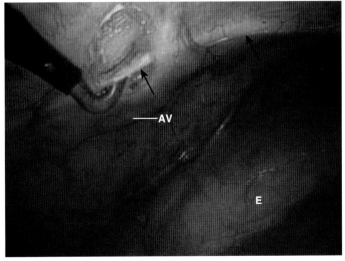

FIGURE 3-6 Dissection of uppermost root of right greater splanchnic nerve *(arrows)* with the hook electrocautery device. AV, azygos vein; E, esophagus.

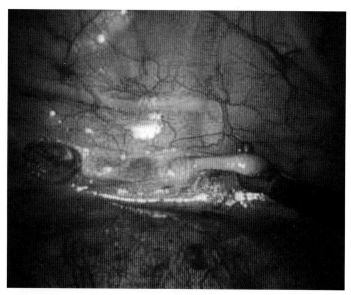

FIGURE 3-7 Elevation of a right splanchnic nerve root with the hook electrocautery device before nerve root division.

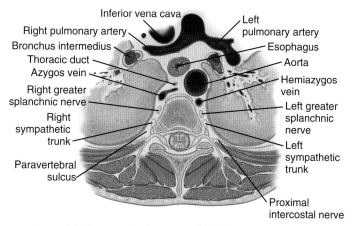

FIGURE 3-8 Cross-sectional anatomy of the chest at the level of T8.

lasts 15 to 20 minutes, is then repeated on the left side with similar technique.

Unilateral or Bilateral Splanchnotomy?

Whether to perform bilateral or unilateral thoracoscopic splanchnotomy remains controversial. Most surgeons would apply the procedure bilaterally. If unilateral thoracoscopic splanchnotomy is preferred, then the left side often is chosen. Unilateral thoracoscopic splanchnotomy has been associated, however, with up to a 40% failure rate at 1-year follow-up, necessitating a contralateral procedure in one out of seven patients. The unilateral procedure typically produces a shorter and more modest response compared with the bilateral procedure.

POSTOPERATIVE CARE

The symptomatic response after surgery is immediate. Opioid analgesia should be weaned over several weeks to minimize withdrawal symptoms. Management by a pain team may be useful. If a chest tube was employed, then it is removed 6 to 8 hours after surgery. A repeat chest radiograph is performed on postoperative day 1 to confirm no residual capnothorax. In uncomplicated cases, most patients are discharged from the hospital on the first postoperative day.

MANAGEMENT OF PROCEDURE-SPECIFIC COMPLICATIONS

In a recent review of the literature, which included 302 patients with chronic pancreatitis, thoracoscopic splanchnotomy was associated with no operative mortality, a morbidity rate of 16.6%, and a conversion rate to open surgery of 1.3%. The most common complications were intercostal neuralgia (7%), pulmonary atelectasis (1.9%), chylothorax (1.3%), and orthostatic hypotension (1.3%). The reoperation rate was 1.3% (thoracotomy $n = 3$, thoracoscopy $n = 1$). The main reasons for reoperation were port site bleeding ($n = 2$) and persistent chylothorax ($n = 2$). Rarely, the procedure may have to be aborted because of extensive pleural adhesions or thickening. The introduction of smaller trocars (5 mm) and the use of the ultrasonic scalpel for division of the splanchnic nerves (instead of electrocautery) have been proposed to reduce the risk for postoperative intercostal neuralgia.

RESULTS AND OUTCOMES

Although the overall success rate of thoracoscopic splanchnotomy in patients with chronic pancreatitis has been 90% in the first 6 months, the rates diminish with longer follow-up. The high success rates reported by some authors came either from short-term follow-up or from series in which stringent patient selection was applied. On the other hand, Maher and colleagues reported a rather disappointing success rate of 20% at 5 years. High rates of postoperative opioid withdrawal in the short term (88% to 100% at 3 to 6 months) markedly declined with time. There are currently no randomized trials to compare thoracoscopic splanchnotomy with celiac plexus block.

The palliation of pain after thoracoscopic splanchnotomy has been associated with weight gain, measurable improvement in quality of life, and return to gainful employment. In addition, thoracoscopic splanchnotomy for a diagnosis of chronic pancreatitis appears to reduce the number of subsequent hospital admissions among responders. Better results are observed with bilateral than unilateral splanchnotomy. Better results also occur when the procedure is applied to cancer patients than to those with chronic pancreatitis because the potential duration of pain relief often is longer than the limited life expectancy of the former patient group. Among patients with small duct chronic pancreatitis, those who have not undergone prior endoscopic or surgical interventions have markedly better results with thoracoscopic splanchnotomy than those who did have prior intervention.

The potential pathophysiologic factors involved in recurrence of abdominal pain after splanchnotomy include (1) technical failure to divide all the splanchnic nerve roots, (2) coexisting somatic pain from involvement of the posterior abdominal wall by the inflammatory process, or (3) the possible existence of pancreatic parasympathetic pain afferents carried by the vagus nerve. The benefits of additional vagotomy, however, remain to be confirmed. Opioid abuse also may contribute to the recurrence of pain for some patients with chronic pancreatitis, and this addiction may interfere with the clinician's ability to evaluate the response to thoracoscopic splanchnotomy. Finally, splanchnotomy may have a placebo effect for some patients, which may explain the relatively large number of patients who experience pain recurrence within 1 year.

Suggested Readings

Ali AS, Ammori BJ: Concomitant laparoscopic gastric and biliary bypass and bilateral thoracoscopic splanchnotomy: the full package of minimally invasive palliation for pancreatic cancer, *Surg Endosc* 17:2028–2031, 2003.

Ammori BJ, Baghdadi S: Minimally invasive pancreatic surgery: The new frontier? *Curr Gastroenterol Rep* 8:132–142, 2006.

Baghdadi S, Abbas MH, Albouz F, et al: Systematic review of the role of thoracoscopic splanchnicectomy in palliating the pain of patients with chronic pancreatitis, *Surg Endosc* 22:580–588, 2008.

Buscher HC, Schipper EE, Wilder-Smith OH, et al: Limited effect of thoracoscopic splanchnicectomy in the treatment of severe chronic pancreatitis pain: A prospective long-term analysis of 75 cases, *Surgery* 143:715–722, 2008.

Cuschieri A, Shimi S, Crosthwaite G, Joypaul V: Bilateral endoscopic splanchnicectomy through a posterior thoracoscopic approach, *J R Coll Surg Edinb* 39:44–47, 1994.

Hammond B, Vitale GC, Rangnekar N, et al: Bilateral thoracoscopic splanchnicectomy for pain control in chronic pancreatitis, *Am Surg* 70:546–549, 2004.

Howard TJ, Swofford JB, Wagner DL, et al: Quality of life after bilateral thoracoscopic splanchnicectomy: Long-term evaluation in patients with chronic pancreatitis, *J Gastrointest Surg* 6:845–852; discussion 853–854, 2002.

Ihse I, Zoucas E, Gyllstedt E, et al: Bilateral thoracoscopic splanchnicectomy: Effects on pancreatic pain and function, *Ann Surg* 230:785–790; discussion 790–791, 1999.

Maher JW, Johlin FC, Heitshusen D: Long-term follow-up of thoracoscopic splanchnicectomy for chronic pancreatitis pain, *Surg Endosc* 15:706–709, 2001.

Makarewicz W, Stefaniak T, Kossakowska M, et al: Quality of life improvement after videothoracoscopic splanchnicectomy in chronic pancreatitis patients: Case control study, *World J Surg* 27:906–911, 2003.

Pietrabissa A, Vistoli F, Carobbi A, et al: Thoracoscopic splanchnicectomy for pain relief in unresectable pancreatic cancer, *Arch Surg* 135:332–335, 2000.

Stone HH, Chauvin EJ: Pancreatic denervation for pain relief in chronic alcohol associated pancreatitis, *Br J Surg* 77:303–305, 1990.

Strickland TC, Ditta TL, Riopelle JM: Performance of local anesthetic and placebo splanchnic blocks via indwelling catheters to predict benefit from thoracoscopic splanchnicectomy in a patient with intractable pancreatic pain, *Anesthesiology* 84:980–983, 1996.

Yim AP, Liu HP: Complications and failures of video-assisted thoracic surgery: Experience from two centers in Asia, *Ann Thorac Surg* 61:538–541, 1996.

Esophagus

LAWRENCE CRIST, BENNY WEKSLER, SHANNON L. WYSZOMIERSKI, AND JAMES D. LUKETICH

Minimally Invasive Ivor Lewis Esophagectomy

The videos associated with this chapter are listed in the Video Contents and can be found on the accompanying DVDs and *on Expertconsult.com.*

The incidence of esophageal adenocarcinoma is increasing rapidly in North America and Western countries. Surgical resection is the best curative therapy for patients with resectable esophageal cancer, but esophagectomy performed by traditional open transthoracic or open trans-hiatal approaches is associated with high morbidity and mortality. To decrease the morbidity and mortality of open esophagectomy, minimally invasive approaches have been adopted and continue to be refined. When performed by experienced surgeons, minimally invasive esophagectomy (MIE) offers a safe and oncologically sound alternative to open esophagectomy.

Minimally invasive techniques for esophageal resection include laparoscopic trans-hiatal esophagectomy, laparoscopic inversion esophagectomy, laparoscopic-thoracoscopic three-hole (McKeown) esophagectomy, and laparoscopic-thoracoscopic (Ivor Lewis) esophagectomy. The approach is usually a matter of surgeon preference but on occasion is dictated by the location of the tumor. For most distal tumors or gastroesophageal junction (GEJ) tumors, an Ivor Lewis approach allows good exposure and adequate margins. After performing MIE for more than 10 years and in more than 1000 patients who had primarily adenocarcinoma of the GEJ, Ivor Lewis MIE has become our preferred technique and is detailed here.

OPERATIVE INDICATIONS

Esophageal resection is the only definitive treatment for esophageal cancer. Most Ivor Lewis MIEs are performed for esophageal adenocarcinoma because of the predominant localization of esophageal adenocarcinoma at the GEJ or distal esophagus. Ivor Lewis MIE is also adequate for most esophageal squamous cell carcinomas in the mid or distal esophagus. Ivor Lewis MIE may not be ideal for upper-third or midesophageal cancers with significant proximal extension because resection with adequate margins may be difficult. In these cases, a modified McKeown MIE may be a good alternative. Distant metastatic disease is also a contraindication for esophagectomy, and careful preoperative and intraoperative assessment for peritoneal and liver metastases is necessary before proceeding with resection.

Esophagectomy may also be performed in patients with Barrett esophagus with high-grade dysplasia. In patients with diagnosis of high-grade dysplasia or early-stage tumors confined to the mucosa (T1a), satisfactory results have also been reported with endoscopic mucosal resection, radiofrequency ablation, and laparoscopic transgastric stripping of esophageal mucosa (see Chapter 6). Thus far, however, there have been only a few reports with good follow-up, and even these only report short- to intermediate-term outcomes. Although endoscopic mucosal resection and radiofrequency ablation offer several immediate benefits to the patient, there are concerns that subsquamous Barrett esophagus may still progress to adenocarcinoma, and continued surveillance endoscopy is required. When endoscopic mucosal resection is performed for early-stage tumors confined to the mucosa, incomplete resection is a concern. Moreover, high-grade dysplasia is often multifocal, and there is a high rate of occult carcinoma in patients who undergo resection for the preoperative diagnosis of high-grade dysplasia. Therefore, we continue to offer MIE for multifocal high-grade dysplasia and early-stage adenocarcinoma. We reserve other ablative therapies for those patients who are unwilling to undergo esophagectomy or are poor candidates for surgery.

Ivor Lewis MIE should be considered as a final option for several benign esophageal conditions when other treatments have been ineffective and the patient's quality of life is significantly affected. These indications include recalcitrant strictures, end-stage achalasia, and gastrointestinal reflux disease that has failed traditional antireflux approaches.

PREOPERATIVE EVALUATION, TESTING, AND PREPARATION

Esophagogastroscopy with biopsy is essential for diagnosis of esophageal adenocarcinoma and for surgical planning but cannot assess the depth of the tumor or lymph node involvement. Computed tomography (CT) and ^{18}F-fluoro-2-deoxy-D-glucose positron emission tomography (PET) scans should be used to assess locoregional lymph node involvement and distant metastasis. The fused PET-CT modality combines metabolic and anatomic information and improves the accuracy of staging. Endoscopic ultrasound (EUS) is the most accurate noninvasive test for locoregional staging of the cancer (T and N classification). Fine-needle aspiration (FNA) can be added as needed to improve accuracy. We routinely assess the depth of the tumor and the nodal involvement by EUS and FNA. Flexible bronchoscopy should be performed in patients with tumors located in the upper and middle thirds of the esophagus to look for tumor infiltration of the airway.

Before esophagectomy, the patient's physiologic status should be thoroughly evaluated to assess the risks of the surgery. This evaluation should include assessments of the patient's cardiovascular and pulmonary function and performance and nutritional status. In most patients, a cardiac stress test should be performed. Baseline pulmonary function tests with arterial blood gas values should be obtained in patients with suspected or documented chronic lung disease. A forced expiratory volume in 1 second (FEV_1) of less than 1 L (about 40% of that predicted for an average man) suggests a higher likelihood of serious pulmonary complications. For selected patients, consultation with cardiology and pulmonary medicine experts may be necessary to develop a treatment plan that balances the risks for cardiac complications with the risk-to-benefit ratio of cardiac intervention, the need for anticoagulation or antiplatelet therapy, and the risk-to-benefit ratio of esophagectomy.

PATIENT POSITIONING IN THE OPERATING SUITE

Patient positioning changes for the three phases of the Ivor Lewis MIE. During the "on-table" esophagogastroduodenoscopy (EGD) before starting resection, the patient is supine. For the laparoscopic portion of the MIE, the patient is positioned supine in steep reverse-Trendelenburg with a footboard in place. The surgeon stands on the patient's right, and the assistant stands on the patient's left. For the thoracoscopic portion of the procedure, the patient is repositioned to the left lateral decubitus position. The surgeon remains to the right of the patient, and the first assistant remains to the left of the patient.

PLACEMENT OF TROCARS

For the laparoscopic portion of the procedure, six abdominal trocars (three 5 mm and three 10 mm) are placed. First, a 10-mm port through a Hasson technique in placed in the right paramedian position. In the average patient, this approximates two thirds the distance from the xiphoid to the umbilicus. In obese patients with a very protuberant abdomen, this two-thirds distance must be reconsidered, and the port likely will have to be moved closer to the upper abdomen. The pneumoperitoneum is established and maintained at a pressure of 15 mm Hg. In patients with cardiopulmonary compromise, the pneumoperitoneal pressure may have to be lowered to under 10 mm Hg. The remaining ports are then placed. A 10-mm port is placed 5 cm to the left of the operating port (30-degree camera port); a 10-mm port is placed 6 cm below the Hasson port to facilitate placement of the jejunostomy tube; and 5-mm ports are placed subcostally on the right and left midclavicular lines (tissue grasper ports). Finally, we place a 5-mm port, for liver retraction, in the right flank, just below the costal margin laterally (Fig. 4-1).

For the thoracoscopic portion of the Ivor Lewis MIE, five ports are used (Fig. 4-2). Correct thoracoscopic port placement is critical because poorly positioned trocars lead to difficulty maneuvering instruments through the rigid chest wall. A 10-mm port is placed in the eighth intercostal space on the posterior axillary line. This is used as the laparoscope port. A 10-mm working port for the ultrasonic shears is introduced in the ninth intercostal space, 6 cm posterior to the posterior axillary

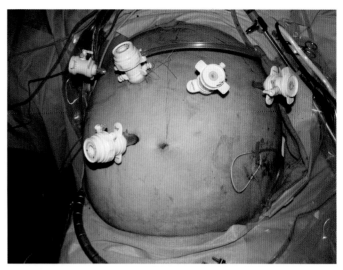

FIGURE 4-1 Port placement for the laparoscopic phase of Ivor Lewis minimally invasive esophagectomy. (From Wizorek JJ, Awais O, Luketich JD: Minimally invasive esophagectomy. In Zwischenberger JB, editor: *Atlas of Thoracic Surgical Techniques*, 1st edition. Philadelphia, 2010, Saunders, pp 305–319.)

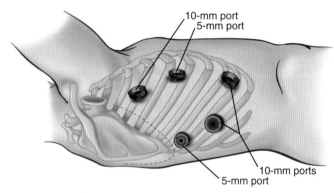

FIGURE 4-2 Port placement for the thoracoscopic phase of Ivor Lewis minimally invasive esophagectomy.

line—just inferior to the tip of the scapula. Ultimately, this port is enlarged to a 5-cm access incision to enable passage of the end-to-end anastomotic stapler and removal of the specimen. A 5-mm port is inserted posterior to the scapular tip, and through this port, the surgeon provides countertraction, using instruments held in his or her left hand. A 10-mm port is inserted in the fourth intercostal space on the midaxillary line, and the surgeon uses this port for retraction during the esophageal dissection. Finally, a 5-mm port is inserted at the midaxillary line near the sixth rib to be used as a suction-irrigator port.

OPERATIVE TECHNIQUE

On-Table Esophagogastroduodenoscopy

After intubation with a double-lumen endotracheal tube, the on-table preoperative EGD is performed with minimal insufflation to avoid gastric and intestinal distention. This EGD is important to confirm the anatomic location and extent of pathology as well as ensure the suitability of the gastric conduit.

Laparoscopic Phase

The laparoscopic portion of the procedure is carried out first. Patient positioning and port placement were described previously. A thorough laparoscopic exploration is performed to evaluate for the presence of occult metastatic disease, and then

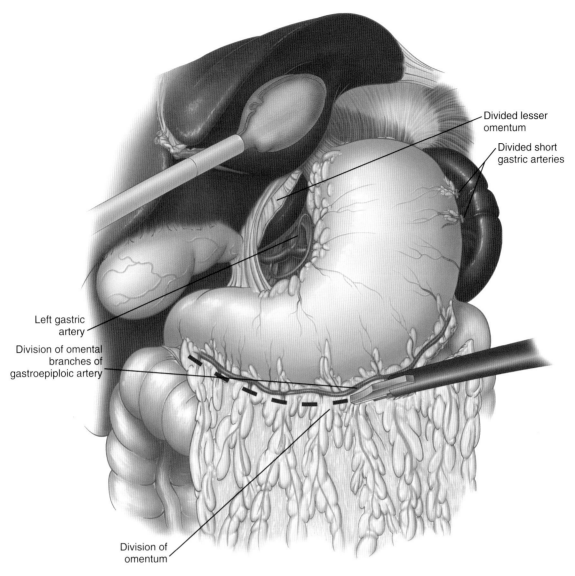

Divided lesser
omentum

Divided short
gastric arteries

Left gastric
artery

Division of omental
branches of
gastroepiploic artery

Division of
omentum

FIGURE 4-3 Gastric mobilization.

gastric mobilization is carried out. The gastrohepatic ligament (lesser omentum) is first divided, and the right and left crura of the diaphragm are dissected. The GEJ is mobilized, and then the esophagus is dissected circumferentially in the lower mediastinum. The greater curvature of the stomach is then mobilized by first dividing the short gastric vessels, followed by division of the gastrocolic omentum while carefully preserving the right gastroepiploic arcade (Fig. 4-3). The mobilized stomach is retracted toward the liver. The mobility of the pylorus can be used as a good guide for the adequacy of dissection. If the pylorus easily reaches the right crus and caudate lobe of the liver, the mobilization is generally adequate. If there is any tension during this maneuver, then remaining attachments between the posterior wall of the stomach and the pancreas may have to be divided. An extensive Kocher maneuver may be necessary to accomplish complete pyloric-antral mobilization. Prior gallbladder surgery frequently limits the pyloric-antral mobility, requiring additional adhesiolysis in this area. Next, a complete celiac lymph node dissection is performed, continuing along the superior border of the splenic artery and pancreas toward the splenic hilum. The lymph node packet is included in the specimen. The left gastric vessels are then identified, dissected, and divided with the use of a laparoscopic stapler with vascular staple load (Fig. 4-4).

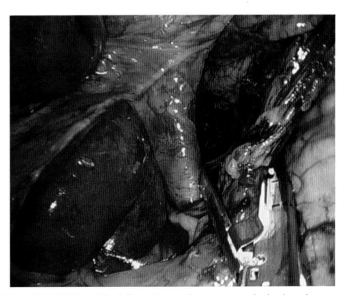

FIGURE 4-4 Division of the left gastric vessels using a vascular load stapler. (From Wizorek JJ, Awais O, Luketich JD: Minimally invasive esophagectomy. In Zwischenberger JB, editor: *Atlas of Thoracic Surgical Techniques*, 1st edition. Philadelphia, 2010, Saunders, pp 305–319.)

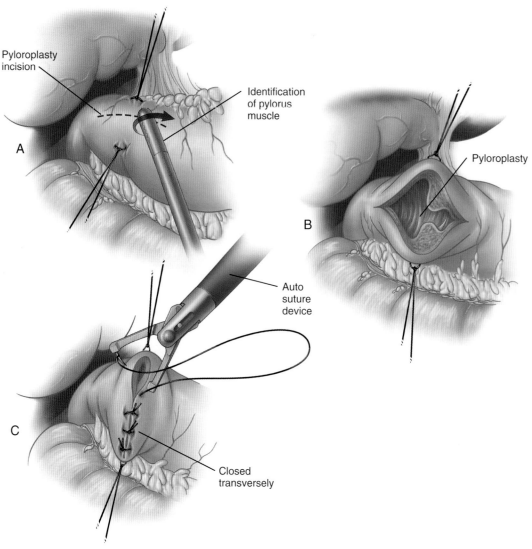

Pyloroplasty
incision

Identification
of pylorus
muscle

A

Pyloroplasty

B

Auto
suture
device

C

Closed
transversely

FIGURE 4-5 Pyloroplasty performed in a Heineke-Mikulicz fashion using the Endo Stitch device.

Attention is then turned to mobilization of the pyloric-antral area and subsequent pyloroplasty. During this mobilization, the surgeon must be diligent in identifying and preserving the right gastroepiploic arcade. The pyloroplasty is started by placing two traction sutures (2-0), one superiorly and one inferiorly, on the pylorus with the Endo Stitch (Covidien, Norwalk, Conn.). The pyloroplasty is performed by opening the pylorus longitudinally with ultrasonic shears and closing it transversely with interrupted sutures using the Endo Stitch device in a Heineke-Mikulicz fashion (Fig. 4-5). A 4- to 5-cm diameter gastric conduit is then constructed. Initially, the very thick and muscular antrum is divided with the use of thick tissue staple loads (4.8 mm). This division begins from the lesser curve above the antrum and proceeds toward the fundus. As this division proceeds cephalad, the thickness of the stomach wall decreases, and 3.5-mm staple loads are more appropriate (Fig. 4-6). To facilitate exposure, staple alignment, and conduit length during this step, the assistant grasps the fundus of the stomach along the line of the short gastric arteries and retracts gently cephalad while another assistant simultaneously grasps the antrum and retracts inferiorly (Fig. 4-7). This essentially elongates the entire stomach and provides the alignment necessary to construct a consistent-diameter gastric conduit. It is recommended that 45-mm staple loads be used in creating the gastric conduit to prevent "spiraling," which

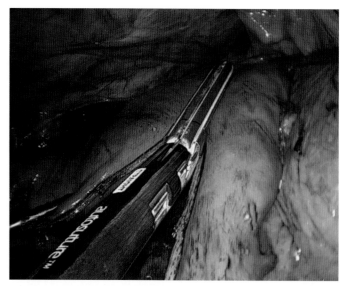

FIGURE 4-6 Construction of the gastric conduit using the Endo GIA stapler. (From Wizorek JJ, Awais O, Luketich JD: Minimally invasive esophagectomy. In Zwischenberger JB, editor: *Atlas of Thoracic Surgical Techniques,* 1st edition. Philadelphia, 2010, Saunders, pp 305–319.)

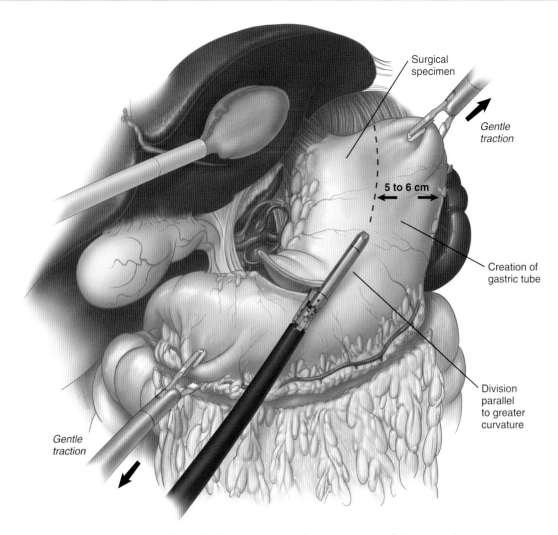

Surgical
specimen

Gentle
traction

5 to 6 cm

Creation of
gastric tube

Division
parallel
to greater
curvature

Gentle
traction

FIGURE 4-7 Retraction of the fundus and antrum during construction of the gastric tube.

may occur with the use of the 60-mm loads. The tip of the gastric conduit is then secured to the specimen using an Endo Stitch. During this step, care is taken to maintain alignment so that subsequent retrieval of the specimen through the hiatus into the chest does not lead to rotation; this maintains perfect anatomic alignment of the gastric conduit, with the short gastric vessels facing the direction of the spleen and the lesser curve staple line facing the right side of the chest.

A feeding jejunostomy is placed next. The camera is switched to the Hasson port. The patient is placed in the Trendelenburg position with the transverse colon and greater omentum retracted cephalad. The ligament of Treitz is identified, and about 30 cm distal to this point, a limb of proximal jejunum is tacked to the anterior abdominal wall in the left middle quadrant with a single 2-0 Endo Stitch. Under direct visualization, a 10-French needle jejunostomy catheter (Abbott, Abbott Park, Ill.) is placed using the Seldinger technique. The catheter position is confirmed by distending the jejunum with 10 mL of air insufflated through the catheter. The jejunum is then tacked circumferentially to the abdominal wall at the catheter entry site using a 2-0 Endo Stitch. A stitch is placed 3 cm distal to the insertion site to prevent torsion and possible strangulation around a single fixed point (Fig. 4-8).

At the completion of the laparoscopic phase, the specimen is tucked into the mediastinum, and the crura are approximated with a single stitch of 0-0 Surgidac (Covidien, Norwalk, Conn.)

to prevent postoperative hernia. The degree of crural closure depends on the size of the hiatal defect and also on the final diameter of the gastric conduit. Care must be taken to avoid undo constriction of the hiatoplasty because this can strangulate the gastric conduit.

On the other hand, a wide open hiatus with a very narrow conduit may be a setup for a delayed hiatal hernia.

Thoracoscopic Phase

After completion of the laparoscopic abdominal stage, the patient is repositioned in the left lateral decubitus position, and thoracoscopic ports are placed as described previously (see Fig. 4-2). An important maneuver at the beginning of the thoracoscopic phase is placement of a 0-0 silk stitch into the central tendon of the diaphragm using the Endo Stitch. The suture is brought out through a 2-mm stab incision using the Endo Close device (Covidien, Norwalk, Conn.) at the lowest part of the costophrenic angle. Traction on this suture pulls the diaphragm inferiorly and improves visualization of the lower esophagus as it nears the diaphragmatic hiatus.

Mobilization of the esophagus is initiated by dividing the inferior pulmonary ligament and retracting the lung medially. The mediastinal pleura is incised anteriorly along the lung edge and up to the azygos vein. The azygos vein is mobilized and divided with a vascular staple load (Fig. 4-9). The phrenic nerve is identified, and the dissection continues by dividing tissue off the

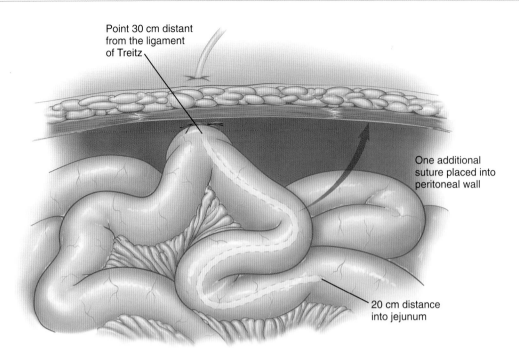

Point 30 cm distant
from the ligament
of Treitz

One additional
suture placed into
peritoneal wall

20 cm distance
into jejunum

FIGURE 4-8 Placement of the needle jejunostomy feeding tube.

pericardium posterior to the phrenic nerve. The dissection then proceeds in a cephalad direction, posterior to the inferior pulmonary vein, and along the pericardium. The right mainstem bronchus is identified, and the subcarinal lymph node packet is dissected en bloc with the specimen. The ultrasonic shears are used for much of the dissection because the sharp blade of this instrument is ideal for a precise dissection plane. The left mainstem bronchus is then identified, and dissection continues superiorly. To avoid thermal injury, care must be taken not to allow an energy-delivering device to come into close proximity or contact with the posterior membranous tracheobronchial tree. The vagi are divided at the level of the azygos vein. Once the azygos is reached, the dissection stays directly on the esophagus to avoid injury to the airway or the recurrent laryngeal nerves. In performing the anterior dissection, it is imperative to identify and be aware of the airway at all times. Once the anterior dissection is complete, the esophagus is mobilized posteriorly off the contralateral pleura. During the posterior dissection, the esophagus is retracted anteriorly, and every effort should be made to avoid injury to the aorta and the thoracic duct. When the circumferential dissection of the esophagus is complete from the hiatus to the thoracic inlet, the specimen and gastric tube are delivered into the chest. The specimen and conduit are separated, and the gastric tube is tacked to the diaphragm with an Endo Stitch. The proximal esophagus is then transected at or above the level of the azygos vein with the ultrasonic sheers. Before dividing the esophagus, one must consider the proximal extent of the tumor or Barrett mucosa and be certain the conduit has adequate length to reach the proximal point of esophageal transection. The exact location for esophageal transection is determined by the preoperative endoscopy. A 4- to 5-cm access incision is then made, and a wound protector (Applied Medical, Rancho Santa Margarita, Calif.) is placed. The specimen is removed and sent for frozen section analysis of the esophageal and gastric margins.

The esophagogastric anastomosis is performed with the use of a 28-mm end-to-end anastomotic (EEA) stapler. The anvil is placed into the proximal divided esophagus through the access incision and secured with a pursestring suture using the 2-0 Endo Stitch. A gastrotomy is made in the tip of the gastric conduit, and the EEA stapler is introduced into the conduit through the access incision (Fig. 4-10). The anastomosis is then created in an end- (proximal esophagus) to-side (gastric conduit) fashion above the level of the azygos vein. When completing the anastomosis, it is important to keep downward pressure on the stapler to avoid a posterior wall disruption. The redundant portion of the gastric conduit is removed using a 60- × 3.5-mm staple load. The chest is then irrigated with copious amounts of warm antibiotic solution to clear any spilled saliva.

An intercostal nerve block is performed with 0.5% bupivacaine (Marcaine). If an omental flap has been harvested, it is wrapped around the anastomosis and secured with an Endo Stitch. A 10-mm Jackson-Pratt drain is placed posterior to the anastomosis along the gastric conduit. The conduit is sutured to the crus at the hiatus with an Endo Stitch to prevent herniation. A 28-French chest tube is placed posteriorly. A nasogastric tube is placed across the anastomosis under direct vision, and the lung is reexpanded. All wounds are closed (Fig. 4-11), and the patient is returned to the supine position. Aggressive oral suctioning is performed, and a toilet bronchoscopy is performed after switching the double-lumen endotracheal tube to a single-lumen endotracheal tube. Every effort is made to extubate the patient in the operating room.

POSTOPERATIVE CARE

The patient is monitored in the ICU for the first night after Ivor Lewis MIE. The head of the bed is elevated to 30 degrees to minimize the possibility of aspiration. Patient-controlled analgesia is administered to optimize respiratory function and early ambulation. Intravenous fluid is maintained judiciously, to optimize tissue perfusion while decreasing fluid overload. Prophylactic anticoagulation and sequential compression devices in the lower extremities are used to prevent thromboembolic complications. The nasogastric tube is flushed with 20 mL of water every

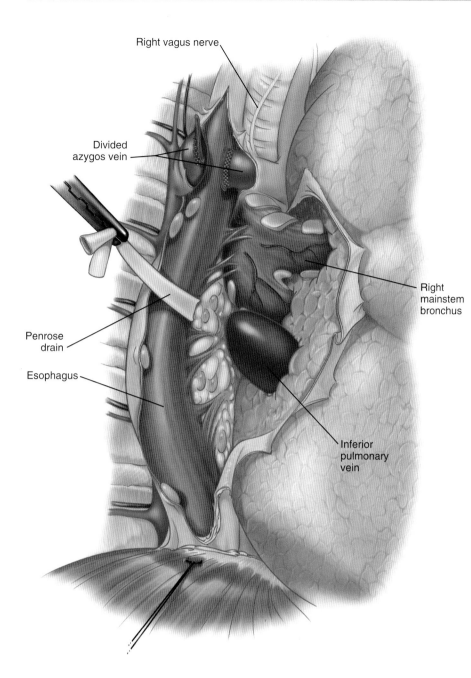

Right vagus nerve

Divided
azygos vein

Penrose
drain

Esophagus

Right
mainstem
bronchus

Inferior
pulmonary
vein

FIGURE 4-9 Mobilization of the esophagus and division of the azygous vein.

6 to 8 hours and kept on low-pressure suction to keep the conduit decompressed.

On the first postoperative day, the patient is transferred from the intensive care unit (ICU) to a monitored floor and begins incentive spirometry at regular intervals during the day with a target of 1 L. Ambulation begins with the aid of a physiotherapist, and the administration of patient-controlled analgesia and intravenous fluids continues. The quality of the patient's voice and effectiveness of the patient's cough are examined because a soft, hoarse voice and ineffective cough are signs of recurrent laryngeal nerve palsy.

On the second postoperative day, the nasogastric tube is removed. Feeding is initiated (20 mL per hour) through the jejunostomy from 3 PM to 9 AM (18-hour schedule). This is increased gradually to the goal tube feed rate (according to the nutritionist's recommendation) based on patient tolerance. The patient is kept NPO until a barium swallow, typically on postoperative day 3, shows that there are no leaks and that the conduit is emptying. After evaluation of the barium swallow, the patient is started on

clear fluids orally (30 mL per hour). If this is well tolerated, the patient is advanced to full liquids, but the volume of oral intake is kept to a minimum (1 to 2 ounces every hour while awake). Early after surgery, nutrition is maintained through the jejunostomy tube. The oral feedings are given for patient comfort and also to begin the gradual transition from jejunostomy tube feeding to an oral diet, which occurs 2 to 3 weeks after surgery.

MANAGEMENT OF PROCEDURE-SPECIFIC COMPLICATIONS

Moderate strictures at the gastroesophageal anastomosis are a common procedure-specific complication and generally can be managed with one or two outpatient dilations. Using the Ivor Lewis approach and a 28-mm EEA stapler, strictures generally are less clinically significant than with a cervical esophagogastric anastomosis or with smaller-diameter EEA, and they respond favorably to dilations. Certain morbidities of esophagectomy

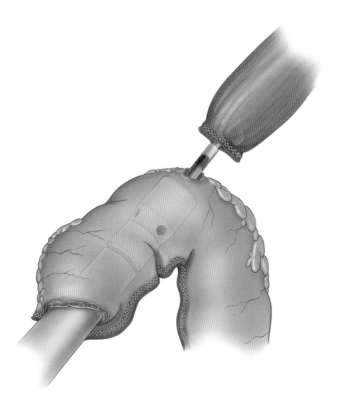

FIGURE 4-10 Thoracoscopic creation of the esophagogastric anastomosis with the EEA stapler.

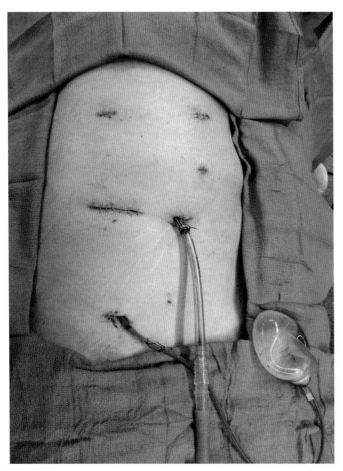

FIGURE 4-11 Skin closure after completion of thoracoscopy. The Jackson-Pratt drain and jejunostomy tube can be seen. (From Wizorek JJ, Awais O, Luketich JD: Minimally invasive esophagectomy. In Zwischenberger JB, editor: *Atlas of Thoracic Surgical Techniques,* 1st edition. Philadelphia, 2010, Saunders, pp 305–319.)

require special attention, namely anastomotic leak, gastric conduit necrosis, and chylothorax. Avoidance and management of these complications are discussed next.

Anastomotic Leak

Anastomotic leak is a frequently reported postoperative complication of esophagectomy. Multiple factors influence the risk for developing an anastomotic leak, including the location and type of anastomosis, anastomotic tension, the quality of the arterial and venous blood supplies near the anastomosis, and the experience of the operating surgeon. Meticulous attention to the handling of the gastric conduit, its blood supply, and the anastomotic technique are all critical determinants of the leak rate and leak severity. It is well recognized that tension at the anastomosis has to be avoided; thus, adequate length of gastric conduit has to be constructed. The use of an appropriately sized conduit also decreases the incidence of leaks. Early in our experience, we discovered that very narrow gastric conduits (2 to 3 cm) were associated with increased anastomotic leaks and gastric tip necrosis; therefore, we now construct wider conduits measuring 4 to 5 cm in diameter. Delayed gastric emptying may cause tension on the anastomosis and result in leaks. The construction of a pyloroplasty and initiation of nasogastric suctioning early postoperatively may help to reduce the incidence of anastomotic leaks. In addition, overly aggressive volumes of oral feedings early in the postoperative period should be avoided. The clinical presentation of patients with anastomotic leak ranges from the relatively asymptomatic, contained leak that requires no intervention to the anastomotic disruption requiring urgent operative intervention.

If the leak is small and contained, no intervention may be required. As the size of the leak increases or the clinical condition of the patient is compromised, a more aggressive diagnostic and planned intervention must be considered. In general, the more stable the patient, the more conservative the approach.

If the Gastrografin swallow, performed on the third or fourth postoperative day, shows a small leak that either is contained or goes directly to the drain and the patient is clinically stable, the patient may be kept under close observation; in some cases, an early diagnostic flexible esophagoscopy to assess the viability of the conduit may be performed. If the leak is not contained or the patient has an otherwise unexplained fever or elevated white blood cell count, one must consider that the leak has led to pleural contamination with free-flowing soilage or to the development of a perianastomotic abscess that may require video-assisted thoracoscopic surgery or open drainage.

In extreme cases, with large areas of necrosis and anastomotic dehiscence, the anastomosis should be taken down, and a proximal esophageal diversion should be carried out. The gastric conduit is reduced into the abdomen, and its viability is assessed; any grossly necrotic areas are resected, and a gastric tube is placed with the plan to return at a later date for conduit reconstruction. Salvage of a few extra centimeters of gastric conduit or proximal esophagus can greatly facilitate later reconstruction.

Some patients may present with a delayed leak from the intrathoracic anastomosis. In this setting, signs and symptoms may include chest pain, dyspnea, and new pleural effusion. The goals of treatment are the same as with any postoperative anastomotic leak: assessment of the conduit at EGD, complete drainage of the leak, complete evacuation of any intrathoracic collections or empyema, and complete lung expansion. Patients who are

Table 4-1 Study Outcomes of Single-Institution Case Series of Ivor Lewis Minimally Invasive Esophagectomy

Study	No. of Subjects	Mortality (%)	Anastomotic Leak (%)	Major Postoperative Complications (%)	LOS (days)
Kunisaki et al, 2004	15	0	13	13	29.6
Bizekis et al, 2006	50	6	6	20	9
Nguyen et al, 2008	51	2	10	12	9.7
Hamouda et al, 2010	51	0	8	19*	16*
Luketich et al, 2012	503	1.2	4.2%	33	8

LOS, length of hospital stay.
*Results in the last 26 of 51 patients who underwent Ivor Lewis minimally invasive esophagectomy.

clinically stable with minimal intrathoracic leaks may be treated conservatively with endoscopy and drain management. In contrast, patients with severe symptoms of sepsis should rapidly be resuscitated and taken to the operating room.

Gastric Conduit Necrosis

Extensive necrosis of the gastric conduit should be a very uncommon event, assuming the conduit and blood supply have been handled with care. But, on occasion, gastric conduit necrosis will be encountered and can be a dreadful complication of esophagectomy. Necrosis can be minimized by avoiding spiraling and twisting of the conduit as it is passed from the abdomen, avoiding constriction at the diaphragmatic hiatus, and avoiding a significantly dilated gastric conduit early postoperatively.

Extensive gastric conduit necrosis should be suspected if the patient exhibits an early and severe leak with fever and tachycardia or metabolic acidosis. If conduit necrosis is suspected, the patient requires urgent esophagoscopy and prompt reexploration to resect the necrotic proximal stomach. When resection of the necrotic portion is necessary, takedown of the gastric tube is almost always required. The viable portion of the distal gastric conduit is returned to the abdomen, and a G-tube is placed. The chest and mediastinum should be widely drained, and a cervical esophagogastrostomy is created. After a period of recovery, rehabilitation, and nutritional optimization, the patient can undergo delayed reconstruction using a colon interposition.

Chylothorax

Chylothorax leads to malnutrition, immunosuppression, and respiratory compromise and can be life-threatening because of ongoing nutritional compromise or immunosuppression. Chylothorax should be an uncommon complication of esophagectomy. It is caused by traumatic injury to the thoracic duct and lymphatic tributaries during esophagectomy and is often the result of technical error. The frequency of chylothorax tends to decrease as surgeon experience with MIE increases. We do not routinely ligate the thoracic duct to avoid chylothorax during esophagectomy but advocate the generous deployment of clips along the right esophageal border to control any ductules arising from the main trunk of the thoracic duct. If an injury is suspected during the primary operation or the dissection has been difficult because of a large tumor or radiation fibrosis, elective ligation should be performed.

Chylothorax presents as persistently elevated chest tube output that increases and becomes milky white after administration of enteral nutrition. A triglyceride level higher than 100 mg/dL in the pleural fluid is associated with a 99% chance of chylous leak, and the presence of chylomicrons is confirmatory. When chylothorax is diagnosed, conservative management, including total parenteral nutrition or medium-chain triglyceride enteral formulas, should be initiated. However, conservative treatment has a high propensity to fail if chest output persists at levels higher than 500 mL per day, and early surgical exploration should be strongly considered. In patients with a high-output leak, we advocate early surgical exploration through a right thorax and mass suture ligation of the thoracic duct at its entry into the thorax. Although this can be performed by a video-assisted thoracoscopic surgery approach, in any situation in which exposure is limited or technical difficulties arise, a thoracotomy should be performed to provide adequate exposure. In some centers, there may be expertise in the Interventional Radiology department to allow lymphatic cannulation and coiling of thoracic duct leaks. This can be a great advantage when the technical expertise is available.

RESULTS AND OUTCOME

There have been several single-institution series published on Ivor Lewis MIE, with the largest published series containing about 50 patients each (Table 4-1). There are also several published case reports on Ivor Lewis MIE, including a case using a colonic conduit with the Ivor Lewis approach and a case of Ivor Lewis MIE in a patient who had previously undergone a Roux-en-Y gastric bypass. Kunisaki and colleagues reported the first series of Ivor Lewis MIE in 2004. There was no operative mortality in this 15-patient series, but the rate of anastomotic leaks was high (13%), and the average hospital stay was lengthy (30 days). In 2008, Nguyen and colleagues reported an updated series of 104 MIEs; 51 were performed using an Ivor Lewis approach. Anastomotic leak occurred in 10% of the patients who underwent Ivor Lewis MIE, and major postoperative complications occurred in 12%. The average hospital stay was 10 days, with an average of 3 days in the ICU.

In 2006, we published our findings in 50 patients who underwent Ivor Lewis MIE, 15 using a totally laparoscopic and thoracoscopic technique and 35 using a laparoscopy with a mini-thoracotomy. The anastomotic leak rate was low (6%). Postoperative complications, seen in 20% of the patients, were less frequent in the patients who underwent a completely laparoscopic and thoracoscopic MIE, and all cases of pneumonia and anastomotic leak occurred in patients who received a mini-thoracotomy. The median hospital stay was 9 days for the patients with the hybrid MIE and only 7 days for the patients with a completely minimally invasive procedure. Median ICU stay was 1 day for both groups. Recently, we presented an updated retrospective series of 503 patients who underwent Ivor Lewis MIE and 477 patients who underwent MIE with a neck anastomosis. In the Ivor Lewis MIE group, our preferred approach now, the anastomotic leak rate was 4.2%, and the 30-day mortality rate was 1.2%. Median hospital stay was 7 days.

In 2010, Hamouda and colleagues published their experience transitioning from open Ivor Lewis esophagectomy to Ivor Lewis MIE. The 51 patients who underwent Ivor Lewis MIE in this series were divided into two groups by time of operation (early group—the first 25 patients, and late group—the next 26 patients). There were no in-hospital deaths in their series. Major postoperative complications were seen in about 19% of patients and were not significantly different between the patients who underwent MIE early and late in the series. Anastomotic leak occurred in 4 patients (8%), with only 1 of the 26 patients (4%) in the late group experiencing this complication. The study of Hamouda and colleagues is the only study to date that directly compares Ivor Lewis MIE with open Ivor Lewis esophagectomy, albeit in a retrospective study rather than a prospective, randomized trial. In their experience, the MIE approach reduced the operative time and the need for blood transfusion, but did not reduce postoperative morbidity.

Recently, with the senior author (JDL) serving as principal investigator and coordinating site, we completed a prospective, phase II, multicenter trial of MIE (Eastern Cooperative Oncology Group [ECOG], 2202), which included both the Ivor Lewis approach and the three-incision McKeown approach. The trial results were reported at the 2009 American Society for Clinical Oncology (ASCO) annual meeting. More than 100 patients were enrolled from 16 institutions across the United States, and 99 patients underwent MIE. Neoadjuvant chemotherapy was administered to 35 patients (33%), and neoadjuvant radiation was administered to 26 patients (25%). The final pathologies included high-grade dysplasia ($n = 11$) and esophageal cancer ($n = 88$). The mortality rate was only 2%, with acceptable morbidity, and a median ICU stay of 2 days. The median lymph node count was 20. At the short-term evaluation, outcomes were acceptable, with an estimated 3-year overall survival for the entire cohort of 50% (95% confidence interval, 35% to 65%). The results of the ECOG 2202 trial are similar to our series of MIE, primarily using the modified McKweon approach, in 222 patients, the largest series of MIE published to date. The final pathologies in the series included high-grade dysplasia ($n = 47$) and esophageal cancer ($n = 175$). The operative mortality rate was only 1.4%. Median ICU stay was 1 day, and median hospital stay was 7 days.

Stage-specific survival, at a median follow-up of 19 months, was similar to published series of open esophagectomy.

There are no published, randomized studies comparing open esophagectomy and MIE, although one is ongoing (the TIME-trial, a multi-institutional study currently enrolling patients in the Netherlands). The outcomes in many series of MIE have been compared with the published outcomes of open esophagectomy and suggest that MIE decreases perioperative morbidity.

MIE is safe and leads to good outcomes, especially when performed in centers with significant experience in MIE and other minimally invasive esophageal procedures. Mortality after the procedure is low. Postsurgical morbidity rates are acceptable, and increasing evidence suggests that MIE reduces morbidity and length of hospital stay compared with open esophagectomy. Although the oncologic outcomes studied to date are limited (3-year survival and lymph node retrieval), the oncologic efficacy of MIE is likely equivalent to that of open esophagectomy.

Suggested Readings

Bizekis C, Kent MS, Luketich JD, et al: Initial experience with minimally invasive Ivor Lewis esophagectomy, *Ann Thorac Surg* 82:402–406, discussion 406–407, 2006.

Hamouda AH, Forshaw MJ, Tsigritis K, et al: Perioperative outcomes after transition from conventional to minimally invasive Ivor-Lewis esophagectomy in a specialized center, *Surg Endosc* 24:865–869, 2010.

Kent M, Luketich JD: Minimally invasive esophagectomy. In Frantzides CT, Carlson MA, editors: *Atlas of Minimally Invasive Surgery*, Philadelphia, 2009, Saunders, pp 3–15.

Kunisaki C, Hatori S, Imada T, et al: Video-assisted thoracoscopic esophagectomy with a voice-controlled robot: The AESOP system, *Surg Laparosc Endosc Percutan Tech* 14:323–327, 2004.

Luketich JD, Alvelo-Rivera M, Buenaventura PO, et al: Minimally invasive esophagectomy: Outcomes in 222 patients, *Ann Surg* 238:486–495, 2003.

Luketich JD, Pennathur A, Awais O, et al: Outcomes after minimally invasive esophagectomy, *Ann Surg* 2012, in press.

Luketich JD, Pennathur A, Catalano PJ, et al: Results of a phase II multicenter study of MIE (Eastern Cooperative Oncology Group Study E2202), *J Clin Oncol* 27:15s(abstr 4516), 2009.

Nagpal K, Ahmed K, Vats A, et al: Is minimally invasive surgery beneficial in the management of esophageal cancer? A meta-analysis, *Surg Endosc* 24:1621–1629, 2010.

Nguyen NT, Hinojosa MW, Smith BR, et al: Minimally invasive esophagectomy: Lessons learned from 104 operations, *Ann Surg* 248:1081–1091, 2008.

Pennathur A, Luketich JD: Minimally invasive esophagectomy: Avoidance and treatment of complications. In Little AG, Merrill WH, editors: *Complications in Cardiothoracic Surgery: Avoidance and Treatment*, ed 2, Hoboken, NJ, 2009, Wiley-Blackwell, pp 247–265.

Sgourakis G, Gockel I, Radtke A, et al: Minimally invasive versus open esophagectomy: Meta-analysis of outcomes, *Dig Dis Sci* 55:3031–3040, 2010.

CONSTANTINE T. FRANTZIDES, SCOTT N. WELLE, MINH B. LUU, AND ANDREW M. POPOFF

Laparoscopic Esophagomyotomy with Nissen Fundoplication

The videos associated with this chapter are listed in the Video Contents and can be found on the accompanying DVDs and *on Expertconsult.com.*

Achalasia is a rare primary esophageal motility disorder characterized by progressive dysphagia. Although the degree may vary among individuals, dysphagia is present in all patients affected by the disorder. Other symptoms, such as chest pain, epigastric pain, odynophagia, regurgitation, vomiting, heartburn, and weight loss, may also be present. Physiologic features include aperistalsis of the esophageal body, normal to high lower esophageal sphincter (LES) resting pressures, and a lack of LES relaxation on swallowing. Treatments are aimed at relieving dysphagia by disrupting the LES musculature or promoting its relaxation. Short-term relief of dysphagia can be achieved with endoscopic botulinum toxin injections or pneumatic dilations. Endoscopic treatment of achalasia was the preferred method in the 1970s and 1980s despite many reports showing the superiority of an esophagomyotomy over dilation. Esophagomyotomy was first described by Heller in 1913 and later modified to a single anterior myotomy. Although the thoracic approach has been widely used to perform the myotomy, the abdominal approach has emerged as the preferred approach by the surgical community. In cases of reoperative myotomy due to incomplete proximal myotomy or a hostile upper abdomen from previous surgeries, the thoracic approach may be useful. Laparoscopic esophagomyotomy was popularized in the 1990s and has become the treatment of choice for patients with achalasia. Long-term relief of dysphagia in the 90% range, minimal postoperative pain, short hospitalization, and overall patient satisfaction contribute to its wide acceptance. Symptoms of postoperative reflux, which can be as high as 60%, can be reduced with the addition of a fundoplication. A balance must be maintained between controlling reflux and avoiding a significant increase in resistance caused by the fundoplication to an aperistaltic esophageal body. The superiority of the complete (Nissen) wrap over partial (Dor, Toupet) wrap in controlling reflux symptoms has been well demonstrated in the treatment of gastroesophageal reflux disease (GERD). The decision to perform a partial versus a complete fundoplication remains controversial, although most fundoplications performed after a myotomy are partial. Several reports show an increased incidence of dysphagia with a complete fundoplication compared with a partial fundoplication. We believe the difference in dysphagia rates represents technical error of the fundoplication rather than a significant difference in the resistance of the complete wrap. We routinely perform a short floppy Nissen fundoplication after an esophagomyotomy with a low incidence of postoperative dysphagia. On the accompanying DVD (as well as on Expert Consult), we have included a video of a laparoscopic esophagomyotomy with Nissen fundoplication as an update and contrast to the procedure described in Chapter 2 of the *Atlas of Minimally Invasive Surgery*, 2009 (see Suggested Readings at the end of this chapter). The fine dissection and tips described here are the result of years of experience of the senior author (CTF), and we hope the viewer will gain the valuable insight necessary to perform the operation successfully.

OPERATIVE INDICATIONS

Dysphagia with manometric findings consistent with achalasia is an indication for surgery. Short-term relief can be achieved with endoscopic injection with botulinum toxin (Botox) or pneumatic dilation. These nonoperative interventions carry a small risk for perforation and may result in scarring, which will increase the risk for mucosal injury during surgical myotomy.

PREOPERATIVE EVALUATION, TESTING, AND PREPARATION

Patients with symptoms of dysphagia should be questioned for the severity, frequency, and concurrent presence of heartburn, chest pain, regurgitation, and significant weight loss. Upper gastrointestinal contrast study may show the characteristic tapering of the distal esophagus (bird's beak deformity). A megaesophagus is indicative of advanced disease and may result in a lower success rate. All patients, especially elderly patients with dysphagia and weight loss, should have an upper endoscopy to evaluate for cancer. Biopsy and further evaluation with endoscopic ultrasound (EUS) should be performed for lesions suspicious for cancer. Esophageal manometry is the gold standard to diagnose achalasia. Manometric findings of tertiary or aperistaltic waveforms, normal to high LES pressures, and high receptive LES pressures are consistent with achalasia. Manometry is especially useful to differentiate achalasia from other esophageal motility disorders such as diffuse esophageal spasm, nutcracker esophagus, and severe GERD. Patients with heartburn who have undergone endoscopic dilation should have a pH study to differentiate pathologic reflux due to dilation from food stasis due to poor esophageal emptying. Nutritional status should be optimized before surgical intervention in patients with a significant weight loss.

POSITIONING AND PLACEMENT OF TROCARS

The patient is placed in modified "French" lithotomy position as shown in Figure 5-1 with 30-degree reverse Trendelenburg. The surgeon stands between the patient's legs, the camera operator stands to the patient's right, and the first assistant stands to the patient's left. Five trocars are placed as shown in Figure 5-2. The initial port (number 1) is placed using the optical trocar in the left midclavicular line subcostally and serves as the surgeon's operating right hand. Subsequent trocars are placed in the order numbered two through five. The basic principles of trocar position and use should be followed: the camera port (number 5) should be in the midline superior to the umbilicus. The surgeon's left-hand working port (number 2) is placed in the right subcostal region in the midclavicular line. The retraction and assistant port (number 3) should be placed in the left midaxillary line caudad to port number 1. Trocar number 4 is used to retract the left lateral lobe of the liver and is placed in the subxiphoid region.

OPERATIVE TECHNIQUE

Exposure

The esophageal hiatus is exposed after the left lateral segment of the liver is retracted anteriorly using a fixed retractor or a hand-held balloon retractor. Use of the fixed retractor avoids the need for an assistant to maintain constant retraction during the case, but insertion and removal of the retractor can be difficult. Alternatively, we prefer to use the balloon retractor, which allows for frequent adjustments to optimize exposure of the esophageal hiatus. We prefer the subxiphoid position for the liver retractor, but a right lateral position of the retractor is an acceptable alternative. Reverse Trendelenburg position to about 30 degrees aids in displacing the omentum, small intestine, and transverse colon to the lower abdomen.

Dissection

Dissection of the esophageal hiatus begins with the division of the gastrohepatic omentum overlying the caudate lobe of the liver. The gastrohepatic omentum is thin and relatively avascular and can be divided using a hook monopolar cautery or the Harmonic scalpel (Ethicon Endo-Surgery, Blue Ash, Ohio). More superiorly, an aberrant or replaced left hepatic artery may be encountered. A small accessory left hepatic artery may be divided, but attempts should be made to preserve a more prominent-appearing left hepatic artery. The peritoneal reflection at the angle of His is incised using the hook electrocautery. Gentle traction by the assistant on the gastrosplenic omentum can aid in the exposure, especially in obese patients. Care should be taken not to cause tearing of the splenic capsule during the retraction of the fundus.

From the angle of His, the dissection continues medially by dividing the phrenoesophageal ligament. The dissection should be superficial to avoid injury to the esophagus or the vagus nerve. We find it useful to place a lighted bougie to aid in the identification of the esophagus. The plane between the esophagus and crura can be developed using blunt dissection with a palpation probe. The remaining attachments of the mediastinum to the esophagus can be divided using a Harmonic scalpel. Care should be taken not to tear the pleura or injure the heart during this phase of the esophageal mobilization.

The anterior vagus nerve appears as a white stringlike structure coursing from the patient's left to right anteriorly. Early identification of the anterior vagus nerve is crucial to prevent injury. Caudal retraction of the stomach is accomplished using the shaft of a grasper from trocar number 2. Alternatively, a Penrose drain can be used to encircle the gastroesophageal junction and retracted from trocar number 3. Adequate mobilization of the esophagus is important in performing a sufficient myotomy.

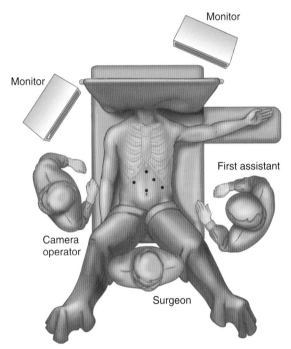

FIGURE 5-1 Patient positioning and operating room layout for the performance of laparoscopic esophagomyotomy.

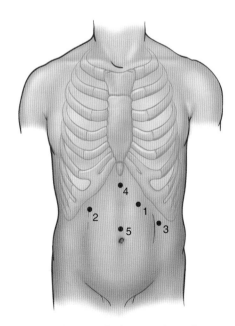

FIGURE 5-2 Port placement for laparoscopic esophagomyotomy.

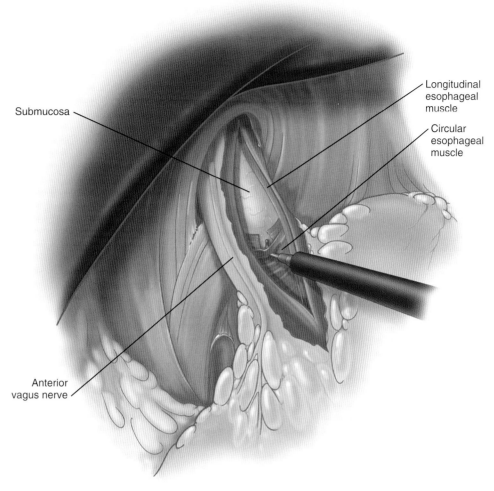

Submucosa

Longitudinal
esophageal
muscle

Circular
esophageal
muscle

Anterior
vagus nerve

FIGURE 5-3 The longitudinal and circular esophageal muscles are divided fiber by fiber using hook electrocautery.

Myotomy

The myotomy begins at the gastroesophageal junction by dividing the pre-esophageal areolar tissue. In obese patients, the pre-esophageal fat pad may need to be excised to adequately expose the gastroesophageal junction. The anterior vagus nerve is identified again, and the planned line of myotomy is chosen just to the patient's left. Along the anterior surface of the distal esophagus, the outer longitudinal muscle fibers are initially divided transversely and subsequently divided along the longitudinal axis of the esophagus. The inner circular muscle fibers are identified and divided. Finding the submucosal plane is a key step to the operation. The vascularity of the mucosa can be illuminated by the lighted bougie and contrasted to the more dense circular muscle fibers. The lighted bougie is pulled back so that the smaller caliber tapered end is at the distal esophagus, allowing more laxity to the muscle fibers. Division of the muscle fibers can be performed using a monopolar hook cautery (Fig. 5-3) or Harmonic scalpel. The lateral back-and-forth movement of the hook will separate the circular layer from the underlying mucosa. The use of a specialized hook with insulation of the posterior surface can help decrease the chance of mucosal injury. Regardless of the instrument used, meticulous dissection of the circular muscle fibers away from the mucosa is necessary before division of the muscle. The use of a Da Vinci robotic system (Intuitive Surgical, Sunnyvale, Calif.) can aid in the precise movements necessary to perform a safe myotomy for those who find this portion of the procedure too difficult. We routinely divide at least 6 cm of esophageal muscle and 2 to 3 cm of gastric muscle fibers (Fig. 5-4). Division of the gastric muscle fibers is more difficult owing to the intertwining of the fibers. However, complete division of these fibers is necessary for the resolution of symptoms. Intraoperative endoscopy may be used to confirm the adequacy of the myotomy and evaluate for potential mucosal injury, especially for surgeons early in the learning curve.

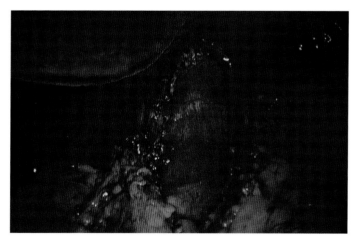

FIGURE 5-4 The laparoscopic view of a completed myotomy.

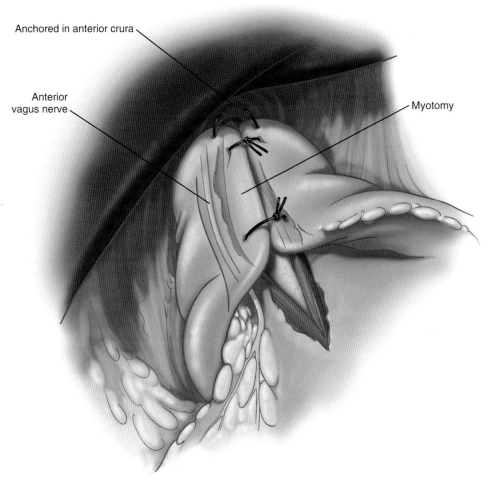

Anchored in anterior crura

Anterior
vagus nerve

Myotomy

FIGURE 5-5 A completed esophagomyotomy with a floppy 360-degree fundoplication.

Reconstruction

The Nissen fundoplication is constructed with the following principles in mind: division of the short gastric vessels, closure of the crural defect (if necessary), use of a bougie, and completion of a short and floppy fundoplication. Division of the short gastric vessels is performed using the Harmonic scalpel starting at the midstomach. Care is taken not to cause thermal injury to the greater curvature of the stomach or the spleen. As the dissection proceeds toward the angle of His, the stomach is progressively retracted to the patient's right using the left-hand working port. Excessive traction of the stomach should be avoided to prevent tearing the splenic capsule. Near the superior pole of the spleen, the fundus of the stomach can come very close to the spleen. Division of the vessels at this point requires a steady hand and fine movements of the Harmonic scalpel. Just before activation of the Harmonic scalpel, traction on the tissue should be decreased to allow better hemostasis. Clear visualization of the left bundle of the right crus indicates a complete mobilization of the fundus. A posterior cruroplasty is performed over the lighted bougie (60 French) using interrupted nonabsorbable sutures. Because of the limited working space around the posterior aspect of the crura, we find it easier to use the Endo Stitch (Covidien, Norwalk, Conn.) with extracorporeal ties secured with a knot pusher. Two to three posterior sutures are used for the primary cruroplasty. The freed fundus is passed posterior to the esophagus and the shoe-shine maneuver is performed to assess the degree of laxity. Using an Endo Stitch with extracorporeal knots,

a 2-cm floppy fundoplication is created with interrupted stitches of nonabsorbable suture (Fig. 5-5). The superior suture incorporates the anterior aspect of the crus to anchor the wrap.

POSTOPERATIVE CARE

Hospitalization averages 1 to 2 days; an upper gastrointestinal Gastrografin study is performed on the first postoperative day to radiographically confirm the adequacy of the myotomy, to evaluate the effectiveness of the fundoplication, and to evaluate for potential leaks. Diet is restricted to clear liquids initially and advanced to soft food.

MANAGEMENT OF PROCEDURE-SPECIFIC COMPLICATIONS

Intraoperative mucosal injury is the most common complication, and, if recognized immediately, it can be primarily repaired. The repaired mucosa should be buttressed with a fundoplication or omentum and drained. Testing of the mucosal integrity can be performed with endoscopic visualization, air insufflation, methylene blue, or a combination. Delayed esophageal or gastric mucosal injuries typically present as persistent tachycardia, chest pain, and fever. When suspected, an esophagogram should be performed to diagnose and assess the extent of the leak. Early small leaks can be repaired by laparoscopy or laparotomy. Extensive inflammation or mucosal damage not amenable to primary repair may require an esophagectomy. A closed drain should be placed near the mucosal repairs and a feeding jejunostomy should be considered.

Pneumothorax can result from tearing of the pleura during the hiatal dissection. Once recognized, communication with the anesthesia team is important to monitor for respiratory compromise. A chest tube is not indicated unless there is a concurrent lung injury. Lowering the pressure limit of the pneumoperitoneum may help respiratory mechanics. Postoperative supplemental oxygen may facilitate the absorption of the capnothorax.

Persistent postoperative dysphagia without a symptom-free interval is a result of a technical error. These errors are due to either an incomplete myotomy or an incorrectly constructed fundoplication. Dysphagia after a prolonged period of symptomatic improvement may represent a natural progression of the disease or the result of chronic GERD. Evaluation with esophagography, endoscopy, manometry, and pH study should be performed before further therapeutic intervention. Postoperative dysphagia can be treated with endoscopic dilation or surgical exploration.

Pathologic reflux can be found in up to 20% of patients studied with pH monitoring after an esophagomyotomy and fundoplication. Interestingly, only half of these patients are symptomatic. In young asymptomatic patients with abnormal reflux, the effects of prolonged contact with gastric refluxate on the esophageal mucosa are unknown. We recommend treating all patients with documented pathologic reflux with acid suppression regardless of symptoms.

RESULTS AND OUTCOMES

Laparoscopic esophagomyotomy for achalasia results in relief of dysphagia in greater than 90% of patients according to most studies. Symptomatic relief and quality of life improvements are durable according to long-term reports. The extent of myotomy, especially onto the gastric muscle fibers, is an important component of short-term outcomes. This assumption stems from studies showing the persistence of hypertrophied muscle extending distally onto the stomach in patients whose symptoms failed to resolve. These findings suggest that division of the crossing fibers of the gastric muscle is crucial in reducing the resistance to the progression of the food bolus. Gastric myotomy to a length of 3 cm has been advocated by Oelschlager and colleagues. Most patients with recurrent dysphagia due to incomplete myotomy can be treated with pneumatic dilation. The few that continue to have symptoms should undergo surgical exploration to determine whether a repeat myotomy is warranted. Sigmoidization of the esophagus has been shown to be associated with only a 50% rate of success with myotomy. Despite the relatively low rate of success, patients with advanced achalasia should be informed of the lower rate of success, and a myotomy should be attempted first. Because of the higher morbidity, an esophagectomy should be reserved for those who have failed both surgical myotomy and pneumatic dilation.

The use of a partial versus complete fundoplication remains controversial. The risk for early postoperative dysphagia must be weighed against the long-term effects of pathologic reflux, especially in younger patients. In a report by Csendes and associates on the long-term results of a myotomy with Dor fundoplication, pathologic reflux and the development of Barrett esophagus

were implicated as the causes of progressive dysphagia after an initial period of success. Youssef and Richards both reported that a partial fundoplication did not result in significant dysphagia. Furthermore, Richards demonstrated that gastric reflux is significantly less with a myotomy and Dor fundoplication compared with myotomy alone. Early reports of laparoscopic esophagomyotomy performed with a complete fundoplication demonstrated high incidences of dysphagia. Wills reported that patients with a myotomy and partial fundoplication experienced less dysphagia than those with a complete fundoplication, but the difference was not statistically significant. In contrast, however, Frantzides and coworkers reported more recently on the superior control of reflux symptoms with a complete 360-degree wrap and demonstrated that a short floppy Nissen properly constructed (i.e., performed over a lighted bougie, avoiding incorporation of the esophagus into the fundoplication, and anchoring the wrap to the crura of the diaphragm) does not increase the incidence of dysphagia compared with a partial wrap. In the same study, a partial wrap resulted in a high incidence of gastroesophageal reflux. A poorly constructed wrap will result in persistent dysphagia regardless of the type of wrap used.

Laparoscopic esophagomyotomy with a concurrent 360-degree fundoplication is a technically demanding operation requiring precise dissection and advanced laparoscopic skills. In experienced and well-trained hands, the results are excellent and durable.

Suggested Readings

Campos GM, Vittinghoff E, Rabl C, et al: Endoscopic and surgical treatments for achalasia: A systematic review and meta-analysis, *Ann Surg* 249:45–57, 2009.

Cowgill SM, Villadolid D, Boyle R, et al: Laparoscopic Heller myotomy for achalasia: Results after 10 years, *Surg Endosc* 24:2644–2649, 2009.

Csendes A, Braghetto I, Burdiles P, et al: Very late results of esophagomyotomy for patients with achalasia: clinical, endoscopic, histologic, manometric, and acid reflux studies in 67 patients for a mean follow-up of 190 months, *Ann Surg* 243:196–203, 2006.

Frantzides CT, Moore RE, Carlson MA, et al: Minimally invasive surgery for achalasia: A 10-year experience, *J Gastrointest Surg* 8:18–23, 2004.

Glatz SM, Richardson JD: Esophagectomy for end stage achalasia, *J Gastrointest Surg* 11:1134–1137, 2007.

Hungness ES, Soper NJ: Laparoscopic esophagomyotomy. In Frantzides CT, Carlson MA, editors: *Atlas of Minimally Invasive Surgery*, Philadelphia, 2009, Saunders, pp 17–22.

Oelschlager BK, Chang L, Pelligrini CA: Improved outcome after extended gastric myotomy for achalasia, *Arch Surg* 138:490–497, 2003.

Rebecchi F, Giaccone C, Farinella E, et al: Randomized controlled trial of laparoscopic Heller myotomy plus Dor fundoplication versus Nissen fundoplication for achalasia: Long-term results, *Ann Surg* 248:1023–1030, 2008.

Richards WO, Torquati A, Holzman MD, et al: Heller myotomy versus Heller myotomy with Dor fundoplication for achalasia: A prospective randomized double-blind clinical trial, *Ann Surg* 240:405–412, 2004.

Rosetti G, Brusciano L, Amato G, et al: A total fundoplication is not an obstacle to esophageal emptying after Heller myotomy for achalasia: Results of a long-term follow-up, *Ann Surg* 241:614–621, 2005.

Schuchert MJ, Luketich JD, Landreneau RJ: Minimally-invasive esophagomyotomy in 200 consecutive patients: Factors influencing postoperative outcomes, *Ann Thorac Surg* 85:1729–1734, 2008.

Wills VL, Hunt DR: Functional outcome after Heller myotomy and fundoplication for achalasia, *J Gastrointest Surg* 5:408–413, 2001.

Youssef Y, Richards WO, Sharp K, et al: Relief of dysphagia after laparoscopic Heller myotomy improves long-term quality of life, *J Gastrointest Surg* 11:309–313, 2007.

Zaninotto G, Costantini M, Rizzetto C: Four hundred laparoscopic myotomies for esophageal achalasia: A single centre experience, *Ann Surg* 248:986–993, 2008.

CONSTANTINE T. FRANTZIDES, SCOTT N. WELLE, JACOB E. ROBERTS, AND TIMOTHY M. RUFF

Laparoscopic Esophageal Mucosal Resection for High-Grade Dysplasia

6

The videos associated with this chapter are listed in the Video Contents and can be found on the accompanying DVDs and *on Expertconsult.com.*

Barrett esophagus is defined as the metaplastic replacement of the normal squamous epithelium of the distal esophagus by columnar epithelium. Three histopathologic subtypes of metaplastic columnar epithelium have been described: two gastric phenotypes and one intestinal type. Because the intestinal type has the greatest risk for malignant transformation, the 2008 guidelines of the American College of Gastroenterology specify that the term *Barrett esophagus* should be restricted to columnar epithelium containing intestinal metaplasia. Estimates of the frequency of Barrett esophagus in the general population have ranged from 0.9% to 4.5%. Gastroesophageal reflux disease is the only known risk factor associated with the development of Barrett esophagus. A recent review of 15 epidemiologic studies in patients with gastroesophageal reflux disease (defined by at least weekly heartburn or acid regurgitation) identified a Barrett esophagus prevalence of 10% to 20% in the West and about 5% in Asia. Barrett esophagus with high-grade dysplasia is considered a premalignant condition. In patients with known Barrett esophagus, the annual risk for developing adenocarcinoma ranges from 0.2% to 2.0%.

The current gold standard for the treatment of Barrett esophagus with high-grade dysplasia is esophagectomy because of the perceived prevalence of invasive carcinoma in such specimens after esophagectomy. Recently, however, a meta-analysis of esophagectomy for high-grade dysplasia revealed invasive adenocarcinoma in only 12.7% of specimens. These data, along with inability or unwillingness to undergo esophagectomy, have further encouraged some patients to pursue more conservative treatment options for high-grade dysplasia. Other treatment options include endoscopic thermal therapy, photodynamic therapy, radiofrequency ablation, and laser ablation. Endoscopic mucosal resection has also been described as successful in treating high-grade dysplasia. One of the drawbacks of endoscopic mucosal resection for high-grade dysplasia or early esophageal cancer in Barrett esophagus has been the high rate of recurrent or metachronous lesions during follow-up in recent series (11% to 30%). Another drawback of endoscopic mucosal resection is that Barrett esophagus affecting segments longer than 2 cm is difficult to treat with endoscopic mucosal resection because piecemeal resection is often necessary. This usually requires a higher level of endoscopic expertise, multiple sessions, and an increased risk for complications. Additionally, it is difficult to be conclusive about the completeness of the resection at the lateral margins. This chapter presents a surgical alternative to esophagectomy and endoscopic management for high-grade dysplasia of the distal esophagus. The senior author (CTF) and colleagues previously published the success of laparoscopic transgastric esophageal mucosal resection; this chapter and the recording on the accompanying DVD (as well as on Expert Consult) are a follow-up to those published reports.

OPERATIVE INDICATIONS

Barrett esophagus with high-grade dysplasia on endoscopic biopsy is an indication for esophageal mucosal resection. A segment of Barrett esophagus longer than 5 cm may require a combined endoscopic and laparoscopic approach.

PREOPERATIVE EVALUATION

The objectives of the preoperative evaluation include (1) confirming the diagnosis of Barrett esophagus with high-grade dysplasia, (2) evaluating for hiatal hernia, (3) evaluating for neoplasm or dysmotility, and (4) determining the patient's suitability for the operation.

A chest radiograph may demonstrate a hiatal hernia and provide information about its size and contents. Concomitant lung disease can be identified as well.

An upper gastrointestinal contrast study will provide information on the anatomy of the esophagus and stomach, which is especially helpful when there is an associated hiatal hernia. In addition, an upper gastrointestinal study can provide direct evidence of the extent of gastroesophageal reflux disease. In the hands of an experienced radiologist, the study can also provide information on the patient's esophageal motility.

An esophagogastroduodenoscopy (EGD) permits direct evaluation of the esophagogastric mucosa. Biopsies of the mucosa can confirm the presence of Barrett esophagus with high-grade dysplasia as well as the presence or absence of cancer. The EGD can also verify the presence of a hiatal hernia.

If the patient has a large hiatal hernia, then a computed tomography scan of the chest is helpful in delineating the anatomy and contents of the hernia sac, including the presence of organs other than the stomach.

POSITIONING AND PLACEMENT OF TROCARS

The patient is placed in a modified French lithotomy position with 30-degree reverse Trendelenburg (see Fig. 5-1 in Chapter

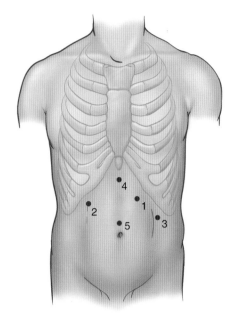

FIGURE 6-1 Port placement for the performance of esophageal mucosal resection.

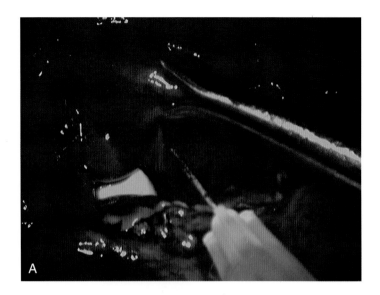

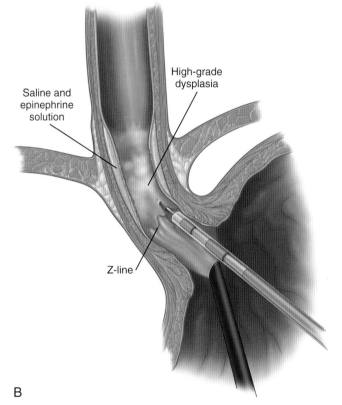

FIGURE 6-2 Submucosal injection of epinephrine and normal saline (1:100,000).

5). The surgeon stands between the patient's legs, the camera operator stands to the patient's right, and the first assistant stands to the patient's left. Five trocars are placed as shown in Figure 6-1. The initial port (number 1) is placed using the optical trocar in the left midclavicular line subcostally and serves as the surgeon's operating right hand. Subsequent trocars are placed in the order numbered two through five. The basic principles of trocar position and use should be followed: The camera port (number 5) is in the midline superior to the umbilicus. The surgeon's left-hand working port (number 2) is placed in the right subcostal region in the midclavicular line. The retraction port for the assistant (number 3) is placed in the left midaxillary line caudad to port number 1. Trocar number 4 is used to retract the left lateral lobe of the liver and is placed in the subxiphoid region.

OPERATIVE TECHNIQUE

The left lobe of the liver is retracted with the use of an inflatable balloon retractor. The esophageal hiatus is visualized. If a hiatal hernia is present, the contents of the hernia are reduced by gentle traction, and the hernia sac is mobilized and excised. The esophagus is circumferentially mobilized and reduced into the abdomen for 3 to 5 cm. In addition, the esophagus is mobilized to an additional 5 cm in the mediastinum. This mobilization of the esophagus allows for a safer dissection of the esophageal mucosa later. If there is an inadvertent esophageal perforation, this may be diagnosed and addressed immediately. Following the circumferential mobilization of the esophagus, a 5-cm transverse gastrotomy is made 4 cm caudad to the gastroesophageal junction. The lumen of the esophagus and the location of the Z-line are visualized through the gastrotomy. A 30-degree laparoscope is indispensible in performing the operation.

A solution of epinephrine and normal saline (1:100,000) is injected with a retractable hypodermic needle system at the Z-line of the distal esophagus to aid in the elevation of the mucosa (Fig. 6-2). The submucosal plane is entered with a modified hook electrocautery instrument; the hook is completely insulated except for the superior edge to allow contact with the underlying

muscular layer and not cause thermal injury (Fig. 6-3). The mucosa is dissected further from the underlying smooth muscle with a curved laparoscopic spatula (Fig. 6-4). The mucosa is circumferentially dissected and excised in four quadrants. The mucosal segment is then excised using hook scissors. The tapered end of a lighted bougie (Medovations Inc., Milwaukee, Wis.) maneuvered by laparoscopic forceps is used as a retractor for exposing the four quadrants of mucosa (Fig. 6-5). The excised mucosa is oriented and marked for proximal and distal pathologic orientation. The raw surface of the esophagus is irrigated profusely, and any bleeding is controlled with cautious use of electrocautery. The esophageal wall in the area of mucosal resection is checked for intactness.

The gastrotomy is approximated with interrupted polyester sutures and then closed with a laparoscopic linear stapler. The

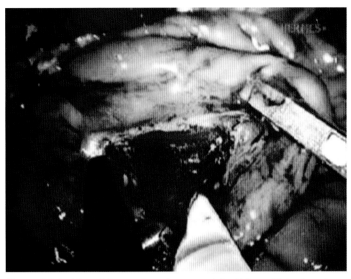

FIGURE 6-3 Incision of the esophageal mucosa at the Z-line with hook cautery.

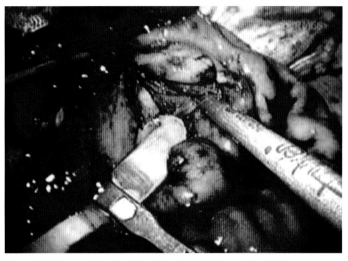

FIGURE 6-5 Maneuvering the lighted bougie with forceps for added exposure; the anterior, medial, and lateral aspects of the esophagus show areas of mucosal resection.

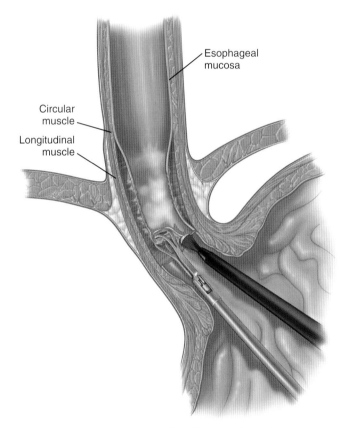

FIGURE 6-4 Diagrammatic representation of transgastric esophageal mucosal resection.

gastroesophageal junction and the gastrotomy site are tested for leaks with both air and methylene blue. A hiatal hernia repair is performed if necessary over a lighted bougie as well as a three-stitch 360-degree Nissen fundoplication, as described in Chapters 3 and 4 of the *Atlas of Minimally Invasive Surgery*, 2009 (see Suggested Readings at the end of this chapter).

POSTOPERATIVE CARE

Hospitalization averages 2 to 3 days; an upper gastrointestinal Gastrografin study is performed on the first postoperative day to evaluate for potential perforation. Diet is restricted to clear liquids initially for 1 week. The patient is evaluated postoperatively at 1 week in the office, and the diet is advanced to soft foods for 1 month before being advanced to a regular diet. Follow-up upper endoscopy is performed at 3, 6, and 12 months, and then annually. Multiple mucosal biopsies and methylene blue staining are performed at each endoscopy.

PROCEDURE-SPECIFIC COMPLICATIONS

In the limited number of procedures performed, no major complications have occurred in the patients; however, the most feared complication is an inadvertent esophageal perforation. If recognized immediately, a small perforation can be primarily repaired. The repaired esophagus should be buttressed with a fundoplication or omentum and drained. Testing of the integrity of the esophagus can be performed with endoscopic visualization, air insufflation, or methylene blue. Delayed injuries typically present as persistent tachycardia, chest pain, and fever. Early small leaks can be repaired by laparoscopy or laparotomy. Perforation with extensive inflammation that is not amenable to primary repair may require an esophagectomy. A closed drain should be placed near the repair, and a feeding jejunostomy may be considered.

Stricture formation after laparoscopic esophageal mucosal resection occurred in 33% of patients (two of six). This stenosis occurred in the early postoperative period and is likely the result of edema and inflammation rather than fibrosis (Fig. 6-6). This complication responded to endoscopic pneumatic dilation without any further sequelae.

Other potential complications that may occur are secondary to the concomitantly performed hiatal hernia repair and Nissen fundoplication, such as bleeding, pneumothorax, and others. For a more thorough discussion of these complications, please refer to the previously mentioned chapters in the *Atlas of Minimally Invasive Surgery*, 2009 (see Suggested Readings at the end of this chapter).

RESULTS AND OUTCOMES

Laparoscopic transgastric esophageal mucosal resection was performed in six patients (all male; median age, 53.5 years; range, 44 to 68 years). All patients had high-grade dysplasia on

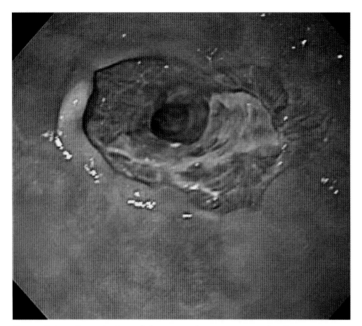

FIGURE 6-6 Endoscopic view of the mucosal resection 2 weeks after surgery in a patient who developed an esophageal stenosis requiring endoscopic pneumatic dilation.

preoperative biopsy. The median length of Barrett esophagus was 4.0 cm (range, 0.5 to 8.0 cm). In the patient with the longest (8.0 cm) segment of Barrett esophagus, the proximal extent of abnormal epithelium could not be reached with the laparoscopic approach. This patient had a complete endoscopic mucosal resection in the early postoperative period. There was no 30-day mortality or morbidity other than the two aforementioned strictures. Five patients had high-grade dysplasia on pathologic examination; one patient had a small region that was reported as carcinoma in situ. The latter patient was offered an esophagectomy, but he elected to undergo surveillance. The patients have been followed for a median of 6.3 years (range, 4.5 to 7.5 years).

All patients regenerated normal squamous epithelium at the site of the mucosal resection 6 months after surgery. One patient developed a recurrence of nondysplastic Barrett epithelium (several small islands) 2 years after resection; he is being managed with surveillance and a proton pump inhibitor. The patient with completion resection has been without recurrence for 6 years.

Laparoscopic esophageal mucosal resection offers advantages over other endoscopic approaches for the treatment of Barrett esophagus with dysplasia: the specimen can be removed with proper orientation for pathology, visualization allows for hemorrhage control and minimal electrocautery use, and a perforation can be diagnosed at the time of surgery and repaired without sequelae. A concomitant hiatal hernia may be repaired if present. Endoscopic modalities are difficult to apply in patients with a large hiatal hernia because accurate placement of probes is challenging and more likely than not will result in inadequate resection. Additionally, the laparoscopic approach allows for the performance of an antireflux procedure that cures

gastroesophageal reflux disease, the main facet of Barrett esophagus genesis. The possibility of a postoperative esophageal stricture exists with any circumferential endoscopic mucosal resection; however, early endoscopy has been valuable in the diagnosis and early treatment of such strictures.

A technical limitation of the laparoscopic mucosal resection is that only up to 5 cm in length of mucosa can be excised because of the technical and mechanical confines of this approach. Additional mucosa can be excised postoperatively with an endoscopic approach. Although early results from this technique are promising, higher patient numbers are necessary for the technique to become mainstream. In addition, the procedure is technically demanding, requiring advanced laparoscopic skills and experience.

Suggested Readings

Conio M, Blanchi S, Lapertosa G, et al: Long-term endoscopic surveillance of patients with Barrett's esophagus. Incidence of dysplasia and adenocarcinoma: A prospective study, *Am J Gastroenterol* 98:1931–1939, 2003.

Dent J, El-Serag HB, Wallander MA, et al: Epidemiology of gastro-oesophageal reflux disease: A systematic review, *Gut* 54:710–717, 2005.

Eli C, May A, Pech O, et al: Curative endoscopic resection of early esophageal adenocarcinomas (Barrett's cancer), *Gastrointest Endosc* 65:3–10, 2007.

Esaki M, Matsumoto T, Hirakawa K, et al: Risk factors for local recurrence of superficial esophageal cancer after treatment by endoscopic mucosal resection, *Endoscopy* 39:41–45, 2007.

Frantzides C, Madan A, Moore R, et al: Laparoscopic transgastric esophageal mucosal resection for high-grade dysplasia, *J Laparoendosc Adv Surg Tech* 14:261–265, 2004.

Frantzides CT, Carlson MA, Keshavarzian A, et al: Laparoscopic transgastric esophageal mucosal resection: 4-year minimum follow-up, *Am J Surg* 200:305–307, 2010.

Frantzides CT, Richards CG: A study of 362 consecutive laparoscopic Nissen fundoplications, *Surgery* 124:651–654, 1988.

Frantzides CT, Carlson MA: Laparoscopic Nissen fundoplication. In Frantzides CT, Carlson MA, editors: *Atlas of Minimally Invasive Surgery*, Philadelphia, 2009, Saunders, pp 23–29.

Frantzides CT, Granderath FA, Granderath UM, et al: Laparoscopic hiatal herniorrhaphy. In Frantzides CT, Carlson MA, editors: *Atlas of Minimally Invasive Surgery*, Philadelphia, 2009, Saunders, pp 31–40.

Konda VJA, Ross AS, Ferguson MK, et al: Is the risk of concomitant invasive esophageal cancer in high-grade dysplasia in Barrett's esophagus overestimated? *Clin Gastroenterol Hepatol* 6:159–164, 2008.

Pech O, Behrens A, May A, et al: Long-term results and risk factor analysis for recurrence after curative endoscopic therapy in 349 patients with high-grade intraepithelial neoplasia and mucosal adenocarcinoma in Barrett's oesophagus, *Gut* 57:1200–1206, 2008.

Prasad GA, Wang KK, Buttar NS, et al: Long-term survival following endoscopic and surgical treatment of high grade dysplasia in Barrett's esophagus, *Gastroenterology* 132:1226–1233, 2007.

Rastogi A, Puli S, El-Serag HB, et al: Incidence of esophageal adenocarcinoma in patients with Barrett's esophagus and high-grade dysplasia: A meta-analysis, *Gastrointest Endosc* 67:394–398, 2008.

Sharma P, Falk GW, Weston AP, et al: Dysplasia and cancer in a large multicenter cohort of patients with Barrett's esophagus, *Clin Gastroenterol Hepatol* 4:566–572, 2006.

Tharavej C, Hagen JA, Peters JH, et al: Predictive factors of coexisting cancer in Barrett's high grade dysplasia, *Surg Endosc* 20:439–443, 2006.

Wang KK, Sampliner RE: Updated guidelines 2008 for the diagnosis, surveillance and therapy of Barrett's esophagus, *Am J Gastroenterol* 103:788–797, 2008.

Yousef F, Cardwell C, Cantwell MM, et al: The incidence of esophageal cancer and high-grade dysplasia in Barrett's esophagus: A systematic review and meta-analysis, *Am J Epidemiol* 168:237–249, 2008.

STAVROS A. ANTONIOU, RUDOLPH POINTNER, AND FRANK A. GRANDERATH

Laparoscopic Revision of Failed Fundoplication and Hiatal Hernia

The videos associated with this chapter are listed in the Video Contents and can be found on the accompanying DVDs and *on Expertconsult.com.*

Laparoscopic fundoplication has been embraced by the surgical community as the procedure of choice for gastroesophageal reflux disease (GERD). After the introduction of laparoscopy in foregut surgery, a significant rise in the number of laparoscopic fundoplications allowed for evaluation of long-term outcomes in large patient series. Hiatal hernia recurrence has been shown to be a significant factor in the failure of antireflux procedures. Patients with failed fundoplication often suffer from persistent, recurrent, or new-onset symptoms.

Redo fundoplication represents one of the most technically challenging procedures in laparoscopic surgery; in addition, complex clinical and diagnostic logistics come into play. Invariably in these cases, the laparoscopic surgeon encounters distorted anatomy, dense adhesions, and fibrotic tissue in proximity to structures such as the esophagus, aorta, liver, and spleen. Success of revisional operations depends on the primary procedure, the patient's symptoms, the results of preoperative tests, and, more important, patient selection.

In this chapter, the absolute and relative indications for revisional fundoplication and hiatal herniorrhaphy and the value of preoperative examinations in selecting the appropriate medical or surgical treatment are discussed. Furthermore, the technique of revisional surgery for failed fundoplication and failed hiatal hernia repair is described, with emphasis on operative risks and pitfalls. Finally, the morbidity and the outcomes of the procedure are outlined.

OPERATIVE INDICATIONS

Patients with "failed fundoplication" may be divided into those with anatomic failure and those with a normal anatomy but persistent foregut symptoms. The latter are subdivided into patients with objective evidence of gastroesophageal reflux, esophageal stenosis, or delayed gastric emptying, and patients with no functional, endoscopic, or imaging evidence that could explain their symptoms.

Anatomic Failure

Seven types of anatomic failure may be encountered.

- *Wrap migration* (44%). A portion of the wrap or the entire wrap has migrated into the mediastinum (Fig. 7-1A). The proposed etiologic factor is inadequate crural closure owing to poor technique or weak tissue, or both; disruption of the cruroplasty results in migration of the wrap into the mediastinum.

- *Slipped hernia* (16%). The gastroesophageal junction has slipped into the mediastinum, whereas the wrap remains below the diaphragm (Fig. 7-1B). It has been postulated to result from the presence of a short esophagus or inadequate mobilization of the esophagus during the primary procedure. The latter is a more probable mechanism.

- *Paraesophageal hernia* (16%). Both the body of the wrap and the gastroesophageal junction remain below the diaphragm, whereas a part of the stomach has migrated into the mediastinum, posterior to the esophagus (Fig. 7-1C). This type of failure is a result of the combination of a loose wrap and a poor crural closure, which allows part of the posterior portion of the wrap to migrate into the mediastinum.

- *Displaced wrap* (10%). The wrap has slipped caudad on the body of the stomach, resulting in formation of a fundal pouch (Fig. 7-1D). The reasons for this type of failure are elusive; inadequate anchorage of the fundoplication may play a role. Retention of food in the herniated pouch may result in an increase of its size and further caudad slippage of the wrap (hourglass stomach).

- *Misplaced wrap* (4%). The plication has been constructed by the fundus and the body of the stomach because of misidentification of the anatomy at the initial operation (Fig. 7-1E).

- *Twisted wrap* (6%). Torsion of the wrap is thought to result from insufficient division of the short gastric vessels and continuous traction counterclockwise (Fig. 7-1F).

- *Disrupted wrap* (4%). A part of the fundoplication or the entire fundoplication has been disrupted. Inadequate construction of the fundoplication (superficially placed sutures) may account for this failure (Fig. 7-1G).

Recurrence usually occurs either during the early postoperative period or in the first 2 years after surgery. Wrap migration is the most common cause for failure. Excessive retching, nausea, and vomiting have been identified as causative factors for failure within the first 2 postoperative weeks; therefore, routine administration of antiemetics after laparoscopic fundoplication has been advocated by many. Early hernia recurrence is considered an indication for revisional fundoplication.

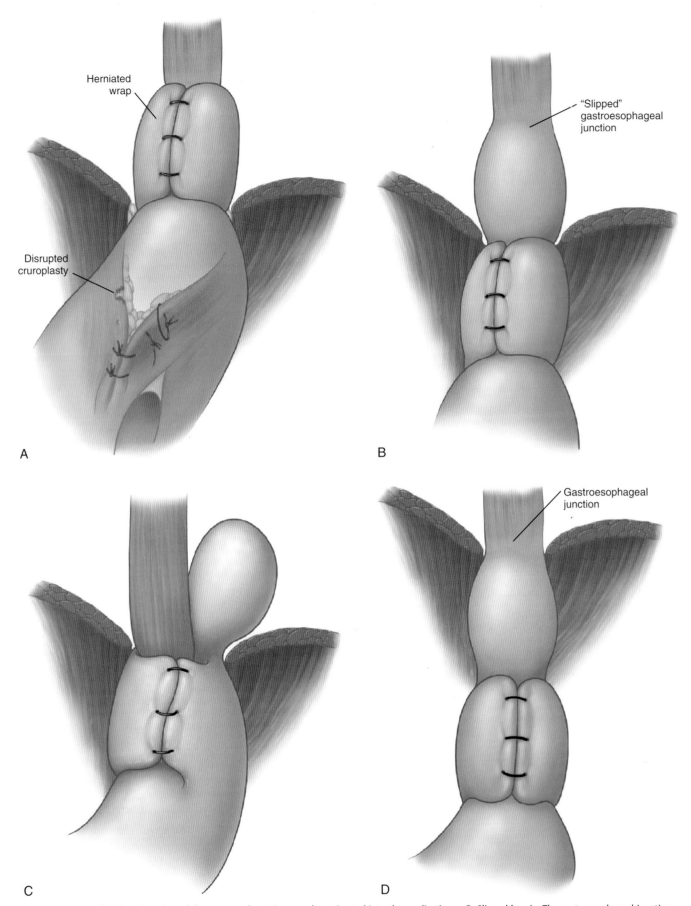

Herniated wrap

Disrupted cruroplasty

A

"Slipped" gastroesophageal junction

B

C

Gastroesophageal junction

D

FIGURE 7-1 **A,** Wrap migration. A portion of the wrap or the entire wrap has migrated into the mediastinum. **B,** Slipped hernia. The gastroesophageal junction migrates into the mediastinum, while the wrap remains intact in the abdomen. **C,** Paraesophageal hernia. A part of the gastric wall, usually posterior to the esophagus, herniates into the mediastinum, while the wrap and the gastroesophageal junction remain in their intra-abdominal position. **D,** Displaced wrap. The wrap has slipped caudal toward the body of the stomach.

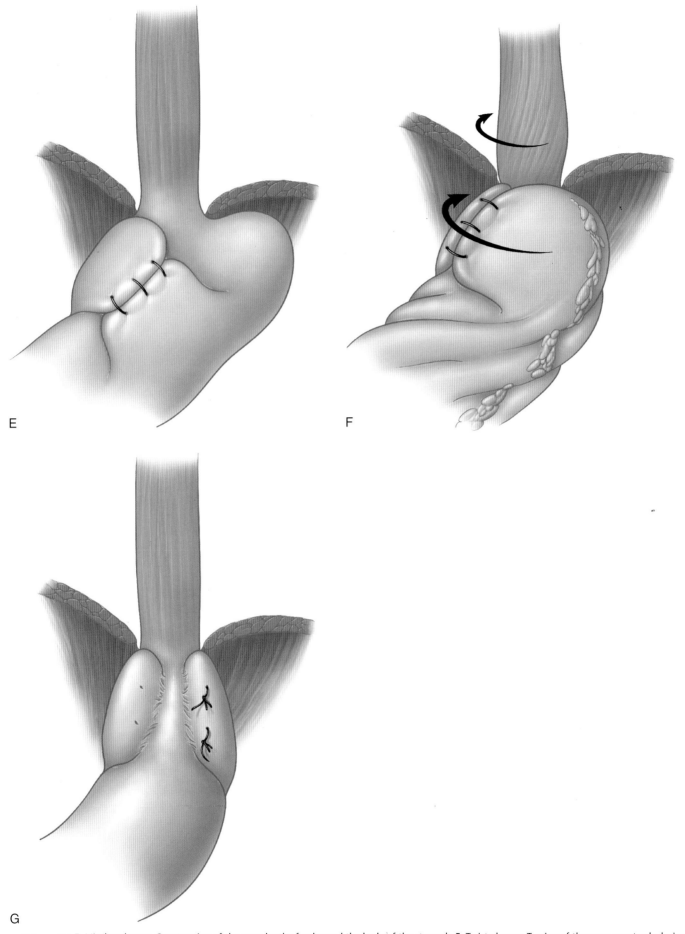

FIGURE 7-1, cont'd **E,** Misplaced wrap. Construction of the wrap by the fundus and the body of the stomach. **F,** Twisted wrap. Torsion of the wrap counterclockwise, owing to traction by the short gastric vessels. **G,** Disrupted/loose wrap.

Late fundoplication failure may present with or without foregut symptoms. The management of symptomatic patients with documented failed fundoplication can be either conservative or operative. Revisional surgery is an effective treatment for individuals with hiatal hernia recurrence and reflux symptoms. Conservative treatment may be considered for high-risk patients or for those with multiple previous abdominal operations. However, patients presenting with hiatal hernia recurrence and dysphagia or gas-bloat syndrome are difficult to manage conservatively.

Foregut Symptoms in the Lack of Anatomic Defect

There are a significant number of patients who complain of persistent, recurrent, or new-onset symptoms without imaging evidence of a distorted anatomy. Most common symptoms include heartburn, regurgitation, dysphagia, and gas-bloating. Manometric and pH studies will distinguish patients with objective evidence of a functional abnormality from those without anatomic or functional evidence of failure; the latter are those who are less likely to benefit from revisional surgery.

Patients with documented anatomic failure of fundoplication with reflux symptoms and an abnormal DeMeester score are excellent candidates for revisional operation. The optimal approach to patients with dysphagia and gas-bloat syndrome without imaging evidence of hernia recurrence is conservative, whereas endoscopic dilation may be necessary in selected cases. Revisional surgery in patients for the previously mentioned symptoms should be the last resort.

PREOPERATIVE EVALUATION, TESTING, AND PREPARATION

A thorough clinical examination and a detailed clinical history are essential for patients with suspected failed fundoplication. Other pathologies of the upper gastrointestinal tract, such as gastritis, peptic ulcer, pancreatitis, cholelithiasis, and cardiac and pulmonary diseases, should be ruled out. Presenting symptoms and the findings of functional and imaging studies should be reviewed carefully. Selective use of barium studies, upper gastrointestinal endoscopy, gastric emptying studies, esophageal pH monitoring, and manometry will determine the form of treatment.

Barium Studies

Barium esophagography is the first diagnostic step in the evaluation of anatomic and functional abnormalities of the upper gastrointestinal tract in patients with failed antireflux procedures. This diagnostic tool delineates the esophageal anatomy and may demonstrate hiatal hernia recurrence or wrap migration, and it provides useful information on the function of the lower esophageal sphincter, esophageal peristalsis, the presence of strictures, and the volume and extent of gastroesophageal reflux. Overview of the gastric and duodenal anatomy may additionally demonstrate pyloric stenosis due to vagal nerve injury.

Gastroscopy

In the absence of a functional or anatomic disorder in barium studies, gastroscopy will identify reflux esophagitis, esophageal strictures due to tight crural closure or mesh erosion, gastritis, and peptic ulcers.

pH Studies

Objective assessment of the presence and severity of pathologic gastroesophageal reflux is provided by esophageal pH monitoring. Such study may be redundant in the presence of a profound anatomic failure and evidence of reflux in barium upper gastrointestinal fluoroscopy.

Manometry

Manometric evaluation of esophageal motility provides a credible assessment of esophageal peristalsis. Furthermore, if barium studies are not diagnostic, manometry may identify a missed esophageal achalasia.

Computed Tomography and Ultrasonography

Barium studies are usually diagnostic in the presence of a profound anatomic failure. Computed tomography is particularly helpful in the diagnosis of wrap migration and disruption or twisting of the wrap. Furthermore, this study provides a detailed preoperative overview of the anatomy and the relation of the herniated tissue to adjacent structures.

In patients with "dyspeptic symptoms," such as vague epigastric pain, colic, nausea, and vomiting, ultrasonography may diagnose cholelithiasis. Injury of the hepatic branch of the anterior vagus nerve during the initial procedure has been implicated as the cause of gallbladder dyskinesia and formation of gallstones; the clinical significance of this hypothesis has yet to be proven.

A diagnostic algorithm based on clinical history, patient complaints, symptom frequency, and severity is essential for the selection of suitable candidates for operative treatment and is presented in Figure 7-2.

Reflux Symptoms

Heartburn and regurgitation following laparoscopic fundoplication are initially evaluated with contrast studies. A barium esophagogram provides an excellent overview of the anatomy and may demonstrate gastroesophageal reflux, hiatal hernia recurrence, esophageal stenosis, or short esophagus. Further diagnostic workup depends on the esophageal and gastric anatomy and the patient's symptoms.

Dysphagia

When dysphagia is the predominant symptom, barium studies may reveal esophageal stenosis, delayed esophageal emptying, anatomic failure of the fundoplication, or esophageal dysmotility. If the differential diagnosis between anatomic stenosis and esophageal achalasia cannot be made, manometry may prove useful. Delayed esophageal emptying may be treated by endoscopic pneumatic dilations; however, this procedure is rarely effective in cases of anatomic failure.

Gas-Bloat Syndrome

Barium esophagogram is the first diagnostic step for patients with excessive gas-bloating. Although symptoms are usually mild

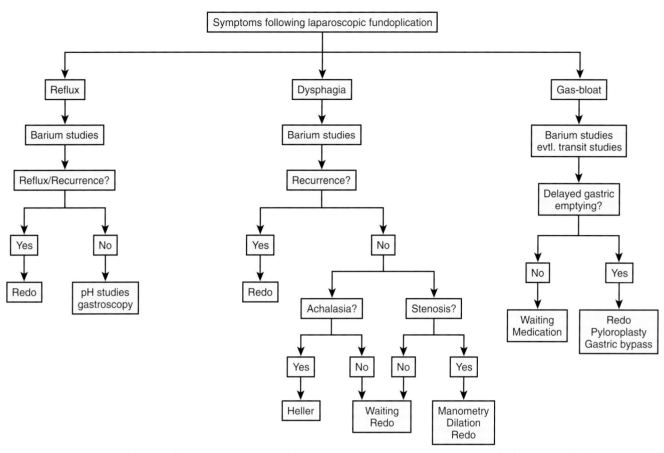

FIGURE 7-2 Treatment algorithm for patients presenting with persisting, new-onset, or recurrent symptoms after laparoscopic fundoplication.

and resolve within the first postoperative year without the need for further treatment, rigorous symptoms are subject to further evaluation. Anatomic failure of the fundoplication or pyloric stenosis may be identified as causative factors. If barium studies suggest a gastric outlet obstruction, transit studies will provide objective evidence of pyloric dysfunction due to vagal nerve injury.

After appropriate diagnostic workup, revisional operation is offered to selected patients. The advantages and potential risks of the procedure, as well as the possibility for new-onset symptoms or worsening of existing symptoms, should be thoroughly discussed with the patient.

PATIENT POSITIONING

The patient is placed in a modified lithotomy split-leg position with the surgeon standing between the patient's legs, or in a supine position with the surgeon to the left of the patient (Fig. 7-3). Because of expected prolonged operative times, the lithotomy position allows for ease in the performance of this procedure. The assistant stands on the right of the surgeon; if necessary, a second assistant operates the camera standing to the left of the surgeon. The monitors are positioned on either side of the head of the operating table. After insertion of the trocars, the reverse Trendelenburg position will allow shifting of the intestine to the lower abdomen.

PLACEMENT OF TROCARS

Trocar positioning follows the principles of standard laparoscopic fundoplication (Fig. 7-4). The incisions of the primary

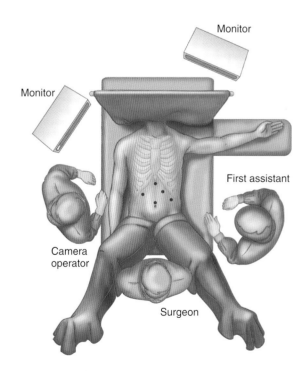

FIGURE 7-3 Placement of the patient on the operating table.

operation may be used, although additional ports may be required during surgery. Pneumoperitoneum is accomplished either with the use of a Veress needle or with an open (Hasson) technique; alternatively, an optical trocar may be used. The rest of the ports are placed under laparoscopic guidance after proper adhesiolysis with the ultrasonic scalpel or electrocautery. A 10-mm port is

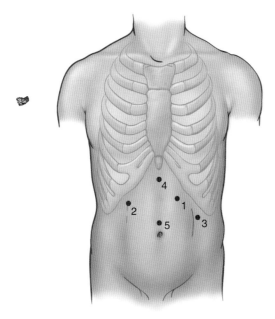

FIGURE 7-4 Positioning of trocars.

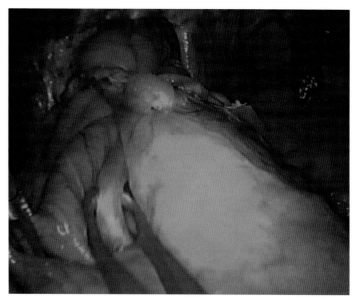

FIGURE 7-5 Traction of the herniated stomach using an atraumatic grasper.

placed 2 to 4 cm above the umbilicus for the camera (port 5). An additional 10-mm port is placed in the left upper abdomen, 2 to 4 cm below the costal margin in the left midclavicular line (port 1). Another 10-mm working port is placed in the right upper abdomen, in the right midclavicular line and 2 to 4 cm below the costal margin (port 2). A 10-mm port is placed below the left costal margin and medial to the left anterior axillary line for retraction of the stomach (port 3). Finally, a 5- or 10-mm port for retraction of the left lobe of the liver (port 4) is placed either 2 cm below the xiphoid (Nathanson retractor, balloon retractor) or 4 to 6 cm below port 2 (snake retractor, fan retractor). Depending on the preferred instruments, 5-mm ports may be used for positions 1, 2, and 4.

OPERATIVE TECHNIQUE

Pressure of the pneumoperitoneum is set at 13 to 15 mm Hg. The anesthesiologist is asked to place a nasogastric tube for decompression of the stomach under laparoscopic guidance. The liver retractor is introduced through port 4 and placed under the left lobe of the liver, applying anterolateral traction. The retractor is either manipulated by the second assistant or held in place with a self-retaining device. The left lobe of the liver is freed up from adhesions to the fundal wrap or to the stomach, or both, with a combined application of blunt and sharp dissection with the hook electrocautery or with the ultrasonic scalpel through port 1. At this point, hemorrhage may occur from the liver parenchyma. Hemostasis is provided by electrocautery and, if persisting, by the application of gauze at the bleeding site; continuous application of pressure by the liver retractor will most likely stop the hemorrhage. Adequate visualization of the stomach, the right crural bundle, and the crural arch should be finally achieved.

After dissection and mobilization of the liver and the stomach have been accomplished, the type of the initial procedure (if the operative report of the first procedure is not available) and the type of failure may become apparent. Two atraumatic graspers are introduced from the working ports, and gentle caudad traction is applied on the body of the stomach. Rarely, the herniated wrap may be reduced into the abdomen with blunt dissection

and gentle traction; more frequently, additional dissection will be necessary. Traction of the body of the stomach with an atraumatic grasper operated by the first assistant through port 3 (Fig. 7-5) allows the surgeon to work through ports 1 and 2. Dissection begins along the lesser curvature and proceeds toward the right crus and the crural arch with application of the ultrasonic scalpel, hook electrocautery, or scissors. Traction of the stomach to the left side with an atraumatic grasper through port 3 facilitates exposure of the right crus. Once the wrap or the esophagus is mobilized 2 to 3 cm cephalad to the level of the crura on the right side, dissection continues anterior to the crural arch. Dismantling of the wrap at this point may be necessary to achieve adequate mobilization of the esophagus. Dissection proceeds to the left side with the assistant pulling the stomach to the right side. The wrap is mobilized from the left crus and the spleen with blunt and sharp dissection. Dense adhesions between the stomach and the left crus or between the stomach and the spleen may render dissection challenging. Division of additional short gastric vessels facilitates greater exposure and safe dissection of the left crus. Creation of a wider retroesophageal window may be necessary. Care must be taken to identify the pancreas to avoid iatrogenic injury to this organ. After the wrap is adequately mobilized from the right, the left, and the posterior aspect, dissection continues dorsally. The crural stitches may be cut with scissors or the ultrasonic scalpel. Care must be taken to preserve the structural integrity of the crura. Attachments of the wrap to the preaortic fascia are usually minimal, so blunt dissection or division with the ultrasonic scalpel allows easy access to the mediastinum.

In cases in which a synthetic mesh was used in the primary procedure, mobilization of the fundus and the esophagus can be technically challenging. If gentle traction and blunt dissection are not effective, integrity of the esophageal or gastric wall should not be jeopardized, and the mesh should be cut with the ultrasonic scalpel.

Further circumferential mobilization of the esophagus allows stepwise traction of the wrap into the abdomen. Additional esophageal mobilization is usually necessary to obtain adequate length of intra-abdominal esophagus. Mediastinal dissection of periesophageal scarred tissue may be the most demanding part of the procedure. The introduction of a lighted 60-French bougie by the anesthesiologist aids in the identification of the esophageal wall and avoids injury to the esophagus and the neighboring structures. Blunt dissection and cautious application of electrocautery, with gentle pushing of the connective tissue fanwise and circumferentially from the esophagus to the surrounding tissue, are preferred at this part of the procedure; if dense adhesions do not allow for safe dissection as described previously, mobilization may be continued with the use of the ultrasonic scalpel close to the esophagus. Inability to obtain adequate abdominal esophageal length without tension may be indicative of a short esophagus, and a Collis procedure may be necessary. Such a procedure has not been necessary in the authors' experience of more than 200 cases. It is our opinion as well as others' that meticulous mediastinal dissection of the esophagus will allow for adequate mobilization, thus obviating the need for an esophageal lengthening procedure.

Once the gastroesophageal junction is restored into the abdomen, the wrap is dismantled by cutting the stitches with scissors and separating the fundic leaves. Several authors prefer to bluntly dissect the fundoplication from the esophagus and cut the wrap with a laparoscopic stapler, whereas others propose leaving the fundoplication in place if the wrap is floppy and intact. Furthermore, it has been reported that in patients in whom the primary preoperative symptom was gastroesophageal reflux, the application of one or two additional fundal sutures may be sufficient for restoring a functional fundoplication. It is our preference to routinely dismantle the wrap, allowing reevaluation of the entire anatomy and thus appropriate operative decision making. Once the anatomic structures of the fundoplication are completely free, the hiatorrhaphy may be reconstructed. The type of closure and the application of a mesh depend on the hiatal defect, the status of the crural pillars, the type of primary failure, and the patient's preoperative symptoms. In the case of a large hiatal defect, in which primary closure would result in repair under tension, the use of mesh should be considered. For this purpose, the mesh should overlap the hiatal defect and the crural pillars for at least 2 cm. It is placed either posterior or anterior to the esophagus and sutured or tacked on the crura without primary closure. Because the hiatus remains open and the crural pillars abducted, care must be taken to avoid injury to the inferior vena cava with the suturing material. After the mesh is placed, it should lie strained on the hiatus without folds.

It should be emphasized that the integrity of the crural tissue may be violated during dissection and adhesiolysis, thus increasing the probability of recurrences for sutured herniorrhaphy. Reinforcement of the hiatal closure in redo fundoplication is therefore strongly encouraged. We prefer to perform primary crural closure and then reinforce the hiatus with a 3- × 5-cm polypropylene mesh. The crura are approximated with two to four nonabsorbable sutures with generous suture bites. The mesh is then introduced and sutured dorsal to the esophagus. Evaluation of the crural arch in relation to the esophagus is carried out, and additional anterior stitches may be placed, if needed. Alternatively, a circular mesh may be used, with a 3-cm keyhole. In this case, the mesh is placed around the esophagus and tacked on the crural pillars and the crural arch (Fig. 7-6).

A wide spectrum of different techniques, mesh materials, and shapes have been evaluated in hiatal hernia repair, and several conclusions may be drawn from current data. The hiatal opening should be sufficiently closed with generous suture bites and

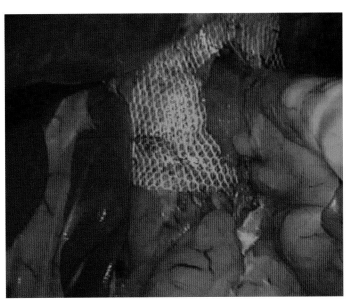

FIGURE 7-6 Reinforcement of the hiatus with a circumferentially placed mesh.

without tension. If such a closure cannot be achieved, or if the structural integrity of the crural pillars is poor, application of a prosthetic material is suggested. This should sufficiently overlap the crural pillars and be sutured to the hiatus with the least possible contact to the esophageal wall, as described in Chapter 4 of the Atlas of Minimally Invasive Surgery, 2009 (see Suggested Readings at the end of this chapter).

Once the crura have been approximated, the fundus should be adequately mobilized for the wrap reconstruction. When reflux symptoms are the primary complaint in the absence of objective evidence of anatomic failure, a tighter fundoplication may be reasonable. The wrap, however, should remain floppy and be constructed around a 60-French dilator. If dysphagia is the primary complaint and the crural closure is not exceedingly tight, a Toupet fundoplication may be justified. Integrity of the esophageal and gastric wall should be evaluated before constructing the wrap with insufflation of air through the nasogastric tube. In the event of a gastric perforation, a laparoscopic repair can be accomplished, and a repeated air insufflation or a methylene blue test may then be performed.

Generous full-thickness suture bites should be applied to the fundus, and anchoring of the fundoplication can be accomplished by incorporating esophageal muscular wall or the anterior arch of the crura. The fundoplication should embrace the gastroesophageal junction, measure 2 to 4 cm in length with three or four nonabsorbable sutures, and be free from any traction from the short gastric vessels. For a more detailed description of the laparoscopic construction of fundoplication, see Chapter 3 of the Atlas of Minimally Invasive Surgery, 2009 (see Suggested Readings at the end of this chapter).

POSTOPERATIVE CARE

During the first postoperative days, mild analgesia is administrated; opioid analgetics are rarely required and should be avoided because of their adverse effects on bowel motility and respiratory function. Although nausea is infrequent, antiemetics may be administered to prevent early recurrence. Upper gastrointestinal fluoroscopy with Gastrografin is advisable the first postoperative day. Such study will evaluate the intactness of the esophagus and stomach and the effectiveness of the fundoplication. Liquid diet is allowed on the first postoperative day. Patients are usually discharged the first or second postoperative day with instructions to remain on soft diet until seen at follow-up in 1 week.

Drinking carbonated beverages and eating gas-producing foods (e.g., beans, broccoli, onions, cauliflower) is discouraged, and meals should be small to avoid gastric distention. Heavy lifting is also discouraged during the first 2 to 3 postoperative weeks. The patient is informed about potential adverse effects during the early postoperative period, including bloating, diarrhea, and dysphagia. More important, patients are educated to report promptly to the surgeon any signs or symptoms of esophageal or gastric perforation, such as fever, abdominal distention, undue abdominal pain, tachycardia, and chest pain.

MANAGEMENT OF PROCEDURE-SPECIFIC COMPLICATIONS

Most common intraoperative complications include esophageal or gastric perforation (14%), pneumothorax (2%), and bleeding (1%). Serosal tears of the stomach are not unusual but are of limited importance once they are recognized, evaluated, and managed, if necessary, with suture repair. In case of a missed esophageal or gastric perforation, the patient may present with fever, chills, epigastric pain, vomiting, or physical and laboratory signs of systemic sepsis. Gastrografin swallow and CT scan with contrast are usually diagnostic of upper gastrointestinal tract perforation.

Gastrointestinal injuries occur during dissection of the stomach, the wrap, or the esophagus from the surrounding tissue or when excising the mesh. Gastric injuries are repaired with 3-0 or 2-0 interrupted sutures. Management of esophageal injuries depends on the extent and the type of perforation. Muscular or full-thickness injuries of 3 cm or less may be repaired with 3-0 absorbable or nonabsorbable sutures. Larger perforations may be subject to esophagectomy because of the possibility of esophageal stenosis or failure of the suture line. Methylene blue test may be useful after suture repair, whereas postoperative Gastrografin swallow is necessary to evaluate the integrity of the esophagus and the stomach. The management of early diagnosed esophageal perforation includes appropriate resuscitation, broad-spectrum antibiotics, placement of a nasogastric tube or temporary endoluminal stent, and monitoring of the vital signs in the intensive care unit. Early reoperation and repair of the injury, or even esophagectomy, may be necessary. Delayed diagnosis of esophageal perforation may result in mediastinitis, mediastinal abscess, and sepsis. Management of this complication is challenging; open procedure with lavage, drainage, and administration of broad-spectrum antibiotics are the treatment of choice.

The incidence of pneumothorax during redo fundoplication is 2% and appears to be similar to primary fundoplication. Adhesiolysis in the mediastinum during revisional operations is challenging. The surgical plane should be close to the esophagus to avoid this complication. A lighted bougie may render dissection safer and help avoid pleural tears. In the event of pneumothorax, the anesthesiologist is asked to evaluate the pulmonary status. If respiratory function is not compromised, the operation may continue laparoscopically. In case of tension pneumothorax with concomitant respiratory compromise, the pneumoperitoneum should be evacuated until oxygenation and respiratory pressures return to normal. Continuation of the laparoscopic procedure may be reattempted with pneumoperitoneal pressures set at

10 mm Hg or lower. If the pneumoperitoneum cannot be tolerated, conversion is the only option. A chest radiograph should be obtained after completion of the operation; placement of a chest tube will rarely be necessary. For more information on how to manage iatrogenic pneumothorax during laparoscopic surgery, see Chapter 4 of the *Atlas of Minimally Invasive Surgery*, 2009 (see Suggested Readings at the end of this chapter).

Hemorrhage occurs in 1.4% of cases. The most common sites of bleeding are the upper pole of the spleen and the short gastric vessels. Minor bleeding from the left lobe of the liver usually occurs during mobilization of the stomach or the wrap. Pressure application by a gauze under the liver retractor may stop the bleeding until the procedure is completed. If persisting, the hemorrhage may be controlled using the spray function of the electrocautery. Division of the short gastric vessels should be performed with the ultrasonic scalpel. This instrument is effective in providing hemostasis; alternatively, clips may be applied for larger vessels. Adhesions to the upper pole of the spleen render dissection hazardous. Hemostatic measures include the use of the ultrasonic scalpel and continuous pressure application with a hemostatic gauze or sponge. Major bleeding sites are the inferior vena cava, the aorta, and branches of the azygos vein. Minor to moderate hemorrhage from abdominal and thoracic veins may be controlled by continuous pressure with a gauze. Persistent bleeding suggests arterial injury, and laparotomy or thoracotomy may be necessary. Fortunately, injury to major vessels occurs rarely; careful dissection, a clear surgical plane, identification of anatomic structures of the mediastinum, and patience may prevent such catastrophic events.

Early wrap migration is perhaps the most frustrating postoperative complication. Retching should be prevented during extubation, and antiemetics should not be spared during the early postoperative period. The patient is instructed to abstain from strenuous physical activities during the first postoperative month. Complaints associated with acute hiatal hernia recurrence include persisting retrosternal or epigastric pain, dysphagia, and heartburn. The symptoms are usually nonspecific and may be attributed to expected postoperative pain. Gastrografin swallow is a well-tolerated and sensitive diagnostic test. Once a hernia recurrence is diagnosed, early reoperation is indicated. The application of a prosthetic material for reinforcement of the cruroplasty under these circumstances is imperative.

Gastric wall necrosis is a rarely encountered complication and results from strangulation of the fundus by the wrap sutures. Symptoms at presentation range from vague epigastric complaints and fever to signs of sepsis. The diagnosis may be established with Gastrografin swallow or computed tomography scan with contrast, or both. Excision of the necrotic tissue with a linear stapler and redo fundoplication are the treatment of choice.

RESULTS AND OUTCOME

Success of the procedure depends highly on appropriate patient selection and the surgeon's experience. Improvement of symptoms is recorded in 80% of patients, and 74% are satisfied with the operative outcome. Furthermore, quality-of-life scores are reported to improve and reach those of the general population for most patients 3 months after surgery. Patients with documented symptomatic anatomic failure are more likely to benefit from revisional operation compared with those without anatomic abnormality. Dysphagia and bloating symptoms in patients without identifiable cause have been recognized as factors for operative failure, and this group of patients should be treated by conservative means as long as possible.

The hernia recurrence rate after laparoscopic redo fundoplication is 13% to 23%. Recurrence rates after a second revisional procedure do not appear to be significantly higher. Laparoscopic redo fundoplication has a conversion rate of 7.4% and a morbidity rate of 16.9%. However, conversion and complication rates are significantly higher following laparoscopic revision for failed open fundoplication. Although laparoscopic redo fundoplication is feasible in 78% of patients after an open procedure, the threshold for conversion should be low.

Suggested Readings

Carlson MA, Frantzides CT: Complications and results of laparoscopic antireflux procedures: A review of 10,489 cases, *J Am Coll Surg* 193:428–439, 2001.

Frantzides CT, Carlson MA: Prosthetic reinforcement of posterior cruroplasty during laparoscopic hiatal herniorrhaphy, *Surg Endosc* 11:769–771, 1997.

Frantzides CT, Carlson M: Laparoscopic fundoplication. In Frantzides CT, Carlson M, editors: *Atlas of Minimally Invasive Surgery*, Philadelphia, 2009, Saunders.

Frantzides CT, Carlson M: Laparoscopic hiatal herniorrhaphy. In Frantzides CT, Carlson M, editors: *Atlas of Minimally Invasive Surgery*, Philadelphia, 2009, Elsevier.

Frantzides CT, Carlson M, Loizides S, et al: Hiatal hernia repair with mesh: A survey of SAGES members, *Surg Endosc* 24:1017–1024, 2010.

Frantzides CT, Madan AK, Carlson MA: A prospective, randomized trial of polytetrafluoroethylene (PTFE) patch repair vs. simple cruroplasty for large hiatal hernia, *Arch Surg* 137:649–652, 2002.

Frantzides CT, Madan AK, Carlson MA, et al: Laparoscopic revision of failed fundoplication and hiatal herniorrhaphy, *J Laparoendosc Adv Surg Tech A* 19:135–139, 2009.

Frantzides CT, Richards CG: A study of 362 consecutive laparoscopic Nissen fundoplications, *Surgery* 124:651–654, 1998.

Granderath FA, Granderath UM, Pointner R: Laparoscopic revisional fundoplication with circular hiatal mesh prosthesis: The long-term results, *World J Surg* 32:999–1007, 2008.

Granderath FA, Kamolz T, Schweiger UM, Pointner R: Failed antireflux surgery: Quality of life and surgical outcome after laparoscopic refundoplication, *Int J Colorectal Dis* 18:248–253, 2003.

Granderath FA, Kamolz T, Schweiger UM, Pointner R: Laparoscopic refundoplication with prosthetic hiatal closure for recurrent hiatal hernia after primary failed antireflux surgery, *Arch Surg* 138:902–907, 2003.

Hatch KF, Daily MF, Christensen BJ, et al: Failed fundoplications, *Am J Surg* 188:786–791, 2004.

Horgan S, Pohl D, Bogetti D, et al: Failed antireflux surgery: What have we learned from reoperations? *Arch Surg* 134:809–817, 1999.

Khajanchee YS, O'Rourke R, Cassera MA, et al: Laparoscopic reintervention for failed antireflux surgery: subjective and objective outcomes in 176 consecutive patients, *Arch Surg* 142:785–792, 2007.

Luketich JD, Fernando HC, Christie NA, et al: Outcomes after minimally invasive reoperation for gastroesophageal reflux disease, *Ann Thorac Surg* 74:328–331, 2002.

Madan AK, Frantzides CT, Patsavas KL: The myth of the short esophagus, *Surg Endosc* 18:31–34, 2004.

Van Beek DB, Auyang ED, Soper NJ: A comprehensive review of laparoscopic redo fundoplication, *Surg Endosc* 25:706–712, 2010.

Stomach

CONSTANTINE T. FRANTZIDES, JOHN G. ZOGRAFAKIS, SCOTT N. WELLE, AND TIMOTHY M. RUFF

Revisional Bariatric Surgery

The videos associated with this chapter are listed in the Video Contents and can be found on the accompanying DVDs and *on Expertconsult.com.*

Operative revision of failed bariatric surgery is not only a technical challenge but also a logistic one. It is of primary importance that strict criteria be followed for considering patients for revisional bariatric surgery. In particular, if the main reason for reoperation is inadequate weight loss, then the burden is to demonstrate a surgically correctable deficiency. Although the rate of revisions may be increasing, this is by no means a new problem. In light of the increasing number of surgical procedures performed, the need for revisional operations is also on the rise.

Historically, the first two widely performed operations for morbid obesity, the jejunoileal bypass (JIB) and stapled vertical banded gastroplasty (VBG), were associated with a high rate of reoperation. The jejunoileal bypass caused nutritional deficiencies and diarrhea. Because of these problems, many patients had to have their jejunoileal bypass revised or reversed. This procedure is no longer being performed and has been replaced by other malabsorptive procedures, including the biliopancreatic diversion (BPD) and the improved variation of the biliopancreatic diversion with or without duodenal switch (DS). The VBG resulted in insufficient weight loss, primarily because of mechanical staple line failure. Over the years, these operations have required revision, conversion to another procedure, or complete reversal. The laparoscopic Roux-en-Y gastric bypass (LRYGB) has emerged as the gold standard for weight loss surgery.

Currently, the most frequently performed operations, LRYGB and laparoscopic adjustable gastric banding, also require revision for complications or unsatisfactory weight loss. The revision rate for the adjustable gastric banding is at least 10% during the first 2 years for either device-related problems or poor weight loss. Similarly, the revision rate for gastric bypass has been shown to be at least 5% to 10% over the first 5 years.

OPERATIVE INDICATIONS

Although the indications to perform primary weight loss surgery for morbid obesity follow the National Institutes of Health guidelines, the indications for performing revisions are vaguely defined. The surgical options are many and may include revision, conversion to another procedure, or complete reversal.

The main indication for revisional surgery is inadequate weight loss after surgery. Eating habits and exercise routines should be reevaluated before pursuing surgical options. It is well recognized that successful weight loss is invariably associated with behavioral and diet modifications and dedicated exercise.

If structural issues, however, are the cause of the failure of the primary operation, further workup is necessary. Obtaining prior operative records may be helpful in future surgical planning; this unfortunately is not always possible. To delineate postsurgical anatomy, esophagogastroduodenoscopy (EGD) and upper gastrointestinal contrast studies are recommended. These diagnostic modalities allow for evaluation of the gastric pouch, the anastomosis, and the presence of staple line disruption, fistulas, ulcers, or strictures. In addition, the presence of a hiatal hernia and gastroesophageal reflux can be shown. Biopsies of the gastric mucosa for *Helicobacter pylori* are recommended. A history of *H. pylori* infection (despite its appropriate eradication) has been shown to lead to postoperative complications.

The most common complications after jejunoileal bypass include chronic renal calculi, malnutrition, bacterial overgrowth, and even renal or hepatic insufficiency. The current recommendation for patients presenting with complications from a previous jejunoileal bypass is to undergo reversal.

After the purely malabsorptive jejunoileal bypass fell out of favor in the 1960s and early 1970s, VBG became the preferred bariatric procedure. The main reasons for reoperation of patients with VBG are dehiscence of the staple line, weight regain, and erosion of the polypropylene mesh or Silastic ring. Options for revision include conversion to an LRYGB or a vertical sleeve gastrectomy (VSG).

Although VBG has historically been abandoned as a primary weight loss operation, it did yield its successor, the laparoscopic adjustable gastric banding (LAGB). The adjustable gastric band has a well-documented reoperative rate exceeding 10% in the first 2 years for complications such as band slippage and migration, band erosion, and port- or catheter-related complications. Options for revision include band repositioning, replacement, or removal with or without conversion to another weight loss procedure. In the case of band erosion, revision may be performed as a staged procedure, initially removing the eroded band with gastric repair followed subsequently by definitive weight loss surgery, or in a single operation.

Indications for surgery after the LRYGB may include weight regain, nonhealing marginal ulcer, stricture at the gastrojejunostomy or jejunojejunostomy, or malnutrition with severe vitamin deficiencies. In addition, complications that may require reoperation include internal hernia and gastrogastric fistula. Revisional surgery options include laparoscopic resection and reconstruction of the gastrojejunostomy, volume reduction of the pouch, revision of the jejunojejunostomy, reduction of internal hernias with closure of the hernia spaces, and lengthening of the Roux or biliopancreatic limbs.

For insufficient weight loss or weight regain, surgical options include lengthening of the biliopancreatic limb, lengthening of the alimentary limb, reduction of the gastric pouch, conversion to a more aggressive hybrid procedure (biliopancreatic diversion with or without duodenal switch), or placement of an adjustable gastric band on the pouch. An endoscopic revision for gastric bypass surgery (StomaphyX, EndoGastric Solutions, Inc., Redmond, Wash.) treats an enlarged gastric pouch or dilated gastrojejunostomy with endoscopic plications. Initial results with the use of this modality are encouraging; however, long-term results are currently unavailable.

Most insurance companies will approve patients for revisional surgery if the procedure will correct surgical complications (e.g., anastomotic ulcer, fistula, internal hernia). This is not the case, however, when it comes to inadequate weight loss. Insurance companies are much more resistant to granting preauthorization for bariatric revisional surgery.

PREOPERATIVE EVALUATION, TESTING, AND PREPARATION

Before a revisional bariatric procedure is performed, the bariatric surgeon will need to determine the cause of failure and evaluate the patient for appropriate treatment options. The bariatric surgeon will need to determine whether failure is due to a complication with the original surgery or the patient's inability to adopt the necessary lifestyle changes. The surgeon should discuss with the patient all of the available options for bariatric revision as well as realistic expectations.

Historically, revisional bariatric surgery has been very high risk. Two decades ago, the overall complication rate with open revisional surgery approached 50%, with a mortality rate of 5% to 10%. With the advent of laparoscopic surgery, these results have improved dramatically during the past decade. Several recent publications have emphasized that laparoscopic experience is associated with improved outcomes.

Patient education is paramount to a good outcome; other components of the preoperative workup may include nutritional and psychological assessments. These consultations may identify patients suffering from untreated psychiatric conditions such as major depressive disorder, binge eating, drug abuse, or alcoholism. Appropriate psychotherapy or counseling may be necessary before surgery.

Routine preoperative testing should be obtained in addition to endoscopy (EGD) and an upper gastrointestinal contrast study. If the patient has a personal or family history of pulmonary embolism (PE) or deep venous thrombosis (DVT), further workup for hypercoagulability may be required. For patients found to have cholelithiasis on preoperative ultrasound, cholecystectomy may be performed concurrently with the revisional surgery.

Preoperative preparation of the patient may include standard mechanical bowel prep with polyethylene glycol electrolyte (PEG) matrix and oral antibiotics (modified Condon-Nichols bowel prep). Perioperative intravenous antibiotics (such as a second-generation cephalosporin and metronidazole) should be initiated before skin incision.

Venous thromboembolism (VTE) prophylaxis can be achieved with lower extremity intermittent pneumatic compression garments. Many surgeons advocate the use of unfractionated heparin or low-molecular-weight heparin routinely. The risks for a VTE event versus hemorrhage (the primary complication of VTE prophylaxis) must be weighed by the surgeon. For patients with a history of PE or DVT, another option to consider is the preoperative placement of a temporary inferior vena cava filter.

PATIENT POSITIONING AND PLACEMENT OF TROCARS

A bariatric operating room table that can be positioned low and in steep reverse Trendelenburg should be used. The table should have appropriate attachments to allow for safe patient positioning, including split-leg attachments as opposed to stirrups. In addition, right-angle footboards are helpful in supporting the weight of a patient placed in steep reverse Trendelenburg. The patient's arms should be extended and padded to prevent tension on the shoulder and brachial plexus.

Two monitors are positioned on either side of the patient's shoulders. Two 40-L high-flow CO_2 insufflators are helpful in maintaining pneumoperitoneum during these technically demanding procedures. In addition to high-resolution camera equipment, a variety of bariatric-length laparoscopes with different viewing angles (0, 30, and 45 degrees) are helpful. Bariatric-length (45 cm) instruments are necessary for performing these revisional surgeries. Atraumatic liver retractors should be used to retract the left lobe of the liver.

Invasive hemodynamic monitoring (i.e., arterial or central venous access) is left to the discretion of the surgeon or anesthesiologist, although often it is unnecessary.

Laparoscopic access to the abdominal cavity is more safely accomplished with the use of an optical trocar placed away from previous incision sites. Most of the revisional bariatric surgeries can be carried out by positioning the trocars as shown in Figure 8-1.

OPERATIVE TECHNIQUE

Revisional bariatric surgery can be technically demanding, and the surgeon should be prepared for all possible scenarios. These operations are best done with the assistance of an additional experienced laparoscopic surgeon. Adhesions from previous open surgeries present a real challenge when proceeding laparoscopically. Identification of correct anatomy is paramount to the success of the operation. Identification of crucial landmarks, including the caudate lobe of the liver, right crus of the diaphragm, gastroesophageal junction, spleen, inferior vena cava, and pancreas, is necessary to reduce the potential for intraoperative complications. The use of a lighted bougie or intraoperative upper endoscopy, or both, may be helpful in identifying the esophagus, pouch, gastroesophageal junction, and any other preexisting anastomoses. Often, a hiatal hernia is present that may have not been identified previously. Such hiatal hernias should be repaired concomitantly with any other procedures.

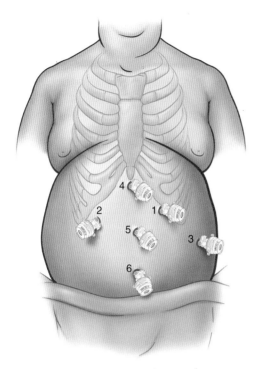

FIGURE 8-1 Trocar placement.

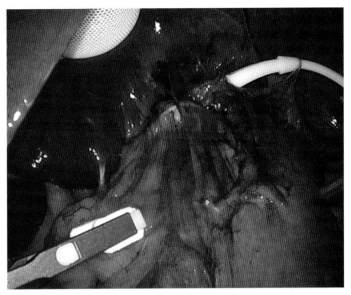

FIGURE 8-2 Laparoscopic view of adjustable gastric band.

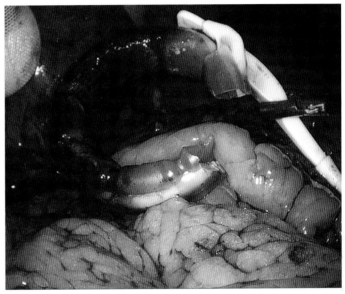

FIGURE 8-3 Appearance of eroded gastric band after removal.

Complications of Adjustable Gastric Banding

Conversion of Eroded LAGB to an LRYGB with Partial Gastrectomy

Upon entering the abdomen, there are often dense adhesions encountered between the left lobe of the liver and the area of the previously placed band. These adhesions are divided sharply, and a liver balloon retractor may facilitate exposure. Once the left lobe of the liver is elevated, the band tubing can be followed to the gastroplasty (Fig. 8-2). Gentle traction on the band tubing would lead the surgeon into the area of the buckle and surrounding reactive capsule. This reactive tissue can safely be divided sharply with scissors or energy source staying to the right of the gastroplasty. Often, because of chronic inflammation from the erosion, this is a very difficult plane to identify and dissect. Once the band is clearly identified, scissors can be used to divide and remove the band from around the stomach (Fig. 8-3). The band is removed, exposing the perforation. It is not necessary to divide the overlying gastroplasty because this tissue will be excised. It is usually easier to approach the dissection and mobilization of the fundus and midstomach rather than continuing the dissection in the right paraesophageal region, which is invariably hostile. Once the fundus is mobilized and the gastroesophageal junction and left bundle of the right crus of the diaphragm are identified, the dissection and gastric mobilization progress to the right. The gastrohepatic omentum is opened widely, and the caudate lobe of the liver, right crus of the diaphragm, and esophageal hiatus are identified. Dissection continues cephalad, to the right bundle of right crus of the diaphragm.

The stomach is retracted caudad, and the gastroesophageal junction and esophagus are completely mobilized. Once all anatomic landmarks are verified, 4.8-mm green staple loads are used to divide the stomach proximal to the eroded band and gastric perforation. If possible, a small cuff of proximal stomach should be kept to allow a more secure anastomosis; it is well recognized that a gastrojejunostomy is a better anastomosis than an esophagojejunostomy. The governing guidelines, however, should be to resect any tissue whose integrity has been compromised by the phlegmon so that the subsequent anastomosis is performed on healthy tissue. The specimen is removed after being placed in a laparoscopic retrieval bag. The gastrojejunostomy or esophagojejunostomy is best accomplished with the transoral placement of the anvil of a 25-mm EEA stapler, as described in Chapter 6 of the *Atlas of Minimally Invasive Surgery*, 2009 (see Suggested Readings at the end of this chapter).

A standard Roux-en-Y reconstruction is performed using the Frantzides-Madan triple-stapling technique, as previously described in Chapter 6 of the *Atlas of Minimally Invasive Surgery*, 2009 (see Suggested Readings at the end of this chapter).

Complications of LRYGB

Laparoscopic Resection of Anastomotic Ulcer with Fistula to the Gastric Remnant

Postoperatively, marginal ulceration at the gastrojejunal anastomosis may lead to acute or chronic blood loss anemia, pain, and vomiting associated with chronic stricture formation. This has been cited to occur as frequently as 7% of cases. Many factors may contribute to this problem, including foreign body reaction, technique, and excessive acid production by the pouch. *H. pylori* infection is a predominant factor in patients who develop postoperative marginal ulceration. Other causes include nonsteroidal anti-inflammatory use, local tissue ischemia, and tobacco exposure (either smoking or oral use). Frequently, these ulcers respond well to proton pump inhibitor therapy.

Peptic digestion of unprotected jejunal mucosa may lead to marginal ulceration. This process may be amplified by secretion of gastric acid from parietal cells found within a large gastric pouch. A large pouch (>50 mL) has been shown to create a higher volume of acid as a result of having a higher number of retained parietal cells that may have unregulated gastric acid secretion. Reducing the size of the gastric pouch has been shown to decrease the frequency of marginal ulceration.

All adhesions to the left lobe of the liver are dissected sharply, exposing the gastrojejunal anastomosis. The pouch is then bluntly and sharply dissected free from the surrounding tissues (i.e., bypassed stomach, gastrosplenic omentum, left lobe of the liver). The proximal portion of the jejunal alimentary limb is likewise mobilized. The dissection then proceeds posterior to the gastrojejunostomy to allow for identification of a potential fistulous tract between the anastomotic ulcer and bypassed stomach (as shown on the accompanying DVD as well as on Expert Consult). The fistula from the anastomosis to the gastric remnant is identified. A window is then created along the lesser curvature of the stomach into the lesser sac and proximal to the gastrojejunal anastomosis. The stomach is then divided cephalad to the gastrojejunostomy using 3.5- or 4.8-mm staple loads, creating a new and smaller gastric pouch. The now-excluded gastrojejunal anastomosis may be adherent posterior to the gastric remnant because of the gastrogastric fistula. Dissection continues by isolating the gastrogastric fistula. The fistula can be divided sharply, and interrupted sutures may be used to oversew the fistula opening on the gastric remnant. The Roux limb is transected, completing excision of the distal pouch, anastomosis, and proximal Roux limb. The specimen can be placed into a laparoscopic retrieval bag and exteriorized. Alternatively, the fistula can be removed en bloc with a partial gastrectomy of the bypassed stomach.

A new gastrojejunostomy is created, as described in Chapter 6 of the *Atlas of Minimally Invasive Surgery*, 2009 (see Suggested Readings at the end of this chapter).

Laparoscopic Revision of Jejunojejunostomy

Stenosis at the jejunojejunostomy, although rare (reported incidence of 2% to 3%), can cause abdominal bloating, colicky abdominal pain, and vomiting, which can be distressing to the patient. The diagnosis of such a stenosis can be difficult. If the stricture is primarily affecting the alimentary limb, it may be visualized with an upper gastrointestinal contrast study. Alternatively, a computed tomography scan with contrast may be used for diagnosis. If the stenosis affects mostly the biliopancreatic limb, the diagnosis may be even more challenging. These patients may present with vague upper gastrointestinal symptoms. The only radiologic findings present may be a dilated gastric remnant or biliopancreatic limb, or both. Because of these subtle radiologic changes, the diagnosis can easily be missed. Consequently, when patients present with these types of symptoms, the surgeon must have a high index of suspicion for a stricture at the jejunojejunostomy or alternatively for an internal hernia, which can also be difficult to diagnose. Revision of this anastomosis will require excising the entire anastomosis and reconstructing the limbs in the correct orientation.

Correct identification of the biliopancreatic limb, afferent alimentary limb, and common channel is crucial. Once identified, these limbs should be marked accordingly. The distal Roux and biliopancreatic limbs are then divided using 2.5-mm white staple loads just proximal to the anastomosis. Resection of the anastomosis is completed by dividing the common channel distally, leaving three blind ends of bowel. The division of the intestine at the jejunojejunal anastomosis should be confined close to the mesenteric border of the intestine, thus avoiding intestinal ischemia.

Two separate anastomoses are necessary for appropriate revision. First, a side-to-side, functional end-to-end anastomosis using 2.5-mm white staple loads is performed connecting the biliopancreatic limb to the common channel, restoring bowel continuity. A traditional double-staple technique may be used for this anastomosis. A 60- × 2.5-mm would create an ample size anastomosis. To decrease the risk for stenosis of the jejunojejunostomy, the alimentary limb is reattached using the Frantzides-Madan triple-staple technique, as described in Chapter 6 of the *Atlas of Minimally Invasive Surgery*, 2009 (see Suggested Readings at the end of this chapter), connecting the limb to the common channel distal to the first anastomosis. All mesenteric defects should be closed to prevent internal herniation.

Laparoscopic Reduction of Internal Hernia

A life-threatening complication of the LYRGB is an internal hernia. Internal hernias can occur in a number of locations after gastric bypass, including a Petersen defect (hernia site between the transverse colon and the mesentery of the alimentary limb), through the mesenteric defect between the jejunojejunostomy, or through the defect of the transverse mesocolon (retrocolic Roux limb placement). Internal herniation may present as acute complete or intermittent small bowel obstruction. Most frequently, this occurs 1 to 2 years after the initial operation, at which time patients experience their greatest weight loss. This weight loss results in thinning of the mesentery, which consequently causes an enlargement of the mesenteric defects.

In the case of a Peterson's hernia, the defect can be identified by retracting the transverse colon cephalad. The intestine will be seen herniating posterior to the mesentery of the afferent alimentary limb and anterior to the transverse mesocolon. The small intestine can then be seen protruding through the defect (Fig. 8-4).

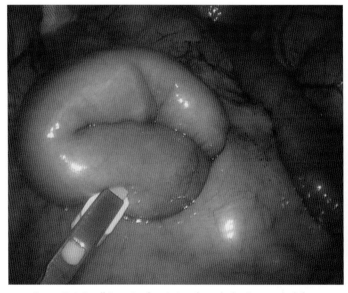

FIGURE 8-4 Small intestine herniating through the Peterson's defect.

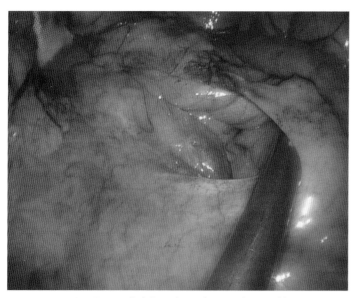

FIGURE 8-5 Peterson's defect after reduction of internal hernia.

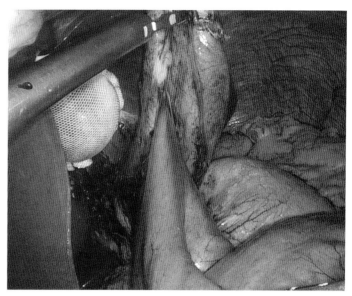

FIGURE 8-7 Large gastric pouch.

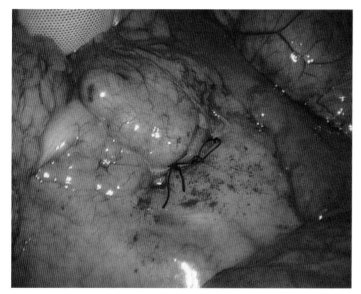

FIGURE 8-6 Completed closure of Peterson's defect.

The intestine in this type of hernia is invariably herniating through the defect from the patient's left to right. The reduction is accomplished by pushing the bowel from right to left through the defect (Fig. 8-5). Care must be taken to ensure that the bowel is reduced in the proper direction. If the bowel is retracted from left to right through the defect, further herniation is induced, which would result in torsion of the mesentery. Any change in the appearance of the intestine (cyanosis) should be a sign of misidentification of the direction of herniation. Once the hernia is reduced, the defect should be closed using nonabsorbable sutures (Fig. 8-6). Likewise, herniations at the jejunojejunostomy mesenteric defect or transmesocolic defect should be identified, the herniated intestine reduced, and the defect closed with nonabsorbable sutures. Once the problematic defect is repaired, it is imperative to identify other defects and close any potential spaces to prevent future hernias.

Bariatric Conversion Procedures

Laparoscopic Reduction of a Large Gastric Pouch
A large dilated gastric pouch can be a potential cause of insufficient weight loss or weight regain. In addition, the presence of a large pouch has been implicated as a potential cause of

anastomotic ulcers, as previously discussed. A large gastric pouch may be the result of chronic overeating or the construction of a large pouch during the primary operation, or both. It is the authors' experience that a large pouch is usually associated with a side-to-side linear stapler gastrojejunostomy rather than with a circular stapler anastomosis. An ample size pouch is necessary when performing a gastrojejunostomy using a linear stapler. This is not the case when the anastomosis is constructed with a circular stapler.

Adhesions to the left lobe of the liver are divided, and the liver is retracted cephalad and to the right for exposure. The right crus of the diaphragm, caudate lobe of the liver, and gastrojejunostomy are identified (Fig. 8-7). The redundant gastric pouch is isolated by dissecting it free from the underlying gastric remnant, the gastrosplenic omentum, and any other adherent tissue until the left bundle of the right crus is visualized. A lighted bougie is placed into the pouch and through the gastrojejunostomy. Using the lighted bougie as a guide, 4.8-mm green staple loads are fired along the bougie starting at the gastrojejunostomy and continuing cephalad to the angle of His, reducing the volume of the stomach (Fig. 8-8). The integrity of the staple line should be evaluated to check for bleeding or leaks (Fig. 8-9).

Laparoscopic Conversion of Failed VBG to LRYGB
Another complex problem requiring revision is a failed VBG with Marlex or Silastic ring gastroplasty. Historically, this procedure was performed in an open fashion, resulting in extensive intraabdominal adhesions.

It is prudent that access to the abdominal cavity be obtained with the use of the optical trocar rather than the blind insertion of the Veress needle and subsequent trocar. After meticulous adhesiolysis, the stomach is identified, and the lateral and medial attachments to the stomach are divided. The gastrosplenic omentum is placed on stretch between two atraumatic graspers and sharply divided with the Harmonic scalpel. Access into the lesser sac is obtained, and division of the short gastric vessels allows for mobilization of the greater curvature and fundus. This dissection and mobilization should be done cautiously to avoid injury to the spleen or pancreas. Further dissection is then carried out between the left lobe of the liver and lesser curvature of the stomach. Dense adhesions are invariably encountered in the area

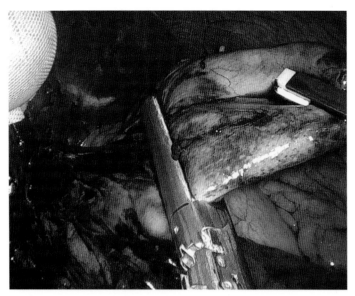

FIGURE 8-8 Stapling of large pouch along a lighted bougie.

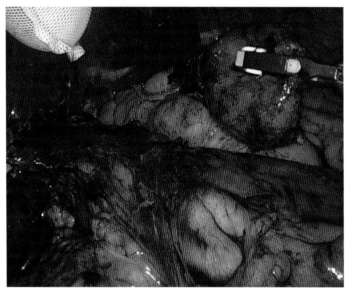

FIGURE 8-9 Transected pouch with intact hemostatic staple line.

of the band. Mobilizing the stomach in this area may be challenging but can be accomplished with meticulous and careful sharp dissection. The gastrohepatic omentum is then divided above the caudate lobe of the liver up to the gastroesophageal junction. The staple line should be identified so that the pouch could be created cephalad to this line. The transection point is then chosen (about 5 cm distal to the gastroesophageal junction), and 4.8-mm green staple loads are used to divide the stomach proximal to the band and previous staple line. Division of the stomach continues cephalad to the angle of His and medial to the vertical gastric staple line, creating a new small pouch, excluding the previous mesh and ring and the fundus of the stomach.

Once the gastric pouch is created, the corpus of the stomach (distal to the band) is divided using 4.8-mm green staple loads, and the proximal stomach is excised. A standard LRYGB using the transoral circular staple technique for the gastrojejunostomy and the Frantzides-Madan triple-staple technique for jejunojejunostomy is then performed as described in Chapter 6 of the *Atlas of Minimally Invasive Surgery*, 2009 (see Suggested Readings at the end of this chapter).

Laparoscopic Conversion of LAGB to LRYGB

The reoperation rate after LAGB has been shown to be as high as 10% at 2 years after band placement. Reasons for reoperation include migration of the band, band slippage, or inadequate weight loss and, as described previously, band erosion. This section of the chapter emphasizes removal of the adjustable gastric band because of failure of the band to produce adequate weight loss. This is technically less demanding than removal secondary to erosion.

The band tubing is followed from the port to the gastroplasty to identify the band. The fibrinous capsule encasing the band is divided, exposing the band. Scissors are used to divide and remove the band, leaving the gastroplasty intact. Atraumatic graspers are placed on either side of the tunnel left behind after removal of the band. This will allow easier identification of the plane of dissection for the reduction of the fundoplasty. The anchoring stitches are identified and divided and the fundoplasty reduced. Care should be taken to prevent injury to the gastric wall. Dissection continues medially and laterally, exposing the right crus of the diaphragm, the esophageal hiatus, and the angle of His.

Hiatal hernia is often a cause of band failure because of improper placement of the band. If such a hernia is present, then a cruroplasty should be performed after mobilization and reduction of the stomach. If at all possible, the pouch should be created proximal to the area of the previously placed band because the tissue integrity may be compromised in the area of the band and fundoplasty. The lesser sac is then entered, and the stomach is divided using 4.8-mm staple loads, creating a small gastric pouch. A standard LRYGB using the transoral circular staple technique for the gastrojejunostomy and the Frantzides-Madan triple-staple technique for jejunojejunostomy is then performed as described in Chapter 6 of the *Atlas of Minimally Invasive Surgery*, 2009 (see Suggested Readings at the end of this chapter).

Laparoscopic Conversion of Miniloop Gastric Bypass to LRYGB

An alternative (yet less favorable) approach to the traditional gastric bypass incorporates a loop anastomosis of the distal jejunum to a gastric pouch, termed the *miniloop gastric bypass* (Fig. 8-10). This procedure, in addition to being restrictive, causes major malabsorption with consequent nutritional deficiencies. Indications for revision of this procedure are usually hypoproteinemic edema, severe iron deficiency anemia, and emaciation.

This procedure can be converted to an LRYGP. The pouch and loop gastrojejunal anastomosis are identified following adhesiolysis. The loop gastrojejunostomy is excised by dividing the tubular gastric pouch and the small intestine proximally and distally to the anastomosis (see Fig. 8-10). Once the anastomosis is excised, a standard LRYGB using the transoral circular staple technique for the gastrojejunostomy and the triple-staple technique for jejunojejunostomy is then performed as described in Chapter 6 of the *Atlas of Minimally Invasive Surgery*, 2009 (see Suggested Readings at the end of this chapter).

POSTOPERATIVE CARE

Routine intensive care unit postoperative care is not usually necessary in these patients. A step-down unit or surgical floor with cardiac telemetry and continuous pulse oximetry monitoring is recommended.

Early ambulation and mobilization are important for VTE prophylaxis. The patient should be instructed to ambulate with

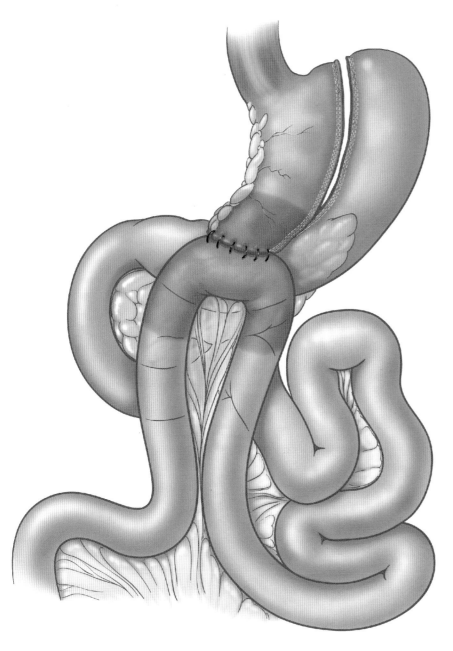

FIGURE 8-10 Miniloop gastric bypass. The distal part of the tubular gastric pouch and the gastrojejunostomy are excised *(shaded area)*.

assistance on the evening of surgery. Many surgeons advocate the use of unfractionated or low-molecular-weight heparin. The risks and benefits of anticoagulation must be weighed by the surgeon. Incentive spirometry and routine respiratory aerosols have been shown to reduce pulmonary complications.

Although the need for a routine upper gastrointestinal contrast study in a primary bariatric surgery in an asymptomatic patient has been debated, a water-soluble Gastrografin upper gastrointestinal swallow is appropriate after revisional bariatric surgery.

A bariatric diet may be started on the first postoperative day following a negative contrast study. Advancing the postoperative diet is at the discretion of the surgeon.

PROCEDURE-SPECIFIC COMPLICATIONS

The most common and feared complication following revisional bariatric surgery is an anastomotic leak at the gastrojejunostomy, which has been reported to occur in up to 20% of cases. Disruptions of the anastomosis may occur early or late in the postoperative period.

Early leaks are invariably secondary to malformation of the staples resulting in gaps in the staple line. The tissue of a previously operated stomach is altered by scar tissue and thickening. Consequently, revisional surgery requires several technical modifications compared with primary bariatric surgery. The correct choice of staple height is imperative. Although a 3.0-mm blue load is acceptable for use in a primary surgery, with reoperations the use of 4.8-mm green staple loads is preferred. Additionally, reinforcement of the anastomotic staple line in primary bariatric surgery is optional (although recommended), but in revisional operations, it is essential. Finally, although routine drainage in initial bariatric operations is often unwarranted, its use should be considered with a revised anastomosis. Any change in the amount or color of the drain fluid should warrant an upper gastrointestinal contrast study to evaluate for a leak.

Late leaks are invariably secondary to tissue ischemia. The blood supply to reoperated tissues is often diminished. Consequently, when revising the gastrojejunal anastomosis, the surgeon must be sure to resect enough stomach to ensure that the new gastrojejunostomy is performed on the healthiest tissue possible. Because these types of leaks occur after the patient has been discharged home, the surgeon must educate the patient to be aware of symptoms consistent with a leak (i.e., fever, tachycardia, and diffuse abdominal pain) and instruct the patient to contact the surgeon if these signs occur.

The other common complication after revisional bariatric surgery is staple-line bleeding. Because the use of larger staples is required for these operations, the incidence of bleeding is increased. Although bleeding at the staple line is often self limited, it may require blood transfusions, endoscopic therapies, or even revision of the anastomosis. The use of staple line buttressing may decrease the incidence of bleeding, although this is somewhat controversial.

RESULTS AND OUTCOMES

Results following revisional bariatric surgery vary. In the hands of an experienced bariatric surgeon, procedures for the correction of complications of the primary operation as well as for failure to lose weight are generally good. Weight loss following revisional procedures is generally less dramatic than after primary bariatric surgery. The results also depend on the original bariatric procedure. Many patients who have failed either VBG or LAGB procedures have fairly good weight loss after conversion to LRYGB. Conversely, patients who fail gastric bypass tend to lose less weight following volume reduction of the pouch or lengthening of the biliopancreatic limb (more malabsorption).

Although the results can vary widely depending on the original procedure and the reason for the revision, it is of utmost importance that candidates for such procedures undergo extensive preoperative evaluation to determine the most appropriate revisional procedure. Because revisional surgery can be more complex and involve more risks than general bariatric surgery, it is important to choose a bariatric surgeon who is experienced and skilled in performing revision bariatric surgery. As with all bariatric procedures, the best weight loss results are achieved by compliant patients.

Suggested Readings

Frantzides CT, Zografakis J: Laparoscopic gastric bypass with Roux-en-Y gastrojejunostomy. In Frantzides CT, Carlson MA, editors: *Atlas of Minimally Invasive Surgery*, Philadelphia, 2009, Saunders, pp 53–66.

Frantzides CT, Zeni TM, Madan AK, et al: Laparoscopic Roux-en-Y gastric bypass utilizing the triple-stapling technique, *J Soc Laparoendosc Surg* 10:176–179, 2006.

Fronza JS, Prystowsky JB, Hungness ES, Nagle AP: Revisional bariatric surgery at a single institution, *Am J Surg* 200:651–654, 2010.

Gagne DJ, Dovec E, Urbandt JE: Laparoscopic revision of vertical banded gastroplasty to Roux-en-Y gastric bypass: outcomes of 105 patients, *Surg Obes Relat Dis* 7:493–499, 2011.

Hedberg J, Hedenström H, Nilsson S, et al: Role of gastric acid in stomal ulcer after gastric bypass, *Obes Surg* 10:1375–1378, 2005.

Iannelli A, Schneck AS, Ragot E, et al: Laparoscopic sleeve gastrectomy as revisional procedure for failed gastric banding and vertical banded gastroplasty, *Obes Surg* 9:1216–1220, 2009.

Morales MP, Wheeler AA, Ramaswamy A, et al: Laparoscopic revisional surgery after Roux-en-Y gastric bypass and sleeve gastrectomy, *Surg Obes Relat Dis* 6:485–490, 2010.

Patel S, Szomstein S, Rosenthal RJ: Reasons and outcomes of reoperative bariatric surgery for failed and complicated procedures (excluding adjustable gastric banding), *Obes Surg* 21:1209–1219, 2011.

Sapala JA, Wood MH, Sapala MA, et al: The micropouch gastric bypass: technical considerations in primary and revisionary operations, *Obes Surg* 11:3–17, 2001.

Radtka JF 3rd, Puleo FJ, Wang L, Cooney RN: Revisional bariatric surgery: who, what, where, and when? *Surg Obes Relat Dis* 6:635–642, 2010.

Rasmussen JJ, Fuller W, Ali MR: Marginal ulceration after laparoscopic gastric bypass: an analysis of predisposing factors in 260 patients, *Surg Endosc* 21:1090–1094, 2007.

Siilin H, Wanders A, Gustavsson S, Sundbom M: The proximal gastric pouch invariably contains acid-producing parietal cells in Roux-en-Y gastric bypass, *Obes Surg* 15:771–777, 2005.

Tevis S, Garren MJ, Gould JC: Revisional surgery for failed vertical-banded gastroplasty, *Obes Surg* 21:1220–1224, 2011.

Zundel N, Hernandez JD: Revisional surgery after restrictive procedures for morbid obesity, *Surg Laparosc Endosc Percutan Tech* 20:338–343, 2010.

BASIL J. AMMORI AND GEORGIOS D. AYIOMAMITIS

Laparoscopic Totally Hand-Sutured Roux-en-Y Gastric Bypass for the Treatment of Morbid Obesity

9

The videos associated with this chapter are listed in the Video Contents and can be found on the accompanying DVDs and on Expertconsult.com.

Morbid obesity or metabolic disorder syndrome is the disease of the modern era. It is associated with numerous cardiovascular, respiratory, metabolic, and arthroskeletal comorbidities, increases the risk for cancer, decreases quality of life, and shortens life span. The same was stated by Hippocrates 2500 years ago: ". . . those naturally fat are more prone to sudden death than the thin."

It is well recognized that no current conservative treatments are capable of producing permanent weight loss in morbidly obese patients. Surgery is currently the only effective treatment for morbid obesity over the long term. A recent meta-analysis confirmed that bariatric surgery is an appropriate therapy for patients who are morbidly obese in whom nonsurgical treatment options have failed. The beneficial effects of bariatric surgery on curing comorbidities, improving quality of life, and prolonging survival are now well established.

Although the laparoscopic approach to Roux-en-Y gastric bypass (LRYGB) is considered a technically highly demanding procedure, it has gained popularity among bariatric surgeons since its introduction in 1994. This procedure is considered the gold-standard approach to surgical correction of morbid obesity because it achieves substantial excess weight loss with durable results in most patients. In addition, it carries a low rate of late complications and metabolic disorders compared with predominantly malabsorptive procedures such as the duodenal switch and biliopancreatic diversion.

INDICATIONS FOR BARIATRIC SURGERY

- The American National Institute of Health, along with European and international guidelines, recommend bariatric surgery in adults with either a body mass index (BMI) of 40 kg/m² or higher or a BMI between 35 and 40 kg/m² with obesity-related comorbidity. The comorbidities attributed to morbid obesity may include type 2 diabetes mellitus, hyperlipidemia, hypertension, coronary heart disease, cardiomyopathy, cerebrovascular disease, obstructive sleep apnea and hypoventilation syndrome, asthma, pseudotumor cerebri, osteoarthritis of spine and weight-bearing joints, female urinary incontinence and infertility, gastroesophageal reflux, cholelithiasis, malignancy (increased risk for colon, ovarian, and endometrial cancer in particular), and psychological disorders.

- Severe cardiorespiratory comorbidities, unless preoperatively remediable, may preclude safe bariatric surgery.

- Severe mental disease not responding to treatment, cognitive retardation, and malignant hyperphagia are generally considered absolute contraindications to bariatric surgery.

- It is advisable to consider patients with inflammatory bowel disease, pelvic or retroperitoneal radiotherapy, or large and complex abdominal wall incisional hernias for a sleeve gastrectomy or adjustable gastric band rather than a gastric bypass.

- A planned pregnancy is not a contraindication to gastric bypass because surgery does not usually affect the course of pregnancy and the health of the baby; however, a 12- to 18-month period of contraception until weight loss stabilizes is recommended.

- Bariatric surgery is available for selected adolescents who approached maturity, but only after extensive multidisciplinary workup; recently, a threshold BMI of 40 kg/m² (with severe comorbidities) or 50 kg/m² (with less severe comorbidities) has been proposed.

- Although there is no fixed age limit that is widely agreed on, consideration should be given to the established comorbidities and the risk for surgery in subjects older than 65 years.

PREOPERATIVE ASSESSMENT

Preoperative assessment for bariatric surgery has to be carried out within a multidisciplinary setup. The team should include an experienced laparoscopic bariatric surgeon, endocrinologist with interest in the management of morbid obesity and diabetes, psychologist, dietitian or nutritionist, pulmonologist, and bariatric anesthesiologist. The bariatric program should have access to a dedicated cardiologist, gastroenterologist, psychiatrist, and radiologist with interest in obesity-related disorders.

- The input of a psychologist or psychiatrist is invaluable to address psychiatric disorders such as psychotic personality, affective disorders, alcoholism, drug abuse, mental retardation, and eating disorders, especially bulimia nervosa and binge-eating disorder.

- Endocrine evaluation should focus on the possible diagnosis of hypothyroidism or Cushing syndrome.

- A history of ischemic heart disease calls for objective assessment such as myocardial perfusion scintigraphy and direct coronary angiography. Evaluation of cardiac function with trans-thoracic, or preferably trans-esophageal, echocardiography when clinically indicated should exclude patients with moderate to severe cardiac dysfunction from undergoing surgery.

- Obstructive sleep apnea and hypoventilation syndrome are common in morbidly obese people, and polysomnography is routine in most bariatric centers. These patients are at increased risk for postoperative complications, especially thromboembolic complications and anastomotic disruption. Patients with severe sleep disorders should be managed preoperatively with respiratory support to improve respiratory function and reduce right heart strain; admission to a high-dependency unit or to a ward with expertise in the management of continuous positive-airway pressure support is advised for the first night after surgery.

- Although routine upper gastrointestinal endoscopy is not necessary, the preoperative detection of iron deficiency—even in the absence of anemia—warrants upper and lower endoscopic or radiologic evaluation to exclude malignancy because the bypass will preclude endoscopic access to the excluded stomach, and morbidly obese patients are at increased risk for colonic malignancy. Although most hiatal hernias could be repaired at the time of the gastric bypass, consideration might need to be given to laparoscopic repair of a very large hiatal hernia as a first stage, with the bypass deferred for 3 to 6 months to reduce tension at the gastrojejunal anastomosis and the potential risk for anastomotic leak.

- Barium upper gastrointestinal fluoroscopy, done preoperatively, may diagnose ailments such as gastroesophageal reflux disease, hiatal hernia, gastric tumors, and duodenal ulcers.

- The role of routine preoperative ultrasonography of the gallbladder and concomitant laparoscopic cholecystectomy for asymptomatic cholecystolithiasis is controversial. At a minimum, symptoms of gallstones should be sought preoperatively and concomitant cholecystectomy carried out if these are confirmed.

- Consideration might need to be given to the insertion of a temporary caval filter, which is then removed 5 to 6 weeks after surgery, in the patient with a history of thromboembolism. Long-term anticoagulation might be a sufficient alternative in patients with recurrent deep venous thrombosis or hypercoagulable hematologic disorders.

PREOPERATIVE PREPARATION

- A preoperative "liver-reducing" diet that is low in carbohydrates and fat is recommended for a minimum of 2 to 3 weeks before surgery and appears to reduce the size of the left lobe of the liver and therefore facilitate laparoscopic access to the stomach.

- Prophylaxis against thromboembolic complications is considered essential by most. Although there is no consensus, commonly applied measures include low-molecular-weight heparin administered preoperatively and continued for 1 to 4 weeks after surgery, graduated-compression stockings for 2 to 6 weeks, and the application of a pneumatic sequential venous compression system to the lower extremities during and after surgery.

- Single-dose intravenous broad-spectrum antibiotic prophylaxis at induction of anesthesia is sufficient for most. However, some surgeons who use the circular stapler for the creation of gastrojejunostomy recommend oral antibiotics (e.g., neomycin and erythromycin) as well as mechanical bowel preparation to "sterilize" the bowel lumen and minimize the risk for wound infection.

OPERATIVE TECHNIQUE

Patient Positioning and Placement of Trocars

The patient is placed in Lloyd-Davies (French) position. Central venous and arterial lines are placed at the discretion of the anesthesiologist but are rarely necessary. We directly access the peritoneal cavity with a bladeless 5-mm-port trocar just below the left costal margin at the anterior axillary line, insufflate the abdomen to 20 mm Hg until five standard ports are safely placed (Fig. 9-1), and then reduce the pneumoperitoneum to 15 mm Hg CO_2. In patients with previous abdominal surgery, once the pneumoperitoneum has been established, the initial 5-mm port can be exchanged with a 10- to 12-mm port, and further ports are placed under vision with a 30-degree laparoscope to enable adhesiolysis; standard ports are subsequently placed as shown in Figure 9-1.

We prefer to first perform the intestinal part of the operation and the jejunojejunal anastomosis (JJA). For that, the surgeon and assistant stand at the head of the table with the surgeon on the patient's right and the assistant on the patient's left. The scrub nurse stands on the patient's right, the monitor is placed over the patient's left knee, and the operating table is kept in a horizontal position. Once the Roux loop has been fashioned and the JJA is completed, the surgeon moves to stand between the legs, the

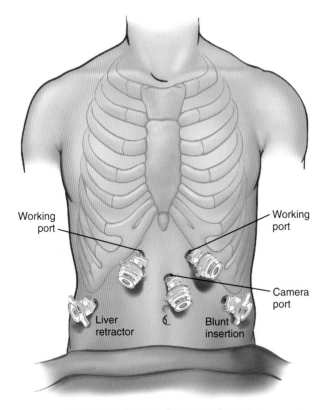

FIGURE 9-1 Schematic illustration of port sites.

assistant stands against the patient's left leg, the scrub nurse remains in the same position to the patient's right, and the monitor is moved over the patient's head and the table tilted into a steep reverse Trendelenburg position. It is very helpful to have an operating table that can be dropped to a fairly low position to reduce surgeon and assistant's shoulder strain.

Construction of the Jejunojejunal Anastomosis

The transverse colon is identified, and the greater omentum is split from its attachment to the colon in a straight line toward the pelvis using an ultrasonically activated scalpel; this line of division runs parallel and often to the right of a constant mid-omental vessel. The intestine is thus exposed, and tension on the antecolic Roux loop is reduced. Upward retraction on the appendices epiploicae of the transverse colon at the point of omental division facilitates exposure of the duodenojejunal flexure. The small intestine is then measured using a marker placed 5 cm from the tips of a pair of atraumatic Yohan graspers.

The length of the biliopancreatic and alimentary limbs will depend on the patient's BMI and comorbidities, although there is no consensus. In patients with BMI of less than 50 kg/m^2, a randomized trial of these conventional lengths (50-cm bilioenteric limb and 100-cm alimentary limb) versus longer limbs (100 and 150 cm, respectively) found no difference in the excess weight loss 12 months after surgery. In patients with a BMI of 50 kg/m^2 or higher, a randomized trial of shorter (50 and 100 cm, respectively) versus longer (100 and 250 cm, respectively) limbs found no significant differences between the two lengths in terms of the excess weight loss at 48 months of follow-up, but significantly greater rates of resolution of type 2 diabetes and lipid disorders were observed when longer limbs were fashioned.

At the chosen distance, the jejunum is divided with an endo-stapler (we prefer 60-mm, 2.5-mm thick, white cartridge load), and the mesentery is split with the Harmonic scalpel down to its root to allow for a tension-free gastrojejunal anastomosis. The distal jejunal loop is marked with a Vicryl suture to avoid confusing it with the proximal end when the jejunojejunostomy is to be constructed and to facilitate its delivery to the gastric pouch for construction of the gastrojejunostomy (Fig. 9-2). The alimentary

limb is measured, and a side-to-side jejunojejunal anastomosis is constructed. We prefer to hand-suture this anastomosis because we had encountered postoperative bleeding from the stapled jejunojejunostomy that necessitated laparoscopic reexploration to evacuate an obstructing hematoma, blood transfusion, and prolongation of hospital stay, as well as intussusception at the stapled jejunojejunostomy that appears to be related to the presence of a staple line acting as a lead point; the authors' experience with both techniques indicates that the sutured anastomosis is safer. A seromuscular layer is fashioned using a 15-cm 3-0 Vicryl suture, the jejunal loops are then opened for approximately 2-cm distance using the Harmonic scalpel (Fig. 9-3), and a second posterior layer is then fashioned using a continuous 26-cm 3-0 Vicryl suture that takes full-thickness bites posteriorly (forming a second posterior layer) and seromuscular bites of a single layer anteriorly (Fig. 9-4). It is difficult to check for leak at the jejunojejunostomy, and we rely on meticulous technique. In the

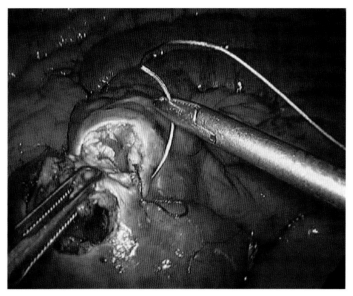

FIGURE 9-3 Parallel jejunal openings with the ultrasonically activated scalpel for the side-to-side jejunojejunal anastomosis.

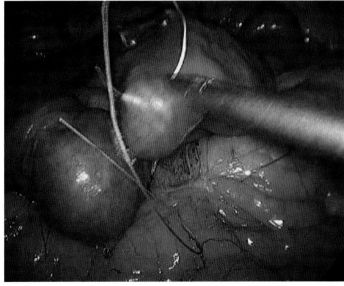

FIGURE 9-2 The distal (Roux) jejunal loop is marked with a suture stitch.

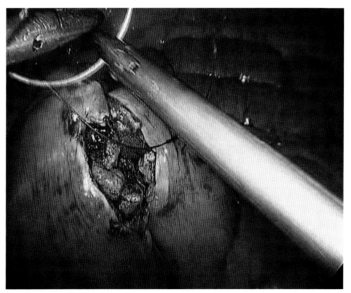

FIGURE 9-4 Suturing of the jejunojejunal anastomosis.

literature, the leak rate of the jejunojejunostomy is extremely low, and we have encountered none.

An alternative option is to double-staple the jejunojejunal anastomosis; this involves firing the stapler (45-mm long, 2.5-mm thick white cartilage) in one direction to fashion a side-to-side jejunojejunostomy, and then firing a second cartilage in the opposite direction before suture-closing or stapling the common enterotomy (the Frantzides-Madan triple-stapling technique is described in Chapter 6 of the *Atlas of Minimally Invasive Surgery*, 2009; see Suggested Readings at the end of this chapter). Double-stapling the jejunojejunostomy avoids stenosis at its proximal end where the alimentary limb joins, but care should be taken to ensure that the second stapler firing crosses the first staple line if a gap within the posterior layer of the jejunojejunal anastomosis is to be avoided with subsequent leak; the posterior staple line should always be inspected for such gap if a stapled technique is employed. It is also imperative to check the stapled anastomosis for bleeding before the common enterotomy is closed.

The mesenteric defect is then suture-closed using a 15-cm continuous 3-0 Vicryl suture (Fig. 9-5). Although some surgeons recommend closure of the defect with a nonabsorbable suture, we have not encountered any herniation at this mesenteric defect—having used absorbable sutures to close it—in more than 1500 cases, and have always found the defect closed at repeat laparoscopy in the occasional patient for investigation of abdominal pain with the intent to look for or exclude internal small bowel herniation.

To prepare for the second (gastric) part of the procedure, the small bowel loops at the jejunojejunostomy are covered with the left half of the greater omentum while the Roux limb is placed—with its suture-marked end—to lie above the transverse colon for ease of its later identification.

Construction of the Gastrojejunal Anastomosis

With the position of the surgeon, assistant, monitor, and operating table adjusted for this part of the procedure (as described previously), the liver is retracted to expose the stomach. We prefer to introduce an 80-mm angled Diamond-Flex Triangular Liver Retractor (Cardinal Health, Dublin, Ohio) through the most right-lateral 5-mm port, and this is fixed in position using a table clamp.

The lesser omentum is dissected close to the lesser curvature of the stomach and about 5 to 7 cm distal to the gastroesophageal junction using the Harmonic scalpel. This involves division of at least two of the neurovascular bundles with preservation of two vessels to supply the gastric pouch and with preservation of the nerve of Latarjet. Once the lesser sac is entered, a 45-mm linear endostapler, loaded with a blue 3.5-mm cartridge, is applied to divide the stomach horizontally (Fig. 9-6). Posterior adhesions to the stomach are divided (Fig. 9-7); failure to do so could result in a much larger pouch than desired. A second 3.5-mm thick 45-mm blue stapler cartridge is then fired cephalad toward the ankle of His (Fig. 9-8). A 32- to 34-French orogastric tube can be used at this stage to create a pouch that is comfortably wide to accommodate it. Attention is then directed to take down the angle of His and mobilize the gastric fundus off the left crus and the diaphragm using the Harmonic scalpel. Posterior mobilization of the gastric fundus then proceeds to create a passage to the left subphrenic space that exposes the left crus; this passage runs medial to a constant posterior short gastric vessel, which we use as a landmark for this dissection (Fig. 9-9). Further

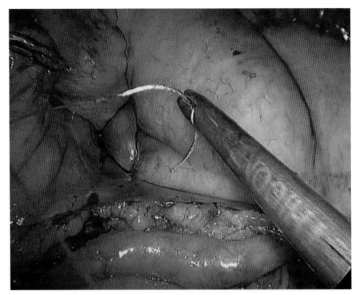

FIGURE 9-5 Suture closure of the small bowel mesenteric defect.

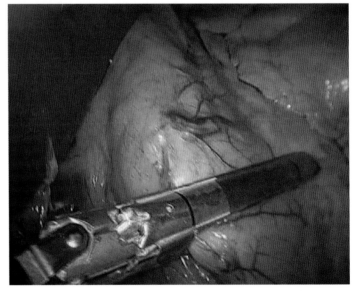

FIGURE 9-6 Horizontal application of 45-mm (3.5-mm blue cartridge) linear endostapler.

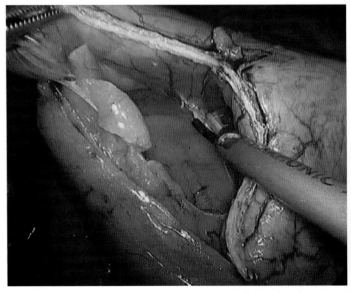

FIGURE 9-7 Adhesions on the posterior gastric wall are taken down.

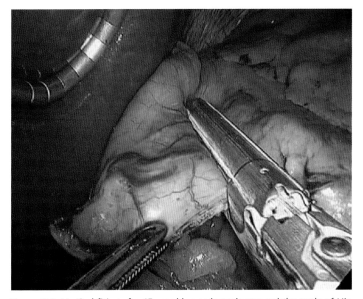

FIGURE 9-8 Vertical firing of a 45-mm blue endostapler toward the angle of His to create the gastric pouch.

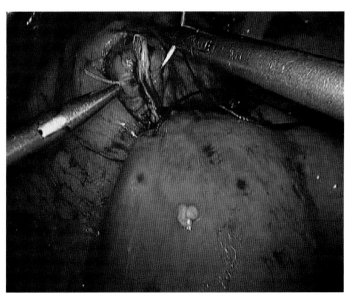

FIGURE 9-10 First posterior layer of the gastrojejunal anastomosis using a 2-0 polyglycolic acid suture in a continuous fashion (the gastric staple line is included in the suturing).

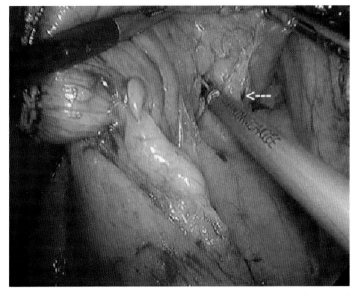

FIGURE 9-9 To complete creation of the gastric pouch, posterior mobilization of the stomach off the left crus of the diaphragm follows a cephalic direction medial to a constant landmark posterior short gastric vessel *(arrow)*, where the stapled division of the stomach will follow.

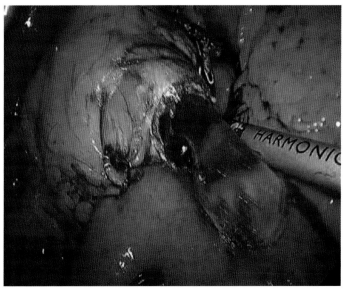

FIGURE 9-11 An approximately 10- to 12-mm anterior gastrotomy is sized over a 32- to 34-French orogastric tube to prepare for the gastrojejunal anastomosis.

vertical divisions of the stomach using 60-mm blue (3.5-mm thick) cartilages takes the division medial to the landmark posterior short gastric vessel and past the left crus to complete the creation of an approximately 30- to 50-mL gastric pouch; the use of a 32- to 34-French orogastric tube aids this division. Clips or figure-of-eight sutures can be used to control bleeding from the staple lines.

The assistant holds the knot of the suture-marked Roux limb and brings it up close to the gastric pouch. Using a 20-cm 2-0 Vicryl suture, a posterior first hand-sutured continuous layer of the gastrojejunal anastomosis is completed about 2 cm from the stapled end of the Roux limb; this suture line should include the posterior wall of the gastric pouch about 2 to 3 mm proximal to the staple line and therefore incorporates the gastric staple line and buries it against the jejunal wall (Fig. 9-10). The anesthesiologist advances the orogastric tube against the transverse staple line of the gastric pouch, and a 10- to 12-mm gastrotomy is created

with the Harmonic scalpel at the anterior wall of the gastric pouch parallel to the staple line and using the 1-cm diameter (32 to 34 French) orogastric tube to size it (Fig. 9-11). A mucosal biopsy from the gastric pouch at the staple line could be obtained with the Yohan grasping forceps for a *Campylobacter*-like organism test to detect *Helicobacter pylori*; we recommend an eradication course to reduce the risk for anastomotic ulceration and perforation.

A parallel enterotomy is made, and a second posterior layer is then fashioned using a continuous 32-cm 3-0 Vicryl suture (Fig. 9-12), which is then continued to complete an anterior single-layer gastrojejunostomy (Fig. 9-13). To ensure a waterproof anastomosis, the Roux limb is clamped with an already fired 45-mm endostapler (Fig. 9-14), the orogastric tube is advanced across the gastrojejunal anastomosis into the Roux limb and a diluted methylene blue (10 mL of the dye in 1 L saline) is injected; the

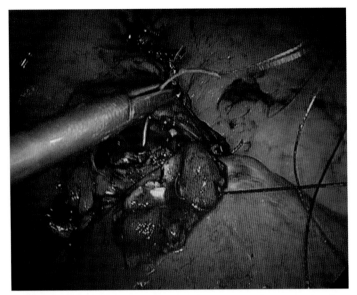

FIGURE 9-12 The second posterior layer of the gastrojejunal anastomosis using a 3-0 polyglycolic acid suture in a continuous fashion.

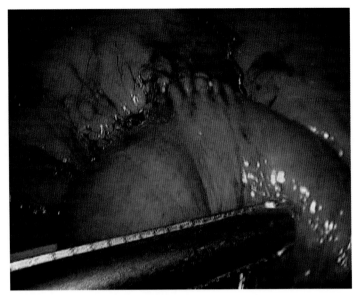

FIGURE 9-14 Occlusion of the Roux limb with an already fired 45-mm endostapler in preparation for the methylene blue leak test.

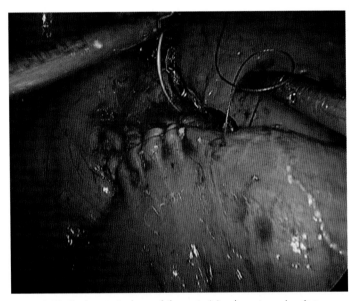

FIGURE 9-13 Single anterior layer of the gastrojejunal anastomosis using continuous 3-0 polyglycolic acid suture.

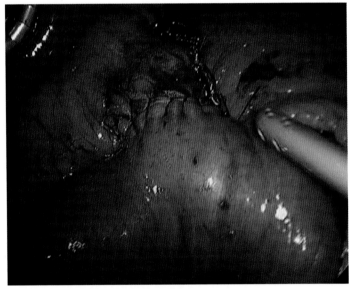

FIGURE 9-15 The completed gastrojejunal anastomosis showing the size of the pouch, the distention of the pouch, and the clamped jejunal Roux loop with absence of anastomotic leakage.

orogastric tube is gradually withdrawn into the esophagus because its presence across the anastomosis and within the pouch might seal a leak from gastrojejunostomy or staple lines of the gastric pouch or Roux limb (Fig. 9-15). Any leak (rare, and would tend to be anterior or at either corner of the gastrojejunal anastomosis) is sutured with an interrupted 3-0 Vicryl, and the leak test is repeated. The methylene blue is then aspirated, and the orogastric tube is removed. More recently, we have been covering the anterior suture line of the gastrojejunal anastomosis with an omental patch in the hope that this will reduce the risk for later perforation of an anastomotic ulcer, which appears to complicate 0.6% to 0.8% of patients after LRYGB.

We do not employ routine nasogastric tube or abdominal drains. Urinary catheters are placed very selectively, such as in patients with impaired renal function, those who are anticipated to have a prolonged procedure due, for example, to previous

abdominal surgery and adhesions, and those considered at high risk for rhabdomyolysis (usually men with high BMI).

During this procedure, we tend to routinely repair any abdominal wall hernia encountered either with laparoscopic or open suturing with nonabsorbable suture or with laparoscopic placement of a temporary Vicryl mesh to avoid intestinal herniation and obstruction with its associated risks for anastomotic leak. Permanent polypropylene mesh should be avoided because of the increased risk for mesh infection; an expensive alterative, however, is to place a permanent porcine collagen mesh.

Closure of the Petersen space between the mesentery of the antecolic Roux loop and the transverse mesocolon is not a universal practice. Internal small bowel herniation may occur in 1% to 7% of patients and could lead to recurrent abdominal colic and small bowel obstruction. If adopted, closure is best carried out after completion of the gastrojejunostomy and therefore requires a return to the theater layout described for the jejunojejunostomy. The assistant retracts the transverse colon cephalically, and a continuous suture closure of the defect proceeds with care to avoid injury to the jejunal vessels and subsequent ischemia and leak at the gastrojejunostomy.

Alternatively, the Roux limb can be brought to the upper abdomen in a retrocolic antegastric or retrogastric approach. The retrocolic and retrogastric approach shortens the distance that the Roux loop has to travel toward the gastric pouch and is therefore useful in tall men in particular, in whom tension at the gastrojejunostomy is more likely. Care should be taken, however, to adequately close the mesenteric defect but to avoid an overzealous closure that could risk obstruction to the Roux loop.

Techniques of Gastrojejunal Anastomosis

Performing the gastrojejunostomy is a critical step during laparoscopic Roux-en-Y gastric bypass. Consequently, different techniques have been described. The circular stapled anastomosis is the most commonly applied technique (see Chapter 6 of the *Atlas of Minimally Invasive Surgery*, 2009; see Suggested Readings at the end of this chapter). Although relatively easy to perform, the anastomosis created by a circular stapler has its drawbacks. Anastomotic stricture and anastomotic leak are well recognized in the field of esophageal or gastric resections. In addition, the introduction and withdrawal of the circular stapler through the abdominal wall and into the intestinal and gastric lumens during the procedure carry a high rate of wound infection. The defect in the abdominal wall created by the stapler is not small and, left unclosed, risks the complication of port-site herniation and the more serious complication of obstruction to the Roux loop with its consequences. Closure of this abdominal wall defect is cumbersome in the morbidly obese patient and is potentially painful.

An alternative technique that is commonly applied to the construction of the gastrojejunostomy is the use of the linear stapler across the posterior wall of the gastric pouch and then suture closure or staple closure of the common gastrotomy-enterotomy. Although this overcomes the problems of abdominal wall complications, anastomotic leak rate (with a recognized average of 1% for all stapled gastrojejunal anastomosis), cost, and adequate sizing of the gastrojejunostomy (often a larger anastomosis than desired is created) are some of the concerns. In addition, stapler malfunction can convert a smooth procedure into a very stressful situation with health risks to the patient. All stapled anastomoses carry a risk for postoperative staple line bleeding, which is at a higher rate than that observed with hand-sutured anastomoses. Although most anastomotic bleeds would resolve with conservative treatment, some would require endoscopic or surgical intervention.

It is the authors' opinion that construction of the gastrojejunal anastomosis using the same approach that has long been applied and tested in open surgery of a hand-sewn anastomosis overcomes many of the shortfalls of the stapled technique. The gastrojejunostomy can also be calibrated to the desired diameter. Although technically more demanding, the skills required and attained are valuable and widely applicable to other laparoscopic procedures. Once the learning curve is overcome, the operating time of the hand-sewn anastomosis is not longer than that of a stapled anastomosis. More importantly, the hand-sewn anastomosis appears to offer a lower leak rate than a stapled gastrojejunostomy.

POSTOPERATIVE CARE

The patient is extubated at conclusion of surgery and transferred to the ward. Although there are no universal criteria for admission to the intensive care unit for the first night after surgery, this should be considered in patients with established severe obstructive sleep apnea, hypoventilation syndrome, coexisting significant cardiac, respiratory or renal comorbidities, very high BMI, or revision of laparoscopic gastric bypass.

Early mobilization is paramount, and sequential compression devices to the lower extremities are maintained when the patient is lying down. If a Foley catheter was inserted, it may be removed once the patient is ambulatory and the renal function is satisfactory. With rare exceptions, a single dose of intravenous antibiotic prophylaxis is sufficient. Limited amounts of water may be allowed on the evening after surgery, free fluids allowed the next morning, and liquid diet for lunch on the first postoperative day assuming satisfactory clinical progress. Most patients may be discharged from the hospital on the evening of the first or the second postoperative day. The main criteria for discharge are that the patient is mobile, can tolerate adequate amount of oral fluids, is comfortable, and does not have tachycardia (heart rate < 100 beats/minute). All patients should be given a contact number to call in case of emergency and should be advised of the classical symptoms of anastomotic leak (triad of severe upper abdominal pain, tachycardia, and sweating). Patients are advised to adhere to a liquid diet for the initial 2 to 3 weeks after surgery and to progress to a pureed diet for a further 2-week period before resuming a solid diet.

Subcutaneous low-molecular-weight heparin is prescribed for 1 to 4 weeks after surgery, and antiembolism stockings are recommended in the authors' practice for 2 to 6 weeks. We advise proton pump inhibitors for a minimum of 2 years after surgery to reduce the risk for perforation of an anastomotic ulcer, which usually occurs within that time frame; however, some recommend it for no more than 3 to 6 months. Daily oral calcium with vitamin D_3 supplements as well as iron and multivitamins should be taken long term, and we recommend that these be started 2 to 3 weeks postoperatively after the gastrojejunostomy has healed. Either vitamin B_{12} should be taken every 3 months as an intramuscular injection of 1 mg, or its blood level should be monitored and supplement given when deficiency is encountered. Alternatively, a sublingual vitamin B_{12} supplement taken once a week would be sufficient. Excess hair loss warrants additional supplementation with oral zinc and selenium supplements for 6 months as well as correction of iron deficiency. Patients who do not tolerate iron supplements can be given intravenous infusion every 3 to 6 months.

Diabetic therapy may be reduced immediately after surgery, and up to 80% of patients may expect remission of their diabetes within 2 years of gastric bypass with discontinuation of drug therapy. Remission of hypertension may also be expected in 60% to 75% of patients within 2 years, and dizziness on standing (i.e., orthostatic hypotension) suggests a need to reduce drug intensity. Patients should receive multidisciplinary follow-up after surgery on a regular and, whenever possible, long-term basis with annual hematologic and biochemical blood monitoring; the general practitioner may take on that role instead once the weight loss has stabilized for 6 months or longer. Outcome assessment after surgery should include weight loss and maintenance, nutritional status, comorbidities, and quality of life. Obesity is a chronic disorder that requires a continuous care model of treatment.

PROCEDURE-SPECIFIC COMPLICATIONS

Postoperative complications of bariatric surgery are not insignificant, and surgeons should be aware that these might have an atypical presentation in obese patients and that early detection and timely management could be life-saving.

- The early clinical features of an anastomotic or staple line leak are severe upper abdominal pain, tachycardia, and sweating. Tachycardia (palpitation) and sweating may, however, be absent in patients receiving β-blockers. An anastomotic leak is a potentially life-threatening postoperative complication and is the most fatal. A negative abdominal drain effluent (if one was placed at surgery) and a negative imaging study do not reliably exclude a leak, and repeat laparoscopy should be considered early if clinical suspicion exists. Repeat laparoscopy should be viewed as an efficient diagnostic modality for which it is wise to adopt a low threshold. The laparoscopic finding of a turbid fluid around the gastric pouch and in the perisplenic area is an early sign, and such patients should be treated as if they have had a leak even if an intraoperative repeat methylene blue leak test was negative. If the leak site is identified within a very small area at the anterior suture line, closure might be attempted over an omental patch. Otherwise, two large abdominal drains should be placed—one from the left to lie next to the gastric pouch and another from the right to lie anterior to the gastric pouch. Further abdominal and pelvic drains might be needed, depending on the extent of contamination. After a thorough lavage, a feeding tube jejunostomy is placed, preferably within the common channel. A nasogastric tube to decompress the pouch is placed under laparoscopic vision. Conversion to a laparotomy is inevitable when there is delay in the diagnosis.

- Postoperative bleeding is either intra-abdominal, usually from the gastric staple line, or more commonly gastrointestinal from the jejunal or gastric staple lines. It often responds to conservative measures and blood transfusion. Rarely, gastroscopy is useful to control bleeding from the staple line. Recurrent bleeding might necessitate a repeat laparoscopy (or laparotomy) and oversewing of all staple lines and anastomoses. Splenectomy is seldom required, and the use of topical procoagulants should facilitate its preservation when there is an injury to the splenic capsule or parenchyma. There is some evidence to suggest that prophylactic low-molecular-weight heparin might contribute to the increased risk for bleeding. Patients who were taking the antiplatelet agent clopidogrel should avoid restarting it (for 2 weeks after surgery) until the anastomoses have healed.

- Acute renal failure secondary to rhabdomyolysis is rare and often complicates prolonged surgery in very large men. These patients should be operated on by the more experienced surgeon to reduce operating time, and their urine output should be monitored for the initial 24 hours. Creatine phosphokinase serum levels should be monitored in such patients in the early postoperative period.

- Stenosis at the gastrojejunostomy is a delayed complication. Endoscopic dilation and, in resistant cases, laparoscopic reconstruction of the anastomosis may be required.

- Peptic ulceration and perforation may complicate about 1% of cases and usually present within the initial 18 months after surgery. These could be related to H. pylori infection, use of nonsteroidal anti-inflammatory drugs, smoking, excess alcohol intake, or idiopathic factors. The most common site is anteriorly at the gastrojejunostomy, although these could also occur within the excluded stomach, duodenum, or jejunum and rarely at the jejunojejunostomy. Presentation is typical with severe acute abdominal pain with or without preceding symptoms of dyspepsia. Laparoscopy, suture closure with an omental patch, and peritoneal lavage are the standard treatment for upper gastrointestinal perforations. Most perforations heal within weeks, and this can be confirmed by contrast studies and careful assessment of the effluent from the abdominal drains. Perforation at the jejunojejunostomy can be managed by tube drainage at the site of perforation that creates a controlled fistula with delayed removal of the tube. Alternatively, the anastomosis can be disconnected, the biliopancreatic limb brought out as an end-jejunostomy, and the alimentary limb brought out as a loop jejunostomy with a feeding catheter placed into its distal limb for enteral feeding, with subsequent restoration of the jejunojejunostomy 6 to 12 months later. Primary closure of the perforation at the jejunojejunostomy may be attempted in low-risk patients, but very careful monitoring for reperforation should follow with alternative reintervention.

- Internal hernias may complicate 1% to 7% of cases after laparoscopic Roux-en-Y. Herniation at the jejunojejunal mesenteric defect is the most common cause if the surgeon did not close that defect, whereas herniation at the Petersen's defect may complicate an antecolic Roux loop, and herniation at the transverse mesocolon may occur in those who had a retrocolic Roux loop. Closure of the mesenteric defects reduces that risk. A long history of symptoms is not uncommon because the hernias tend to spontaneously reduce and recur. These hernias often elude radiologic detection, and the classic finding of mesenteric swirl on computed tomography is rarely seen. A diagnostic laparoscopy is warranted in the presence of unexplained and clinically significant abdominal colic. Reduction of the hernia with closure of the defect is often laparoscopically feasible when the condition is chronic (see Chapter 8), whereas laparotomy is warranted in the acute situation in which there is gross intestinal distention and ischemic bowel.

- Vitamin and mineral deficiencies and protein malnutrition may ensue over the long-term in 5% to 10% of patients following gastric bypass with varied severity. The sequelae may be neurologic (e.g., ataxia, Wernicke encephalopathy), hematologic (e.g., iron deficiency or megaloblastic anemia), metabolic (e.g., osteopenia, osteoporosis, and pathologic fractures), nutritional (e.g., protein malnutrition, bacterial overgrowth, and protein-losing enteropathy), and psychological (e.g., anorexia nervosa). Long-term vitamin and mineral supplements are necessary for prevention, and measurement of micronutrients (vitamins B_1, B_6, B_{12}, D, and E, folate, calcium, magnesium, phosphorus, selenium, and copper) is mandatory. Some of the consequences, particularly neurologic disorders, may not be fully reversible following replacement therapy. Bacterial overgrowth can be confirmed with a glucose-hydrogen breath test and is treatable with antibiotics (we adopt a 2-week course of ciprofloxacin and a 4-week course of metronidazole as first-line therapy). Anorexia nervosa can be quite difficult to manage and requires a multidisciplinary approach of pharmacotherapy, psychotherapy, cognitive therapy, and family therapy.

RESULTS AND OUTCOME

Large centers, including the authors', report an operative mortality rate with laparoscopic Roux-en-Y gastric bypass in the region of 0.2%, although this figure could be as high as 1% in some departments depending on their patient mix. Gastric bypass results in 60% to 80% excess weight loss within 18 to 24 months of surgery, and this is a recognized predictor of remission of comorbidities such as type 2 diabetes. Weight regain, however, may be encountered in 10% to 15% of patients within 5 to 10 years of surgery.

Based on the authors' experience, leak from the gastrojejunostomy appears to be less common after hand-sutured than stapled anastomotic technique and is the most common cause of death. Higa and colleagues reported no leaks in a series of 1040 laparoscopic gastric bypass patients, whereas we encountered it in four patients (who were high-risk candidates with significant comorbidities, high BMI, and older age) in just over 1500 procedures (0.27%). A 1% leak rate is commonly recognized with stapled gastrojejunostomy. When compared with the stapled gastrojejunostomy, the hand-sutured technique avoids complications such as bleeding from the staple line, as well as those specific to the use of the circular stapler such as stapler malfunction, pharyngeal perforation (for the transesophageal placement of the anvil), and port wound infection and herniation at the site of introduction of the stapler gun into the peritoneal cavity. The hand-sutured technique may also offer cost savings through reduction in cost of staplers, and in experienced hands it can be completed within a comparable operative time to that of a stapled anastomosis.

The laparoscopic totally hand-sutured Roux-en-Y gastric bypass is surgically feasible and is safe in the hands of the experienced laparoscopic bariatric surgeon, with low associated morbidity. There is a learning curve to be overcome, and this could stretch between 50 and 100 cases, depending on the surgeon's established laparoscopic expertise.

Suggested Readings

Atchison M, Wade T, Higgins B, Slavotinek T: Anorexia nervosa following gastric reduction surgery for morbid obesity, *Int J Eat Disord* 23:111–116, 1998.

Ballesta-Lopez C, Poves I, Cabrera M, et al: Learning curve for laparoscopic Roux-en-Y gastric bypass with totally hand-sewn anastomosis: analysis of first 600 consecutive patients, *Surg Endosc* 19:519–524, 2005.

Berger JR: The neurological complications of bariatric surgery, *Arch Neurol* 61:1185–1189, 2004.

Frantzides CT, Carlson MA, Schulte WJ: Laparoscopic gastric stapling and Roux-en-Y gastrojejunostomy for the treatment of morbid obesity: an experimental model, *J Laparoendosc Surg* 5:97–100, 1995.

Frantzides CT, Zeni TM, Madan AK, et al: Laparoscopic Roux-en-Y gastric bypass utilizing the triple stapling technique, *JSLS* 10:176–179, 2006.

Frantzides CT, Zeni TM, Mahr C, et al: Value of preoperative upper endoscopy in patients undergoing laparoscopic gastric bypass, *Obes Surg* 16:142–146, 2006.

Frantzides CT, Zografakis J: Laparoscopic Roux-en-Y gastric bypass. In Frantzides CT, Carlson MA, editors: *Atlas of Minimally Invasive Surgery*, Philadelphia, 2009, Saunders.

Gentileschi P, Kini S, Catarci M, Gagner M: Evidence-based medicine: open and laparoscopic bariatric surgery, *Surg Endosc* 16:736–744, 2002.

Gonzalez R, Lin E, Venkatesh KR, et al: Gastrojejunostomy during laparoscopic gastric bypass: analysis of 3 techniques, *Arch Surg* 138:181–184, 2003.

Hamade AM, Butt I, Balbisi B, et al: Closed blunt-trocar 5 mm-port for primary cannulation in laparoscopic surgery: A safe technique, *Surg Laparosc Endosc Percutan Tech* 16:156–160, 2006.

Hamza N, Abbas MH, Darwish A, et al: Predictors of remission of type 2 diabetes mellitus after laparoscopic gastric banding and bypass, *Surg Obes Relat Dis* 7:691–696, 2011.

Higa KD, Boone KB, Ho T, Davies OG: Laparoscopic Roux-en-Y gastric bypass for morbid obesity: Technique and preliminary results of our first 400 patients, *Arch Surg* 135:1029–1033, discussion 1033–1034, 2000.

Inabnet WB, Quinn T, Gagner M, et al: Laparoscopic Roux-en-Y gastric bypass in patients with BMI <50: A prospective randomized trial comparing short and long limb lengths, *Obes Surg* 15:51–57, 2005.

Koffman BM, Greenfield LJ, Ali II, et al: Neurologic complications after surgery for obesity, *Muscle Nerve* 33:166–176, 2006.

Kramer LD, Locke GE: Wernicke's encephalopathy: Complication of gastric placation, *J Clin Gastroenterol* 9:549–552, 1987.

Madan AK, Harper JL, Tichansky DS: Techniques of laparoscopic gastric bypass: on-line survey of American Society for Bariatric Surgery practicing surgeons, *Surg Obes Relat Dis* 4:166–172, discussion 172–173, 2008.

Pinheiro JS, Schiavon CA, Pereira PB, et al: Long-long limb Roux-en-Y gastric bypass is more efficacious in treatment of type 2 diabetes and lipid disorders in super-obese patients, *Surg Obes Relat Dis* 4:521–527, 2008.

Ruiz de Adana JC, Hernández Matías A, Hernández Bartolomé M, et al: Risk of gastrojejunal anastomotic stricture with multifilament and monofilament sutures after hand-sewn laparoscopic gastric bypass: a prospective cohort study, *Obes Surg* 19:1274–1277, 2009.

Ruiz de Adana JC, López-Herrero J, Hernández-Matías A, et al: Laparoscopic hand-sewn gastrojejunal anastomoses, *Obes Surg* 18:1074–1076, 2008.

Sauerland S, Angrisani L, Belachew M, et al: Obesity surgery: evidence-based guidelines of the European Association for Endoscopic Surgery (EAES), *Surg Endosc* 19:200–221, 2005.

GEORGE S. FERZLI, SEAN RIM, AND MICHAEL F. TIMONEY

Laparoscopic Roux-en-Y Gastric Bypass with Medial Rotation of the Left Hepatic Lobe

10

The videos associated with this chapter are listed in the Video Contents and can be found on the accompanying DVDs and *on Expertconsult.com.*

The laparoscopic Roux-en-Y gastric bypass has now become the most commonly performed bariatric procedure. It has well-established benefits in promoting weight loss and in significantly reducing comorbidities like diabetes and hypertension. One of the crucial steps in performing this procedure is gaining access to the angle of His. In the bariatric population, steatosis of the liver is prevalent. This condition can significantly impair clear visualization of this anatomic region, resulting in a technically difficult and unsafe operation. In the authors' practice, all patients are required to lose 10% of their body weight during the preoperative period and to maintain a low-calorie diet for 14 days preceding surgery. This is done to reduce liver volume. However, as described in a paper by Morris and colleagues, body mass index (BMI) and outer abdominal fat may not be as reliable in predicting morbidity and mortality as is a measure of intra-abdominal fat. They suggest using a computed tomography (CT) scan to quantitate the amount of perinephric fat as a measure of intra-abdominal fat in patients undergoing liver resection. These findings may perhaps be applied to the correlation between intra-abdominal fat measurements and liver volume.

Traditionally, visualization of the angle of His is obtained by retracting the left lobe of the liver cephalad and anteriorly. The triangular ligament is left in place, and retraction is performed with a fan or a Nathanson retractor, or a laparoscopic grasper. In most cases, this technique should provide sufficient exposure of the angle of His to create the gastric pouch. However, in patients having excessive liver bulk, adequate exposure may not be possible with this method. In the past, two-stage procedures have been described to deal with these situations. Either a sleeve gastrectomy or a Roux-en-Y bypass with a larger pouch is performed in the first stage, and the patient returns for revision. In the authors' experience, we have found that medial rotation of the left lobe of the liver with antehepatic gastrojejunostomy creation is the safest and most effective technique in those whose excessive liver bulk would otherwise preclude a one-stage procedure.

OPERATIVE INDICATIONS

Currently, the standard criteria for undergoing bariatric surgery are a BMI of greater than 40 kg/m^2 or greater than 35 kg/m^2 with obesity-related comorbidities (e.g., obesity hypoventilation, obstructive sleep apnea, diabetes, hypertension, cardiomyopathy, or musculoskeletal dysfunction). Patients must also have

demonstrated a failure of weight loss under a medically supervised diet. The type of procedure chosen is determined by patients' weight-loss goals, their comorbidities, and their eating habits. This is a decision shared by the patient and the surgeon. It has been demonstrated by level one evidence that gastric bypass is the gold standard by which other bariatric procedures are measured.

PREOPERATIVE ASSESSMENT AND PREPARATION

A multidisciplinary approach is necessary for preoperative evaluation and optimization of the bariatric patient. A dedicated team of internists, cardiologists, pulmonologists, gastroenterologists, nutritionists, and psychologists is used in the preoperative evaluation and preparation of the bariatric patient for surgery (Table 10-1). Any medically reversible causes of obesity such as hypothyroidism are investigated and treated. A careful history of all medications is obtained, including over-the-counter and herbal supplements.

Patients also undergo a thorough psychiatric evaluation to ensure that they do not have an underlying eating disorder or a psychotic illness. It is vital that they understand the emotional and mental stress that may occur with the changes in their diet. Support groups in which those being evaluated for bariatric surgery meet with each other, as well as with postoperative patients, to share their experiences and concerns may help to better prepare them for surgery.

Patients with obstructive sleep apnea and obesity hypoventilation routinely undergo pulmonary function tests and respiratory therapy to minimize postoperative respiratory complications.

Preoperative evaluation of the upper gastrointestinal tract is also performed endoscopically to ensure that there are no abnormalities like ulcer disease, masses, *Helicobacter pylori* infection, or hiatal hernia. A sonogram is also obtained to rule out cholelithiasis. Positive findings like *H. pylori* may need to be addressed preoperatively or, like cholecystectomy, at the time of surgery. Finally, there should be a low threshold for cardiac evaluation and optimization, given this high-risk patient population.

All patients older than 50 years are required to undergo colonoscopy, and men older than 50 years must have a prostate-specific antigen test. Women older than 35 years must be

Table 10-1 Preoperative Assessment Team

Psychologist	Mental health assessment
Nutritionist	Low-calorie diet program
Physical therapist	Exercise program
Internist	Complete blood count, metabolic panel, liver function tests, iron studies, prostate-specific antigen level for males >50 years old
Endocrinologist	Thyroid function tests, parathyroid hormone, vitamins A, D, B_{12} levels
Gastroenterologist	Upper endoscopy, colonoscopy for patients >50 years old
Pulmonologist	Pulmonary function test, sleep apnea study
Cardiologist	Echocardiogram, stress test
Radiologist	Gallbladder sonogram, venous duplex, inferior vena cava filter for high-risk patients, mammogram for women >40 years old
Gynecologist	Papanicolaou test for women >35 years old

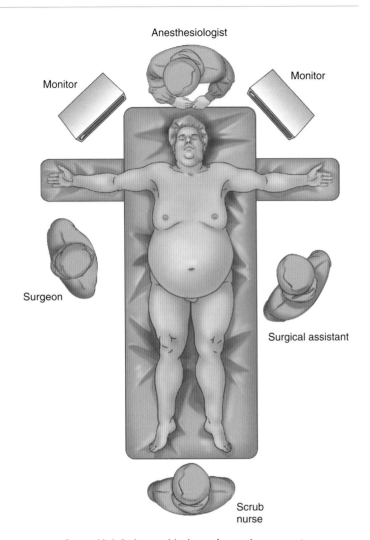

FIGURE 10-1 Patient positioning and operating room setup.

evaluated by a gynecologist and undergo a Papanicolaou test. Women older than 40 years are required to be up to date with their screening mammography. Women of child-bearing age are advised not to get pregnant for 18 months following surgery. Preoperatively, they are urged to stop oral contraceptives for 6 weeks, owing to the risk for increasing coagulability. A venous duplex is obtained in all patients, and an inferior vena cava filter is placed in those considered at high risk for venous thromboembolism.

Under the guidance of the internist, patients are mandated to lose 10% of their body weight preoperatively. This is done in conjunction with the nutritionist and physical therapist. Monthly documentation of vital signs, weight, and behavioral intervention to reinforce healthy eating and exercise habits is required for a minimum of 6 consecutive months preoperatively. All possible information about bariatric surgery, including preoperative preparation, risks, complications, and postoperative care, is given to patients. The morning of surgery, patients are started on proton pump inhibitors and subcutaneous heparin injections, and they are given a dose of intravenous antibiotics before incision.

PATIENT POSITIONING

The patients are placed supine on the operating room table with both arms extended (Fig. 10-1). The Lloyd-Davies position can also be employed, with the surgeon standing between the legs. However, we feel the supine position with the surgeon at the patient's right side reduces stress on the patient's legs. A Foley catheter is not routinely placed, and patients are asked to void just before entering the operating room. Before induction of anesthesia, they are given a dose of broad-spectrum antibiotics, and intermittent pneumatic compression devices are placed on both legs. A foot board is placed, but with the authors' technique, we have never required the use of a steep reverse Trendelenburg position. The bariatric anesthesiologists routinely employ a fiberoptic laryngoscope that greatly facilitates endotracheal intubation.

PLACEMENT OF TROCARS

The authors' choice of access is the Veress needle, which is usually placed at the umbilicus, unless there is a hernia or a concern for adhesions. In these cases, we place it either at the Palmer point

or at the site of the first trocar. An open technique is rarely used. Once pneumoperitoneum is established, a 10-mm trocar is placed 16 to 18 cm below the angle of His. The surgeon calculates this location by placing the base of the palm just above the left costal margin and making the incision at the tip of the third finger. A 10-mm 30-degree laparoscope is placed through this trocar, and the Veress needle and its trajectory are visualized to ensure that there has been no injury on insertion. The needle is removed under direct visualization, and the insufflator is connected to the trocar. A 5-mm trocar is inserted just below and to the right of the xiphoid process. This trocar is angled toward the patient's left shoulder so that it comes through the falciform. Through this trocar, the left lobe of the liver is retracted anteriorly and cephalad, making it possible to visualize the angle of His and determine the approach. Once this is done, the remaining trocars are triangulated around the angle of His, as illustrated in Fig. 10-2.

OPERATIVE TECHNIQUE

Creating the Biliopancreatic Limb

The greater omentum is swept cephalad to reveal the transverse mesocolon, which is retracted superiorly by the assistant with atraumatic graspers. The ligament of Treitz is then identified, keeping in mind its relatively constant anatomic location at the intersection between lines drawn from the left shoulder to the umbilicus and the xiphoid to the left anterior-superior iliac spine (Fig. 10-3).

The small bowel is then measured 80 to 120 cm distally by running it in a clockwise fashion. The assistant then releases the transverse mesocolon and grasps the small bowel at this distance. An enterotomy is created with hook electrocautery just proximal to the planned transection point to facilitate its recognition as the biliopancreatic limb when later making the jejunojejunostomy. The window in the mesentery is bluntly created, and the small bowel is transected using a laparoscopic linear stapler with a 60-mm cartridge of 2.5-mm staples (Fig. 10-4).

Jejunojejunal Anastomosis

The small bowel is measured another 150 cm by running it counterclockwise. At this point, the assistant retracts distally and toward the patient's left. The surgeon grasps the bowel proximally and retracts medially to create an enterotomy in between. This bowel is brought up to the stapled end of the biliopancreatic limb at the site of the prior enterotomy, and a side-to-side stapled jejunojejunostomy is created (Fig. 10-5). The enteroenterostomy is closed with interrupted figure-of-eight 2-0 silk sutures (Fig. 10-6). The mesenteric defect is closed in a similar fashion,

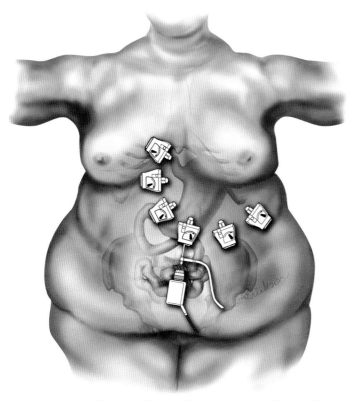

FIGURE 10-2 Placement of trocars. (Copyright Anne Erickson CMI.)

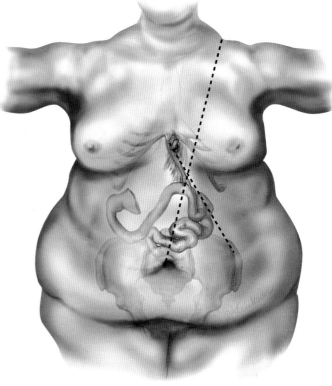

FIGURE 10-3 Projection of the ligament of Treitz. (Copyright Anne Erickson CMI.)

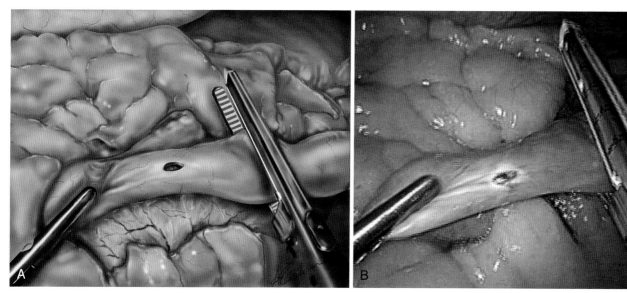

FIGURE 10-4 Enterotomy and transection of the biliopancreatic limb. (A, Copyright Anne Erickson CMI.)

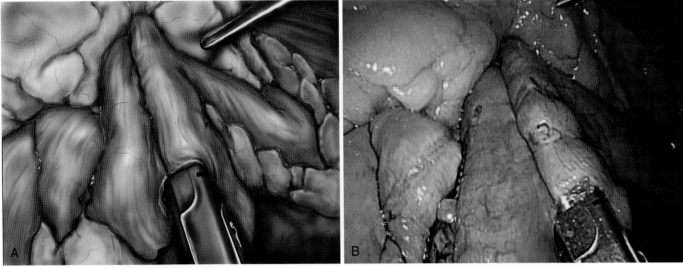

FIGURE 10-5 Feeding the stapler into the bowel. (**A**, Copyright Anne Erickson CMI.)

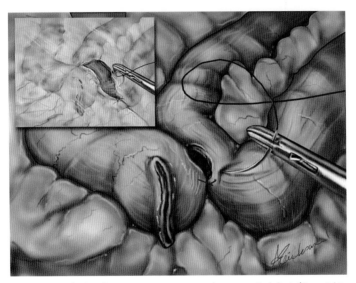

FIGURE 10-6 Closing the enteroenterostomy and mesenteric defect. (Copyright Anne Erickson CMI.)

starting from its root. The small bowel serosa is incorporated with the last stitch to prevent jejunojejunal intussusception.

Creation of the Gastric Pouch with Medial Rotation of the Left Hepatic Lobe

A laparoscopic grasper is inserted through the subxiphoid port to retract the left lobe of the liver from below. Ideally, the left side of the right crus just above the gastroesophageal junction is identified and clamped with the grasper to maintain retraction (Fig. 10-7). Alternatively, a fan or a Nathanson retractor can be used to access this space. It is imperative to exercise extreme caution here because such a liver can be friable, and excessive retraction can result in a large tear of the capsule or even a fracture of the parenchyma. In addition, the left lobe of the liver may become ischemic from the pressure caused by the retractor, in which case the retraction must be released periodically. Finally, peak airway pressures must be closely monitored because cephalad retraction may compromise adequate ventilation. Regardless of technique, a bulky liver can prevent satisfactory exposure of the angle of His. In these instances, simply taking down the triangular ligament of

the liver and rotating its left lobe medially may be all that is required to proceed safely.

The ligament is incised from a lateral to medial direction with an energy source (Fig. 10-8). Care must be taken to avoid injuring the spleen because the large left hepatic lobe and the ligament can be wrapped around the upper pole of the spleen. A key principle when incising the triangular ligament is to stay as close to the liver as possible. A moist sponge can also be placed behind the triangular ligament during its division to protect the stomach and the spleen. Once the left lobe is reflected off the spleen, the greater curvature of the stomach is at risk for injury as the incision is carried medially. Again, this can be avoided by staying close to the liver surface. The medial edge of the esophagus signifies the limit of dissection. Finally, careful attention must be paid to the fat pad of Belsey, which must not be encroached as it overlies the gastroesophageal junction. So long as the liver is not cirrhotic and friable, the left lobe can now be folded inferiorly and medially onto itself. A laparoscopic grasper is then used to maintain retraction by grasping the fatty tissue of the lesser curvature by the pars flaccida.

Once adequate exposure is obtained, we begin dissection of the lesser curvature at the level of the first coronary vein. The avascular connective tissue plane overlying the gastric serosa is peeled away without the need of energy devices. By staying directly on the serosa, we avoid injury to the vagus and its branches. Dissection of the posterior stomach is performed bluntly with closed graspers, being careful to stay in the correct plane because adhesions are often encountered here. To facilitate this maneuver, the assistant should fan out the stomach by grasping the greater curvature of the stomach at two points (Fig. 10-9).

At this point, it is essential to confirm that there is nothing in the stomach or esophagus, such as an orogastric tube or temperature probe. A 45-mm cartridge of 3.5-mm staples is fired horizontally across the stomach to create the distal margin of the gastric pouch. A calibrating tube is inserted orally and is advanced to the staple line under laparoscopic visualization. Traditionally, the gastric pouch is sized by inflating the balloon to 15 to 30 mL. Alternatively, the terminal branches of the coronary vein are fairly constant and thus may serve as an excellent landmark for creating the lateral staple line.

The posterior dissection of the stomach is continued cephalad by inserting closed graspers under the lateral edge of the first

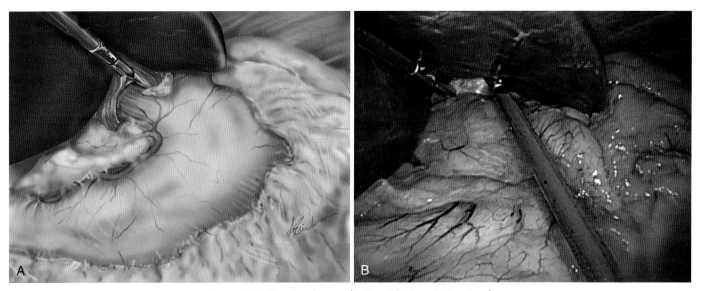

FIGURE 10-7 Clamping the crus. (**A**, Copyright Anne Erickson CMI.)

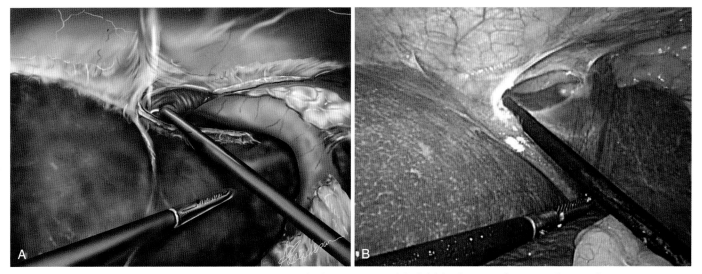

FIGURE 10-8 Incising the triangular ligament and inferior retraction of the left lobe. (**A**, Copyright Anne Erickson CMI.)

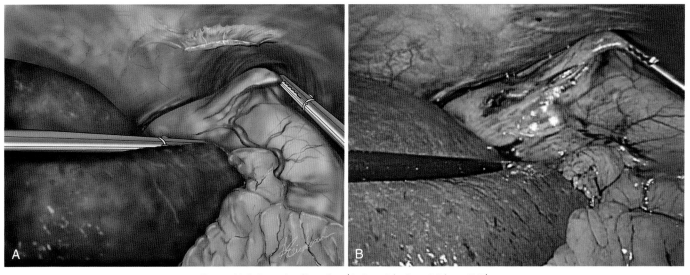

FIGURE 10-9 Posterior dissection. (**A**, Copyright Anne Erickson CMI.)

staple line. Once this space is created, a second load of staples is fired toward the angle of His, parallel to the calibrating tube and along the edges of the coronary vein branches. It is the authors' preference to use reinforced staples for the remainder of the transections because we have noted significantly reduced bleeding and hematoma formation at the staple line with their use. The first two applications are done without reinforcement because the synthetic absorbable film hinders one's ability to suture the gastrojejunostomy. As the angle of His is reached, it is imperative to visualize the upper pole of the spleen, which may be adherent to the posterior wall of the stomach. A window between the stomach and the spleen is carefully created at the angle of His, staying lateral to the Belsey fat pad. Once this is accomplished, a final row of staples can be fired to complete the transection. It is important that a small rim of gastric tissue is left lateral to the Belsey fat pad to prevent the narrowing of the gastroesophageal junction (Fig. 10-10). A different sort of pitfall here is leaving a bridge of undivided gastric tissue between the pouch and the bypassed stomach, which will inevitably lead to symptoms similar to a gastrogastric fistula.

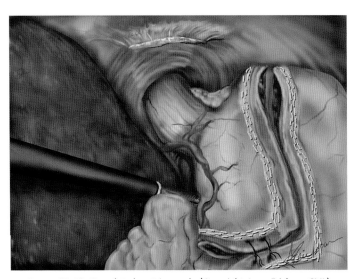

FIGURE 10-10 Completed gastric pouch. (Copyright Anne Erickson CMI.)

Antehepatic Gastrojejunostomy

The alimentary limb is brought up to the gastric pouch over the transverse colon by the assistant and held in place with the staple line facing laterally (Fig. 10-11). If there is excessive tension on the limb, the omentum can be divided vertically with either a Harmonic scalpel or LigaSure device (Covidien, Boulder, Colo.). We do not recommend dividing the mesentery because this may compromise the blood supply to the anastomosis. The anastomosis is fashioned with interrupted 2-0 silk sutures in a single layer. The posterior layer is created from left to right, with four to five figure-of-eight sutures spaced several millimeters apart. The staple line of the gastric pouch is incorporated into this layer (Fig. 10-12).

The calibrating tube is then pushed in slightly to create a point of tension on the gastric pouch just above the suture line, and a small gastrotomy is made with the use of hook electrocautery. The calibrating tube is pushed through to ensure an adequately sized lumen and is then retracted. An enterotomy of similar size is created on the Roux limb, also by electrocautery, with care taken not to burn the posterior wall. Meticulous technique is obligatory with the corner sutures because these locations are known to be susceptible to leakage during intraoperative testing with methylene blue. The suturing of the gastrojejunal anastomosis begins at the lateral corner by taking a full-thickness outside-in forehand bite of the small bowel from the left-sided 10-mm trocar. The serosa of the small bowel can be retracted gently with the left hand to ensure that the posterior wall is not incorporated in the stitch. Through the same left-sided trocar, a full-thickness bite of the stomach wall is taken in a backhanded fashion from inside-out. This maneuver is repeated to complete the figure-of-eight suture. The right-sided corner is then sutured in a mirror-image fashion. The small bowel is taken backhanded from the left-sided trocar, and the gastric wall is taken forehanded. Four to five simple sutures are then placed in between without tying, to allow for visualization of the posterior wall. The sutures are grasped upward on either side of the anastomosis, and the calibrating tube is passed into the Roux limb to ensure a patent lumen before the sutures are tied (Fig. 10-13).

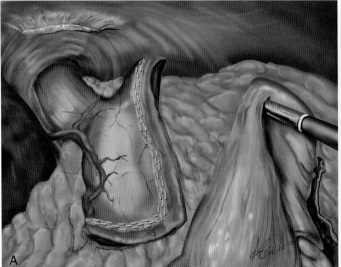
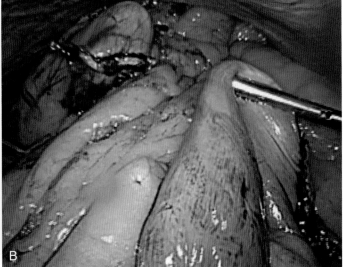

FIGURE 10-11 Antehepatic orientation of the alimentary limb. (A, Copyright Anne Erickson CMI.)

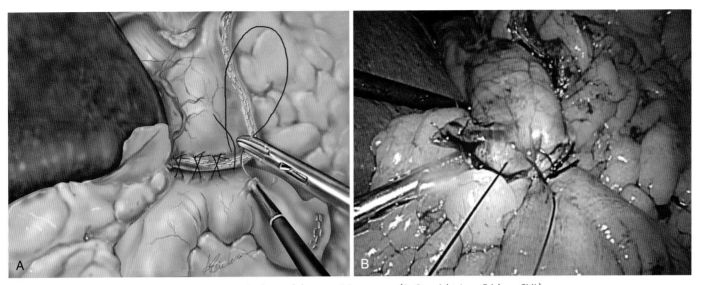

FIGURE 10-12 Posterior layer of the gastrojejunostomy. (**A**, Copyright Anne Erickson CMI.)

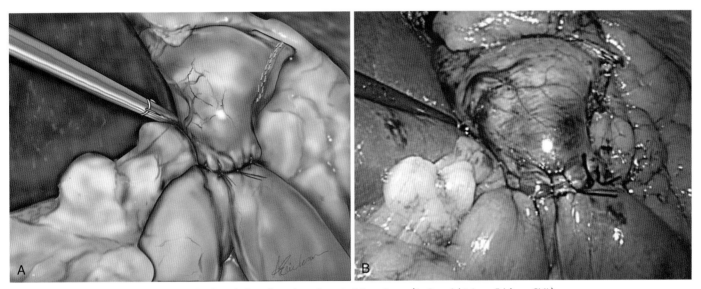

FIGURE 10-13 Completion of antehepatic gastrojejunostomy. (**A**, Copyright Anne Erickson CMI.)

To perform a leak test, the Roux limb is occluded 10 to 15 cm distally, and 150 mL of methylene blue is injected into the open port of the calibrating tube. The anterior suture line must be inspected with great care, after ensuring adequate distention of both the gastric pouch and the proximal Roux limb. To assess the posterior suture line, the small bowel serosa is gently grasped laterally and medially and rotated in both directions. If a leak is found, it is suture-repaired with the lumen distended to minimize the risk for incorporating the opposite wall into the stitch. The test is repeated until no leak is observed, after which the methylene blue is suctioned from the calibrating tube. The anastomosis is then tested under water with insufflation of air into the pouch. The left lobe of the liver is then carefully flipped over the gastrojejunostomy, restoring the normal anatomy. A 10-French Jackson-Pratt drain is placed along the staple line and anastomosis. The tubing is brought out through the left-sided 5-mm trocar site, avoiding another incision. The remaining ports are removed under direct visualization, and the skin incisions are closed with staples.

POSTOPERATIVE CARE

Patients are extubated after the procedure and transferred to an intensive care unit. Pneumatic compression devices and subcutaneous heparin are continued for venous thromboembolism prophylaxis. Proton pump inhibitors are also administered as a measure of gastrointestinal prophylaxis. Early ambulation is emphasized, and physical therapy is initiated immediately. A combination of narcotics and nonsteroidal anti-inflammatory agents is administered intravenously for analgesia.

Nothing by mouth is instituted until patients undergo an upper gastrointestinal study on postoperative day 1. If no edema or leakage is noted, and patients have no nausea, fever, pain, or tachycardia, they are started on a sugar-free, noncarbonated clear liquid diet. If tolerated, they are discharged later that evening on proton pump inhibitors, with sucralfate prescribed for at least 90 days. They are advanced to a pureed diet in the second to third week, and then to a soft diet by weeks 3 to 4. Regular diet is usually resumed by the third month. Patients are instructed to contact the surgeon in case of a body temperature higher than 38° C (100° F), a sustained heart rate higher than 100 beats/minute, new-onset abdominal or back pain, nausea, vomiting, redness, swelling, or foul-smelling discharge at the incision sites.

Patients are seen in the office 7 days after surgery. They are required to meet with the surgeon, internist, nutritionist, physical therapist, and psychologist monthly for the first 3 months, then every 3 months for the first year. From then on, they are seen every 6 months to keep a log of their weight, resolution of comorbidities, medications, and laboratory values. According to the Endocrine Society Guidelines, specific blood tests required are iron, vitamin B_{12}, folate, calcium, 25-hydroxyvitamin D, phosphorous, parathyroid hormone, and alkaline phosphatase. These should be measured every 6 months after surgery for the first 2 years, then yearly. Patients are instructed to begin taking oral calcium and multivitamins within several weeks of their surgery. They are also advised to follow-up closely with their primary care physicians as well as their cardiologist, pulmonologist, and gastroenterologist as needed, and they are encouraged to continue attending support group sessions.

PROCEDURE-SPECIFIC COMPLICATIONS

Postoperative complications include anastomotic leak, bleeding, internal herniation, anastomotic stricture, anastomotic ulcer, and nutritional deficiencies. If leakage is suspected clinically, early diagnosis and treatment are the most important factors in patient survival. A CT scan with oral contrast must be obtained as soon as possible. A controlled leak can be managed conservatively with continued closed-suction drainage as long as the patient remains in stable condition. On the other hand, a sick patient with or without radiographic studies mandates an emergent return to the operating room. If the leak is identified, it can be treated with a buttressed repair, placement of large-caliber drains, and placement of a feeding tube distally. In cases in which the leak site is not apparent with a methylene blue test, treatment should still consist of drainage and placement of a feeding tube.

Postoperative bleeding can usually be managed conservatively in stable patients who respond to fluid challenges and blood transfusions. Possible sources include the port sites, anastomoses (less common with the hand-sutured technique), and staple lines. Endoscopy may be necessary in cases of persistent gastrointestinal bleeding, but this is rare. Also uncommon are the spleen, liver, omentum, and mesentery as sources of delayed bleeding. Regardless of the suspected source, unstable patients should be brought back to the operating room immediately.

Internal herniation can occur in an acute or chronic fashion, through the mesenteric defect at the site of the jejunojejunostomy or through the Petersen's space. Patients often present with abdominal or back pain, and a CT scan may or may not be helpful because the classic sign of mesenteric swirling is rarely present. In fact, the herniated loop often reduces spontaneously, and there may be no abnormal findings on a CT scan. Persistent symptoms without an obvious source warrant a diagnostic laparoscopy (see Chapter 8). Prevention is the key, through meticulous closing of mesenteric defects during the initial operation.

Anastomotic strictures can be managed with repeat endoscopic dilation. A revision of the anastomosis is rarely required. Marginal ulcer formation is another late complication and can be prevented by promoting smoking cessation, prescription of long-term proton pump inhibitors, and avoidance of nonsteroidal anti-inflammatory agents. In addition, patients should be screened for *H. pylori* preoperatively. A new-onset ulcer near the anastomotic site should raise the suspicion of a gastrogastric fistula, particularly if the patient has stopped losing or has begun regaining weight (see Chapter 8). Diagnosis is confirmed by an upper gastrointestinal study or endoscopy. The treatment is reoperation if symptoms are refractory to medical or endoscopic therapy. Nutritional and vitamin deficiencies are prevented by prophylactic supplementation and close monitoring of laboratory tests and weights during postoperative visits. The most common deficiencies observed are protein, iron, vitamin B_{12}, and vitamin D.

RESULTS AND OUTCOMES

Patients generally lose 60% to 80% of their excess body weight within the first year following surgery. There is also a significant resolution of obesity-related comorbidities such as hypertension, diabetes, and gastroesophageal reflux disease. Mortality rates after laparoscopic Roux-en-Y gastric bypass are less than 1% in most centers and close to 0.3% in centers of excellence. Overall morbidity rates related to complications such as anastomotic leak, infection, bleeding, and stenosis are about 15%.

In the authors' center, we have now performed a total of 25 Roux-en-Y gastric bypasses with medial rotation of the left hepatic lobe and antehepatic gastrojejunostomy (23 females and 2 males). There were no intraoperative or acute postoperative complications. The mean operative times and lengths of stay were not statistically different from those not undergoing an antehepatic approach. During the authors' long-term follow-up of these patients, we have also noted no deviation from the norm in terms of complications or weight loss.

In our experience, medial rotation of the left hepatic lobe provides a safe and effective method of completing a Roux-en-Y gastric bypass in those with excessively bulky livers. Other options include staged operations or aborting the procedure altogether. Our technique allows completion of the planned procedure without increased risk, avoiding the necessity of a second operation in which adhesions may further increase the difficulty. The only additional steps required are division of the triangular ligament and medial rotation of the left hepatic lobe. We do, however, recognize the limitations of this technique in patients whose livers are tense and friable. We strongly advise sound judgment and meticulous surgical techniques when such cases are encountered.

Suggested Readings

Ahmed S, Morrow E, Morton J: Perioperative considerations when operating on the very obese: tricks of the trade, *Minerva Chir* 65:667–675, 2010.

Carrodeguas L, Szomstein S, Soto F, et al: Management of gastrogastric fistulas after divided Roux-en-Y gastric bypass surgery for morbid obesity: analysis of 1,292 consecutive patients and review of literature, *Surg Obes Relat Dis* 1:467–474, 2005.

Daellenbach L, Suter M: Jejunojejunal intussusception after Roux-en-Y gastric bypass: a review, *Obes Surg* 21:253–263, 2011.

Ferzli G, Edwards ED: Ante-hepatic gastrojejunostomy, *Am J Surg* 195:708–710, 2008.

Ferzli G, Fingerhut A: Trocar placement for laparoscopic abdominal procedures: a simple standardized method, *J Am Coll Surg* 198:163–173, 2003.

Frantzides CT, Carlson MA, Moore RE, et al: Effect of body mass index on nonalcoholic fatty liver disease in patients undergoing minimally invasive bariatric surgery, *J Soc Laparoendosc Surg* 8:849–855, 2004.

Frantzides CT, Zografakis J: Laparoscopic Roux-en-Y gastric bypass. In Frantzides CT, Carlson MA, editors: *Atlas of Minimally Invasive Surgery*, Philadelphia, 2009, Saunders.

Ludman EJ, Ichikawa LE, Simon GE, et al: Breast and cervical cancer screening specific effects of depression and obesity, *Am J Prev Med* 38:303–310, 2010.

Morris K, Tuorto S, Gönen M, et al: Simple measurement of intra-abdominal fat for abdominal surgery outcome prediction, *Arch Surg* 145:1069–1073, 2010.

Nguyen N, Longoria M, Gelfand DV, et al: Staged laparoscopic Roux-en-Y: a novel two-stage bariatric operation as an alternative in the super-obese with massively enlarged liver, *Obes Surg* 15:1077–1081, 2005.

Pratt GM, Learn CA, Hughes GD, et al: Demographics and outcomes at American Society for Metabolic and Bariatric Surgery Centers of Excellence, *Surg Endosc* 23:795–799, 2009.

Schauer PR, Ikramuddin S, Gourash W, et al: Outcomes after laparoscopic Roux-en-Y gastric bypass for morbid obesity, *Ann Surg* 232:515–529, 2000.

Zeni TM, Frantzides CT, Mahr C, et al: Value of preoperative upper endoscopy in patients undergoing laparoscopic gastric bypass, *Obes Surg* 16:142–146, 2006.

Laparoscopy-Assisted Distal Gastrectomy for Cancer

SEIGO KITANO, YOHEI KONO, AND NORIO SHIRAISHI

11

The videos associated with this chapter are listed in the Video Contents and can be found on the accompanying DVDs and *on Expertconsult.com.*

Gastric cancer is one of the most common cancers worldwide with about 989,600 new cases and 738,000 deaths per year, accounting for about 8% of new cancers. Early gastric cancer (EGC) is defined by the Japanese Gastric Cancer Association guidelines as the cancer contained to the gastric mucosa or submucosa despite lymph node (LN) metastasis. Recently, the incidence of EGC has increased in Asian countries, presumably because of advances in diagnostic modalities (endoscopy technology and examination technique) and the popularity of mass screening (e.g., yearly barium meal study). The incidence of stage I gastric cancer is 1.5 times higher than that of other gastric cancer in Japan. The main strategy against gastric cancer, including EGC, is surgical removal of the cancer cells. For the treatment of gastric cancer with the risk for LN metastasis, gastrectomy with LN dissection is routinely performed in Asian countries.

Laparoscopy-assisted distal gastrectomy (LADG) with dissection of regional LNs for the treatment of EGC was developed in 1991. Since then, the number of LADGs has rapidly increased because of the high incidence of gastric cancer located in the distal stomach, especially in Asian countries. This chapter will focus on LADG. The rapid popularization of LADG has been based on advances in surgical technique and the development of several laparoscopic surgical instruments, such as laparoscopic coagulation shears and a laparoscopic vessel-sealing system. In Japan, more than 34,600 patients with EGC underwent laparoscopic gastrectomy between 1991 and 2009, and in 2009 alone, more than 5500 patients with gastric cancer underwent LADG.

Laparoscopic techniques have several disadvantages compared with traditional open surgical techniques, including loss of touch sensation and the necessity of using long forceps in a two-dimensional work environment. Previously it had seemed difficult to apply laparoscopic techniques to gastrectomy for cancer across a large number of hospitals. Several study groups in Japan and Korea, however, have conducted numerous conferences and organized training courses to standardize the techniques of LADG with less invasiveness. As a result, LADG with LN dissection is now performed safely in patients with gastric cancer, especially those with EGC, in many centers across Asia. Herein we discuss the present status of LADG in Japan, including the indications for and techniques of LADG.

OPERATIVE INDICATIONS

The indication for LADG is EGC with risk for LN metastasis and advanced gastric cancer (AGC) without serosal invasion, all located in the distal two thirds of stomach. The incidence of LN metastasis in EGC is about 5% to 20%. With the development of endoscopic submucosal dissection (ESD) techniques, EGC without risk for LN metastasis is treated by ESD. The Japanese Gastric Cancer Association guidelines define EGC with a risk for LN metastasis as follows: (1) well-differentiated mucosal cancer of more than 2.0 cm in diameter, (2) well-differentiated mucosal cancer with ulceration, (3) poorly differentiated mucosal cancer, and (4) submucosal cancer. LADG is applied to these conditions, which are diagnosed by endoscopic examination, barium meal examination, and computed tomography (CT) findings as ECG with risk for LN metastasis.

The indication of LADG for advanced cancer remains controversial because of the lack of clinical evidence of oncologic safety. Most surgeons who perform open surgery worry about the possibility of an increased incidence of port-site recurrence and peritoneal metastasis. Therefore, LADG in Japan is applied to AGC without serosal invasion and lymph node status of N2 or higher. The extent of LN dissection in Japan is determined according to the predicted frequency of LN metastasis. The Japanese Gastric Cancer Association guidelines indicate the following: D1 or D1+ for EGC, and D2 for AGC (see definitions in Fig. 11-1 and Tables 11-1 and 11-2).

PREOPERATIVE EVALUATION, TESTING, AND PREPARATION

Preoperative evaluation should stage the gastric cancer and the patient's systemic tolerance to surgical stress. Gastric tumor staging as defined by the American Joint Committee on Cancer (AJCC) is shown in Table 11-3. For the staging of gastric cancer, endoscopic examination (with biopsy and ultrasound) and barium meal study are used to evaluate the location, histologic type, size, and depth of wall invasion of the gastric cancer. Ultrasound examination and CT are used to evaluate invasion to other organs, nodal metastasis, hematogenous metastasis, and peritoneal dissemination. AGC without serosal exposure (T2) is

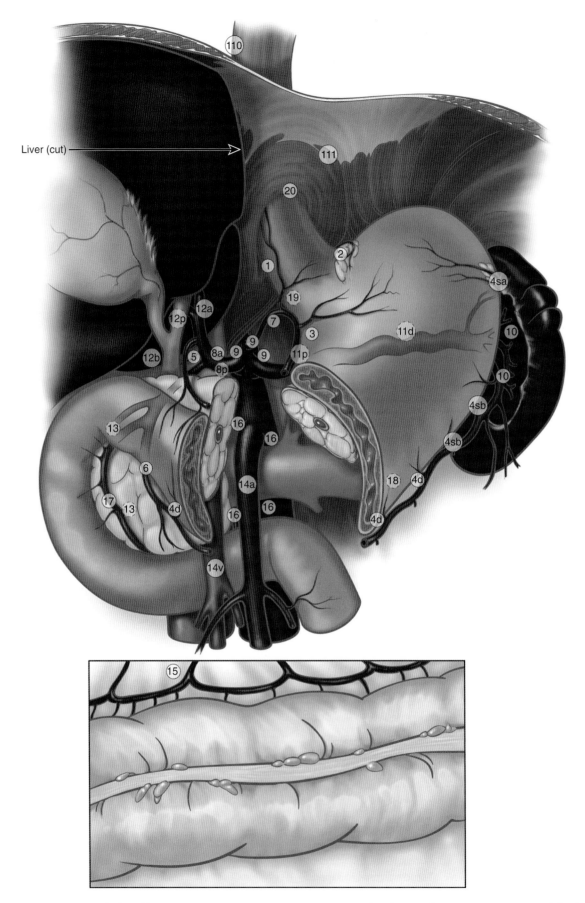

Liver (cut)

Figure 11-1 Regional lymph nodes. (Adapted from Japanese Gastric Cancer Association: Japanese classification of gastric carcinoma, 2nd English edition. *Gastric Cancer* 1:10–24, 1998.)

Table 11-1 Lymph Node Stations of the Japanese Classification System for Gastric Cancer*

No.	Description
1	Right paracardial LN
2	Left paracardial LN
3	LN along the lesser curvature
4sa	LN along the short gastric vessels
4sb	LN along the left gastroepiploic vessels
4d	LN along the right gastroepiploic vessels
5	Suprapyloric LN
6	Infrapyloric LN
7	LN along the left gastric artery
8a	LN along the common hepatic artery (anterosuperior group)
8p	LN along the common hepatic artery (posterior group)
9	LN around the celiac artery
10	LN at the splenic hilum
11p	LN along the proximal splenic artery
11d	LN along the distal splenic artery
12a	LN in the hepatoduodenal ligament (along the hepatic artery)
12b	LN in the hepatoduodenal ligament (along the bile duct)
12p	LN in the hepatoduodenal ligament (behind the portal vein)
13	LN on the posterior surface of the pancreatic head
14v	LN along the superior mesenteric vein
14a	LN along the superior mesenteric artery
15	LN along the middle colic vessels
16a1	LN in the aortic hiatus
16a2	LN around the abdominal aorta (from the upper margin of the celiac trunk to the lower margin of the left renal vein)
16b1	LN around the abdominal aorta (from the lower margin of the left renal vein to the upper margin of the inferior mesenteric artery)
16b2	LN around the abdominal aorta (from the upper margin of the inferior mesenteric artery to the aortic bifurcation)
17	LN on the anterior surface of the pancreatic head
18	LN along the inferior margin of the pancreas
19	Infradiaphragmatic LN
20	LN in the esophageal hiatus of the diaphragm
110	Paraesophageal LN in the lower thorax
111	Supradiaphragmatic LN
112	Posterior mediastinal LN

*See Fig. 11-1 for illustration of station positions.
Data from Japanese Gastric Cancer Association: Japanese classification of gastric carcinoma, 2nd English edition. Gastric Cancer 1:10–24, 1998.

Table 11-2 Extent of Lymph Node Dissection (D Type) with Respect to Gastric Tumor Stage for Distal Gastrectomy*

Type	Stations	Applicable Tumor Stage
D1	1, 3, 4sb, 4d, 5, 6, 7	T1a tumor without indication for endoscopic resection; well-differentiated T1b tumor smaller than 1.5 cm with cN0
D1+	D1 stations, plus 8a, 9	T1 tumor with cN0 (other than listed above)
D2	D1 stations, plus 8a, 9, 11p, 12a	T1 tumor with cN(+); resectable T2 (or deeper) tumor

*See Fig. 11-1 and Table 11-1 for definition of lymph node stations; see Table 11-3 for tumor staging.

Table 11-3 TNM Staging for Gastric Cancer

T Stage	N Stage (No. of Nodes)				
	N0	N1 (1-2)	N2 (3-6)	N3a (7-15)	N3b (≥16)
T1 (mucosa/submucosa)	IA	IB	IIA	IIB	IIB
T2 (muscularis propria)	IB	IIA	IIB	IIIA	IIIA
T3 (subserosa)	IIA	IIB	IIIA	IIIB	IIIB
T4a (serosa)	IIB	IIIA	IIIB	IIIC	IIIC
T4b (surrounding organs)	IIIB	IIIB	IIIC	IIIC	IIIC
Any T or N, M1	IV				

From Edge SB, Byrd DR, Compton CC, et al: AJCC Cancer Staging Manual, ed 7, New York, 2009, Springer, pp 117–126.

diagnosed by laparoscopic examination under the same anesthetic as LADG. An algorithm of treatment selection for various subtypes of EGC and AGC is shown in Figure 11-2. To determine systemic tolerance to surgical stress, heart, respiratory, liver, and kidney function are evaluated in the same manner as with open surgery.

As of 2011, there is no convincing evidence that neoadjuvant chemotherapy for gastric cancer produces a clinically relevant improvement in survival. A phase III study of neoadjuvant chemotherapy involving bulky T3-4 gastric cancer is ongoing in Japan. Currently, adjuvant chemotherapy with S-1 (a formulation containing tegafur, gimeracil, and oteracil) is recommended for patients in Japan with stage II or III advanced gastric cancer after resection. There is no special preoperative preparation for LADG. Because the morbidity rate associated with LADG may be increased with obese patients (BMI >30 kg/m^2), the relative merits of LADG in the obese patient should be carefully

considered. Prophylactic antibiotics are administered only on the operative day (30 minutes before skin incision, every 3 hours through the operation, and then one more dose several hours after the procedure).

PATIENT POSITIONING IN THE OPERATING SUITE

A gastric tube is inserted before the induction of general anesthesia. After general anesthesia, the patient is placed in the low lithotomy position, with 10 degrees of reverse-Trendelenburg tilt (Fig. 11-3A). Both of the patient's arms are extended. The operator stands between the patient's legs (Fig. 11-3B). The camera operator stands on the patient's right side, and the operative assistant stands on the patient's left side.

POSITIONING AND PLACEMENT OF TROCARS

A Hasson cannula is placed in the subumbilical position in an open manner, and a CO_2 pneumoperitoneum of 10 mm Hg is created. Four additional trocars are then placed in the upper abdomen: two 10-mm trocars are inserted superior to the umbilicus just lateral to each rectus sheath, and then two 5-mm trocars are inserted superior and lateral to the 10-mm ports, into the left and right upper quadrants (Fig. 11-4).

OPERATIVE TECHNIQUE

The basic steps of LADG include a laparoscopic gastric resection (distal two thirds) and LN dissection, followed by extraction of

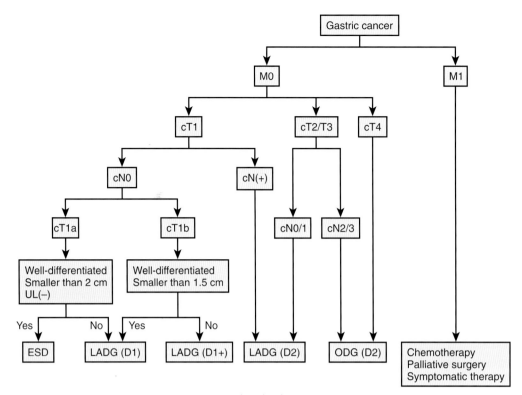

FIGURE 11-2 Treatment algorithm for gastric cancer in Japan.

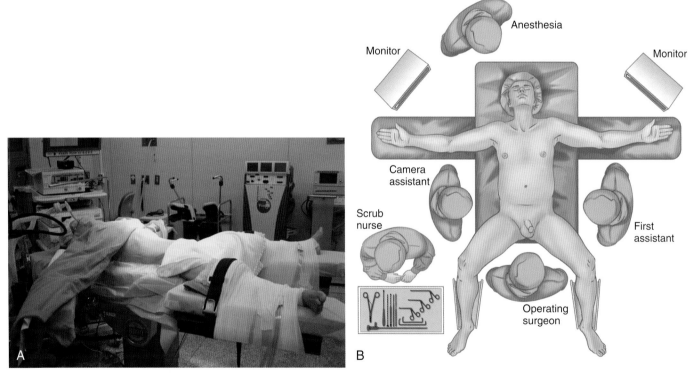

FIGURE 11-3 **A,** Patient positioning for laparoscopy-assisted distal gastrectomy. **B,** Positioning of operating team and monitors.

the specimen and creation of the anastomosis through a small incision (5 cm), with a final repeat laparoscopy for irrigation and drainage of the abdominal cavity. In this narrative, we describe a D2 lymph node dissection (see Table 11-2 for definition). All references to numbered lymph node stations are described in Figure 11-1 and Table 11-1.

1. Dissection of the Greater Omentum (LN Station 4d) and the Left Gastroepiploic Vessels (LN Station 4sb)

The stomach is retracted superiorly by the assistant, and the gastrocolic ligament of the greater omentum is divided 3 cm away from and parallel to the gastroepiploic vessels, using the

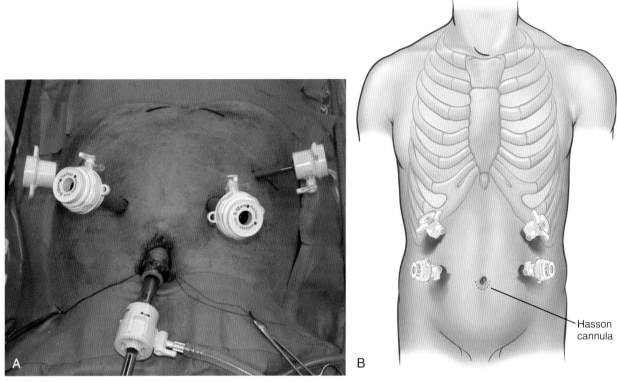

FIGURE 11-4 Port placement for laparoscopy-assisted distal gastrectomy.

laparoscopic ultrasonic coagulation shears (LCS) or the vessel sealing system (Fig. 11-5). The division of the gastrocolic ligament is performed from the inferior pole of the spleen to the infrapyloric area (LN station 4d). Because the left gastroepiploic vessels are located posterior to the gastrocolic ligament, dissection of the connective tissue is performed from the outside layer to identify these vessels. The left gastroepiploic vessels are divided at their origin from the splenic artery by clipping and then cutting with the LCS (LN station 4sb); see Figure 11-6.

2. Dissection of the Right Gastroepiploic Vessels (LN Station 6)

In dissection of the station 6 nodes, it is important to release the adhesions between the gastric antrum and the mesocolon and between and antrum and the anterior head of the pancreas. The antrum is retracted superiorly by the assistant. After the surface of the pancreatic head is exposed, the right gastroepiploic vein is easily identified. This vein is clipped and cut distal to the branching of the anterosuperior pancreaticoduodenal vein, which allows collection of the infrapyloric nodes (LN station 6) (Fig. 11-7). The right gastroepiploic artery is then exposed at its origin from the gastroduodenal artery, on the anterosuperior surface of the pancreas. The right gastroepiploic artery is clipped and divided such that the superior pancreaticoduodenal artery is preserved. Infrapyloric vessels from the gastroduodenal artery also are identified and divided (see Fig. 11-7A).

3. Dissection of the Lesser Omentum (LN Station 3) and Nodes along the Proper Hepatic Artery (LN Station 12a) and Division of the Right Gastric Vessels (LN Station 5)

For dissection of nodal stations 3, 5, and 12a, the liver is lifted with a snake retractor (Fig. 11-8). The lesser omentum is divided

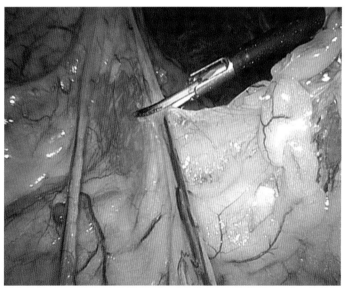

FIGURE 11-5 Division of the gastrocolic ligament of the greater omentum (LN station 4d).

using the LCS from the left side of the hepatoduodenal ligament to the right side of the gastroesophageal junction (LN station 3). The assistant places the right gastric vessels on gentle stretch, and a nonvascular area is identified above the duodenal bulb. This area is opened, and the connective tissue along the right side of the right gastric vessels is dissected to expose the origin of right gastric artery from the common hepatic artery. The connective tissue along the left side of the proper hepatic artery (LN station 12a) is dissected and swept toward the specimen. The right gastric vessels are clipped and divided at their origin (see Fig. 11-8), thus collecting the suprapyloric nodes (LN station 5) with the specimen.

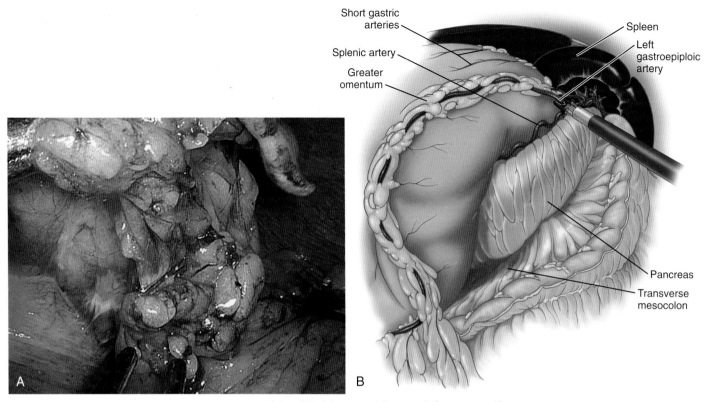

FIGURE 11-6 Division of the left gastroepiploic vessels (LN station 4sb).

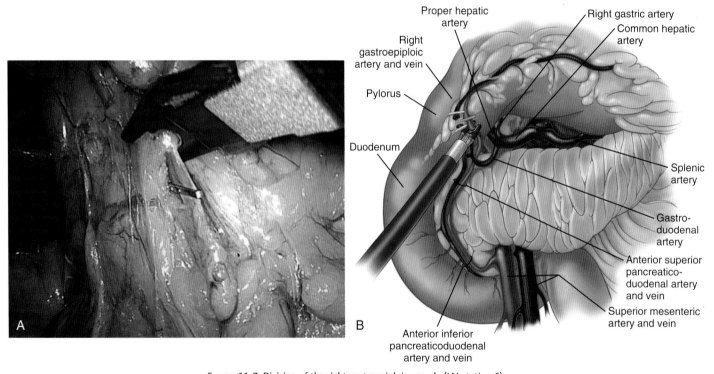

FIGURE 11-7 Division of the right gastroepiploic vessels (LN station 6).

4. Transection of the Duodenum

We prefer to employ a Roux-en-Y reconstruction after distal gastrectomy. If the tumor is not located near the duodenum, then the duodenum is transected at the proximal bulb with a laparoscopic linear stapler-cutter (Fig. 11-9), typically with a blue cartridge (normal staple length). If the duodenum appears thickened (e.g., from previous peptic disease), then a green stapler cartridge (long staple length) may be employed.

5. Nodal Dissection along the Common Hepatic and Celiac Arteries (LN Stations 8a and 9)

The peritoneum overlying the common hepatic artery is elevated, and the upper margin of the pancreas is identified. The peritoneum is opened along the upper margin of the pancreas, from the distal end of the common hepatic artery to the origin of the celiac artery. The portion of the connective tissue that surrounds the celiac artery (LN stations 8a and 9) is dissected from anterior

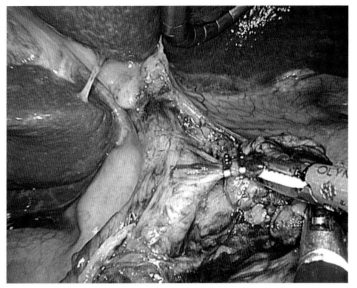

FIGURE 11-8 Division of the right gastric vessels (LN station 5).

to posterior (Fig. 11-10). During this dissection, the left gastric vein is identified, clipped, and cut at the superior margin of the pancreas.

6. Division of the Left Gastric Artery (LN Station 7)

After the peritoneum is opened along the upper margin of the right crus, the origin of the left gastric artery from the celiac axis may be dissected. The connective tissue on the left side of the left gastric artery is swept toward the stomach and resected en bloc with the specimen. Gerota fascia will be apparent during this step. The left gastric artery is clipped and divided at its origin (Fig. 11-11), thereby collecting LN station 7 with the specimen.

7. Nodal Dissection along the Splenic Artery (LN Station 11p)

During the dissection of the origin of the left gastric artery, the origin of the splenic artery from the celiac axis also will be

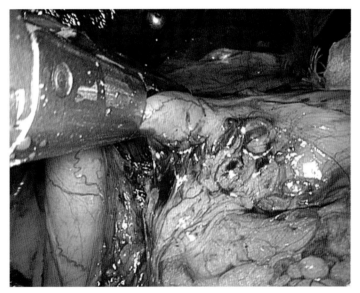

FIGURE 11-9 Transection of the duodenum.

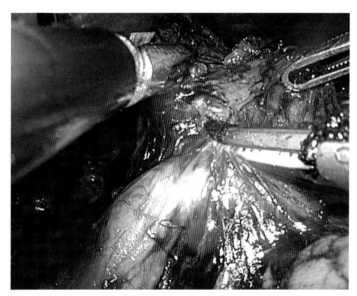

FIGURE 11-10 Dissection of nodal-bearing tissue along the common hepatic and celiac arteries (LN stations 8a and 9).

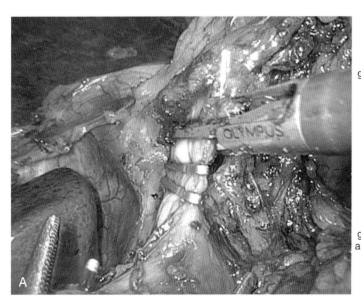

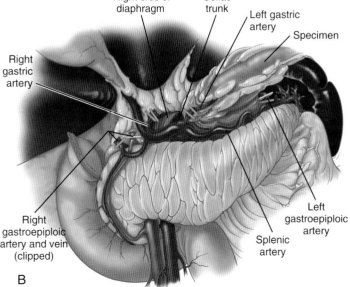

FIGURE 11-11 Division of the left gastric artery (LN station 7).

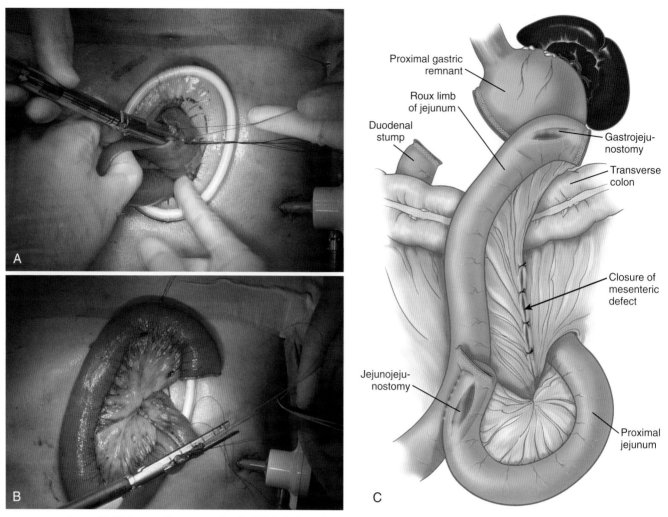

FIGURE 11-12 Roux-en-Y reconstruction for LADG. **A,** Gastrojejunostomy. **B,** Jejunojejunostomy. **C,** Completed reconstruction.

exposed. After the peritoneum at the upper margin of the distal pancreas is opened, the LNs along the splenic artery (LN station 11p) are dissected with forceps and LCS, swept toward the stomach, and resected en bloc with the specimen.

8. Dissection of the Left Cardiac and Superior Gastric Nodes (LN Stations 1 and 3)

The stomach is pulled inferiorly, placing the upper lesser curvature on stretch. The left cardiac and superior gastric nodes (stations 1 and 3) are dissected with the LCS from both the anterior and posterior sides of the stomach, swept toward the gastric corpus, and resected en bloc with the specimen. During the dissection of stations 1 and 3, both trunks of the vagus nerve are cut.

9. Mini-Laparotomy and Roux-en-Y Reconstruction

After the mobilization and nodal dissection are performed laparoscopically, a 5-cm incision is created in the upper midline. The wound is protected with a wound protector. The distal stomach is exteriorized through the mini-laparotomy, and the oral margin of the cancer is confirmed by palpation and/or a clip that was attached to the gastric mucosa as a marker during a preoperative endoscopy. The distal gastrectomy is then completed with a linear stapler-cutter, using a blue cartridge. After the specimen is removed, the wound protector is occluded with a glove, and

the abdomen is reinsufflated. A loop of jejunum 30 cm from the ligament of Treitz is identified and pulled out through the mini-laparotomy. The jejunum is transected at this point with the linear stapler-cutter, and a gastrojejunostomy is created with a functional end-to-end anastomosis, as is done during open surgery (Fig. 11-12A and C). A jejunojejunostomy is then performed 30 cm distal to the gastrojejunostomy in a similar fashion (see Fig. 11-12B and C) to complete the Roux-en-Y reconstruction. The edge of the efferent jejunal mesentery is fixed to the transverse mesocolon to prevent internal hernia (see Fig. 11-12C). The tip of nasogastric tube is placed into the remnant stomach.

10. Irrigation, Drainage, and Closure of the Operative Wound

On completion of the anastomoses, the abdomen is reinsufflated again, and hemostasis is evaluated. The efferent limb of jejunum is checked for any twisting. After irrigation of the abdominal cavity, a closed-suction drain is placed below the liver, and the incisions are closed.

POSTOPERATIVE CARE

Although postoperative pain typically is mild because of the short length of the laparotomy, epidural anesthesia is routinely used for 2 days after LADG. On the first postoperative day, the nasogastric tube is removed, drinking water is permitted, and ambulation is encouraged. The urinary catheter is removed on postoperative day 2.

Recent data have suggested that the recovery of gastrointestinal activity after LADG is faster than after open distal gastrectomy (OGD). Flatus usually is observed on postoperative day 2. A regular diet usually is given on postoperative day 4, at which time the drainage tube may be removed. The average hospital stay in Japan after LADG is 14 days. Although this length of stay appears to be longer compared with the stay after the similar procedure in American and European hospitals (which also have different medical insurance systems), in Japan the length of stay after LADG is shorter than after OGD.

MANAGEMENT OF PROCEDURE-SPECIFIC COMPLICATIONS

According to the 10th national survey by the Japan Society of Endoscopic Surgery, the rates of intraoperative and postoperative complications associated with LADG are 1.1% and 7.5%, respectively (Table 11-4). The most frequent intraoperative complications include bleeding and injury to other organs (particularly the pancreas), and the most frequent postoperative complications are related to anastomosis, such as anastomotic stenosis and leakage.

During the operation, hemorrhage can occur secondary to connective tissue injury caused by the grasping forceps, anatomic misrecognition of vessel branches, and incomplete vessel sealing with the LCS. In particular, bleeding from the left gastroepiploic vessels, the cardiac branches of the left gastric artery, and the small branches supplying LN station 8 can occur. In most cases, bleeding can be stopped with clipping, vessel sealing, or other laparoscopic techniques. If bleeding cannot be controlled laparoscopically, then open conversion should be performed. Injury to other organs, especially to the pancreas, can occur from rough

handling of the tissues or inappropriate use of the instruments. The surgeon should take care to avoid mechanical injury caused by the tips of the forceps and the LCS and thermal injury caused by cavitation and heat from the active blade of the LCS.

Most anastomoses in LADG are created using the linear stapler-cutter. The B-shaped formation of the staple is critical during creation of a gastrointestinal anastomosis. An anastomotic stenosis can be caused by a mismatch in size between a circular stapler and intestinal diameter, intestinal twisting near the anastomotic site, and local ischemia. Management of complications, including anastomotic leak, stenosis, and pancreatic injury, is performed similarly to open surgery.

RESULTS AND OUTCOME

Comparisons of short-term outcome between LADG and ODG for EGC have been reported in a number of retrospective studies and several randomized controlled trials. In contrast, there have been only a few studies on long-term outcome after LADG for AGC.

Short-Term Outcome after LADG

In regard to operative findings, blood loss in LADG was lower than that in ODG, but operative times were longer with LADG. The additional time required in LADG is dependent on patient body mass index and surgical experience. Because a learning curve is involved with gaining the necessary skill required to perform LADG safely, the importance of the establishment of standard techniques, the improvement of operative instruments, and the development of an education and training system have been emphasized to decrease LADG operation time. With the technique described in this chapter, an operative experience of 50 cases appears to be needed to achieve optimal proficiency.

The technical safety of LADG for EGC is accepted worldwide. LADG has been shown to have several advantages over ODG, including earlier recovery of intestinal movement, lower frequency of analgesic requirement, and shorter hospital stay. The types of operation-specific morbidity in LADG essentially are the same as with ODG, but overall, the morbidity and mortality rates in LADG appear to be similar to or lower than those in ODG. The risk factors for surgical complications of LADG for EGC have been related to the degree of the nodal dissection and relative surgical experience.

Long-Term Outcome after LADG

There have been few studies published on long-term outcome after LADG. The oncologic feasibility of LADG for EGC can be evaluated by survival benefits. The Japanese Laparoscopic Surgery Study Group, in which 16 surgical units participate, reviewed the long-term results of 1294 ECG patients who had undergone laparoscopic gastrectomy. This group showed a 99.7% 5-year disease-free survival rate for stage IA disease, 98.7% for stage IB, and 85.7% for stage II. The Korean Laparoscopic Gastrointestinal Surgery Study (KLASS) group reported on the recurrence rate in 1485 patients who had undergone LADG for gastric cancer at 10 institutions. This study showed that the incidence of recurrence in EGC after LADG was only 1.6%, and these data suggest that LADG is oncologically feasible for the treatment of EGC. LADG appears to cause no explicit long-term operation-specific complications. The possibility that LADG might be associated with a

Table 11-4 Perioperative Complications in 10,355 Cases of Laparoscopy-Assisted Distal Gastrectomy

Complication	No.	Percentage of Total
Intraoperative		
Bleeding	79	0.8
Injury to other organ	23	0.2
Instrument failure	60	0.6
Other	14	0.1
TOTAL	176	1.7
Postoperative		
Anastomotic leak	113	1.1
Anastomotic stenosis	206	2.0
Intra-abdominal abscess	76	0.7
Pancreatic leak	130	1.3
Wound infection	77	0.7
Ileus	36	0.3
Bleeding	47	0.5
Other	47	0.5
TOTAL	732	7.1

Data from Japan Society for Endoscopic Surgery: Nationwide survey on endoscopic surgery in Japan [Japanese]. J Jpn Soc Endosc Surg 15:557–679, 2010.

lower frequency of intestinal obstruction compared with ODG has been reported. In addition, 1-year weight loss may be less in patients after LADG compared with ODG. Further studies to clarify the long-term outcomes of LADG for EGC will be necessary.

Suggested Readings

Hosono H, Arimoto Y, Ohtani H, et al: Meta-analysis of short-term outcomes after laparoscopy-assisted distal gastrectomy. *World J Gastroenterol* 12:7676–7683, 2006.

Japanese Gastric Cancer Association: Japanese classification of gastric carcinoma, 2nd English edition. *Gastric Cancer* 1:10–24, 1998.

Japanese Gastric Cancer Association: *Guidelines for the Treatment of Gastric Cancer*, Tokyo, 2001, Kanahara.

Japan Society for Endoscopic Surgery: Nationwide survey on endoscopic surgery in Japan [Japanese]. *J Jpn Soc Endosc Surg* 15:557–679, 2010.

Jemal A, Bray F, Center MM, et al: Global cancer statistics. *CA Cancer J Clin* 61:69, 2011.

Kim HH, Hyung WJ, Cho GS, et al: Morbidity and mortality of laparoscopic gastrectomy versus open gastrectomy for gastric cancer: An interim report. A phase III multicenter, prospective, randomized trial (KLASS trial). *Ann Surg* 251:417–420, 2010.

Kitano S, Iso Y, Moriyama M, et al: Laparoscopy-assisted Billroth I gastrectomy. *Surg Laparosc Endosc* 4:146–148, 1994.

Kitano S, Shiraishi N, Uyama I, et al: A multicenter study on oncologic outcome of laparoscopic gastrectomy for early cancer in Japan. *Ann Surg* 245:68–72, 2006.

Melon MA, Khan S, Yunus RM, et al: Meta-analysis of laparoscopic and open distal gastrectomy for gastric carcinoma. *Surg Endosc* 22:1781–1789, 2008.

National Cancer Center: Cancer statistics in Japan. Available at: http://ganjoho.jp/data/professional/statistics/hosp_c_registry/2008_report_0804.pdf. Accessed April 14, 2011.

Noshiro H, Shimizu S, Nagai E, et al: Laparoscopy-assisted distal gastrectomy for early gastric cancer: Is it beneficial for patients of heavier weight? *Ann Surg* 238:680–685, 2003.

Sakuramoto S, Sasako M, Yamaguchi T, et al: Adjuvant chemotherapy for gastric cancer with S-1, an oral fluoropyrimidine. *N Engl J Med* 357:1810–1820, 2007.

Song J, Lee HJ, Cho GS, et al: Recurrence following laparoscopy-assisted gastrectomy for gastric cancer: A multicenter retrospective analysis of 1,417 patients. *Ann Surg Oncol* 17:1777–1786, 2010.

DENNIS C. T. WONG

Laparoscopic Repair of Perforated Peptic Ulcer

The videos associated with this chapter are listed in the Video Contents and can be found on the accompanying DVDs and on Expertconsult.com.

The overall incidence of peptic ulcer disease has declined significantly over the past few decades owing to the introduction of histamine-2 receptor blockers in the 1970s and proton pump inhibitors in the 1990s. The successful treatment of *Helicobacter pylori* also played an important role in its decline, and studies have shown that ulcer recurrence after treatment is low. Despite these dramatic epidemiologic changes, the incidence of complications arising from peptic ulcer disease has not declined. In fact, perforated peptic ulcer has been on an increasing trend, particularly in elderly people, with the popularized use of nonsteroidal anti-inflammatory agents being the most likely culprit. The importance of ulcer perforation cannot be underestimated because it is associated with major morbidity and accounts for more than 70% of all peptic ulcer mortality. It is the second most common perforated viscus following perforated appendicitis.

Currently, perforated peptic ulcers can be effectively treated with simple closure with omental patch without the need for additional procedures for acid reduction. This is the result of the effective medical treatment using proton pump inhibitors together with complete eradication of *H. pylori*. Compared with traditional treatment by Graham-Steele patch closure or gastrectomy, this is a straightforward procedure that is ideally performed using minimally invasive techniques. The first laparoscopic suture repair of duodenal ulcer perforation was reported in 1990, and this procedure has been widely adopted since. Our institution first reported the technique of laparoscopic single-stitch omental patch repair in 1997, and the technique has been routinely practiced since 2004. Our experience has shown that this technique is safe and reliable.

OPERATIVE INDICATIONS

All perforated peptic ulcers warrant immediate treatment. Most should be treated with urgent surgery. We recommend the routine use of laparoscopy for all cases of suspected perforated peptic ulcer that present with typical history of sudden-onset epigastric pain and signs of generalized peritonitis. In the absence of free air under the diaphragm (about 30%), an urgent abdominal computed tomography scan may be performed to exclude other causes of acute abdomen. Cases in which laparoscopy may not be considered include patients with previous abdominal surgeries, clinical evidence of concomitant bleeding ulcer, or gastric outlet obstruction. These patients should undergo conventional repair by upper midline laparotomy. Iatrogenic (following endoscopic procedures) ulcer perforation is not an absolute contraindication to laparoscopic repair but should be performed with caution because these perforations tend to be quite sizeable and difficult to treat with omental patch alone, and open conversion is often necessary. Other indications for conversion to an open procedure are unidentifiable site of perforation, nonpyloroduodenal perforation, perforation larger than 10 mm, and technically difficult repair. There is controversy about whether patients with a clinically sealed-off perforated ulcer should receive surgery because there is evidence suggesting that conservative management can be successful. The diagnosis of sealed-off perforation should be suspected if the patient does not present with severe sepsis or generalized peritonitis and there is no extravasation of contrast during radiologic upper gastrointestinal studies. When conservative treatment is chosen, the patient must be closely monitored. A low threshold for immediate laparoscopy is warranted if the patient's condition changes.

PREOPERATIVE EVALUATION, TESTING, AND PREPARATION

Perforated peptic ulcer is a surgical emergency and operation should be swiftly arranged to reduce morbidity and mortality. A thorough preoperative assessment by an experienced anesthetist is essential. The general assessment should include the American Society of Anesthesiology classification status. Any existing electrolyte imbalance should be corrected.

Preoperatively, the patients are kept NPO, and a nasogastric tube is inserted to reduce further peritoneal contamination. They are started empirically on a second-generation cephalosporin (ciprofloxacin if penicillin allergy) and intravenous proton pump inhibitor. Patients with risk for thromboembolic events should also receive prophylactic anticoagulation, usually low-molecular-weight heparin given intramuscularly.

Informed consent should include explanation of risks of surgery in general, but more specifically, surgeons should mention the rate of open conversion (about 30%), morbidity rate (about 25%), and overall mortality rate (about 10%). The need for postoperative intensive care unit admission should be anticipated for patients who are elderly, are hemodynamically unstable, or have multiple medical comorbidities.

PATIENT POSITIONING

The patient is placed in the modified lithotomy (Lloyd-Davies) position. The surgeon stands between the patient's legs and the assistant on patient's right side, with the monitors positioned on either side of the head of the table (Fig. 12-1). Care is taken to ensure that all pressure points are adequately padded.

OPERATIVE TECHNIQUE

Placement of Trocars

The initial 10-mm port is inserted by the Hasson technique through a curvilinear infraumbilical incision for the use of a 30-degree laparoscope. Pneumoperitoneum is established and maintained at 12 mm Hg. Two 5-mm working trocars are positioned on either side along the midclavicular line and at the level of the umbilicus (Fig. 12-2). If the liver or gallbladder is obscuring the operative field, an additional 5-mm port is placed at the subxiphoid region for retraction. It is important that all these additional trocars are inserted under direct laparoscopic guidance to avoid organ injury.

Identification of Site of Perforation

Because most perforations occur at the pyloroduodenal region, laparoscopic localization is usually not difficult (Fig. 12-3). Situations in which laparoscopic localization may be problematic include perforation at atypical sites, such as gastric ulcers located on the posterior wall, lesser curve, or greater curve, and ulcers located at the posterior duodenal wall. Identification of these

ulcers often requires further dissection, including dissection into the lesser sac, division of short gastric vessels, or mobilization of the duodenum. The concomitant use of intraoperative endoscopy may help in localization; it should be done, however, with caution and minimal insufflation. Conversion to open surgery is usually recommended if difficulty is encountered. Detailed description of management of these atypically located ulcers is beyond the scope of this chapter.

Peritoneal Washing

The degree of peritoneal contamination varies, and it is generally related to delay in presentation and size of perforation. The peritoneal cavity is thoroughly irrigated with copious amount of warm saline, at least 5 to 6 L or whatever volume required until it is completely cleared. Particular attention should be paid when irrigating the perihepatic spaces, bilateral paracolic gutters, and pelvis. Appropriate patient positioning will often help in achieving this goal.

Omental Patch Repair

A healthy "tongue" of omentum is selected for patch repair. It is brought up to the site of perforation to ensure adequate length without undue tension. It is the author's preference to use the laparoscopic single-stitch technique as opposed to the traditional Graham repair in open surgery. A 15-cm length of 2-0 absorbable suture is used for repair. The needle should enter the tissue at least 5 mm adjacent to the ulcer perforation and then exit through the perforation itself (Fig. 12-4). A generous bite of the selected tongue of omentum is taken using the same needle (Fig. 12-5).

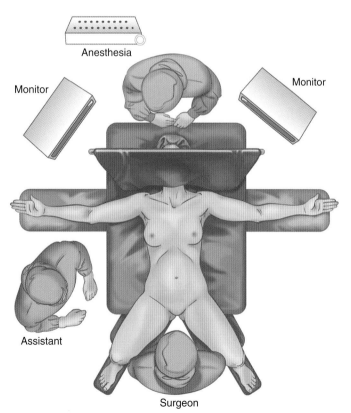

FIGURE 12-1 Operating room setup for laparoscopic repair of perforated peptic ulcer. The patient is in the modified lithotomy position with operating surgeon adopting the French position and assistant on patient's right side.

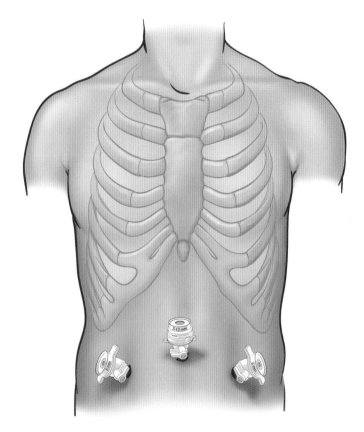

FIGURE 12-2 Trocar positioning includes a 10-mm subumbilical port and two 5-mm ports on either side at the midclavicular line.

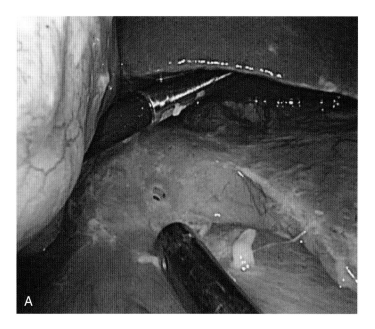

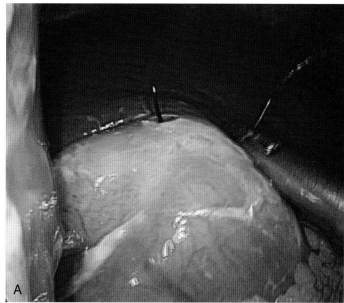

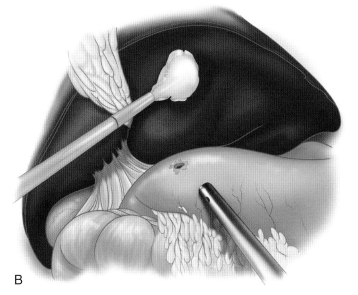

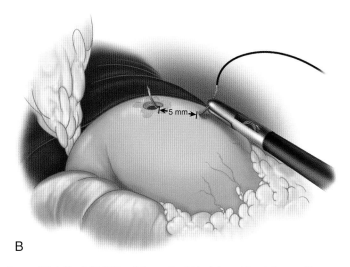

FIGURE 12-4 The initial bite of tissue should be taken at least 5 mm adjacent to the ulcer edge, exiting through the perforation itself with 2-0 absorbable suture.

FIGURE 12-3 A, Perforation identified at the pyloroduodenal region. **B,** Diagrammatic representation of perforated duodenal ulcer.

The needle is then reintroduced into the perforation and exits at least 5 mm on the opposite side. The suture is tied using the intracorporeal technique (Fig. 12-6). The author's experience has shown that the success of repair is determined by how well this suture is tied: tying the suture with excessive force may result in suture cut-through and ischemia of the omentum; in contrast, tying the knot loosely may cause failure of adequate closure of the perforation by the omentum. If there is doubt concerning the integrity of the repair, an air leak test can be performed either by the nasogastric tube or by gentle insufflation using an endoscope. An abdominal drain is usually not required unless the surgeon has concerns about the repair or there is gross contamination of the peritoneal cavity.

POSTOPERATIVE CARE

A successful repair is reflected by a typical recovery phase. The overall septic picture of the patient should improve within the first 24 to 48 hours after surgery. The patient is kept NPO with a nasogastric tube in situ for decompression and drainage of gastric secretions for the first 2 postoperative days. Intravenous proton pump inhibitors and antibiotics can be switched to the oral route when the patient is allowed liquid diet, usually on the third postoperative day. The patient can be discharged home after resolution of postoperative ileus. A full 1-week course of antibiotic is prescribed together with a proton pump inhibitor until follow-up (peritoneal sampling for culture and sensitivity should guide the antibiotic treatment). An upper endoscopy is performed 6 to 8 weeks later to check *H. pylori* status by CLO testing for duodenal ulcer perforation and to assess for healing in gastric ulcer perforation.

MANAGEMENT OF PROCEDURE-SPECIFIC COMPLICATIONS

The most important specific complication related to this operation is leakage. This means failure of the omentum to effectively seal off the perforation. The patient presents with recurrence of

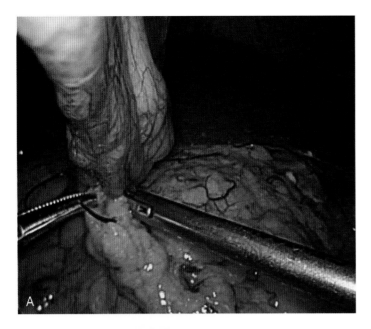

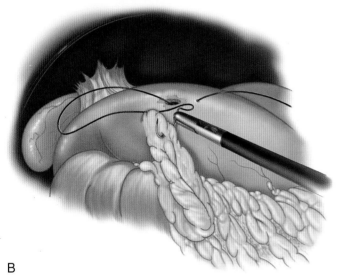

Figure 12-5 A generous bite of a healthy tongue of omentum is selected for patch repair.

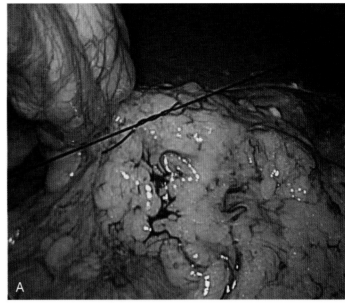

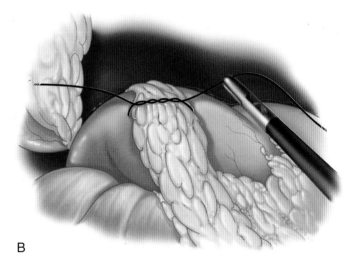

Figure 12-6 Intracorporeal knot tying to secure the omental patch.

peritonitis in the first 1 to 2 days after surgery, or if still intubated and sedated, the clinical sepsis persists or worsens. There should be high index of suspicion for this complication if the patient's recovery is not as expected. For patients who have abdominal drains inserted, the presence of bile would be indicative of repair failure. These patients should undergo immediate repeat laparoscopy. Whether to re-repair laparoscopically or to convert to an open procedure is at the discretion of the operating surgeon.

Intra-abdominal abscess may occur at the subphrenic or subhepatic space or in the pelvis. Drainage of the collection should be performed either surgically or under radiologic guidance. It is important to thoroughly irrigate the peritoneal cavity with at least 5 L of warm saline or an amount adequate to achieve complete clearance.

RESULTS AND OUTCOME

Most of the current evidence on laparoscopic versus open repair of perforated peptic ulcers is from nonrandomized prospective and retrospective studies of varying methodologies with overall small sample sizes. Although few studies have shown advantages of the laparoscopic technique, findings were inconsistent and therefore inconclusive. Only three randomized prospective trials have been published to date, but even these differ considerably in terms of the laparoscopic technique employed. The results from these randomized controlled trials on laparoscopic versus open repair are summarized in Table 12-1.

Our institution had conducted a randomized controlled trial in 2002 in which 130 patients were recruited over a 3-year period. Similar to the other two randomized trials, we found that patients who underwent laparoscopic repair had significantly less postoperative pain requiring fewer intramuscular injections (0 vs. 6, $P < .001$) and shorter hospital stay (6 days vs. 7 days, $P = .004$). However, in addition, our laparoscopic group required significantly less operating time (42 vs. 52.3 minutes, $P = .025$), fewer respiratory infections (0 vs. 7, $P = .005$), and earlier return to daily activities (10.4 vs. 26.1 days, $P = .001$) compared with the open group. In our accumulated experience of more than 300 cases of laparoscopic repair, the rate of conversion to open repair was 30%, with an overall mortality rate of 9%.

Table 12-1 Summary of All Recent Randomized Controlled Trials on Laparoscopic versus Open Repair of Perforated Peptic Ulcer

Study	No. of Subjects	Procedure	Operation Time (min)	Conversion	Analgesic Use	Hospital Stay (days)	Return to Activity/ Work (days)	Overall Morbidity	Mortality
Lau et al, 1995	93	*Laparoscopic:*	94.3 ± 40*	29%	No difference on POD 1	5	Within 4 wk 80%*		
		Omental patch—24						5	0
		Sutureless fibrin glue—24						6	2
		Open:	53.7 ± 42	17%		5	77%*		
		Omental patch—24						5	1
		Sutureless fibrin glue—21						5	0
Siu et al, 1997	121	Omental patch repair:		14%	Significantly less on PODs 1 and 3 in laparoscopic group			Less respiratory infection	
		Laparoscopic—63	42 ± 25*			6 (4-35)*	10.4 (6.9)*	(0 vs. 7)*	1.6%
		Open—58	52.3 ± 24*			7 (4-39)*	26.1 (15.1)*		5.2%
Bertleff et al, 2009	101	*Laparoscopic:* Suture/omental patch—52	N/A	4%	Significantly less pain PODs 1, 3, and 7	6.5 (9.3)	N/A	12 (23%)	4%
		Open: Suture/omental patch—49				8.0 (7.3)		24 (49%)	8%

*Significant difference; data shown in mean (range).
POD, postoperative day.

Suggested Readings

Bertleff MJOE, Halm JA, Bemelman WA, et al: Randomized clinical trial of laparoscopic versus open repair of the perforated peptic ulcer: The LAMA trial, *World J Surg* 33:1368–1373, 2009.

Crofts TJ, Park KGM, Steel RJC, et al: A randomized trial of non-operative treatment for perforated peptic ulcer, *N Engl J Med* 320:970–973, 1989.

Lau WY, Leung KL, Kwong KH, et al: A randomized study comparing laparoscopic versus open repair of perforated peptic ulcer using suture or sutureless technique, *Ann Surg* 224:131–138, 1996.

Lau WY, Leung KL, Zhu XL, et al: Laparoscopic repair of perforated peptic ulcer, *Br J Surg* 82:814–816, 1995.

Lunevicius R, Morkevicius M: Systematic review comparing laparoscopic and open repair for perforated peptic ulcer, *Br J Surg* 92:1195–1207, 2005.

Nathanson LK, Easter DW, Cuschieri A: Laparoscopic repair/peritoneal toilet of perforated duodenal ulcer, *Surg Endosc* 4:232–233, 1990.

Sanabria A, Villegas MI, Morales Uribe CH: Laparoscopic repair for perforated peptic ulcer disease, *Cochrane Database Syst Rev* 4:CD004778, 2005.

Siu WT, Leong HT, Law BKB, et al: Laparoscopic repair for perforated peptic ulcer: A randomized controlled trial, *Ann Surg* 3:313–319, 2002.

Siu WT, Leong HT, Li MKW: Single stitch laparoscopic omental patch repair of perforated peptic ulcers, *J R Coll Surg Edinb* 42:92–94, 1997.

Wong DCT, Siu WT, Wong SKH, et al: Routine laparoscopic single-stitch omental patch repair for perforated peptic ulcer: Experience from 338 cases, *Surg Endosc* 23:457–458, 2009.

Hepatobiliary System

ALEXANDER ROSEMURGY, HAROLD PAUL, NATALIE DONN,
KENNETH LUBERICE, MICHELLE VICE, AND SHARONA ROSS

Laparoscopic Single-Site Cholecystectomy

13

The videos associated with this chapter are listed in the Video Contents and can be found on the accompanying DVDs and on Expertconsult.com.

Rapid change is occurring in surgery and specifically in minimally invasive surgery. Concepts only imagined 20 years ago are now within our grasp, such as "scarless" laparoscopy. Scarless laparoscopy ensures that the postoperative scar is hidden within the umbilicus.

This evolutionary approach to laparoscopy is given many names with many associated acronyms, such as laparoendoscopic single-site (LESS) surgery, single-incision laparoscopic surgery (SILS), and single-port access (SPA) surgery, to mention but a few. Although this approach is new, adoption is occurring quickly and broadly, and many different operations have been undertaken using this approach. Because the term *LESS surgery* has been introduced into the domain of common use, it is the authors' choice for denoting this approach. We believe that LESS surgery will become the standard approach for laparoscopic operations in the years to come and is quickly finding its role as a favored approach for cholecystectomy.

Transumbilical laparoscopic single-site operations should not violate the tenets of conventional laparoscopy and should be performed with the same safety and efficacy.

OPERATIVE INDICATIONS

The advent of LESS surgery has not changed the indications for cholecystectomy. Cholecystectomy is generally considered for patients with symptomatic cholelithiasis, cholecystitis, biliary dyskinesia, and malignancy.

Cholelithiasis and Chronic Cholecystitis

Chronic cholecystitis is gallbladder inflammation virtually always occurring with cholelithiasis. The primary presentation of chronic cholecystitis is pain. Ranging from constant discomfort to episodes weeks and months apart, the frequency of attacks is quite variable. Lasting usually hours, attacks are distinct and significant enough that many patients accurately recall them.

Other symptoms of chronic cholecystitis may include nausea and vomiting with each episode, along with bloating and belching. Patients with asymptomatic gallstones account for two thirds of patients with cholelithiasis. Asymptomatic gallstones are generally not an indication for cholecystectomy unless the patient is undergoing another abdominal procedure (e.g., bariatric surgery).

Choledocholithiasis

Choledocholithiasis may be detected during an assessment for biliary tract symptoms, during cholecystectomy (with intraoperative cholangiogram), or after cholecystectomy. Diagnosed preoperatively, the bile duct should be cleared by endoscopic sphincterotomy, unless laparoscopic common bile duct exploration is in the surgeon's armamentarium, followed by LESS cholecystectomy. If undocumented choledocholithiasis is determined by cholangiography during LESS cholecystectomy, various options can be undertaken, including the following:

- Conversion to open cholecystectomy with common bile duct exploration
- LESS or laparoscopic cholecystectomy and common bile duct exploration
- LESS cholecystectomy with postoperative endoscopic sphincterotomy and stone extraction

Patients diagnosed with choledocholithiasis after undergoing cholecystectomy are best treated with endoscopic sphincterotomy and stone extraction.

Acute Cholecystitis

Acute cholecystitis occurs in two forms: acalculous and calculous. The latter form is much more common and occurs when the cystic duct becomes obstructed and gallbladder drainage or emptying ceases. Patients generally present with right upper quadrant pain and elevated white blood cell count with an excess number of early forms of polymorphonuclear leukocytes (i.e., bands). Clinically, patients with acute cholecystitis will also have fever and anorexia.

It is still a controversy whether patients with acute cholecystitis should promptly undergo cholecystectomy or should undergo the procedure after a period of treatment with systemic antibiotics.

Acalculous cholecystitis is a consequence of systemic hemodynamic collapse, or at least diversion of necessary blood flow away from the gallbladder such that patchy focal necrosis (or more) of the gallbladder results. Occasionally, acalculous cholecystitis can be temporized by drainage of the gallbladder so that pressures in the gallbladder can be reduced to promote blood flow throughout the gallbladder wall. In more extreme cases, a necrotic gallbladder can be drained percutaneously.

Biliary Dyskinesia

Gallbladder dyskinesia can lead to bothersome symptoms. Usually these symptoms are postprandial and involve right upper quadrant pain or epigastric pain and, with time, can lead to weight loss. The hallmarks of biliary dyskinesia are the lack of cholecystolithiasis on imaging of the gallbladder and a diminished gallbladder ejection fraction on study with biliary scanning and stimulation of the gallbladder with cholecystokinin (CCK).

PREOPERATIVE EVALUATION, TESTING, AND PREPARATION

Ideal operative candidates for LESS cholecystectomy do not have acute cholecystitis, are without notable comorbidities, are not morbidly obese, are not excessively tall, and do not have a history of prior abdominal surgery. Although some of these parameters describing the ideal patient are general and ill defined, some are readily obvious.

Testing specific for gallbladder pathology or disease is an essential prerequisite to cholecystectomy. Given appropriate indications, such as symptoms consistent with biliary dyskinesia or chronic cholecystitis, an ultrasound of the gallbladder and right upper quadrant is a minimum in the evaluation process and may be all that is necessary given documentation of gallstones, gallbladder sludge, or similar findings. Other imaging studies, such as computed tomography and magnetic resonance imaging, can show stones or the equivalent in the gallbladder but are beyond the necessary ultrasound unless being obtained for reasons other than documentation of chronic gallbladder pathology.

For patients with suspected acalculous biliary dyskinesia, a biliary scan with CCK analog administration is appropriate to determine gallbladder filling and ejection fraction. As previously noted, an ejection fraction of less than 35% is abnormal, but an ejection fraction of less than 25% is generally considered an indication for cholecystectomy, if consistent with the patient's symptoms.

No discussion of testing for gallbladder disease would be complete without mentioning the need for a thorough physical examination. Notable findings on physical examination indicative of liver disease, gastrointestinal bleeding, or other diseases or disorders should lead to further evaluation. Similarly, a laboratory profile, including liver function tests, complete blood count, urine analysis, and a chemistry profile, is warranted. An electrocardiogram is indicated for most patients older than 40 years and for selected younger patients.

Before the cholecystectomy, a thorough informed consent should be obtained. Given the intent to undertake LESS cholecystectomy, a consent should be obtained for single-incision laparoscopic cholecystectomy through the umbilicus, possible multiple-incision laparoscopic cholecystectomy, possible open cholecystectomy, and possible intraoperative cholangiogram. Conversion from the LESS approach to another approach, including a conventional laparoscopic approach or an open cholecystectomy, is not to be interpreted by the patient as failure but rather as good judgment.

Patients are counseled to shower the morning of the cholecystectomy. Patients void before transport to the operating suite, and a bladder catheter is not generally employed. Preoperative antibiotics are given with induction of anesthesia and patients are prepped with alcohol. A povidone-iodine-impregnated barrier is applied as the patient is draped.

POSITIONING AND PLACEMENT OF TROCARS

Patients are placed supine on the operating room table with the arms extended. The operating surgeon stands on the patient's left side, and the assistant stands on the patient's right, or left side, whichever is more ergonomic for the assistant. The assistant may be a scrub technician, a nurse, or a surgeon.

After injection of dilute solution of 0.5% bupivacaine with epinephrine, a vertical incision is made in the umbilicus. This incision never violates the ring of skin around the umbilicus, and thus the postoperative scar should not be apparent. The incision is about 1.2 cm in length and is vertical in orientation. For a very small umbilicus that will not permit a 1.2-cm incision, a shorter cruciate incision is employed. Once the skin incision is made, the dissection continues down to the fascia, everting the umbilicus as the incision and dissection are undertaken. Only a limited dissection is required before a small incision is made on the lineal alba to allow entry into the peritoneal cavity. The incision is then enlarged as needed. If a single multitrocar port is to be used, larger fascial access must be obtained (Fig. 13-1A and B). If multiple 5-mm trocars are to be used (Fig. 13-1C), the fascial opening should not be enlarged to avoid air leak.

If a multitrocar single port is to be used, the facial defect is then enlarged as necessary to accommodate the port. Water-soluble lubricant is liberally applied at the umbilicus to facilitate placement of a single multitrocar port (see Fig. 13-1A and B).

If LESS cholecystectomy does not involve placement of a single multitrocar port, but rather uses two to several 5-mm trocars, the small fascial defect at the umbilicus is not enlarged. The first 5-mm trocar is then placed through this defect, and after pneumoperitoneum is established, a second 5-mm trocar is placed adjacent to the first but through its own fascial puncture. It is usually best to place the trocars side by side with one trocar in the natural umbilical defect (see Fig. 13-1C).

OPERATIVE TECHNIQUE

Exposure

If two 5-mm trocars are used to perform LESS cholecystectomy, adjunctive sutures will be necessary to obtain exposure. Polypropylene sutures (2-0) are used on a Keith needle. With the 5-mm camera through one 5-mm trocar and a needle holder through the other, the adjunctive sutures for exposure are placed. The first needle with suture is placed into the peritoneal cavity over the fundus of the gallbladder and is grasped by the needle holder. The needle is placed through the gallbladder fundus and is then returned through the abdominal wall near its entrance site. This allows the surgeon or assistant to lift the gallbladder up toward the abdominal wall (Fig. 13-2A). A second suture is then placed subxiphoid into the peritoneal cavity. The exposure accomplished by the first suture allows for the second suture to be placed at the infundibulum of the gallbladder in a figure-of-eight fashion. This second suture is then brought to the abdominal wall along the anterior axillary line at the subcostal margin. Pulling on one end of the second suture or other end allows the gallbladder to be "puppeteered" back and forth as necessary to obtain exposure through a left twist or a right twist. The operation then unfolds in a standard fashion.

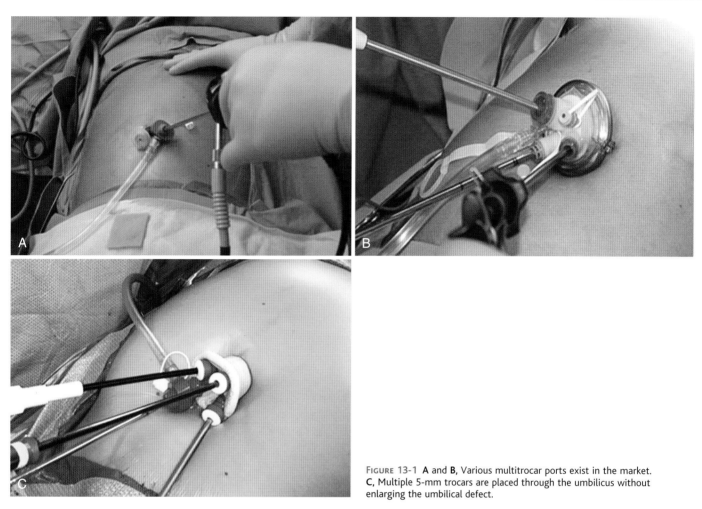

FIGURE 13-1 **A** and **B**, Various multitrocar ports exist in the market. **C**, Multiple 5-mm trocars are placed through the umbilicus without enlarging the umbilical defect.

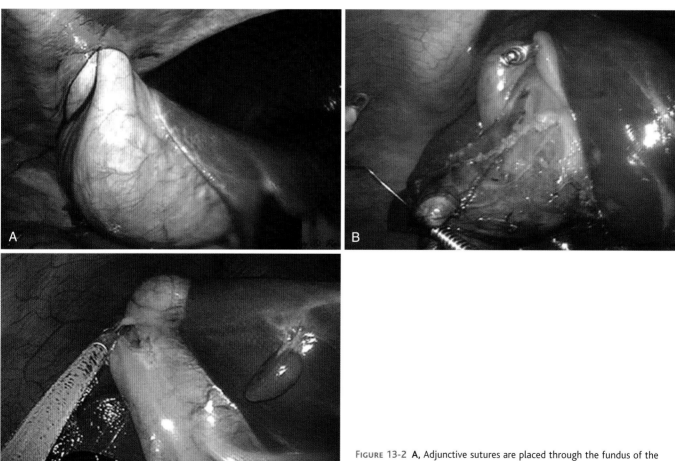

FIGURE 13-2 **A**, Adjunctive sutures are placed through the fundus of the gallbladder to obtain proper exposure. **B**, An EndoGrab device is used for retraction. **C**, Rigid locking and bent graspers are used for cephalad retraction of the fundus and lateral retraction of the infundibulum.

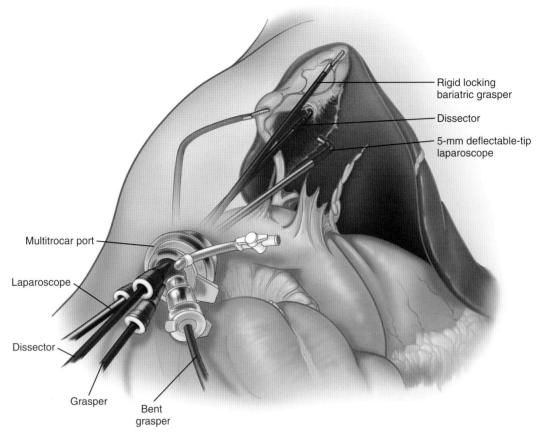

FIGURE 13-3 Proper placement of instruments within a multitrocar port.

It is possible to supplant adjunctive sutures with EndoGrab devices. These are placed through a 5-mm trocar and can effectively grasp the gallbladder and retract it to close proximity to the abdominal wall, which is securely grasped with the device (Fig. 13-2B). If necessary, the devices can be relocated to improve exposure.

If a single multitrocar port is used (i.e., a SILS port or TriPort), the use of graspers can also replace the use of adjunctive sutures for gallbladder retraction (Fig. 13-2C). For the safe and expeditious performance of the procedure, it is important that each port is used for the appropriate instrument (Figs. 13-3 and 13-4). A 5-mm deflectable-tip laparoscope is placed through port number 1, a rigid locking bariatric grasper is placed in port number 2, a bent grasper is placed in port number 3, and finally number 4 is the working port (see Figs. 13-3 and 13-4). With the grasping instruments, the gallbladder is retracted cephalad and maneuvered lateral or medial as needed (see Figs. 13-2C and 13-3). The grasper used to retract the infundibulum can be a bent, reticulating, or articulating grasper. An articulating grasper is shown in Figure 13-2C, and a bent grasper is shown in Figures 13-3 and 13-4.

Mobilization and Removal of the Gallbladder

With appropriate exposure, it is best to begin the dissection up around one third to one half the distance from the infundibulum to the fundus along the medial side of the gallbladder. After a window is developed between the infundibulum of the gallbladder and the liver, the cystic duct and artery become more apparent (Fig. 13-5A). The dissection proceeds with the separation of the cystic artery and cystic duct, and a "critical view" is obtained

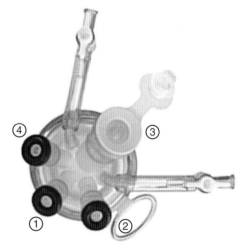

FIGURE 13-4 A 5-mm deflectable-tip laparoscope is placed through port number 1, a rigid locking bariatric grasper is placed through port number 2, a bent grasper is placed through port number 3, and finally the dissecting instruments are placed through port number 4.

(Fig. 13-5B). The cystic duct and the artery are then individually doubly clipped. Once these key structures have been clipped and divided, the gallbladder is freed from the gallbladder fossa. Before the gallbladder is disengaged from the liver, the operative field and gallbladder fossa are inspected for bleeding or bile leaks. Exposure will be lost once the gallbladder is completely detached from the liver. The gallbladder is then removed after it has been placed in a retrieval bag (Fig. 13-6). Extraction of the gallbladder with a large stone may require extension of the umbilical incision.

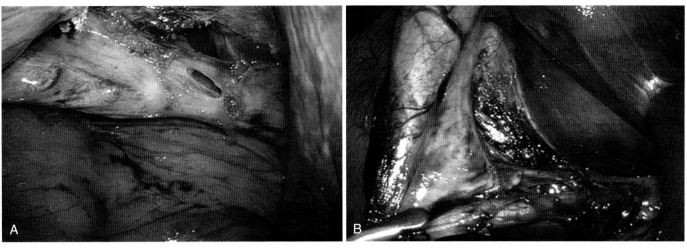

FIGURE 13-5 The critical view demonstrating the cystic duct and artery.

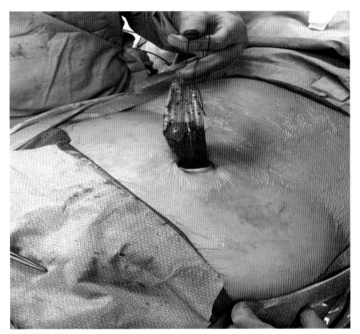

FIGURE 13-6 The gallbladder is extracted through the umbilical defect.

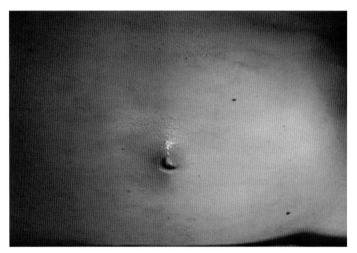

FIGURE 13-7 Closure of umbilical defect at the end of the operation.

Closure of the Incision and Wound Care

After the gallbladder is removed, the facial defect is closed in a figure-of-eight fashion using monofilament absorbable suture. The knot is buried. After the fascial incision is closed, the skin is approximated with absorbable running subcuticular suture (Fig. 13-7).

POSTOPERATIVE CARE

After undergoing LESS cholecystectomy, patients can be discharged as soon as they recover from anesthesia, tolerate liquids, and are able to void. If the patient is required to stay overnight, it is usually the result of comorbid conditions requiring further hospital care, a "hangover" from prolonged anesthesia, prolonged postoperative nausea, or urinary retention.

Postoperative pain is minimal, and most patients require no more than one postoperative injection of narcotic analgesia. Patients can generally be sent home with 6 to 10 tablets of a class II narcotic analgesic. Patients with more severe pain need to be evaluated for possible complications and, as a minimum, observed in the hospital.

Postoperative follow-up is within 7 to 10 days of the operation, and most patients are ready to return to normal activities within 7 days.

MANAGEMENT OF PROCEDURE-SPECIFIC COMPLICATIONS

Complications associated with laparoscopic cholecystectomy occur in fewer than 5% of all operations. The LESS approach should not lead to increased morbidity. Relative to laparoscopy, LESS cholecystectomies should have equivalent rates of intraoperative complications. It has been estimated that 80% to 85% of notable biliary and vascular injuries are a result of direct injury to the biliary and vascular structures by surgical instruments during dissection. A minority of injuries are related to thermal injury while monopolar electrocautery is in use. Furthermore, about half of all injuries during laparoscopic cholecystectomy occur in the most complex cases and are associated with inflammation, excessive scarring, or abnormal anatomy. Operations lasting longer than 3 hours are at particular risk for injury to biliary or vascular structures. Converting to a multitrocar operation or an open procedure is not a failure but rather reflects good judgment.

Early identification and management of intraoperative injuries, such as bile duct injuries, may prevent serious consequences. Most patients with biliary injury present with persistent abdominal pain, bloating, distention, nausea, vomiting, fever, or jaundice in the early postoperative period. A small number of patients will present months or years later with recurrent cholangitis or cirrhosis as a consequence of previous bile duct injury with biliary stricture.

Intraoperative bile duct injuries are associated with various factors, including severely inflamed gallbladders, obesity, bleeding, anatomic variations, and surgical technique. Inadequate exposure and failure to correctly identify the anatomic structures before ligating or dividing them are the most common causes of injury to the biliary system.

The routine use of intraoperative cholangiography as a preventative measure for bile duct injury is controversial. Nonetheless, in the case of a suspected bile duct injury, it is important that an intraoperative cholangiography be performed to assess the integrity of the biliary tree.

Management of a biliary injury is determined by various factors, including whether the injury is discovered during the operation, the type of injury, and the level and extent of the injury. Small biliary laceration may be managed with primary closure or better yet with the placement of a T-tube.

Major bile duct injuries, such as transection of the common hepatic or the common bile duct, are managed with Roux-en-Y bilioenteric anastomosis. Cystic duct leakage can be managed with percutaneous drainage and concomitant endoscopic biliary stenting. More extensive coverage of procedure-specific complications is provided in Chapter 20 of the *Atlas of Minimally Invasive Surgery*, 2009 (see Suggested Readings at the end of this chapter).

RESULTS AND OUTCOMES

It is the authors' opinion that LESS cholecystectomy will replace the traditional multitrocar approach to cholecystolithiasis as the new gold standard of surgery for selected patients. The few studies completed have shown that LESS cholecystectomy results in an even shorter length of hospital stay, less postoperative pain, and a quicker return to normal bowel function. In addition, there is greater patient satisfaction with the single-incision approach than with the conventional multiple-incision technique because of superior cosmesis with the former. The skeptics, however, caution that the indiscriminate use of LESS cholecystectomy may result in a higher number of biliary tree complications and incisional hernias.

Suggested Readings

Aprea G, Bottazzi E, Guida F, et al: Laparoendoscopic single site (LESS) versus classic video-laparoscopic cholecystectomy: A randomized prospective study, *J Surg Res* 166:e109–e112, 2011.

Bucher P, Morel P: Development of laparoscopic single-site cholecystectomy mandates critical view of safety dissection and routine intraoperative cholangiography, *J Am Coll Surg* 212:422–423, 2011.

Bucher P, Ostermann S, Pugin F, Morel P: Female population perception of conventional laparoscopy, transumbilical LESS, and transvaginal NOTES for cholecystectomy, *Surg Endosc* 25:2308–2315, 2011.

Carlson MA, Frantzides CT, Ludwig KA, et al: Routine or selective use of intraoperative cholangiography in laparoscopic cholecystectomy, *J Laparoendosc Surg* 3:31–37, 1993.

Duron V, Nicastri G, Gill P: Novel technique for a single-incision laparoscopic surgery (SILS) approach to cholecystectomy: Single-institution case series, *Surg Endosc* 25:1666–1671, 2011.

Elsey J, Feliciano D: Initial experience with single-incision laparoscopic cholecystectomy, *J Am Coll Surg* 210:620–626, 2010.

Frantzides CT, Sykes A: A re-evaluation of antibiotic prophylaxis in laparoscopic cholecystectomy, *J Laparoendosc Surg* 4:375–378, 1994.

Frantzides CT, Carlson MA: Laparoscopic cholecystectomy. In Frantzides CT, Carlson MA, editors: *Atlas of Minimally Invasive Surgery*, Philadelphia, 2009, Saunders, pp 155–159.

Gill IS, Advincula AP, Aron M, et al: Consensus statement of the Consortium for Laparoendoscopic Single-Site Surgery, *Surg Endosc* 24:762–768, 2010.

Hernandez J, Morton C, Ross S, et al: Laparoendoscopic single site cholecystectomy: The first 100 patients, *Am Surg* 75:681–685, 2009.

Hernandez J, Ross S, Morton C, et al: The learning curve of laparo-endoscopic single site (less) cholecystectomy: Definable, short, and safe, *J Am Coll Surg* 211:652–657, 2010.

Hodgett S, Hernandez J, Morton C, et al: Laparoendoscopic single site (LESS) cholecystectomy, *J Gastrointest Surg* 13:188–192, 2009.

Ito M, Asano Y, Horiguchi A, et al: Cholecystectomy using single-incision laparoscopic surgery with a new SILS port, *J Hepatobiliary Pancreat Sci* 17:688–691, 2010.

Podolsky E, Rottman S, Curcillo P: Single port access (SPA) cholecystectomy: Two year follow-up, *J Soc Laparoendosc Surg* 13:528–535, 2009.

Toomey P, Ross S, Albrink M, Rosemurgy A: Increasing the relevance of laparoendoscopic single-site (LESS) surgery, *Asian J Endosc Surg* 23:62–65, 2010.

Way LW, Stewart L, Gantert W, et al: Causes and prevention of laparoscopic bile duct injuries: Analysis of 252 cases from a human factors and cognitive psychology perspective, *Ann Surg* 237:460–469, 2003.

ERIC S. HUNGNESS AND NATHANIEL J. SOPER

Natural Orifice Transluminal Endoscopic Cholecystectomy

14

The videos associated with this chapter are listed in the Video Contents and can be found on the accompanying DVDs and *on Expertconsult.com.*

Cholecystectomy for gallbladder disease is one of the most common general surgical procedures with about 750,000 procedures performed per year. Up until the 1980s, open cholecystectomy was the norm, but laparoscopic cholecystectomy revolutionized surgery and is now the recognized gold standard. This is based on the reduction in overall morbidity with less postoperative pain, decreased hospital stay, and quicker return to work compared with open surgery. Despite the minimally invasive nature of laparoscopic cholecystectomy, some morbidity does exist. The usual four incisions do cause pain and scarring and can get infected, and incisional hernias may occur. As a result, potentially less invasive options for cholecystectomy have been developed over the past 5 years, including single-incision laparoscopy (SIL) and natural orifice transluminal endoscopic surgery (NOTES).

Single-incision laparoscopic cholecystectomy is usually performed with one umbilical skin incision, but it can include either a single or multiple fascial incisions depending on the technique and equipment used. The umbilical skin and fascial incisions may actually be longer than usually made during laparoscopic cholecystectomy and may not decrease pain or result in quicker return to normal functioning for patients. The long-term rate of incisional hernia is also a concern.

NOTES cholecystectomy may offer a less morbid minimally invasive surgical option by greatly reducing or eliminating skin and fascial incisions. The NOTES concept is to use a body's natural orifice (i.e., mouth, vagina, anus) as the entry point into the peritoneal cavity, by making a hole in a hollow viscus (i.e., stomach, vagina, rectum), passing flexible or rigid instruments into the peritoneal cavity, performing a procedure, and closing the viscus. Transvaginal (TV) cholecystectomy has been performed much more frequently than transgastric (TG) cholecystectomy. All TG and most TV NOTES cholecystectomies have been performed in a hybrid fashion, with at least a 5-mm laparoscope inserted at the umbilicus to ensure safe peritoneal access, assist in dissection, and offer a traditional laparoscopic view should orientation become difficult.

The main advantage of the TG approach is that is it applicable to both sexes, but several disadvantages exist. First, retroflexion of a flexible endoscope to the right upper quadrant is required and can result in spatial disorientation. Steerable overtubes can help overcome this drawback, but this equipment is expensive and requires small-caliber specialized flexible endoscopic

equipment. Most reported cases also recommend liberal laparoscopic dissection and additional retraction ports. The risk for gastrotomy leak and specimen extraction must also be considered. The cricopharyngeus is the narrowest point of the esophagus and can be a limiting factor if attempting to extract gallbladders with multiple gallstones or single stones larger than 1 cm in diameter. Esophageal perforation during TG cholecystectomy has been reported.

The TV approach offers several advantages for female patients needing cholecystectomy. First, most gallbladder disease occurs in women. Second, TV access to the pelvis is a standardized procedure in gynecologic surgery that is performed under direct visualization, allowing for easy closure. The gallbladder is also a "straight shot" from the vagina to the right upper quadrant, allowing for better spatial orientation. TV cholecystectomy is usually performed in a hybrid fashion; however, pure NOTES cholecystectomy has been described. The TV approach also allows for the use of rigid instrumentation and thus more accurate force transmission and precision. In fact, most TV cholecystectomies (>1000) have been performed in Germany using rigid instruments. There are several concerns about the TV approach, including dyspareunia, fertility, and hollow-organ injury. The gynecologic literature suggests that the risk for dyspareunia after TV surgery is less than 1%. TV surgery has also been used by infertility experts and poses little risk to fertility. Hollow-organ injury (bladder and rectum) has been reported as a complication of TV cholecystectomy. Regardless of the approach, at this time NOTES cholecystectomy must be considered an investigational procedure, and institutional review board approval should be obtained.

PREOPERATIVE EVALUATION, TESTING, AND PREPARATION

Patients being considered for TG or TV cholecystectomy should have a benign disease of the gallbladder necessitating cholecystectomy and should be worked up in standard fashion. Patients with acute cholecystitis or known choledocholithiasis should be excluded because of the expected inflammation or adhesions in the triangle of Calot.

Right upper quadrant ultrasound with gallstone sizing is mandatory, especially when considering TG cholecystectomy owing

Table 14-1 Exclusion Criteria

Transvaginal
  Prior abdominal or pelvic surgery
  Severe endometriosis
  History of vaginal trauma
  Gallstone diameter >3 cm
  Existing dyspareunia
  Positive Papanicolaou test
  Cervical cancer
Transgastric
  Prior esophageal or stomach surgery
  Large hiatal hernia
  Gallstone diameter >1.5 cm
  Indeterminate gallstone size with wall-shadow complex
  Esophageal stricture or web

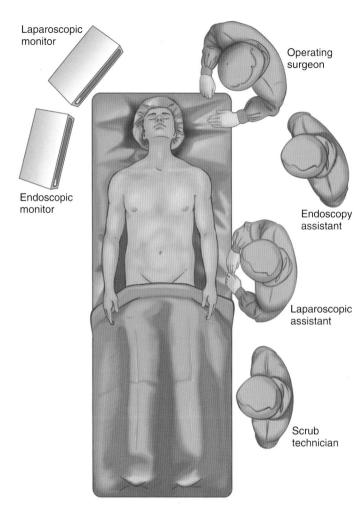

FIGURE 14-1 Patient positioning and operating room layout for transgastric cholecystectomy.

to the possibility of large specimens becoming stuck at the cricopharyngeus. If the largest gallstone cannot be measured and a wall-shadow sign is encountered, the gallbladder is most likely filled with multiple small stones that may act as one stone too large for removal. These patients, as well as those with gallstones larger than 1.5 cm in diameter, should not be offered the TG approach. For the TV approach, gallstones larger than 2 to 3 cm in diameter may cause a tearing of the vaginotomy and should be considered a relative contraindication.

Routine preoperative laboratory tests consistent with institutional outpatient surgery guidelines, routine use of a single preoperative dose of intravenous antibiotics, and prophylaxis for deep venous thrombosis are recommended. Patients undergoing TV cholecystectomy should also have a preoperative vaginal bimanual examination by a gynecologist, have a negative Papanicolaou test within the prior 12 months, and undergo bladder catheterization and a povidone-iodine vaginal prep. Other exclusion criteria for both TG and TV cholecystectomy are listed in Table 14-1. Female patients with a contraindication to the TV approach may be considered for the TG approach.

PATIENT POSITIONING IN THE OPERATING SUITE

NOTES cholecystectomy requires multiple surgical teams and access to both endoscopic and laparoscopic equipment with the ability to project both images simultaneously to closely placed monitors. Careful planning, communication, and coordination are required among the surgical team, operating room nursing staff, and anesthesia team to ensure proper positioning and visualization.

Patients undergoing TG cholecystectomy are placed in a supine position with a flexible anode tube for tracheal intubation. A bite block should be used to help with esophageal intubation with the endoscope or a flexible overtube, or both. The operating surgeon is positioned at the head of the bed cephalad to the left shoulder, with the endoscopy assistant to the left. The laparoscopic assistant is positioned on the patient's left side with the scrub technician to his or her left. Depending on the type of retraction used, an additional assistant on the patient's right is helpful. With this setup, all members of the team have good visualization of both the endoscopic and laparoscopic monitors that are positioned on the patient's right side toward the head (Fig. 14-1).

Patients undergoing the TV approach are positioned in a low lithotomy position with the hips not flexed, similar to the

position for a laparoscopic sigmoid colectomy. This will minimize any laparoscopic instrument interference with the patient's left thigh. Careful attention is given to ensuring minimal pressure on the patient's calves to avoid peroneal nerve injury. The operating surgeon is seated between the patient's legs, with the endoscopy assistant to the left. The laparoscopic assistant is positioned on the patient's left side, with the scrub technician to his or her left. The monitors are positioned similarly to the TG approach (Fig. 14-2).

POSITIONING AND PLACEMENT OF TROCARS

A hybrid approach is currently recommended for all NOTES cholecystectomies. We prefer a 5-mm umbilical port placed after Veress needle insertion and insufflation of carbon dioxide gas to an upper limit of 12 mm Hg. A 5-mm port is required to accommodate a laparoscopic clip applier, and the EndoGrab (Virtual Ports Ltd., Richmond, Va.) device is used for gallbladder retraction. Currently, there are no endoscopic clips that are appropriate for cystic duct and artery ligation. An additional right upper quadrant port (2, 3, or 5 mm, depending on the availability of 2- or 3-mm laparoscopic instruments) is helpful, particularly with the TG approach given the need for the endoscope to retroflex to the right upper quadrant, and for gastrotomy closure.

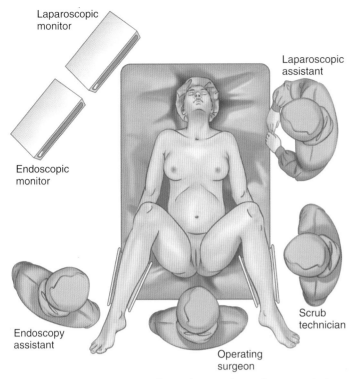

FIGURE 14-2 Patient positioning and operating room layout for transvaginal cholecystectomy.

OPERATIVE TECHNIQUE

Exposure

TV access is performed in the standard fashion with laparoscopic visualization to ensure safe access to the peritoneum. Briefly, a speculum is placed into the vagina, and a uterine sound is placed transcervically followed by a uterine manipulator. The uterus is anteverted, and the vaginal mucosa is elevated posterior to the cervix and scored with electrocautery. Under laparoscopic visualization, scissors are placed through the cul-de-sac anterior to the rectum and posterior to the uterus. The defect is extended to accommodate a 15-mm trocar, and anchoring Vicryl sutures are placed with the needles left on to facilitate closure. The trocar, followed by the endoscope, is then placed under direct laparoscopic vision into the peritoneum (Fig. 14-3). An alternative method has been described in the literature whereby after the uterine manipulator is placed, a nonbladed laparoscopic trocar is directly inserted in the pouch of Douglas between the uterosacral ligaments.

Although safe TG access for human NOTES procedures has been described, we feel that it should always be performed under laparoscopic visualization for cholecystectomy to ensure proper placement of the gastrotomy. The optimal location for the gastrotomy is on the anterior aspect of the stomach at the level of the incisura, slightly toward the lesser curvature (Fig. 14-4). If the

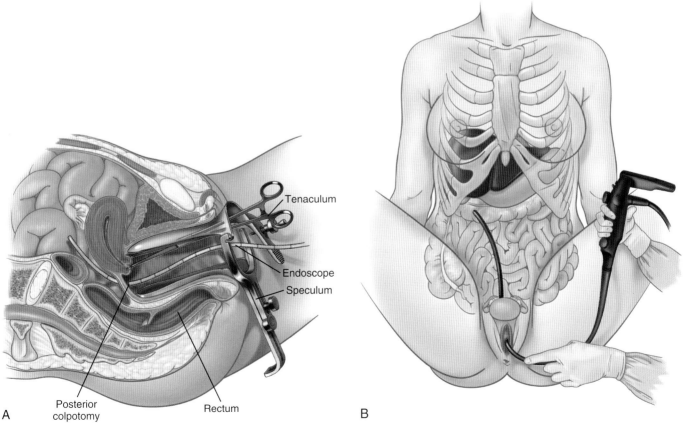

A   B

FIGURE 14-3 **A,** Introduction of the endoscope through a posterior colpotomy. **B,** Transvaginal cholecystectomy.

see through the balloon), and then the entire balloon and endoscope unit is advanced into abdomen. The gallbladder is then targeted with retroflexion to the right upper quadrant. Visualization is then switched entirely to the endoscope so that the 5-mm umbilical port can be used for retraction.

Retraction

As with single-incision laparoscopic cholecystectomy, gallbladder retraction is critical and can be challenging in NOTES cholecystectomy. A variety of techniques have been described, including the use of a percutaneous 2-mm grasper, suture retraction, or the addition of an additional laparoscopic trocar. We now use the EndoGrab device for internal retraction of the gallbladder. One end of this 5-mm laparoscopic device grasps onto the gallbladder. The other end, connected by a nitinol wire, grabs the peritoneum suspending the gallbladder. We usually use two devices, the first for cephalad retraction of the fundus and the second for anterolateral retraction of the infundibulum. The TV approach offers an additional option for gallbladder retraction. A second long laparoscopic instrument can be placed alongside the vaginal trocar or can be placed through the trocar alongside the endoscope if a 15-mm trocar is used.

Dissection

The principles of dissection for NOTES cholecystectomy mirrors that of laparoscopic cholecystectomy. Varying amounts of dissection can be accomplished with the use of 5-mm laparoscopic instruments through the umbilical port. One cautionary aspect of the NOTES dissection is that the view from the endoscope is generally more posterior and inferior compared with that of laparoscopic cholecystectomy. It is important to be confident in the anatomy, obtaining the "critical view of safety" before clipping the cystic duct or artery. Omental adhesions are bluntly taken down, followed by retraction of the gallbladder. The medial and lateral peritoneal attachments are then dissected and cauterized with commercially available "hot" biopsy graspers or snare cautery with just the distal tip exposed. Once the critical view of safety has been achieved, cystic duct and artery clipping through the laparoscopic port proceeds. At this time, there are no endoscopic clips that are designed for reliable tissue approximation. It should be remembered that control of hemorrhage with only one laparoscopic port may be difficult; therefore, slow, careful dissection should be done to decrease the chance of bleeding. The gallbladder is then carefully dissected off the liver bed in standard fashion using the tip of a snare cautery device.

Specimen Retrieval

TV specimen retrieval with a snare cautery placed around the infundibulum of the freed gallbladder is straightforward and should be done under laparoscopic visualization. Gallstones greater than 3 cm may pose a risk to tear the vaginotomy. The TG specimen retrieval is riskier because it must be brought out through the relatively narrow esophagus, particularly at the level of the cricopharyngeus. Excessive tension should not be used, minimizing the chance of esophageal perforation. It is also helpful to pass a guidewire into the peritoneum before specimen retrieval to maintain visualization of the gastrotomy. Once the specimen and endoscope are brought into the stomach, the intragastric air is released, significantly decreasing visualization.

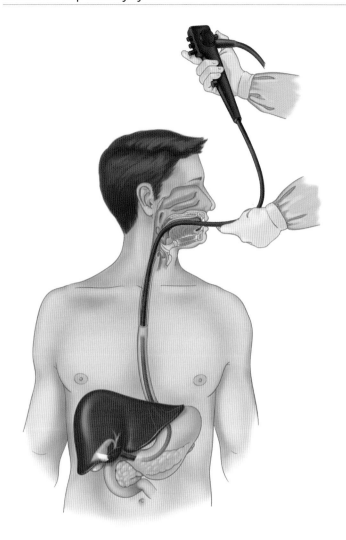

FIGURE 14-4 Transgastric cholecystectomy.

gastrotomy is too close to the lesser curvature, bleeding may occur, and if too far lateral, it may be difficult to retroflex to the right upper quadrant. A diagnostic upper endoscopy with a standard, single-channel therapeutic endoscope is then performed to rule out any gastric pathology, to aspirate gastric contents, and to cover the stomach mucosa with dilute bacitracin wash using a commercially available spray catheter.

The endoscope is removed and replaced by the Endosurgical Operating System (EOS) if available. The current generation of this platform has an outer diameter of 16 mm and two 6-mm and two 4-mm working channels. An Olympus N-180 scope is placed into one of the 6-mm working channels, and the entire unit is passed into the stomach under direct endoscopic visualization. Care is taken to avoid pharyngeal or esophageal injury. Carbon dioxide insufflation tubing is connected to one of the working ports, and the stomach is insufflated.

After the optimal location for gastrotomy is determined using laparoscopic guidance, a needle knife (using the endoscope accessory channel or EOS 4-mm port) is used to make a small puncture that is followed by an 18- to 20-mm CRE wire-guided balloon that is passed down one of the other working channels. The midpoint of the balloon is positioned at the gastric wall, and the balloon is slowly filled with saline to the desired diameter according to the manufacturer's recommendations. Once dilated, the scope is positioned up against the balloon (so you can actually

Closure

The guidewire inserted before specimen retrieval is used to locate the gastrotomy and is the first step in closure. The dilation balloon is then inserted through the gastrotomy, inflated, and drawn back to temporarily seal the gastrotomy allowing for the pneumogastrium to reaccumulate. If the endosurgical operating system is used for the case, the g-Prox device (USGI Medical, San Clemente, Calif.) can be used for the closure of the gastrotomy. A helix grasper is screwed into the gastric mucosa at the corner of the gastrotomy to draw tissue into the g-Prox device, which is then clamped. A hollow-tipped needle is passed through the tissue, and the helix is removed. Anchoring baskets are then deployed and cinched. Multiple g-Prox firings are deployed to successfully close the gastrotomy. Additional laparoscopic sutures are placed to reinforce the closure but require at least two ports and extracorporeal knots. The closure is then tested for leaks with air insufflation.

Vaginotomy closure is much easier to perform than closure of the gastrotomy because it is easily visualized after speculum insertion. The previously placed stay sutures are used to identify the edges and inspect for lateral tearing. The vaginotomy is then closed with running Vicryl suture with long conventional needle drivers.

POSTOPERATIVE CARE

Transvaginal

Pain at the umbilicus or right upper quadrant after the TV approach is minimal and is usually adequately controlled with acetaminophen or a mild narcotic. Most women do not complain of any perineal or vaginal discomfort after TV cholecystectomy. Patients may experience some mild spotting, so wearing a feminine pad is advised. No sexual intercourse, tampon insertion, or douching is recommended for 1 month after the procedure. Patients may advance their diet as tolerated and are usually discharged the day of the procedure.

Transgastric

Pain control for the TG approach is similar to that of TV patients; however, TG patients usually have at least one additional right upper quadrant port. They also typically complain of a sore throat similar to that of having an endoscopy. Patients are kept NPO overnight and are started on clear liquids on the morning of postoperative day 1.

MANAGEMENT OF PROCEDURE-SPECIFIC COMPLICATIONS

Bleeding

Bleeding may occur during access or dissection when using either the TG or TV approach. Bleeding during the gastrotomy is usually a result of dissecting too close to the lesser curvature. It can also occur during dissection of the triangle of Calot because of the less precise dissection tools used. Management of hemorrhage during NOTES cholecystectomy is theoretically more difficult than during traditional laparoscopic cholecystectomy for this same reason. It is generally easier to control the bleeding with the umbilical laparoscopic port using either a laparoscopic clip applier or hot forceps with endoscopic visualization than to deploy endoscopic tools or clips. If bleeding is not quickly controlled, additional trocars should be placed to control the bleeding laparoscopically.

Bile Tract Injury

Bile tract injury is the most feared complication of cholecystectomy and is thought to occur in 0.4% to 0.6% of laparoscopic cholecystectomies. The same principles for reducing the chance of bile track injury for laparoscopic cholecystectomy should be used for NOTES cholecystectomy. The medial and lateral peritoneal attachments are dissected, allowing the infundibulum to move right to left. Careful dissection in the triangle of Calot is used to demonstrate the critical view of safety before clipping and cutting the cystic duct and artery. It needs to be reemphasized that the endoscopic view for NOTES cholecystectomy is more inferior and posterior than during traditional laparoscopic cholecystectomy and can be disorienting during the TG approach because of retroflexion. Conversion to laparoscopic cholecystectomy is necessary if the anatomy is ambiguous and should not be considered a failure. Intraoperative cholangiogram can also be performed to help identify the biliary tree.

Gastrotomy Leak

One of the most concerning aspects of TG cholecystectomy is the possibility of a gastrotomy leak, although none has been reported in the literature. Reinforcement of the gastrotomy closure with laparoscopic sutures may reduce this risk and is recommended in all cases. If a leak is suspected, Gastrografin swallow is recommended. There should be a low threshold to reexplore the patient if leak is suspected.

Bowel and Bladder Injury

Bowel and bladder injury have been described for TV cholecystectomy. Laparoscopic visualization during vaginotomy and for all TV instrument exchanges is recommended with the help of a uterine manipulator to reduce this risk. Injuries identified intraoperatively are handled in standard fashion after conversion to full laparoscopic or open technique. Delayed presentation of the injury is possible; therefore, a high index of suspicion is needed to quickly diagnose this potentially life-threatening complication.

Esophageal Perforation

As mentioned previously, esophageal perforation has been described as a major complication of TG cholecystectomy and has occurred during specimen impaction. Gallstone diameter larger than 1.5 cm or indeterminate gallstone size on right upper quadrant ultrasound should be considered a contraindication to TG cholecystectomy. Endoscope intubation is also a potential cause of perforation; therefore, good technique with advancement only under direct visualization is advised.

RESULTS AND OUTCOME

More than 2000 human NOTES hybrid cholecystectomies have been performed to date around the world, with most using TV access. A few pure TV cases have been performed, with the first reported by Bessler, but technology is lacking at this time for wide advancement of totally incisionless cholecystectomy. Less than

100 TG cholecystectomies have been performed, with all having at least one laparoscopic trocar inserted. At this time, feasibility of both approaches has been demonstrated, but it is unclear what advantage exists aside from less scarring and improved cosmesis.

The largest published series comes from Zornig and associates and the German registry, where hybrid TV cholecystectomies were performed with rigid instruments. Of the 551 patients, 3% had serious complications, including bladder and bowel perforation. No biliary tract injury was described, whereas almost 5% of cases were converted to laparoscopic or open. Older and obese patients were more likely to suffer a complication. Other, smaller studies from centers using flexible endoscopic equipment have shown similar complication and conversion rates. A more recent matched comparison from Zornig and colleagues with laparoscopic cholecystectomy patients showed only a longer operative time for the TV approach, but no difference in terms of complications, hospital length of stay, analgesia use, or return to work.

Results for hybrid TG cholecystectomy are more sparse, with the largest published series from Zorron and associates ($N = 10$). Complications rates are higher for this approach, and peritonitis and esophageal perforation have been reported. Misinterpretation of biliary anatomy resulting in a near-miss bile tract injury has also been reported with TG cholecystectomy. As a result, liberal laparoscopic assistance is advocated by our group and others.

Additional data and long-term follow-up are needed to fully evaluate the place that NOTES will have in the armamentarium of treating gallbladder disease. Randomized trials are now under way, including the Natural Orifice Surgery Consortium for Assessment and Research (NOSCAR) multicenter clinical trial.

Suggested Readings

Auyang ED, Hungness EH, Vaziri K, et al: Human NOTES cholecystectomy: Transgastric hybrid technique, *J Gastrointest Surg* 13:1149–1150, 2009.

Bessler M, Stevens PD, Milone L, et al: Transvaginal laparoscopically assisted endoscopic cholecystectomy: A hybrid approach to natural orifice surgery, *Gastrointest Endosc* 66:1243–1245, 2007.

Federlein M, Borchert D, Muller V, et al: Transvaginal video-assisted cholecystectomy in clinical practice, *Surg Endosc* 24:2444–2452, 2010.

Horgan S, Cullen JP, Talamini MA, et al: Natural orifice surgery: Initial clinical experience, *Surg Endosc* 23:1512–1518, 2009.

Nau P, Anderson J, Happel L, et al: Safe alternative transgastric peritoneal access in humans: NOTES, *Surgery* 149:147–152, 2011.

Perretta S, Dallemagne B, Donatelli G, et al: The fear of transgastric cholecystectomy: misinterpretation of the biliary anatomy, *Surg Endosc* 25:648, 2011.

Salinas G, Saavedra L, Agurto H, et al: Early experience in human hybrid transgastric and transvaginal endoscopic cholecystectomy, *Surg Endosc* 24:1092–1098, 2010.

Santos BF, Auyang ED, Hungness ES, et al: Preoperative ultrasound measurements predict the feasibility of gallbladder extraction during transgastric natural orifice translumenal endoscopic surgery cholecystectomy, *Surg Endosc* 24:1168–1175, 2011.

Zornig C, Siemssen L, Emmermann A, et al: NOTES cholecystectomy: Matched-pair analysis comparing the transvaginal hybrid and conventional laparoscopic techniques in a series of 216 patients, *Surg Endosc* 25:1822–1826, 2010.

Zorron R, Palanivelu C, Galvao Neto MP, et al: International multicenter trial on clinical natural orifice surgery—NOTES IMTN study: Preliminary results of 362 patients, *Surg Innov* 17:142–158, 2010.

Veeraiah Siripurapu, Tzu-jung Tsai, Pavlos Papavasiliou, and Andrew A. Gumbs

Laparoscopic Radical Cholecystectomy

The videos associated with this chapter are listed in the Video Contents and can be found on the accompanying DVDs and on Expertconsult.com.

Gallbladder cancer is a disease process that has a diverse worldwide variation. It has a very high incidence in parts of northern India, Pakistan, Bolivia, Peru, and Ecuador. It also has a notable presence in South Asia and some central and eastern European countries. Females have a higher incidence, with factors such as cholelithiasis, obesity, and infections related to *Salmonella paratyphi* and *typhi* showing a higher relative risk. It has been estimated that approximately 1% of patients with gallstones in Western countries will develop gallbladder cancer. In areas of high risk such as Ecuador, this increases to 5% to 10% and may be as high as 20% in Bolivia and Peru. A subset of patients with cholelithiasis will develop porcelain gallbladder, which is a consequence of a chronically inflamed wall. However, not every patient with a porcelain gallbladder will develop gallbladder cancer, with the risk more in the range of 10% to 20%. Despite these possible etiologic factors, the exact pathway behind gallbladder cancer remains veiled and likely multifactorial.

As an anatomic structure, the gallbladder lies below hepatic segments IVB and V with close proximity to the portal structures. Because it has only one muscle layer, the tumor has easier access to the serosa of adjacent organs, and its close proximity to the structures of the hepatoduodenal ligament often make surgical resection difficult or impossible. Of note, the gallbladder has an adventitial layer along its attachment to the liver and a serosa only along its extrahepatic portion. The first-echelon nodes of drainage are the cystic and pericholedochal nodes, with connection further to portal and common hepatic artery nodes, making their dissection a critical part of any surgical resection. The disease process often frustrates because of delays in diagnosis, resulting in presentation at an advanced stage and incurability. For those who present at an earlier stage, surgery remains the only chance of cure, with the consideration of postoperative chemotherapy and radiation.

In the era of laparoscopic cholecystectomy, the incidental identification of gallbladder cancer represents the majority of presentations for this disease process. Gallbladder cancer is a relatively rare disease, with the incidence rate in the United States estimated to be approximately 1.2 cases per 100,000 per year. It is associated with a poor prognosis, with 5-year survival rates for gallbladder cancer being reported at 5% to 10% in recent years and with a median survival of 3 to 6 months from the time of diagnosis. This has been improving, however, with groups reporting median survival of 50 months for those amenable to surgical resection. Since George Pack first suggested in 1955 a radical liver resection for gallbladder cancer, there is consideration of partial hepatectomy ranging from wedge resection to formal hepatectomy. The advent of laparoscopy to the field of hepatobiliary surgery has further added to the surgical approach and bears discussion.

CONTROVERSIES REGARDING THE PROPER SURGICAL MANAGEMENT

Currently, there are multiple controversies regarding the proper surgical management of gallbladder cancer: choice of initial procedure for preoperatively suspected gallbladder cancer, timing of re-resection, extent of resection for T1b or greater lesions (including number of lymph nodes needed, extent of parenchymal resection, and need for routine excision of the common bile duct), and the appropriateness of the minimally invasive approach. Although laparoscopic cholecystectomy was one of the first minimally invasive procedures of the gastrointestinal tract and still one of the most common, the suspicion or diagnosis of gallbladder cancer has been considered a contraindication to laparoscopy. Regardless, most gallbladder cancers are diagnosed after routine laparoscopic cholecystectomy; when found to be a T1a lesion, the therapeutic management is considered complete. When the postoperative pathologic examination, however, reveals a T1b to T3 lesion, most patients are referred to tertiary oncology centers and undergo open re-resection. Patients found to have T4 lesions or metastatic disease are considered inoperable and only offered palliative chemotherapy. Neoadjuvant chemoradiation is considered for large T2 lesions that would warrant a formal hepatectomy in an effort to decrease the tumor burden, for all T3 lesions, and when there are concerns for bile leakage during initial cholecystectomy.

PREOPERATIVELY SUSPECTED GALLBLADDER CANCER

When patients are found to have gallbladder polyps or mass greater than 1 cm or less than 1 cm with the presence of blood flow, porcelain gallbladder, or evidence of invasion into the gallbladder hepatic parenchymal bed, gallbladder cancer should be suspected. Currently, at most centers, when there is no evidence of metastatic disease or concerns for a T4 lesion, most patients undergo a laparoscopic cholecystectomy followed by either intra-operative frozen-section analysis and open completion radical cholecystectomy at the same operation or a second operation after final histopathologic review.

ADVENT OF THE LAPAROSCOPIC APPROACH

Surgeons have been reluctant to apply minimally invasive techniques to the surgical management of gallbladder cancer because of the perceived difficulty of laparoscopically dissecting tumors off the structures of the portal triad. As a result, laparoscopic radical cholecystectomy has been one of the last minimally invasive procedures performed. Gumbs and colleagues reported the first laparoscopic radical cholecystectomy in 2009 on a patient with the preoperative suspicion of gallbladder cancer due to a 4-cm mass seen on abdominal ultrasound and cross-sectional imaging. Despite a negative preoperative serum immunoglobulin G4 (IgG4) level, the postoperative diagnosis was consistent with autoimmune cholecystitis. Nonetheless, the patient was discharged home tolerating a regular diet on the second postoperative day.

The next patient with the preoperative suspicion of gallbladder cancer was found to have a 7.5-cm malignant mass in the dome of the gallbladder, with intraparenchymal invasion during the laparoscopic radical cholecystectomy; as a result, a formal resection of hepatic segments IVB and V was required to obtain an R_0 resection. In addition, the cystic duct stump at the confluence with the common bile duct was found to have disease. A laparoscopic common bile duct excision was then performed and the biliary tree reconstructed with a laparoscopic Roux-en-Y choledochojejunostomy. Because of the success with these patients, we began to approach patients who had undergone previous cholecystectomy and were found to have gallbladder cancers.

POSTOPERATIVELY DIAGNOSED GALLBLADDER CANCER

The need for re-resection following an incidentally diagnosed gallbladder cancer depends on the final pathologic stage of the tumor. By definition, T1a tumors only invade the *lamina propria.* A cholecystectomy with negative margins done laparoscopically or by open techniques is considered curative because re-resection of the gallbladder fossa with or without lymphadenectomy has never been proved to yield a survival benefit. Re-resection, however, is advised in patients with T1b to T3 tumors because of improved overall survival. Patients with incidentally diagnosed gallbladder cancer often have a better prognosis because most are early lesions (T1 to T2). Patients found to have incidental gallbladder carcinomas who undergo re-resection may actually have improved survival compared with those with non-incidentally diagnosed cancer. T2 lesions make up the majority (67%) of incidentally diagnosed gallbladder carcinomas and are associated with a 5-year survival rate of greater than 60%, compared with less than 20% for those treated with cholecystectomy alone. Patients with T3 disease, which is defined as a tumor that invades into the serosa and/or the liver and/or an adjacent organ, are at a higher risk for peritoneal carcinomatosis. Formal re-resection and hepatoduodenal lymphadenectomy may provide a survival benefit in patients without evidence of peritoneal disease. Patients with improperly treated T3 disease have a 5-year survival rate of 0 to 15% compared with 25% to 65% for

T3 patients who undergo completion radical cholecystectomy re-resection. The extend of liver resection for gallbladder malignancy is still ill defined.

Because of the authors' success with these patients and the ability to spare patients unnecessary laparotomy, all resectable patients with preoperatively suspected gallbladder cancer and patients found to have T1b to T3 disease after cholecystectomy are now approached laparoscopically.

OPERATIVE INDICATIONS

Operability in gallbladder cancer relies heavily on preoperative staging and considerations of findings during the initial laparoscopy or as part of a preoperative staging workup. The American Joint Committee on Cancer (AJCC) in its seventh edition has established subcategories for stage IV gallbladder cancer. Stage IVA is defined by tumor invasion into the main portal vein, the hepatic artery, or two or more extrahepatic structures. The presence of metastases to the periaortic, pericaval, or superior mesenteric artery or celiac nodes or of distant metastases further defines stage IVB (Table 15-1). As mentioned previously, the extent of liver resection needs strong consideration and is

Table 15-1   TNM Staging of Gallbladder Cancer

Primary Tumor	
Tx	Primary tumor cannot be assessed
T0	No evidence of primary tumor
Tis	Carcinoma in situ
T1a	Tumor invades lamina propria
T1b	Tumor invades muscle layer
T2	Tumor invades perimuscular connective tissue, no extension beyond serosa or into liver
T3	Tumor perforates serosa or directly invades the liver or other adjacent organs or structure (stomach, duodenum, colon, pancreas, omentum, extrahepatic bile ducts)
T4	Tumor invades main portal vein or hepatic artery or invades two or more extrahepatic organs or structures.

Regional Nodes	
Nx	Regional nodes cannot be assessed
N0	No regional lymph node metastasis
N1	Metastases to nodes along the cystic duct, common bile duct, hepatic artery, and/or portal vein
N2	Metastases to periaortic, pericaval, superior mesenteric artery, and/or celiac artery lymph nodes

Distant Metastasis	
Mx	Distant metastasis cannot be assessed
M0	No distant metastasis
M1	Distant metastasis

Stage 0	Tis	N0	M0
Stage I	T1	N0	M0
Stage II	T2	N0	M0
Stage IIIA	T3	N0	M0
Stage IIIB	T1-3	N1	M0
Stage IVa	T4	N0-1	M0
Stage IVb	Any T	N2	M0
	Any T	Any N	M1

From Edge SB, Byrd DR, Compton CC, et al., editors: AJCC Cancer Staging Manual, ed 7, New York, 2010, Springer, pp 215–217.

controversial, with differing opinions regarding the suitability of nonanatomic resections of the gallbladder bed versus complete resection of segments IVB and V and even extended right hepatectomy (segments IV to VIII). We consider major hepatectomy or even extended hepatectomy only when this is necessary to achieve an R_0 resection because there has been no conclusive difference noted in overall survival between minor and major hepatectomy.

Nodal disease stretching down the portal chain posterior to the pancreas or duodenum may present a challenge. For disease that is not invading vascular structures, dissection is often achieved satisfactorily; however, larger nodes may not be removed successfully without a pancreatoduodenectomy. This must be taken with due caution in terms of morbidity and mortality when performing such a procedure allied with a radical cholecystectomy.

Powered analysis suggests that involvement of the common bile duct is associated with advanced T stage and is an independent prognostic factor in survival. Positive margins at the cystic duct mandate further resection of the common bile duct to achieve R_0 resection, which, although a poor prognosticator, is associated with a better survival outcome than R_1 resection.

PREOPERATIVE EVALUATION

Routine preoperative workup includes chest radiography, electrocardiography (ECG), serum complete blood count, chemistries, liver function studies, and serum tumor markers consisting of carcinoembryonic antigen and CA 19-9 levels. In addition, serum IgG4 levels are measured routinely in all patients before surgery to rule out the presence of autoimmune cholecystitis. Unfortunately, as noted previously, this test has a significant false-positive rate. The indocyanine green test is routine in Asia because the high rate of hepatitis-related cirrhosis may influence the extent of hepatic resection. All formal hepatectomies must be assessed for residual liver volume and Child-Pugh classification and should be followed by pathologic examination for underlying liver cirrhosis grade, especially if the liver is not chemotherapy naïve.

Ultrasound is limited in the diagnosis of early lesions and as such is unreliable for staging. In some 20% to 30% of cases, gallbladder cancer may present as an asymmetrical wall thickening that has an expanded differential diagnosis ranging from cholecystitis, adenomyomatosis, acute hepatitis, or portal hypertension to congestive heart failure. Gallbladder cancer arising on a background of chronic inflammation certainly makes radiologic interpretation more difficult. Asymmetrical wall thickening with persistent arterial enhancement or isodensity during the hepatic venous phase should, however, heighten suspicion. In cases in which a mass-occupying lesion is noted, as occurs in some 40% of patients, ultrasound that shows a heterogenous and hypoechoic tumor is classic.

Although ultrasound is often the first imaging technique performed in those undergoing cholecystectomy for unsuspected gallbladder cancer, high-resolution imaging in the form of computed tomography (CT) or magnetic resonance imaging (MRI) is most often used to help identify residual tumor burden or metastatic disease. CT scan with intravenous contrast is used to delineate the hepatic vasculature and rule out evidence of vascular invasion, such as portal vein or hepatic arterial narrowing or frank invasion. Abdominal MRI with gadolinium is used in an effort to ascertain the extent of intraparenchymal involvement.

In cases of recent cholecystectomy, it may be difficult or impossible to differentiate hepatic invasion from enhancement because of scarring from the recent surgery.

The role of ^{18}F-fluorodeoxyglucose positron emission tomography (FDG-PET) in gallbladder cancer is still in flux. Because gallbladder cancer is highly PET avid, studies have suggested that FDG-PET may change the operative decision in 25% of cases. In up to 50% of cases of incidentally found gallbladder cancer, metastatic spread was shown by FDG-PET. Although this is highly suggestive of a role for FDG-PET, false-positive results may be noted in areas of inflammation from recent laparoscopic cholecystectomy, with recent data also noting FDG-PET to have a negative predictive value of 65%, suggesting a greater extent of residual disease that might be missed. It may be that the role of FDG-PET is best served to rule out distant spread, whereas residual disease is best assessed by intraoperative laparoscopic ultrasound and reexploration.

VALUE OF STAGING LAPAROSCOPY

With the advent of laparoscopic cholecystectomy, distinct situations may arise concerning laparoscopy and gallbladder cancer. The detection of gallbladder cancer during or after the initial procedure remains the main method of incidental diagnosis. It may, however, present as an unsuspected finding during laparoscopic or open cholecystectomy. In addition to these considered events, the role of staging laparoscopy with intraoperative laparoscopic hepatic ultrasound is increasingly important. Gallbladder cancer has a rate of peritoneal metastases that ranges from 25% to 70%, with T stage being a strong correlate. It is unfortunate that despite high-quality preoperative imaging, up to 20% to 50% of laparoscopies reveal the presence of peritoneal carcinomatosis. As a preoperative tool, it is unlikely to be warranted when a recent laparoscopic cholecystectomy detecting gallbladder cancer has been performed and adequate thought has been given to a peritoneal and hepatic survey by the initial surgeon.

PATIENT POSITIONING

The authors place their patients in a modified lithotomy position, the so-called French position, with both arms out and the legs almost extended (Fig. 15-1). The patient is on a beanbag with a lower strap across the pelvis to stabilize the patient when extended reverse Trendelenburg positioning is needed. For formal right hepatectomies, a bump below the right upper quadrant is placed to elevate the liver. The surgeon stands between the patient's legs, and monitors are placed at the head of the operating table, with the second monitor for the assistant (Fig. 15-2). Depending on the patient's anatomy, the assistant stands either to the right or to the left of the patient.

PLACEMENT OF TROCARS

Entry into the abdomen is achieved either with a Veress needle in patients with virgin abdomens or abdominal obesity or by using the open technique in those with recent abdominal surgery or prior surgery in the right upper quadrant. The Veress needle is positioned under the right subcostal cage, with the skin held taut by a bullet clamp pierced through the umbilicus. Entry is confirmed by initial aspiration and then verification of intra-abdominal pressure. After establishing pneumoperitoneum to 12

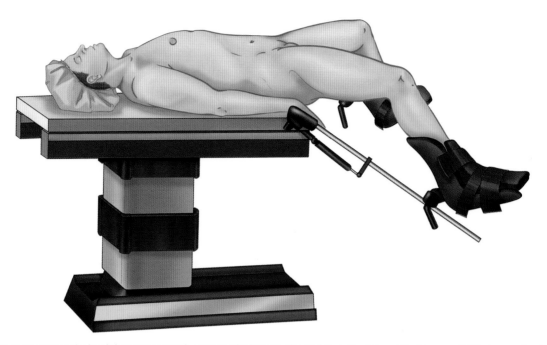

FIGURE 15-1 Patient positioning in the low lithotomy or French position. The legs are almost fully extended, and the hips are slightly hyperextended. (Knees are slightly lower than the hips.)

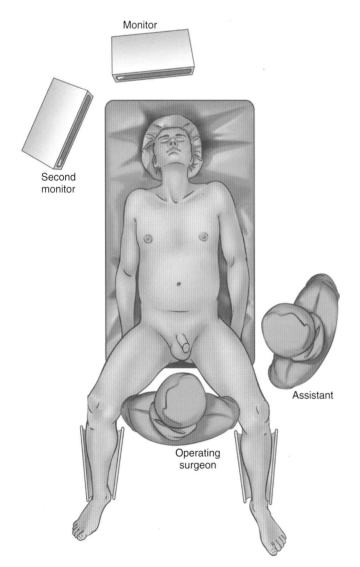

FIGURE 15-2 Operating room setup; the surgeon stands between the patient's legs with the assistant on either side of the patient. The monitors are at the head of the bed.

to 15 mm Hg, a 12-mm trocar is placed one handbreadth below the right subcostal margin in the midclavicular line (Fig. 15-3). This is achieved through a modified open technique with dissection to the anterior fascia, using needle aspiration to confirm lack of adhesions. Having done so satisfactorily, a 10-mm, 30-degree camera is used to identify appropriate placement of the other trocars. The trocars are generally placed in a curved line extending across the midline with a 10- to 12-mm port placed four fingerbreadths aside the entry port and a further 10- to 12-mm port on the opposite side. A 5-mm port is placed on the medial aspect, subxiphoid, along the curvilinear line. Generally, four trocars are necessary and are fashioned so that these incisions can be used for conversion if necessitated.

OPERATIVE TECHNIQUE

Exposure

The abdomen is initially inspected for evidence of peritoneal carcinomatosis. Any suspicious lesions are biopsied and sent for frozen section. Positive biopsy results preclude resection. The operation proceeds if there is no evidence of carcinomatosis. For preoperatively or intraoperatively diagnosed lesions, peritoneal lavage is performed, and intraoperative results are obtained before continuing with the radical cholecystectomy. While awaiting results, the laparoscopic hepatoduodenal lymph node dissection may begin. Adhesions to the gallbladder fossa are preserved, whereas other adhesions are lysed using ultrasonic shears (Harmonic scalpel, Ethicon Endo-Surgery, Cincinnati, Ohio). Hepatic ultrasound is performed to evaluate the liver for metastasis and to locate the extent of parenchymal disease to ensure a margin-free transection and to identify the relation of the cancer to the portal structures. The patient is placed in reverse Trendelenburg position, and the liver is retracted superiorly through the assistant's port. A laparoscopic liver retractor is used for exposure, and every effort is made not to touch the gallbladder and to ensure no spillage of bile.

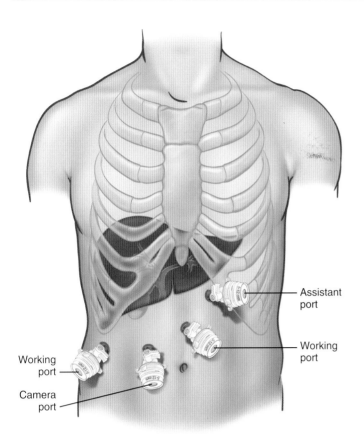

FIGURE 15-3 Trocar positioning. The first trocar is placed one handbreadth below the right subcostal margin; two working trocars are placed to the left and right of the primary trocar. A trocar is placed in the left upper quadrant and subxiphoid region or right flank for the assistant. The assistant's trocar is placed in the left upper quadrant. All ports are 10 mm in diameter, except for the assistant's trocar, which can be 5 mm.

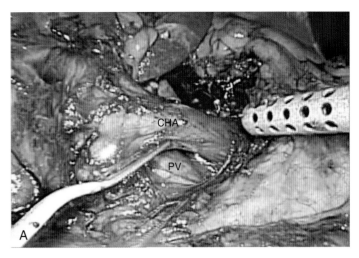

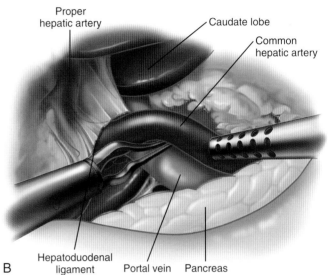

FIGURE 15-4 The laparoscopic hepatoduodenal lymph node dissection begins at the common hepatic artery (CHA) and proceeds toward the bifurcation. The portal vein (PV) is found in a triangle bordered by the CHA, the gastroduodenal artery, and the superior border of the portal vein.

Dissection

Using the ultrasound dissector in one hand and a laparoscopic bipolar device (Medtronic, Jacksonville, Fla.) in the other hand, the *pars lucida* of the lesser omentum is incised to expose the common hepatic artery. Lymphadenectomy begins at the common hepatic artery lymph node and proceeds toward the *porta hepatis* (Fig. 15-4). All lymphatic tissue is dissected, from the superior portion of the duodenum to the liver hilum, exposing the gastroduodenal artery, proper hepatic artery, and bifurcation of the right and left hepatic arteries (Figs. 15-5 and 15-6). During this dissection, the portal structures are assessed for invasion by tumor (Fig. 15-7). Vascular reconstructions are not carried out for gallbladder cancer. If the patient has enlarged lymph nodes posterior to the head of the pancreas or along the aortocaval region, an extended Kocher maneuver is performed laparoscopically, and these lymph nodes are sampled first.

If the patient had a cholecystectomy previously and the cystic duct margin was assessed and negative for malignancy, the liver parenchymal dissection is initiated. If the cystic duct margin was not assessed in the previous operation, it is imperative that the cystic duct be identified, resected, and sent to pathology for frozen section (Fig. 15-8). A positive cystic duct margin warrants resection of the common bile duct with reconstruction to achieve negative margins, which can be done laparoscopically. When the cystic duct stump cannot be found, the procedure is converted to open. If the cystic duct still cannot be found,

resection of the common bile duct is then performed, followed by reconstruction.

Parenchymal Transection

Wedge resection of the gallbladder bed is begun by confirming the extent of resection with the laparoscopic ultrasound (Fig. 15-9). If the gallbladder is still present, it is left attached to the gallbladder fossa for en bloc resection. Before embarking on the hepatic parenchymal transection, it is paramount that the patient's central venous pressure be low. The patient should be given as little intravascular volume as possible before and during the procedure.

Hepatic parenchymal transection is performed with the ultrasonic shears in one hand and the laparoscopic bipolar device in the other. Glisson capsule is scored with the active blade of the ultrasonic shears or with the monopolar cautery. The assistant's role during parenchymal transection involves retraction and suction with the laparoscopic aspirator. Larger segmental branches in the hepatic parenchyma can be severed with the ultrasonic shears if they are smaller than 5 mm; if they are larger, they are clipped before their transection. The active blade of the ultrasonic shears can be used with the blades open to hasten

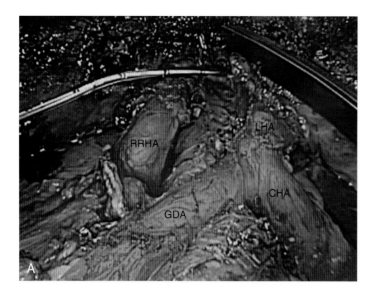

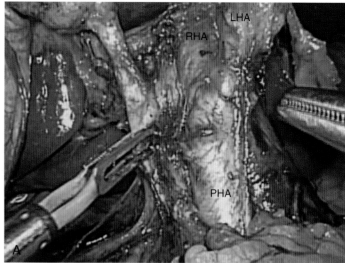

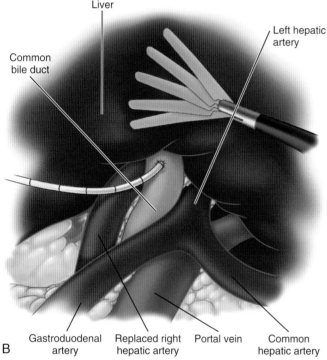

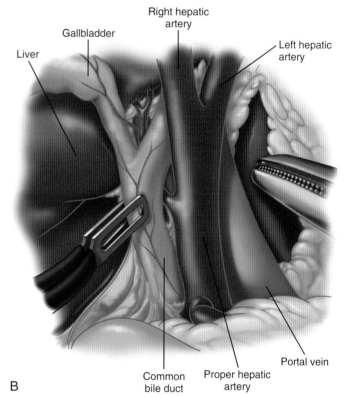

FIGURE 15-5 Patient with replaced right hepatic artery (RRHA); the common hepatic artery (CHA), gastroduodenal artery (GDA), and left hepatic artery (LHA) are also seen. A 5-French pediatric feeding tube has been placed in the patient's common bile duct and is used during the creation of the choledochojejunostomy to prevent inadvertent closure of the biliary tree. A laparoscopic liver retractor can also be seen in the upper right hand corner of the image.

FIGURE 15-6 The proper hepatic artery (PHA) and bifurcation of the right (RHA) and left hepatic arteries (LHA) are shown.

dissection around these intraparenchymal structures. The laparoscopic ultrasound can be used to identify the middle hepatic vein in the superior aspect of the gallbladder bed before transection.

The laparoscopic bipolar device helps to achieve hemostasis during parenchymal transection and also along the structures of the portal triad. Alternatively, topical hemostatic agents (Surgicel, Ethicon Biosurgery, Somerville, N.J.) are used to obtain hemostasis along the hepatic parenchyma or along the structures of the hepatoduodenal ligament. Sometimes, during the hepatic resection, holes are created deep into the parenchyma. These holes can be particularly difficult to control if they begin to bleed. Injectable expanding hemostatic agents (Surgiflo, Ethicon Biosurgery, Somerville, N.J.) can be useful to obtain hemostasis. For

patients who need to remain on antiplatelet therapy during the procedure, fibrin glue (Evicel, Ethicon Biosurgery, Somerville, N.J.) is placed along the raw edge of the hepatic parenchyma to reduce the risk for postoperative bleeding.

The specimen is then placed in a specimen retrieval bag and removed from the abdomen. It is sent to pathology for frozen section analysis of the cystic duct margin and hepatic parenchymal margins. Additional parenchymal margins are taken laparoscopically if pathology reveals a positive margin.

Choledochojejunostomy

If the cystic duct margin is positive for malignancy, a resection of the common duct can be performed laparoscopically. The common bile duct is dissected circumferentially and transected just below the confluence of the right and left hepatic ducts. The

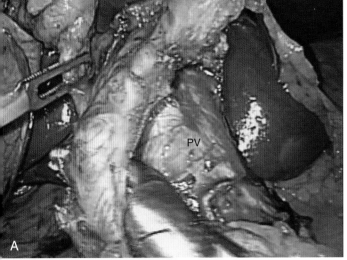

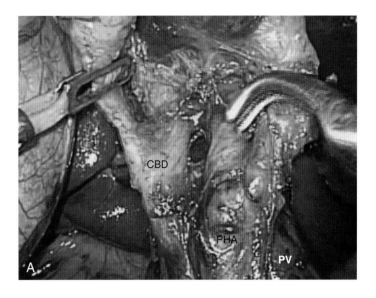

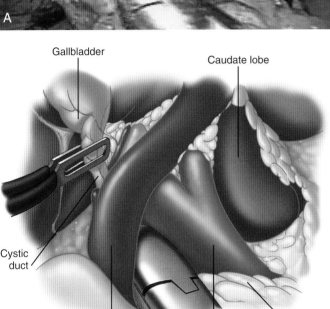

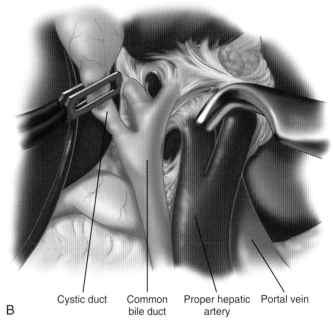

FIGURE 15-7 Laparoscopic hepatoduodenal lymphadenectomy. The portal vein (PV) is skeletonized and seen as it courses behind the hepatic artery.

FIGURE 15-8 The structures of the portal triad. The confluence of the common bile duct (CBD) and cystic duct are highlighted in green. The proper hepatic artery (PHA) and portal vein (PV) are also labeled.

free end of the common bile duct is grasped, retracted anteriorly and inferiorly, and transected at the most distal extrapancreatic portion of the duct using a laparoscopic vascular stapler. Alternatively, it can be oversewn laparoscopically. If frozen section analysis of the common bile duct reveals negative margins, reconstruction is done laparoscopically by a Roux-en-Y choledochojejunostomy. If the distal margin is positive, a pancreatoduodenectomy is performed. If the proximal margin is positive, both the right and left ducts are sampled and sent to pathology. If only one duct is positive, that corresponding hepatic lobe is removed. If both ducts are positive, then bilateral external transhepatic stents are placed for postoperative brachytherapy and right and left hepaticojejunostomies created. Unless the hepatic ducts are enlarged to at least 5 mm, these anastomoses should probably be done through open techniques.

To reconstruct the biliary tree, the ligament of Treitz is identified, and the small bowel is transected approximately 45 cm distal using a laparoscopic GIA stapler device (Tri-Staple, Covidien, Norwalk, Conn.). The Roux limb is positioned adjacent to the common bile duct to assess whether the anastomosis is tension free (Fig. 15-10). The jejunum can be further mobilized

by dividing a small portion of the mesentery using the ultrasonic shears. An enterotomy is made in the Roux limb using the ultrasonic shears. A 5-French pediatric feeding tube is placed across the biliary anastomosis to prevent inadvertent closure of the lumen during construction of the anastomosis. Posteriorly, a single running layer anastomosis is fashioned using a 3-0 or 4-0 absorbable suture. Care is taken to keep the knots extraluminal. The anterior layer of the anastomosis is created either in a running fashion for larger common bile ducts or using interrupted stitches for common bile ducts smaller than 5 mm.

The jejunojejunostomy is created using a laparoscopic linear stapler in a side-to-side fashion. The common enterotomy is closed with two layers of running 3-0 silk suture.

EXCISION OF PREVIOUS TROCAR SITES

When the use of a specimen retrieval bag cannot be confirmed from the previous operative report or upon discussions with the operating surgeons, or in cases in which bile leakage occurred,

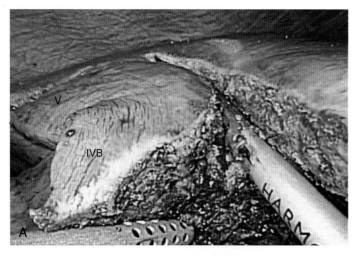

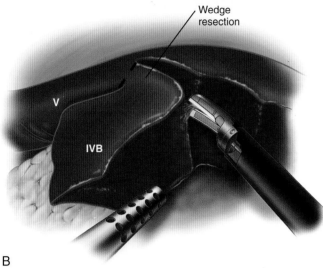

FIGURE 15-9 The hepatic parenchymal transection of the gallbladder bed (hepatic segments IVB and V) is performed with the ultrasonic shears.

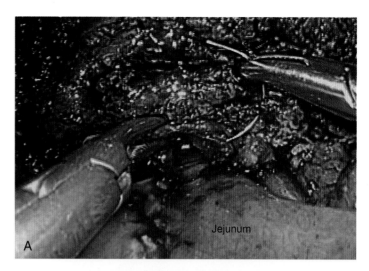

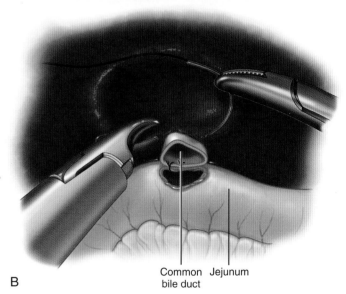

FIGURE 15-10 Laparoscopic choledochojejunostomy. The common bile duct and jejunum are shown as the anterior layer of the choledochojejunostomy is created.

the skin and fascia around the trocar used for specimen retrieval are excised. This site is then used for removal of the hepatic parenchymal specimen and closed with interrupted suture. The skin is closed with running monofilament absorbable suture. When the extraction site cannot be confirmed, all trocar sites are similarly excised and closed.

POSTOPERATIVE CARE

Patients are monitored overnight in the intensive care unit only if they have significant comorbidities or if there are concerns for postoperative hemorrhage. Low-molecular-weight heparin is started on the first postoperative day unless there are signs of bleeding or evidence of coagulopathy. If a significant amount of liver was resected, coagulation levels are checked for the first 3 postoperative days and low-molecular-weight heparin continued if these remain within normal limits. Phosphate levels are checked routinely in the postoperative phase because of the increased risk for phosphatemia after liver resection, which is due to liver regeneration. Liver function tests are checked only when there are concerns for hepatic failure.

Nasogastric tubes are discontinued on the first postoperative day unless residual drainage is greater than 250 mL over 4 hours. Early ambulation is encouraged, as is incentive spirometry. Diet is advanced as tolerated.

PROCEDURE-SPECIFIC COMPLICATIONS

Bleeding

The major source of bleeding during this procedure arises from injury to the middle hepatic vein during parenchymal transection of segments IVB and V. This can be avoided through the use of intraoperative ultrasonography to identify the location of the middle hepatic vein or other large intraparenchymal vessels such as segmental veins. If bleeding persists from the middle hepatic vein after transection, control is obtained with gentle pressure and use of a local hemostatic agent. Large veins encountered during parenchymal resection can be transected using either clips or a linear stapler with a vascular load.

Hepatic parenchymal bleeding is controlled with a combination of techniques, including the use of laparoscopic bipolar forceps, maintaining low central venous pressures during parenchymal transection, and meticulous dissection. The liver is inspected for bleeding after decreasing the pneumoperitoneal pressure.

As mentioned, topical hemostatic agents can reduce the risk for intraoperative or postoperative hemorrhage. Expanding topical agents can be used to obtain hemostasis in holes created in the hepatic parenchyma, and fibrin glue is used along the raw liver surface of patients on antiplatelet therapy. When a major hepatectomy is required, however, all antiplatelet medication is stopped.

Bile Leak

At the conclusion of hepatic resection, the transected liver surface should be inspected carefully for signs of bile drainage. Any areas of bile leak can be oversewn laparoscopically. Prevention of bile leak is through meticulous dissection and understanding of liver anatomy. Postoperative bilomas are treated with percutaneous drainage and endoscopic biliary stent placement. After common bile duct excisions, the Roux-en-Y choledochojejunostomy can be stented transhepatically.

PORT SITE RECURRENCE

It is well recognized that aerosolization of tumor cells can cause implantation of such cells at the trocar sites. This can be minimized with the evacuation of the pneumoperitoneum while the trocars are still in place. In addition, all specimens should be extracted through a wound protector or placed in a specimen retrieval bag before removal.

RESULTS AND OUTCOME

Although laparoscopic cholecystectomy is the accepted standard of care for T1a gallbladder cancer, with negative margins on final pathologic analysis and no intraoperative bile leak, the laparoscopic management of gallbladder cancer staged T1b to T3 remains controversial. The surgical goal is to achieve an R_0 oncologic outcome even if adjacent organ resection is required. As

surgeons continue to acquire and perfect their laparoscopic skills, and as technologic advancements in laparoscopic instrumentation and visualization modalities for liver resection come into play, laparoscopic radical cholecystectomy will ultimately replace open surgery.

Suggested Readings

Furlan A, Ferris JV, Hosseinzadeh K, Borhani AA: Gallbladder carcinoma update: multimodality imaging evaluation, staging and treatment options. *AJR Am J Roentgenol* 191:1440–1447, 2008.

Gumbs AA, Hoffman JP: Laparoscopic radical cholecystectomy and Roux-en-Y choledochojejunostomy for gallbladder cancer. *Surg Endosc* 24:1766–1768, 2010.

Gumbs AA, Hoffman: Laparoscopic completion radical cholecystectomy for T2 gallbladder cancer. *Surg Endosc* 24:3221–3223, 2010.

Gumbs AA, Milone L, Geha R, et al: Laparoscopic radical cholecystectomy. *J Laparoendosc Adv Surg Tech* 19:519–520, 2009.

Hueman MT, Vollmer CM, Pawlik TM: Evolving treatment strategies for gallbladder cancer. *Ann Surg Oncol* 16:2101–2115, 2009.

Shukla PJ, Barreto SG, Arya S, et al: Does PET-CT scan have a role prior to radical re-resection for incidental gallbladder cancer? *HPB (Oxford)* 10:439–445, 2008.

Shirai Y, Ohtani T, Tsukada K, et al: Combined pancreaticoduodenectomy and hepatectomy for patients with locally advanced gallbladder carcinoma: long term results. *Cancer* 80:1904–1909, 1997.

Shirai Y, Yoshida K, Tsukada K, et al: Identification of the regional lymphatic system of the gallbladder by vital staining. *Br J Surg* 79:659–662, 1992.

Shirai Y, Yoshida K, Tsukada K, et al: Radical surgery for gallbladder carcinoma: long-term results. *Ann Surg* 216:565–568, 1992.

Takasaki K, Kobayashi S, Muto H, et al: Our experiences (5 cases) of extended right lobectomy combined with pancreato-duodenectomy for the carcinoma of the gall bladder. *J Biliary Tract Pancreas* 1:923–932, 1980.

Tsukada K, Hatakeyama K, Kurosaki I, et al: Outcome of radical surgery for carcinoma of the gallbladder according to the TNM stage. *Surgery* 120:816–821, 1996.

Yamaguchi K, Chijiiwa K, Saiki S, et al: Retrospective analysis of 70 operations for gallbladder carcinoma. *Br J Surg* 84:200–204, 1997.

WAN YEE LAU, ERIC C. H. LAI, AND STEPHANIE HIU YAN LAU

Laparoscopic Cholecystectomy for Acute Cholecystitis

16

The videos associated with this chapter are listed in the Video Contents and can be found on the accompanying DVDs and on Expertconsult.com.

Although laparoscopic cholecystectomy is now the gold standard operation for symptomatic gallstones, its role in the management of acute cholecystitis has only been accepted in the past one to two decades. It is still considered a relative contraindication for some patients and for surgeons who are not experienced in laparoscopic surgery.

In acute calculous cholecystitis, acute inflammation can result in considerable distortion of the biliary and vascular anatomy, putting the common bile duct and the hepatic artery at a higher risk for injury. This distortion is especially prominent around the triangle of Calot, where a stone is usually impacted at the cystic duct, causing distention and thickening of the gallbladder. Edema, as a consequence of inflammation, makes the dissection of the triangle of Calot difficult. The cystic duct might become so edematous and thickened that it cannot be secured with the standard clips used for elective laparoscopic cholecystectomy. Also, if the inflammation resolves rapidly after gallbladder removal, the clips might loosen and become dislodged. Therefore, alternative methods like using an Endoloop (Ethicon Biosurgery, Cincinnati, Ohio), suturing, or a linear stapler may have to be considered in these situations. In severe cases, the cystic duct and the cystic artery may not be visualized. The greater omentum and sometimes the adjacent organs such as the duodenum and the colon become adherent to the inflamed gallbladder. These structures are highly friable because of the inflammation and can be easily injured if handled without care. The inflamed gallbladder often proves difficult to grasp and maneuver because the tissues are too edematous and friable, or the gallbladder may simply be too distended to allow the grasping forceps to obtain an adequate grip. The acutely inflamed gallbladder is also more easily torn, resulting in bile or stone spillage.

Bleeding is a common reason for conversion from laparoscopic to open surgery, either because the laparoscopic view is obscured or because the bleeding cannot be stopped laparoscopically. There are many potential sources of intraoperative bleeding. Torn mesenteric or omental vessels may occur during dissection of inflammatory adhesions away from the gallbladder and ductal structures. Bleeding can also arise from an injured or torn cystic artery because of the difficult dissection. Often, the most difficult to avoid is bleeding from the gallbladder fossa. These injuries occur because it is difficult to dissect the posterior wall of the inflamed gallbladder from the gallbladder fossa and to adequately coagulate the small vessels within the liver bed. Bile leaks may also occur in the gallbladder fossa if the dissection has been carried out too deeply into the liver. Finally, extraction of the gallbladder specimen from the peritoneal cavity can be difficult because of the thickened gallbladder wall.

The pathophysiology in the initiation of acute calculous cholecystitis is believed to be due to obstruction to the cystic duct by a stone. This causes distention of the gallbladder and stretching of the gallbladder wall. This stimulates the synthesis of prostaglandins I_2 and E_2, which mediate the inflammatory response, resulting in chemical cholecystitis with inflammation and edema. Secondary bacterial infection with enteric organisms (most commonly *Escherichia coli*, *Klebsiella* species, and *Streptococcus faecalis*) sets in usually after 2 to 3 days if the attack of acute cholecystitis is not resolved. This can further progress to gangrenous changes and perforation of the gallbladder. The omentum usually adheres to the gangrenous or perforated site, and the infection is confined. At times, when the omentum fails to contain the gangrenous and perforated site, bile peritonitis follows. If untreated, the patient develops septicemia.

The pathogenesis of acute acalculous cholecystitis is a paradigm of complexity. Ischemia and reperfusion injury, or the effects of eicosanoid proinflammatory mediators, appear to be the central mechanisms. Bile stasis, gallbladder distention due to prolonged fasting, total parenteral nutrition, opioid therapy, and positive-pressure ventilation have all been implicated. Patients who are hypotensive, old, or diabetic and those who are immunocompromised are especially prone to developing this condition.

OPERATIVE INDICATIONS

Diagnosis of Acute Calculous Cholecystitis

The presumptive diagnosis of acute calculous cholecystitis is based mainly on clinical grounds, with fever, persistent right upper quadrant abdominal pain, tenderness, and guarding in the right upper abdomen and a positive Murphy sign. These patients should be admitted to a hospital and investigated further. Routine blood tests show leukocytosis with a white cell count usually greater than $10,000/mm^3$. Liver function tests usually show normal bilirubin and alkaline phosphatase. Abdominal ultrasound should be a routine investigation carried out soon after hospital admission. The sensitivity and specificity of ultrasound are 85% and 95%, respectively, for diagnosing acute cholecystitis, and normal liver function tests and a normal common bile duct on ultrasonographic examination would effectively rule out choledocholithiasis. An ultrasound diagnosis of acute cholecystitis is made with the following findings:

- Presence of gallstones with a distended gallbladder
- Thickened gallbladder wall
- Pericholecystic fluid (double-wall sign)
- Positive ultrasonic Murphy's sign

Note that these ultrasonic signs should be interpreted carefully and should be taken together and interpreted with the clinical presentations of the patient. The presence of gallbladder stones alone without the other ultrasonic and clinical features of acute cholecystitis might suggest that the patient is suffering from an attack of biliary colic. The presence of gallbladder sludge is nonspecific and may be observed during prolonged fasting and during parenteral nutrition. Gallbladder distention may be present in the setting of prolonged fasting, parenteral nutrition, prior vagotomy, or distal common bile duct obstruction. It may not be present when prior inflammation and fibrosis limit the distensibility of the gallbladder. The finding of pericholecystic fluid alone is not sensitive in diagnosing acute cholecystitis, and it may even be absent in the early stages of inflammation. It is also nonspecific and may occur in patients with pancreatitis, ascites, or peritonitis. A positive sonographic Murphy's sign is very specific for acute cholecystitis, but it can still be masked by the heavy use of narcotics. A combined use of the clinical features, ultrasound, and laboratory testing would give an accuracy rate of more than 95% in diagnosing acute cholecystitis.

In case of doubt, computed tomography (CT) can be added to improve the diagnostic accuracy. The CT features of acute cholecystitis include a distended gallbladder with thickened wall, pericholecystic inflammatory changes, and fluid. Gallstones may or may not be visualized. Transient hepatic attenuation difference in the adjacent liver, especially with the use of intravenous contrast, may be detected because of the hyperemia caused by the adjacent inflammation. Biliary scintigraphy can also be used to enhance the accuracy rate of acute cholecystitis.

The finding of common bile stones in patients with acute cholecystitis is extremely uncommon. Patients who have a strong suspicion of associated choledocholithiasis, including patients with dilated common bile duct on ultrasonography, abnormal liver function with elevated bilirubin and/or alkaline phosphatase, and elevated pancreatic enzymes (i.e., amylase or lipase) should be further investigated with magnetic resonance cholangiopancreatography or endoscopic retrograde cholangiopancreatography (ERCP). The management of patients with associated choledocholithiasis is beyond the scope of this chapter.

Diagnosis of Acute Acalculous Cholecystitis

Acute acalculous cholecystitis accounts for 5% to 14% of all cases of acute cholecystitis. It develops in critically ill, aged patients or patients who have severe multitrauma. However, the development of acute acalculous cholecystitis is not limited to severely ill patients or patients who are treated in the intensive care unit. There is an association between acute acalculous cholecystitis and patients with diabetes, malignant disease, abdominal vasculitis, congestive heart failure, atherosclerotic disease, shock, and cardiac arrest. In children, it is associated with a postviral attack.

The mortality rate approaches 50%, and death is due to delay in diagnosis in a poor-risk patient. The clinical diagnosis can be difficult in severely ill patients. Ultrasonographic diagnosis of acute acalculous cholecystitis in critically ill patients is controversial, and there is evidence that ultrasound may not be a reliable routine screening tool for acute acalculous cholecystitis. The role of laparoscopic surgery is also controversial. In a high surgical risk patient, however, early diagnosis with rapid intervention is crucial in managing this disease if outcomes are to be improved. Percutaneous cholecystostomy appears to be a logical treatment for those patients who have no evidence of gallbladder perforation and bile peritonitis. If the diagnosis is made late with bile peritonitis, open cholecystectomy may be the preferred treatment for critically ill patients.

The remainder of this chapter concentrates only on laparoscopic cholecystectomy for acute calculous cholecystitis.

PREOPERATIVE EVALUATION, TESTING, AND PREPARATION

The patient is well hydrated, and any electrolyte imbalances are corrected. Broad-spectrum antibiotics (usually a second-generation cephalosporin) are administered, the pain is alleviated, and the patient is kept NPO. A nasogastric tube is used if there is evidence of ileus; otherwise, a nasogastric tube is inserted during surgery after induction of general anesthesia. Cardiopulmonary workup is carried out in those patients who have a past history of heart or lung diseases, and correction of associated morbidities (e.g., diabetes and hypertension) is done. A thorough explanation of the diagnosis and the various therapeutic alternatives are discussed with the patient.

CHOICE OF THERAPIES

The gold standard of treatment for a low-risk patient with acute cholecystitis is cholecystectomy, either early or delayed. However, for patients who are critically ill and those who are too frail or too old for cholecystectomy, ultrasound- or CT-guided percutaneous cholecystostomy is an effective treatment, without any evidence of gallbladder perforation and bile peritonitis. Percutaneous cholecystostomy can be used as a definitive treatment or as a temporizing measure in critically ill patients, allowing for delayed definitive surgical treatment when the patient's condition improves.

Laparoscopic versus Open Cholecystectomy for Acute Cholecystitis

Studies have shown that laparoscopic cholecystectomy, carried out in experienced hands, offers significant advantages compared with open cholecystectomy in terms of morbidity, hospital stay, and return to normal activity. The quality of life after laparoscopic cholecystectomy is excellent, which includes physical activities and social function.

Timing of Laparoscopic Cholecystectomy: Early versus Delayed

The controversy over the optimal timing for laparoscopic cholecystectomy in patients with acute cholecystitis has now been more settled because recent studies have shown that early laparoscopic surgery has advantages over delayed surgery. Until

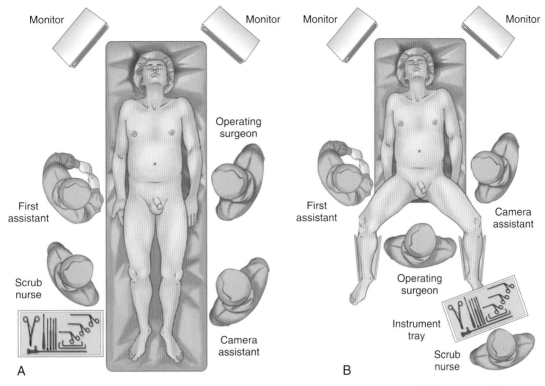

FIGURE 16-1 **A,** Operating room layout with the patient in supine position. **B,** Operating room layout with the patient in lithotomy position.

recently, the management of a patient with acute cholecystitis was nonoperative as far as possible, and an interval cholecystectomy was to be carried out 4 to 6 weeks after the acute cholecystitis had settled down with conservative treatment. Randomized comparative studies have shown that early laparoscopic cholecystectomy by experienced surgeons results in better outcomes than delayed laparoscopic cholecystectomy (4 to 6 weeks later). These recent studies have also shown that the optimal timing for laparoscopic cholecystectomy in patients with acute cholecystitis is within 2 to 3 days of onset of symptoms. A delay in laparoscopic cholecystectomy of more than 48 hours (in some studies, 72 hours) increases the difficulty of the operation and results in a higher conversion rate to open surgery. The main aim of early intervention is to operate during the edema phase when the tissues are easily separable and the tissue planes are better visualized. Increased vascularity, adhesions, fibrosis, and sometimes gangrene and perforation are encountered in delayed surgery; all these factors account for the increase in conversion rate. A patient with acute cholecystitis who is fit for surgery should be treated as a semi-emergency and operated on within 24 hours of hospital admission.

POSITIONING AND PLACEMENT OF TROCARS

The patient may be placed in either the supine or lithotomy position. The operating room setup and the patient positioning are depicted in Figure 16-1.

General endotracheal anesthesia is induced, and the nasogastric and urinary catheters are inserted. Sequential compression devices for prevention of deep venous thrombosis are used routinely.

Pneumoperitoneum is established using the open Hasson technique through a small subumbilical incision. After the insertion of the umbilical port, pneumoperitoneum is established

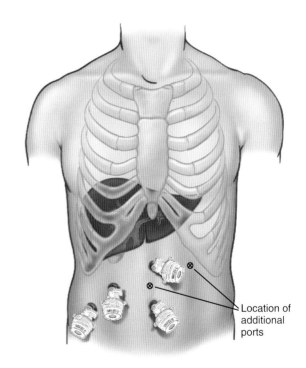

FIGURE 16-2 Location of commonly used and additional ports.

and pressure is kept at 10 mm Hg. A 30-degree-view laparoscope is introduced with an attached video camera, and the peritoneal cavity is examined. The three accessory trocars are then inserted through the abdominal wall under laparoscopic guidance. Sometimes it is necessary to insert a fifth trocar to obtain adequate exposure. The location of the ports is shown in Figure 16-2.

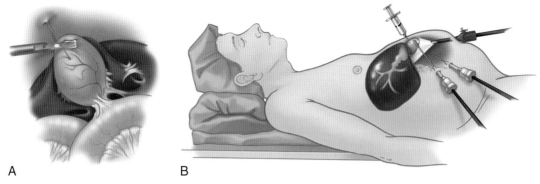

A   B

FIGURE 16-3 Percutaneous decompression of a distended gallbladder with a needle.

OPERATIVE TECHNIQUES

Laparoscopic cholecystectomy for acute cholecystitis is technically more difficult than elective cholecystectomy for symptomatic gallstones, and it should only be carried out by surgeons who are experienced in laparoscopic surgery. The technique varies with the level of the technical difficulty.

Usual Acute Cholecystitis

This is the most commonly encountered scenario. The acutely inflamed gallbladder is usually covered by the greater omentum. When the gallbladder is completely covered, the initial approach is to identify the gallbladder wall. The gallbladder is identified easily when the dissection is commenced on the medial wall of the gallbladder adjacent to the liver. Dissection can be commenced using a blunt-tipped suction nozzle. Dense or vascular adhesions are controlled with short bursts of monopolar cautery energy and then sharply dissected. Special care must be taken when separating the inflamed gallbladder from the colon and duodenum to avoid mechanical or thermal injuries to these structures. Placing the patient in a 20- to 30-degree reverse Trendelenburg and 20- to 30-degree left-tilt position will help to better identify the gallbladder.

After freeing the fundus of the gallbladder of all adhesions, the fundus is grasped and retracted cephalad toward the right shoulder of the patient in a manner similar to that used for simple cholecystectomy. Unfortunately, the inflamed gallbladder often proves difficult to grasp and hold with a routine 5-mm grasper. In this situation, 10-mm atraumatic forceps may be required to allow for a secure grip and retraction. If the gallbladder is tensely distended, it should be decompressed before further attempts to retract it with atraumatic forceps. Decompression can be accomplished using a 16-gauge or larger angiocatheter introduced percutaneously into the dome of the gallbladder (Fig. 16-3). The puncture site can then be occluded by applying a grasping forceps over it (Fig. 16-4) or with a suture (Fig. 16-5).

The greater omentum is further freed from the gallbladder until the gallbladder is fully exposed. Attention should then be paid to dissecting the triangle of Calot. If the triangle of Calot is difficult to dissect because of inflammation and edema, dissection should start on the lateral lower aspect of the gallbladder using a combination of electrocautery and ultrasonic instruments. This approach allows for safe mobilization of the lateral lower third of the gallbladder and exposes the cystic duct–common duct junction. In a difficult cholecystectomy, the gallbladder should then be freed from the liver bed on the medial

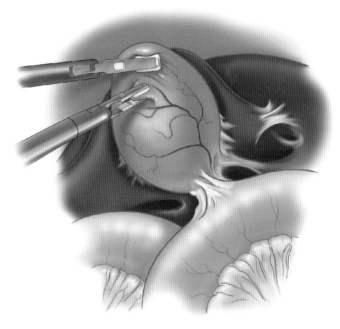

FIGURE 16-4 The puncture site is occluded with the grasping forceps.

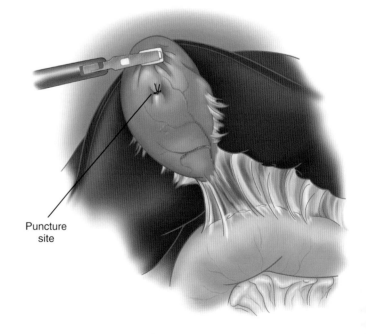

Puncture site

FIGURE 16-5 The puncture site is suture closed.

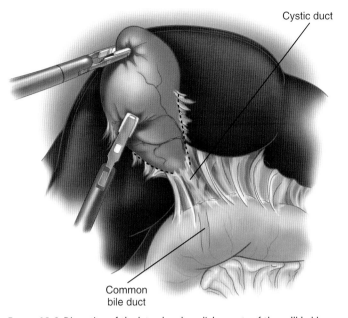

FIGURE 16-6 Dissection of the lateral and medial aspects of the gallbladder.

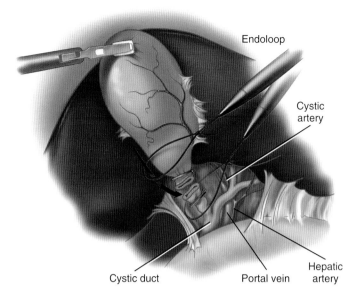

FIGURE 16-7 Division of the cystic duct between clips and ligation of the cystic duct stump with a pre-tied laparoscopic suture.

side by using a similar method of dissection (Fig. 16-6). The division of the peritoneal reflection of the medial and lateral aspects of the gallbladder allows for mobilization of the infundibulum and facilitates the safe dissection and identification of the cystic duct and artery.

The use of intraoperative cholangiography in laparoscopic cholecystectomy for acute cholecystitis is still controversial. The authors do not routinely perform intraoperative cholangiography because the incidence of choledocholithiasis is very low in patients with acute cholecystitis. They resort to investigating patients with high risks for choledocholithiasis preoperatively by using magnetic resonance cholangiopancreatography or ERCP and planning treatment for these patients according to the preoperative findings. Intraoperative cholangiography, however, is imperative in those cases in which the anatomy is in doubt and in patients with impacted stone at the cystic duct or elevated liver function tests.

The main trunk and the anterior and the posterior branches of the cystic artery are carefully identified. The cystic artery is divided after clipping with Hem-o-lok clips (Weck Pilling, Research Triangle Park, N.C.). An atraumatic forceps is used to milk the impacted stone at the cystic duct back into the gallbladder. The standard clips used in elective cholecystectomy are usually not suitable for acute cholecystitis because of the inflammation and edema. Two large laparoscopic Hem-o-lok clips are used to ligate the cystic duct. The cystic duct is divided between the Hem-o-lok clips, and an Endoloop is placed around the cystic duct stump and tightened in the cystic duct stump as shown in Figure 16-7. Alternatively, a linear stapler may be used for the secure ligation and division of the thickened and inflamed cystic duct.

In some cases, the cystic artery may not be visible because of the inflammation and edema. In such cases, it may be necessary to divide the cystic duct before gaining control of the artery. However, the operating surgeon needs to be very careful because the cystic artery or one of its branches may be torn or avulsed after the cystic duct is divided. This is one of the most common causes of significant intraoperative bleeding during emergent laparoscopic cholecystectomy.

The gallbladder is then dissected from the liver bed. The dissection is again best carried out using a combination of electrocautery and ultrasonic instruments as described previously. It is useful to carry out the "right-left twist" to expose the medial and lateral aspects of the gallbladder (Fig. 16-8).

In acute cholecystitis, the inflamed gallbladder is friable, and it is easily torn. A tear into the gallbladder should be controlled as rapidly as possible. If the tear is small, it can be controlled by simply reapplying the same forceps over the puncture site. Large tears require closure with either an Endoloop or a suture (Fig. 16-9).

Stones that have dropped into the peritoneal cavity should be retrieved if possible. Small stones can be aspirated with an irrigation-suction cannula. Large stones can be retrieved using a bag (Endobag, Covidien, Norwalk, Conn.).

Before complete dissection of the gallbladder from the liver, the peritoneal cavity should be copiously irrigated with saline and the operative field examined for any signs of persistent bleeding or bile leaks, which should be properly dealt with. The authors usually place a drain in the subhepatic space after completely detaching the gallbladder from the liver. The gallbladder specimen is then placed inside a specimen bag, and the specimen is extracted through the umbilical wound.

Difficult Acute Cholecystitis

There are multiple reasons why laparoscopic cholecystectomy for acutely inflamed gallbladder is technically more difficult than elective cholecystectomy for simple cholelithiasis, which have been outlined in the introduction. It should be emphasized that the purpose of laparoscopic cholecystectomy, compared with open cholecystectomy, is to hasten convalescence and cause less pain. These goals must not be substituted for safety. If intraoperative progress is slow and dubious, if the anatomy of the biliary tree is uncertain, and if there is a feeling of uneasiness and uncertainty, conversion to open cholecystectomy is in order. The decision to convert to open surgery should be viewed as a good clinical judgment, rather than a failure. The following technical laparoscopic approaches can be applied to deal with some

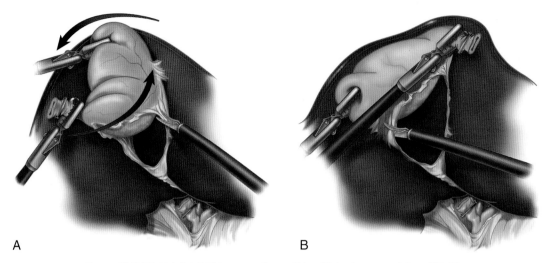

A   B

FIGURE 16-8 "Right-left twist" to expose the medial and lateral aspects of the gallbladder.

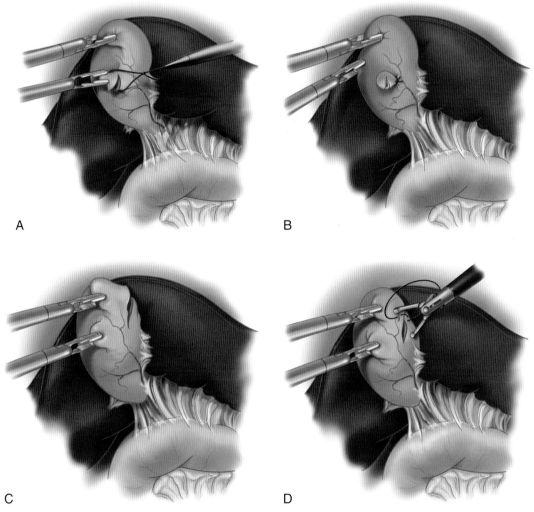

A   B

C   D

FIGURE 16-9 Large tears in the gallbladder are closed with pre-tied laparoscopic suture or suturing.

particular situations encountered in a difficult laparoscopic cholecystectomy for acute cholecystitis.

Bleeding

Meticulous and gentle dissection of the gallbladder from the surrounding tissues and from the liver bed is important to avoid excessive bleeding. Often the most difficult source of bleeding comes from the gallbladder fossa. Any bleeding should be controlled immediately rather than waiting until the entire operative field is obscured by blood. The judicious use of electrocautery and ultrasonic energy devices can reduce bleeding from the gallbladder fossa during dissection of the gallbladder from the liver. Although some surgeons find laser to be useful on the raw liver bed left after cholecystectomy, we find compression to be very useful in achieving hemostasis in the gallbladder fossa. A 2- × 2-inch laparoscopic gauze with radiopaque thread can be used. Compression is achieved by the surgeon's left hand holding a forceps with the gauze at the tip. This forceps with the gauze can be used to push the liver upward for better exposure of the gallbladder fossa. The right hand is free to insert the irrigation-suction device to make sure that the area is clean. A hemostatic tool can be used to replace the irrigation-suction device to ensure hemostasis using the right hand, and usually a monopolar electrocautery is enough to control the bleeding point.

For control of bleeding from a main named vessel, the surgeon should never attempt to clip a bleeding major vessel blindly within a pool of blood because damage to adjacent vital structures can occur. Simple compression with a 2- × 2-inch gauze sometimes is helpful. If compression is useless, the bleeding site and its surrounding area can be compressed with the gentle application of the jaws of an atraumatic clamp. The same procedure as mentioned earlier is then followed: cleaning, aspiration, irrigation, and application of either a clip or electrocautery, depending on the situation, after the bleeding site is clearly identified.

Hostile Triangle of Calot

It is sometimes difficult to dissect the inflamed and edematous structures within the triangle of Calot. A stroking or twisting motion with a cherry swab stick may prove very helpful. This stick helps to separate and expose the tissue planes surrounding the cystic duct and artery. If the cystic duct and artery are not easily dissected free from the surrounding tissues, the only remaining alternatives are retrograde laparoscopic cholecystectomy or conversion to open cholecystectomy.

Retrograde cholecystectomy (fundus-first cholecystectomy) is carried out by putting traction and countertraction on the gallbladder and liver to provide the necessary exposure. The gallbladder is dissected from the fundus to the infundibulum using the electrocautery unit or an ultrasonic energy device. This procedure leaves the cystic duct and the cystic artery as the last two structures remaining to be identified and secured (Fig. 16-10).

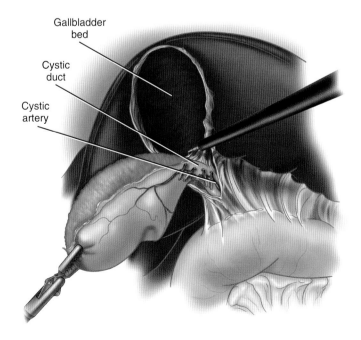

Gallbladder bed

Cystic duct

Cystic artery

FIGURE 16-10 Retrograde laparoscopic cholecystectomy (fundus to infundibulum laparoscopic cholecystectomy).

Thickened Cystic Duct

In acute cholecystitis with a cystic duct impacted with a stone, the inflammation and edema can be so severe that even after milking the impacted stone back into the gallbladder, the cystic duct is too large to be secured with an endoscopic clip. One solution is retrograde laparoscopic cholecystectomy, after which the cystic duct is ligated using an Endoloop both proximal and distal. The cystic duct can then be divided between the ligatures without spillage of the contents from the gallbladder. Alternatively, a linear stapler-cutter can be used.

POSTOPERATIVE CARE

The postoperative management of laparoscopic cholecystectomy for acute cholecystitis is quite straightforward. If there is no ileus before the surgery and if the patient is hemodynamically stable, the nasogastric tube and the urinary catheter can be removed at the end of the surgery. The drain is usually removed on the first postoperative day, and the patient is discharged home on the second or the third postoperative day when the patient is afebrile and tolerating a normal diet. If the drainage is bilious, it is prudent to delay removal of the drain until the source of bile leak has been identified and controlled.

COMPLICATIONS—PREVENTION AND MANAGEMENT

The complication rates for laparoscopic cholecystectomy for acute cholecystitis are definitely higher than for simple symptomatic cholelithiasis. The common major specific complications after laparoscopic cholecystectomy for acute cholecystitis are discussed next.

Bile Leaks

Because acute cholecystitis is associated with edematous inflamed and friable tissue, there is an increased risk for bile leaks. There can also be accidental tearing of tissues during the dissection. Thermal injury to the bile duct wall or injury to the intrahepatic bile ducts due to deep dissection into the liver parenchyma may result in bile leaks. It is advisable to aspirate any collection of bile in the operative field and to address the bile leaks appropriately during surgery.

Postoperatively, bile leaks can result in biliary peritonitis. A drain is usually placed in acute cholecystitis so that any bile leak can be identified early and investigated. Bile leaks can also be due to injury to an aberrant biliary anatomy or injury to the common bile duct, which is the most dreaded complication of laparoscopic cholecystectomy. Proper identification of the anatomy, attention to details in the surgical technique including the avoidance of excessive dissection, excessive traction to the cystic duct, and excessive use of electrocautery are means to prevent common bile duct injury. When the surgeon is faced with a phlegmonous gallbladder and with an uncertain anatomy, an intraoperative cholangiography may be considered. Bile leaks from the cystic duct are possible, especially in cases with wide edematous cystic ducts where clips are placed. This can be effectively prevented by applying Endoloops or by the use of staplers as previously described. ERCP with sphincterotomy to decompress the biliary system is the most common approach to deal with this complication and is usually successful.

Bleeding

Diffuse oozing is usually encountered from the liver bed during dissection, and adequate hemostasis should be ensured at the end of the operation. If the patient continues to bleed postoperatively, the usual sites of bleeding are (1) the omentum after adhesiolysis, (2) the cystic artery, (3) major vascular injury, such as common hepatic or right hepatic artery, and (4) gallbladder bed. The treatment is close monitoring, correction of coagulopathy, and replacement of lost blood. If bleeding continues, reoperation is necessary. Laparoscopic exploration may be used as the initial attempt to identify the location of the bleeding and manage it. If the bleeding site cannot be identified or the bleeding rate is too fast, a laparotomy is necessary.

Septic Complications

Intraperitoneal abscess usually is a result of infection of a collection of bile or blood. Treatment is antibiotics and drainage (either percutaneous under ultrasound guidance or with open surgery). Infection commonly occurs in the umbilical wound where the gallbladder specimen is retrieved.

To avoid such complications, stones spilled into the peritoneal cavity are removed, and the infected gallbladder is exteriorized in a retrieval bag. The peritoneal cavity is profusely irrigated after completion of the procedure.

RESULTS AND OUTCOME

Various studies have shown that laparoscopic cholecystectomy is safe and effective for the management of acute cholecystitis. The overall reported complication rate is about 20%, and the mortality rate ranges from 0 to 0.9% The common bile duct injury rate is 0.3% to 0.6% for noninflamed gallbladder, but a higher incidence of 1.5% has been reported for laparoscopic cholecystectomy for acute cholecystitis. The rates of conversion to open surgery for acute cholecystitis operated within and after 72 hours of onset of symptoms were 12% and 30%, respectively, emphasizing the importance of an early operation.

In conclusion, laparoscopic cholecystectomy can be carried out safely in patients with acute cholecystitis, provided the surgeon is experienced in laparoscopic surgery. The surgeon should maintain a low threshold for conversion to open surgery.

Suggested Readings

Frantzides CT, Carlson MA, Luu M: Laparoscopic cholecystectomy. In Frantzides CT, Carlson MA, editors: *Atlas of Minimally Invasive Surgery*, Philadelphia, 2009, Saunders, pp 155–159.

Glavic Z, Begic L, Simlesa D, et al: Treatment of acute cholecystitis: A comparison of open vs laparoscopic cholecystectomy. *Surg Endosc* 15:398–401, 2001.

Kiviluoto T, Sirén J, Luukkonen P, et al: Randomized trial of laparoscopic versus open cholecystectomy for acute and gangrenous cholecystitis. *Lancet* 351:321–325, 1998.

Kum CK, Eypasch E, Lefering R, et al: Laparoscopic cholecystectomy for acute cholecystitis. Is it really safe? *World J Surg* 20:43–48, 1996.

Lai PB, Kwong KH, Leung KL, et al: Randomized trial of early versus delayed laparoscopic cholecystectomy for acute cholecystitis. *Br J Surg* 85:764–767, 1998.

Lo CM, Liu CL, Lai EC, et al: Early versus delayed laparoscopic cholecystectomy for treatment of acute cholecystitis. *Ann Surg* 223:37–42, 1996.

Mahmud S, Masaud M, Canna K: Fundus-first laparoscopic cholecystectomy. *Surg Endosc* 16:581–584, 2002.

Petelin JB: Laparoscopic common bile duct exploration and intraoperative cholangiography. In Frantzides CT, Carlson MA, editors: *Atlas of Minimally Invasive Surgery*, Philadelphia, 2009, Saunders, pp 161–167.

Serralta AS, Bueno JL, Planells MR, et al: Prospective evaluation of emergency versus delayed laparoscopic cholecystectomy for early cholecystitis. *Surg Laparosc Endosc Percutan Tech* 13:71–75, 2003.

ROBERT C. G. MARTIN II, CHARLES R. ST. HILL, AND RUSSELL E. BROWN

Laparoscopic Liver Resection

17

The videos associated with this chapter are listed in the Video Contents and can be found on the accompanying DVDs and *on Expertconsult.com.*

Hepatic resection for metastatic disease has been practiced for decades. Lortat-Jacob described right hepatectomy for secondary malignancy in 1952. Initial anecdotal success has been followed by continued improvements in survival. The progressive success of colorectal liver metastasis resection can be attributed to improvements in multimodality therapy, including systemic chemotherapy and targeted therapies, as well as efforts to increase the proportion of patients eligible for resection. Additional improvements in surgical and anesthetic techniques, as well as postoperative care, have made hepatic surgeries safe at specialized centers.

Laparoscopic liver resections have been reported since 1992, with formal anatomic resections described in 1996. In contrast to many intra-abdominal procedures, the laparoscopic approach to hepatic resection has been adopted more cautiously. This is largely a result of concerns regarding difficulty in liver mobilization, parenchymal transaction, the perceived risks for hemorrhage, and the size of the specimen to be exteriorized. Carbon dioxide gas embolism, tumor dissemination, and inferior oncologic results were also among early fears. However, hepatobiliary units are increasingly reporting success with this approach. Their patients have benefited from a reduction in blood loss, reduced postoperative morbidities, and shorter hospital stay with equivalent rates of negative margins. Careful analysis of outcomes and establishment of training paradigms are necessary to benefit the population at large. With this, there is expected growth in the use of laparoscopic liver resection for benign, malignant, and transplantation applications.

This chapter focuses on laparoscopic liver resection from the perspective of metastatic disease because this is the most common indication for the general surgeon. The principles discussed can be applied to resection for other causes. The laparoscopic technique for right hepatectomy is described in detail in this chapter; the same principles, however, apply to other anatomic resections.

OPERATIVE INDICATIONS

The Louisville Statement, based on an international consensus meeting, concluded that laparoscopic liver resection is well accepted for solitary lesions measuring 5 cm or less that are located in segments 2 to 6. Multiple lesions, larger lesions, and those in the more challenging segments 1, 7, and 8 may also be resected; however, this should be limited to specialized centers and surgeons with significant experience in this field.

In considering the types of lesions amenable to resection, there are many, including benign and malignant neoplasms. Hepatic adenomas, when large, symptomatic, or with concerning features on imaging studies, can be resected using laparoscopic techniques. Adenomas larger than 4 cm may have increased risk for hemorrhage and are appropriate for resection. If the tumor is smaller than 4 cm but causing significant symptoms, it can also be resected. Because of the low malignant potential of a small symptomatic lesion, ablation techniques should also be considered in their management.

Several series have reported results equivalent to open resection for both hepatocellular carcinoma and colorectal liver metastasis. Hepatic resection, when feasible, is the only treatment associated with long-term survival. Based on a review of actual 10-year survivors who underwent resection before 1994 (i.e., before the use of "modern" chemotherapy), we can postulate current 10-year survival in at least one out of six patients after resection of colorectal liver metastasis.

Laparoscopic live-donor hepatectomy is becoming more prevalent but remains controversial. This should be performed only by experienced surgeons and under the auspices of a worldwide registry.

ALTERNATIVE THERAPIES

One of the most widely accepted nonresection techniques for addressing hepatic tumors is local tumor ablation. The rationale underlying the use of local ablative therapies for metastatic colorectal cancer rests largely on the observed survival benefit after resection of colorectal liver metastasis, and three theoretical concepts: (1) tumor consolidation, (2) oligometastases, and (3) the Norton-Simon hypothesis. After highly effective systemic therapy, micrometastases are eradicated, leaving behind stable macrometastatic tumor burden. This concept, known as *tumor consolidation,* leads to the thought that elimination of this "consolidated" tumor may yield a survival benefit. The oligometastases theory assumes that a subgroup of patients are identified to have a focal area of metastatic disease that is not yet widely disseminated. This subgroup may benefit from complete ablation of this metastatic focus. Finally, the Norton-Simon hypothesis states that effectiveness of chemotherapeutics is proportional to tumor growth rate. Decreasing the overall tumor burden by "debulking" will result in a smaller volume of more rapidly dividing metastatic cells that are more chemosensitive.

Nonresectional liver-directed therapies can be broadly categorized as catheter based (e.g. transarterial chemoembolization, drug-eluting bead therapy, and radioembolization) or intraparenchymal ablative techniques. The two most widely used intraparenchymal ablative modalities for colorectal liver metastasis by surgeons are radiofrequency ablation (RFA) and microwave ablation (MWA). A discussion of cryoablation and of emerging ablative technologies (e.g., laser interstitial thermal therapy, irreversible electroporation, and high-intensity focused ultrasound) is also included.

Hyperthermic Ablative Technologies

Modern hyperthermic ablative technologies rely on exposure of tumors to supranormal temperatures to ablate intrahepatic tumors. This takes advantage of the tumor's inability to dissipate heat by augmenting blood flow that is found in healthy tissues. In contrast to cryotherapy, which is used for tumors that are more resistant to freezing than normal cells, malignant cells are more sensitive to hyperthermic damage than normal cells.

For most tumors, exposure to temperatures above 42° C results in low-level thermal injury, with more effectiveness noted with increased exposure time and temperature. At progressively higher temperatures, there is an exponential and inverse relationship between treatment temperature and the exposure time needed to achieve cell death; thus, higher treatment temperatures require less exposure time for successful ablation. Temperatures above 60° C lead to cell death through complex interactions involving apoptosis, microvascular damage, ischemia-reperfusion injury, Kupffer cell activation, altered cytokine expression, alterations in the immune response, RNA and DNA destruction, dissolution of lipid bilayers, and protein denaturation. Thermal coagulation begins in the range of 70° C, and tissue desiccation occurs at about 100° C.

Radiofrequency Ablation

RFA achieves local hyperthermia using high-frequency alternating electric current in the radiofrequency range (100 to 500 kHz). Local hyperthermia results from ionic vibration and frictional heating of surrounding tissues. RFA gained popularity in the 1990s and serves as the prototypical ablation platform for most clinicians today.

Radiofrequency current is applied through an electrode that is deployed within the tumor, using ultrasound, computed tomography (CT), or magnetic resonance imaging (MRI) guidance. RFA probes were initially developed as single-needle electrodes but have evolved to multiprobe and internally cooled arrays with attendant increases in treatment volumes and more reliable geometric ablation zones. Several devices are marketed worldwide, and none has emerged as superior with regard to ablation size, reproducibility, or local tumor control.

Percutaneous, laparoscopic, and open surgical approaches have been successfully used for RFA treatment, each with inherent advantages and disadvantages. The choice of approach should be individualized based on tumor anatomy, extent of disease, and patient comorbidities. An open surgical approach to RFA is preferable for patients with large tumors, multiple tumors, and tumors near large blood vessels that may otherwise be inadequately ablated because of heat-sink effects. Hepatic inflow occlusion (Pringle maneuver) diminishes the heat-sink effect from large intrahepatic vessels and is easier with open surgery compared with laparoscopic surgery. An open approach also allows for extremely accurate intraoperative ultrasound, which facilitates ablation of large tumors near blood vessels or in difficult anatomic regions of the liver. Peripherally situated tumors may be safely ablated by packing adjacent organs away from the liver, thus providing a layer of protection difficult to achieve with other approaches. Thoracic transdiaphragmatic approach to tumors near the dome of the liver has also been described, and this technique may be useful for patients in whom multiple prior surgical procedures have resulted in prohibitive perihepatic scar tissue.

Laparoscopic RFA is an option for patients with tumors for which percutaneous RFA is not feasible or safe, such as peripherally situated tumors near adjacent organs like the stomach or colon. Patients may benefit from the decreased incisional morbidities and faster recovery times afforded by a laparoscopic approach. However, prudent surgical judgment must be exercised in selecting patients for whom the laparoscopic approach is appropriate, and oncologic principles should not be compromised intraoperatively. Modern endoscopic optics and laparoscopic ultrasound probes permit excellent visualization, making this approach increasingly attractive.

Percutaneous RFA is well suited for patients with colorectal liver metastasis who are not good candidates for more invasive procedures because of comorbid conditions. In general, percutaneous RFA requires tumor sizes and locations that can be accessed without damaging adjacent organs or vascular structures. Although CT-guided RFA is relatively easy for small tumors in the lower segments of the liver, tumors along the periphery of the liver can pose a challenge for safe access. Artificially induced ascites or pleural effusions by injection of dextrose solution has been reported as a means of "separating" vulnerable nearby organs, thus potentially expanding the application of this modality. Cirrhotic patients and those with limited intrahepatic recurrences after hepatectomy are examples of patients who may be best served by a percutaneous approach.

Regardless of the device or approach used, attention to RFA probe placement is critical to successful tumor ablation. Careful assessment of preablation imaging studies (CT or MRI) and thorough ultrasound examination of both the tumor and surrounding hepatic anatomy during treatment assist with successful probe placement. Ultrasonography can monitor the progression of the ablation during RFA. Gas bubbles generated by an ablation may interfere with accurate ultrasonography of tissues deep to the electrode, which can hinder repositioning of the electrode for overlapping ablation zones when treating larger tumors. Initial ablation of the deepest portions of the tumor, followed by serial redeployment as the electrode is withdrawn, may mitigate this effect. Imaging-related difficulties may be more pronounced with the percutaneous approach; however, an immediate post-RFA CT can be readily performed to assist with the assessment of the ablation zone.

Complication rates associated with RFA are low, ranging from 2.4% to 27%, depending on the threshold for defining complications. By compiling more than 1300 patients from 18 different studies, Scaife and Curley reported an overall mortality rate of 0.5%, a major complication rate of 2%, and a minor complication rate of 6% after hepatic RFA. The risk for hepatic failure is quite low following RFA, even in patients with abnormal hepatic parenchyma. For this reason, RFA seems particularly attractive for cirrhotic patients. Monopolar RFA requires careful placement of grounding pads before ablation because inadequate electrical grounding has been implicated in full-thickness skin burns. Other potential complications following RFA include wound infections, intra-abdominal abscess, renal failure, hepatic abscess, biliary tract injury, pleural effusion, fever, pain, and minor hemorrhage. A "postablation syndrome" has also been described and is characterized by low-grade fever, malaise, chills, myalgia, delayed pain, and nausea and vomiting. This syndrome is usually self-limited and resolves within 10 days but must be differentiated from more serious postoperative complications. Both RFA and MWA can be safely performed in patients with implanted cardiac devices but require coordination with cardiologists and perioperative device interrogation.

Because there are no published randomized controlled trials comparing RFA and resection, the effectiveness of RFA in colorectal liver metastasis is largely based on several single-arm, retrospective, or prospective studies. These studies have inherent flaws related to selection bias, differing end points, and varying definitions of eligibility for RFA or resection. However, available data suggest that RFA is an effective treatment modality in improving survival in colorectal liver metastasis. In a clinical evidence review, Wong and associates noted the wide variability in reported 5-year survival rates (14% to 55%) and local recurrence rates (3.6% to 60%) following RFA, which are indicative of variability in selection criteria, treatment experience or technique, and end points across multiple institutions.

Despite the variability in study designs, the preponderance of evidence supports the superiority of resection over RFA and the benefit of RFA over systemic chemotherapy alone. Abdalla and associates compared 368 patients who underwent potentially curative procedures (resection only, resection with RFA, and RFA only) with 70 patients with liver-only disease who received only regional or systemic chemotherapy. Importantly, this series used patients with unresectable disease confirmed at laparotomy as the control group, rather than historical controls. They noted significant differences in both overall recurrence rates of 52% (resection only), compared with 64% (resection + RFA) and 84% (RFA only), and 4-year survival rates of 65%, 36%, and 22% for resection, resection + RFA, and RFA only, respectively.

Abdalla and associates noted a survival advantage for patients undergoing either resection with RFA or RFA alone compared with chemotherapy only ($P = .0017$). Also, in a series by Berber and colleagues, 135 unresectable patients were treated with laparoscopic RFA. Their median survival of 28.9 months was compared with the historical survival of 11 to 14 months using chemotherapy alone, showing significant improvement with RFA. These data suggest that RFA, although not superior to resection, does expand the armamentarium of surgeons. It allows for treatment options beyond chemotherapy alone for patients not amenable to resection, with the potential for improved survival.

Tumor number has been shown to affect both survival and recurrence rates; patients with solitary colorectal liver metastasis have a better outcome than those with multiple metastases. Tumor size is an important factor affecting the rate of local recurrence following RFA, with multiple groups associating colorectal liver metastasis tumor diameter of 4 cm or greater with increased rates of local recurrence. Whether this is a function of unfavorable tumor biology or a limitation of current ablative technologies is a matter of ongoing debate. The relationship between increasing tumor size (or number) and increasing risk for local recurrence highlights the need for early detection and intervention for low-volume colorectal liver metastasis.

Choice of treatment approach (open, laparoscopic, or percutaneous) may also influence local recurrence risk. Eisele and Kuvshinoff and their colleagues showed lower rates of local recurrence for open and laparoscopic RFA compared with a percutaneous approach. Improvements in hepatic exposure and the increased sensitivity of intraoperative ultrasound allowed by an open or laparoscopic RFA approach likely contribute to the lower local recurrence rates after operative compared with percutaneous RFA. Additionally, open and laparoscopic approaches allow for visual inspection of the liver surface for occult lesions and of the peritoneal cavity for extrahepatic disease. The apparent superiority of operative RFA is most likely due to better visualization, better control of surrounding structures, and more sensitive inspection of the peritoneal cavity.

Microwave Ablation of Colorectal Liver Metastasis

MWA, like RFA, is a hyperthermic ablative modality used in the treatment of colorectal liver metastasis. MWA uses microwave frequencies ($\geq$900 MHz) to stimulate water molecules in target tissues, with resultant heat generation and thermal ablation. Although RFA uses ionic agitation to produce heat, MWA induces rotation of water molecules with resultant rapid increases in temperature. MWA was first developed as a hemostatic adjunct to parenchymal transection during hepatectomy. It gained in popularity (largely in the Eastern hemisphere) for the treatment of hepatocellular carcinoma, and later for liver metastases. Recent approval for MWA devices has led to increased use within the United States.

In clinical practice, MWA is similar to RFA in many respects, namely in selection of candidates, the device safety profile, and the approach to probe placement. Advantages of MWA include speed (median ablation times of 10 minutes), the ability to simultaneously ablate with multiple antennae, and lack of grounding-pad complications. Other advantages have been suggested with regard to larger active (as opposed to conductive) heating zones and avoiding the limitations of increased impedance around RFA probes. Probes for MWA include single- and multiple-antenna arrays as well as loop antennae for expanded ablation zones. As with RFA, MWA can be performed through percutaneous, laparoscopic, or open surgical approaches. The reasons for choosing one approach over another parallel the rationale for RFA discussed previously.

Although data are limited, survival and local recurrence rates after MWA appear to be comparable to those associated with RFA. The authors have reported on 50 patients with unresectable colorectal liver metastasis treated by MWA. At a median follow-up of 3 years, recurrences at the ablation site were noted in 6% of patients, with a median disease-free survival of 12 months and a median overall survival of 36 months. As with RFA, MWA has also been employed in combination with hepatic resection for patients with colorectal liver metastasis not amenable to one-stage resection. Tanaka and coworkers reviewed 53 patients with five or more bilobar metastases who underwent either resection or resection plus MWA. At a median follow-up of 21 months, they noted no significant difference between the two groups with respect to overall, disease-free, or hepatic recurrence-free survival. The 3-year overall survival was similar for patients who required combined resection-ablation and those who underwent hepatectomy alone.

Laser-Induced Thermotherapy

Laser-induced thermotherapy (LITT) is another thermal ablative technology that uses low-intensity lasers (diode or N-YAG) to emit photons. These photons are then absorbed by natural molecular chromophores present in all human cells and converted into heat, resulting in cell death. LITT has indications similar to those for RFA, namely, unresectable primary and secondary liver tumors. Like RFA, it can be performed by percutaneous, laparoscopic, or open surgical approaches. As with other thermal ablative techniques, LITT ablation volumes can be increased by inflow occlusion, serial ablation, or placement of multiple laser fibers into the target tissue, resulting in overlapping zones of ablation.

An advantage of LITT is its compatibility with MRI guidance. Unlike RFA or MWA, LITT does not interfere with MRI. Ultrasound or CT may be used for tumor targeting and placement of the laser fibers, followed by MRI of ablation progression. Real-time temperature monitoring is another potential advantage of LITT in conjunction with MRI guidance because it allows the clinician to ensure that temperatures are high enough for successful ablation and low enough in surrounding tissue to minimize collateral damage. However, at present, the limited availability of LITT, MRI guidance, and thermal mapping has precluded widespread use of LITT.

Few large-scale studies of LITT in the treatment of colorectal liver metastasis have been published. Vogl and coworkers, in a review of 603 patients with colorectal liver metastasis, reported a median survival of 3.5 years and a 5-year survival rate of 37% after diagnosis of metastases. Pech and colleagues reported on 117 colorectal metastases in 66 patients treated by MRI-guided LITT. At a relatively short median follow-up of 8.7 months, a median progression-free survival of 6.1 months and a median overall survival of 23 months were noted. An analysis of the complications associated with the LITT in 899 patients with 2520 lesions (primary and metastatic) concluded that the procedure had an acceptably low morbidity, comparable to other thermal ablative modalities.

Currently, LITT is available in only a few centers worldwide. Further multi-institutional studies are warranted to refine the feasibility, safety, durability, and efficacy of LITT in the treatment of colorectal liver metastasis.

Cryoablation

Cryoablation was described early in the evolution of liver ablative technologies and involves placement of a cryoprobe into liver metastases by open surgical, laparoscopic, or percutaneous approaches. The cryoprobe tip is then rapidly cooled using liquefied gases and, over sequential freeze-thaw cycles, forms an "ice ball" encompassing the colorectal liver metastasis and a rim of normal liver. The progression of the ice ball can be easily monitored by ultrasound. Tissue destruction follows by multiple mechanisms, including membrane rupture, dehydration, protein denaturation, vascular stasis, and electrolyte disturbances.

Hepatic cryoablation has some significant limitations. Heat-sink effects may limit effective treatment of colorectal liver metastasis in close proximity to intrahepatic vascular structures, which may not allow for sufficiently low treatment temperatures. This raises the potential risk for incomplete ablation, which may result in a higher risk for local recurrence. In addition, little intrinsic hemostasis is achieved by cryoablation, and hemorrhage has been reported as a result of cracking of the ice-ball formation. A potentially lethal cytokine-mediated systemic inflammatory response termed *cryoshock* has been described following cryoablation with a frequency of 1%. Perioperative mortality after cryoablation is estimated at 1.5%. These complications, as well as reports of inferior results compared with other ablative technologies, have limited the use of cryoablation for colorectal liver metastasis at most centers.

High-Intensity Focused Ultrasound

High-intensity focused ultrasound (HIFU) is an emerging, noninvasive thermal ablative technology that focuses acoustic energy within solid organs, resulting in temperature elevation and coagulative necrosis. Mechanical effects (inertial cavitation) are also observed in HIFU and contribute to cell death. HIFU transducers deliver intensities and compression-rarefaction pressures that are much higher than those seen in diagnostic ultrasound transducers.

HIFU is most successful in situations with good acoustic coupling between the ultrasound probe and the tumor (e.g., prostate ablation or open surgical applications in the kidney). For hepatic HIFU, coupling between the skin and intervening tissues is suboptimal and has resulted in skin burns as well as rib necrosis. The ablation zone after a single HIFU is typically cigar shaped and measures 1 to 3 mm × 8 to 15 mm. Treatment of larger volumes requires precise "painting" of the target lesion and can lead to difficulties in treating larger tumors in mobile organs, such as the liver. As with all thermal ablative modalities, the potential for incomplete ablation secondary to heat-sink effect exists. Potential advantages of HIFU are largely related to its completely noninvasive approach. Continued refinements in techniques and technologies, as well as prospective evaluations of efficacy in colorectal liver metastasis, may show it to be a viable treatment option in the future.

Irreversible Electroporation

Irreversible electroporation (IRE) is an emerging intraparenchymal ablative technology that is based on the application of short-duration (microsecond to millisecond) high-voltage (1000 to 3000 V) pulses to target tissues, with the formation of nanoscale defects in the lipid bilayer and resultant cell necrosis. IRE probes can be placed using open surgical, laparoscopic, or percutaneous approaches, and multiprobe arrays can be used to achieve increased ablation volumes.

IRE is unique in two respects: First, it accomplishes ablation through nonthermal means and is not hindered by heat-sink effect. Second, it appears that IRE preferentially ablates parenchymal tissues, with relative sparing of bile ducts and blood vessels. These properties make IRE an attractive technology for patients with hepatic tumors in close proximity to vascular or biliary structures associated with a risk of incomplete ablation or vascular and biliary injury with thermal ablative techniques.

Ongoing multi-institutional prospective evaluations of safety, efficacy, and durability of IRE treatments are necessary to define the patient populations most likely to benefit from this technology and to compare it with other ablative modalities.

Although hepatic resection remains the gold standard therapy for hepatic malignancy, many patients will continue to benefit from ablative therapies. Further refinements in techniques and technologies will continue to expand the ablative options available to patients with colorectal liver metastasis. Continued analysis is required to delineate the biology and define the optimal role of ablation in the multidisciplinary treatment of colorectal liver metastasis.

PREOPERATIVE EVALUATION, TESTING, AND PREPARATION

The central tenets in the preoperative evaluation of patients for potential surgical resection of hepatic malignancy are (1) evaluation of the patient's fitness for operation, (2) anatomic and functional determination of tumor resectability, and (3) estimation of an individual's "tumor biology."

All patients with colorectal liver metastasis benefit from evaluation by a multidisciplinary team composed of physicians (surgeons, medical oncologists, radiologists, pathologists) as well as nurses, social workers, and research coordinators. Based on the authors' experience, this approach has been invaluable in terms of reaching efficient consensus on patient treatment plans among specialties. Multidisciplinary conferences and clinics minimize delays in treatment, improve communication between specialties, and allow for the identification of those "unresectable" patients who may, in fact, benefit from surgical resection, ablation, or catheter-based therapies.

A careful evaluation of a patient's physiologic capability to tolerate hepatic resection is necessary to ensure favorable outcomes after hepatectomy. In addition to a deliberate cardiopulmonary evaluation and the attention to medical comorbidities required for major abdominal surgery, a thorough consideration of the patient's liver function is required. The decision for hepatectomy relies largely on history, physical examination, and routine laboratory studies (complete blood count, liver function testing, and coagulation studies) to screen for underlying liver dysfunction. Preoperative imaging studies may also help to identify those patients with underlying hepatic disease.

Resectability of colorectal liver metastasis has been well defined by the AHPBA/SSAT/SSO in a 2006 consensus statement as an expected margin-negative (R_0) resection. The remnant liver must preserve at least two contiguous hepatic segments with adequate inflow, outflow, and biliary drainage with a functional liver remnant volume of more than 20% (for healthy liver).

Determination of resectability is primarily based on preoperative imaging. High-quality cross-sectional imaging is critical for gauging the extent of disease, response to preoperative therapy, and operative planning. Patients should be routinely reimaged after any course of systemic therapy, preferably within 4 weeks of planned resection. Currently, the triple-phase helical CT is thought to be the most useful modality for defining intrahepatic anatomy and resection planes. Ultrasound and MRI are reserved as adjuncts for further characterization of small or equivocal lesions noted on three-phase CT. Fusion positron emission tomography has demonstrated high sensitivity (95% on a per-patient basis, 76% on a per-lesion basis) and has been found to be beneficial in assessing extrahepatic disease burden.

Meticulous preoperative attention to the relationships of colorectal liver metastasis to arterioportal inflow, biliary drainage, and hepatic venous outflow are necessary and allows for an informed and efficient hepatectomy. At present, this level of anatomic detail is only evident using either three-phase CT or dynamic MRI. Positron emission tomography has insufficient resolution to make these preoperative determinations. Vascular and biliary anomalies are common and should be anticipated

before resection. If necessary, CT arterial reconstruction and magnetic resonance cholangiopancreatography may be useful in clarifying anatomic variants.

Given the potential morbidity and devastating consequences of postoperative liver insufficiency, much attention has been given to the functional liver remnant, which remains after extended (≥5-segment) hepatectomy. CT volumetry has been used to quantify the functional liver remnant by standardized methods. Safety of extended hepatectomy has been demonstrated for functional liver remnant volumes exceeding 20% for patients with normal liver parenchyma. Those patients with underlying liver disease require more conservative limits of functional liver remnant (i.e., 30% for moderate fibrosis, 40% for cirrhosis).

Besides delineating intrahepatic anatomy, preoperative cross-sectional imaging may also help to identify the presence of concomitant parenchymal disease (e.g., fibrosis or cirrhosis, portal hypertension, steatohepatitis) or extrahepatic disease. Identification of concomitant hepatic pathology or extrahepatic metastases requires a careful search for the presence of hepatic atrophy, "beaking" of the liver edge, liver nodularity, splenomegaly, ascites, varices, omental "caking," peritoneal nodules, and porta hepatis or aortocaval lymphadenopathy.

Diagnostic laparoscopy has a role in staging those patients in whom preoperative imaging or high-risk scores suggest a high likelihood for finding intra-abdominal extrahepatic disease or for patients with indeterminate intrahepatic lesions that may be best characterized by intraoperative ultrasound. Occasionally, laparoscopy can be useful in assessing the status of the remnant liver. In those patients whose history, laboratory studies, or imaging predicts marginal liver function, diagnostic laparoscopy can be employed to visually examine the liver as well as to perform biopsies before proceeding with hepatectomy.

PATIENT POSITIONING

The patient is placed in the supine position with steep reverse Trendelenburg and rotated slightly left or right depending on the segment of liver to be resected. The operating surgeon stands to the left of the patient and the assistant and/or camera operator on the right. This may be reversed depending on the location of the tumor and liver segment to be resected. Two monitors are placed, one on each side of the patient near the head of the bed at the surgeon's eye level for reduced fatigue and neck strain. Use of high-definition equipment is paramount for the optimal visualization necessary to dissect highly vascular structures encountered during this procedure successfully.

PLACEMENT OF TROCARS

Ports are placed according to the specific procedure. For a right hepatic lobectomy, a 12-mm port is first placed superior to the umbilicus, and CO_2 insufflation is achieved (port number 1, Fig. 17-1). This port can be converted for hand-assist access or extended to extract the specimen following a totally laparoscopic approach. Next, a 5-mm port is placed just inferior to the right costal margin laterally (port number 2; see Fig. 17-1). A 12-mm port is then placed in the right midclavicular line just inferior to the umbilicus (port number 3; see Fig. 17-1). If necessary, an additional 5-mm port can be placed in the subxiphoid region for improved visualization during mobilization of the dome of the right liver from the diaphragmatic and

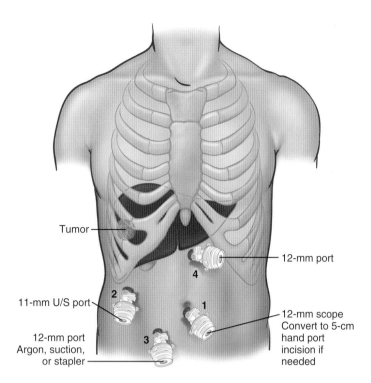

FIGURE 17-1 Trocar placement. Port 1: 12-mm vertical incision for 10-mm, 30-degree laparoscope. This can be extended for placement of a hand-assist port or specimen extraction. Port 2: 5-mm transverse incision in the right lateral, subcostal region for blunt retractor and flexible liver retractor. Port 3: 12-mm transverse incision in the midaxillary line, just inferior to the umbilicus for dissection, hemostasis and tissue sealing, and stapling devices. Port 4: 5-mm transverse incision in the subxiphoid region for additional retraction or 5-mm laparoscope to aid in visualization during mobilization of the posterior liver attachments.

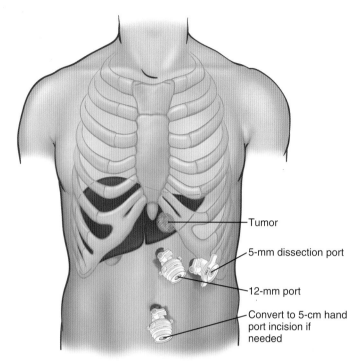

FIGURE 17-2 Port placement for left hepatectomy.

retroperitoneal attachments (port number 4; see Fig. 17-1). Alternatively, for left hepatic lobectomy, three ports are used that mirror the first three placed in a right hepatectomy. A 12-mm port is placed just superior to the umbilicus and a second 12-mm port just superior to the supraumbilical port in the right midclavicular line. Finally, a 5-mm port is placed laterally just inferior to the left costal margin (Fig. 17-2). Again, the supraumbilical port may be converted for hand assistance or specimen extraction.

OPERATIVE TECHNIQUE

The overriding principles of laparoscopic hepatic resection are identical to those described for open hepatectomy. The abdomen is explored laparoscopically, and the liver is mobilized and surveyed using laparoscopic ultrasound. The line of transection is identified and marked with electrocautery. Inflow may be occluded through intermittent Pringle application, while the liver parenchyma is transected using a combination of hemostatic assist devices, clips, and vascular staplers. In most of the authors' cases, inflow and outflow are controlled intraparenchymally during parenchymal transection.

We employ a permissive hypotensive technique with continuous communication with the anesthesiologist to minimize blood loss during mobilization and parenchymal transection. Systolic blood pressure is kept higher than 90 mm Hg, and central venous pressure is maintained at less than 5 mm Hg. Once the specimen is removed, crystalloid is administered intravenously to achieve euvolemia. Blood transfusions are used sparingly and only when clinically justified.

The description of the procedure is divided into distinct stages: (1) exploration, (2) liver mobilization, (3) intraoperative ultrasonography, (4) inflow control, (5) outflow control, (6) parenchymal transection, and (7) hemostasis and biliostasis and specimen extraction.

Exploration

Peritoneal spread of metastatic disease would prompt termination of the procedure, although biopsy or further evaluation with laparoscopic ultrasound may be appropriate.

Liver Mobilization

For right hepatic lobectomy, the first part of the procedure consists of adequate mobilization. The falciform ligament is freed from its anterior abdominal wall attachments with the use of the harmonic shears placed through port number 3 and a blunt retractor through port number 2 (see Fig. 17-1). An Endoloop (Ethicon Endo-Surgery, Cincinnati, Ohio) is then placed over the transected edge of the falciform ligament and brought out through a separate, 2-mm stab incision in the anterior abdominal wall on the left lateral side using a Carter-Thomason needle suture passer (CooperSurgical, Trumbull, Conn.). This is used to create traction for the remainder of the dissection.

Any adhesions to the inferior surface of the gallbladder and liver are lysed using a combination of a hemostatic assist and tissue sealing device, electrocautery, and blunt dissection. The blunt dissector through port number 2 (see Fig. 17-1) may be replaced with a flexible laparoscopic liver retractor for improved visualization and countertraction. Familiarity with laparoscopic adhesiolysis is essential in performing this step. Because of inflammation from the tumor, there may also be dense adhesions along the lateral edge of the liver to the abdominal wall that must be addressed. Dissection continues along the triangular ligament between the liver and diaphragm and continues into the

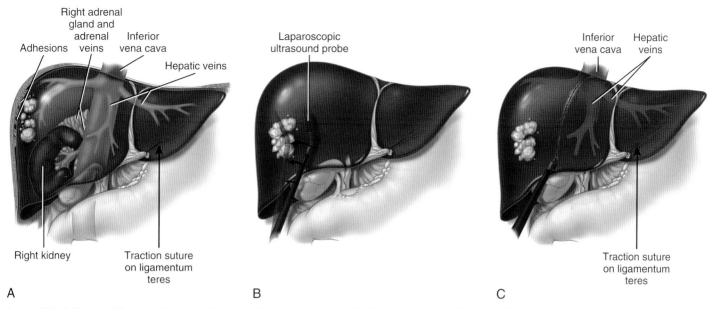

Right adrenal
gland and
adrenal   Inferior
Adhesions   veins   vena cava
Inferior vena cava
Hepatic veins

Right kidney   Traction suture
on ligamentum
teres

A

Laparoscopic
ultrasound probe

B

Inferior   Hepatic
vena cava   veins

Traction suture
on ligamentum
teres

C

FIGURE 17-3 **A**, Liver mobilization. Inferior attachments and lateral adhesions to the diaphragm are carefully lysed with a tissue sealing device or electrocautery. The triangular ligament is also taken down while being mindful of the right renal and adrenal vasculature when the retroperitoneum is approached. **B**, Intraoperative ultrasound. A laparoscopic ultrasound probe is used to define the size and extent of the tumor as well as the biliary, venous, and arterial hepatic anatomy. **C**, A search for occult metastases and masses is performed, and the transection plane is then scored using electrocautery.

retroperitoneum. Care must be taken to protect the adrenal vasculature during this portion of the procedure. If a hand-assist port is used, the surgeon's hand is used to ensure that these vessels are preserved. Endo Shears (United States Surgical Corporation, Norwalk, Conn.) (port number 3; see Fig. 17-1) are used for fine dissection surrounding the vena cava, which should be extended for an arc of about 90 degrees (Fig. 17-3A).

Intraoperative Ultrasonography

After the liver is completely mobilized, a thorough intraoperative ultrasound examination is performed. The laparoscopic ultrasound probe is placed through port number 3 (see Fig. 17-1). Evaluation of the relationship and proximity of intrahepatic metastases to arterioportal, biliary, and hepatic venous structures is reconciled with the preoperative imaging. An active search for occult intrahepatic lesions is undertaken. At this point, several critical decisions must be made before committing to parenchymal transection. Change in the lesion size, development of new lesions, or discovery of occult lesions will dictate the next step. These new findings are minimized when preoperative imaging is performed close to the time of the procedure; however, lesions below the detection limit may be appreciated with laparoscopic ultrasound. A lesion in the contralateral lobe may prompt biopsy or termination of the procedure. Significant changes in size may require change in the extent of resection (Fig. 17-3B).

After the ultrasound evaluation, the cystic duct and artery are dissected free. When the duct and artery are adequately visualized, two hemostatic clips are placed proximally and one clip distally on each structure, and they are transected. An atraumatic grasper (port number 2; see Fig. 17-1) is placed on the dome of the gallbladder and used in conjunction with the falciform Endoloop to create traction and countertraction. At this point, laparoscopic ultrasound may also be employed to assist in determining the plane of resection. It will generally bisect the gallbladder fossa and extend to the middle hepatic vein. The surface of the liver is delineated with electrocautery as a guide (Fig. 17-3B).

Inflow, Outflow, and Parenchymal Transection

The inflow and outflow within the parenchyma are controlled using a laparoscopic linear stapler that is temporarily clamped on the porta hepatis. There is no need to perform extrahepatic dissection of these structures. A second Endoloop is placed over the dome of the gallbladder and brought out through a small 2-mm incision on the right lateral abdominal wall using a Carter-Thomason needle suture passer. Transection of the liver parenchyma is performed using a hemostatic assist and tissue sealing device and vascular stapling devices to control large vessels and ducts. Hemostatic clips are also used to control hemorrhage if necessary. The blunt tips of the hemostatic assist device are advanced into the liver gently to find a low-resistance path. If resistance is encountered, the angle of entry should be adjusted to avoid injury to hepatic vessels causing hemorrhage. Careful dissection will avoid time wasted controlling hemorrhage and possible loss of visualization. As the retroperitoneum is approached, extra caution is warranted to avoid injury to the vena cava. Hand assistance can be prudent at this juncture. The right and middle hepatic veins are transected with vascular staples, and the remainder of the parenchyma is divided (Fig. 17-4).

Hemostasis, Biliostasis, and Extraction

After the parenchyma is completely transected, the cut surface of the remnant liver is cauterized using argon-beam coagulation (Fig. 17-5). This technique should not be attempted on large vessels because argon embolism is possible. Some groups also advise decrease in pneumoperitoneum pressure to avoid embolization. An absorbable hemostatic agent is sprayed onto the cut surface to aid in detection of any occult hemorrhage or oozing biliary ducts. The specimen is placed in a bag of adequate size for extraction through the hand-assist port or after extending the supraumbilical 12-mm port site. The Endoloop attached to the falciform is returned to its anatomic position by stapling to

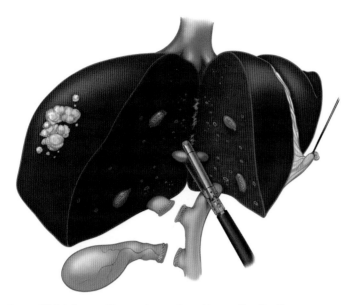

FIGURE 17-4 Inflow, outflow, and parenchymal transection. Traction-countertraction is achieved using the Endoloops over the falciform, and the gallbladder is pulled through the respective lateral abdominal wall. Parenchymal transection proceeds along the previously marked plane. A combination of devices is used with larger vessels and ducts transected with stapling devices or surgical clips and Endoshears. The hepatic veins are transected using a stapling device before complete parenchymal transection. Care must be taken to avoid injury of the retrohepatic vena cava during this maneuver.

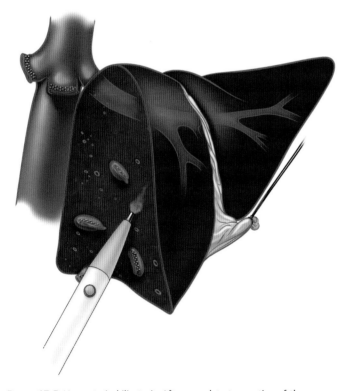

FIGURE 17-5 Hemostasis, biliostasis. After complete transection of the parenchyma, hemostasis and biliostasis are obtained. Argon-beam coagulation is used on the cut surface and for small-diameter vessels. Larger vessels or ducts are controlled with surgical clips, suture ligature, or hemostatic and tissue sealing devices.

the anterior abdominal wall. This maneuver protects against torsion of the remnant left lobe, potentially causing thrombosis of the left hepatic vein. The pneumoperitoneum is evacuated, and the trocars are removed under direct visualization. Fascial closure stitches are placed at 12-mm port sites to avoid incisional hernias.

POSTOPERATIVE CARE

Patients are monitored closely postoperatively for signs of hemorrhage, biliary leak, infection, and hepatic failure. They can expect length of stay as short as a few days; preparation of the patient and family for possible complications and extended stay is prudent. The laparoscopic approach minimizes the need for postoperative analgesics and, as noted later in the text, significantly decreases the median hospital stay to about 3 days. Early ambulation is encouraged, and regular diet is resumed quickly.

MANAGEMENT OF PROCEDURE-SPECIFIC COMPLICATIONS

Clinically significant CO_2 embolism has been reported during laparoscopic liver resection using CO_2 pneumoperitoneum. This must be recognized and treated promptly to avoid significant morbidity and possible mortality. The advantage of CO_2 pneumoperitoneum over oxygen or air is its relatively higher solubility in blood, minimizing the occurrence of hemodynamically significant gas embolism. Additional care should be taken when employing argon-beam coagulation during laparoscopic liver resection. Increase in insufflation pressure occurs during its use, and the potential for embolism is increased because it is 17 times less soluble than CO_2 in blood.

Gas embolism should be suspected after an abrupt decrease in end-tidal CO_2 followed by a decrease in systolic blood pressure. The appropriate response after diagnosis is to evacuate the pneumoperitoneum and change the patient's position from steep reverse Trendelenburg to Trendelenburg in left lateral decubitus. The central venous pressure line can be aspirated in an attempt to remove the gas that may collect in the right atrium, causing the hemodynamic alterations. Definitive diagnosis is by transesophageal echocardiography.

Significant intraoperative hemorrhage from a major hepatic vessel or the inferior vena cava in most series is comparable to or decreased compared with open procedures. However, it remains a significant concern because it may take considerable time to convert to an open approach and adequately control bleeding. Incorrect orientation is a common cause of inadvertent transection of a major vessel leading to intraoperative hemorrhage. To avoid such complications, adequate liver mobilization during the initial phase of the operation is important. Intraoperative ultrasound after mobilization also ensures proper orientation and is of most importance when employing a totally laparoscopic approach. It is prudent when facing difficulty to convert early in anticipation of, rather than in response to, an ensuing problem.

If significant hemorrhage is encountered, an attempt should be made to control or at least temporize it before conversion to open because this will take some time. Some groups isolate the portal triad and loosely place a vascular loop that may be used to apply the Pringle maneuver temporarily. Alternatively, a linear stapler may be clamped temporarily on the porta hepatis, as mentioned earlier. This allows most vessels to be controlled laparoscopically, and in the event conversion to open is necessary, it significantly decreases blood loss while opening. Obviously, during a hand-assist procedure, the Pringle maneuver or direct pressure should be applied when needed.

Bile duct leakage is another possible complication of hepatic resection. Reports suggest that this is no more common with a laparoscopic versus an open approach, occurring in less than 2% of patients. Important points to consider in avoiding this complication include appreciation of aberrant anatomy and meticulous inspection and control of leakage from the raw surface of the remnant liver at the time of surgery. Aberrant anatomy should be noted on preoperative imaging, reinforcing the importance of high-quality images. Intraoperative ultrasound is helpful in planning an appropriate plane of resection to avoid damaging major biliary ducts. After transection, care should be taken to visualize the entire cut surface of the remnant liver after the patient is adequately volume-resuscitated and pneumoperitoneal pressure is reduced. Both of these factors may mask biliary leak as well as venous oozing during the procedure. Leaks are controlled preferably with direct visualization of ducts and placement of hemostatic clips or suture ligature. Electrocautery, ultrasonic sheers, and laparoscopic staples are alternative methods.

RESULTS AND OUTCOME

Several studies have compared the results of laparoscopic with open hepatectomy. Over time, the results of laparoscopic hepatic resection have improved because of increasing surgeon experience, improved instrumentation, appropriate patient selection, and improved imaging. Although large prospective randomized trials are lacking, comparative trials consistently show equivalence to an open approach with the inherent advantages of laparoscopy.

The authors recently compared their experience over the past 10 years with laparoscopic lobectomy to a matched group of patients undergoing open hepatectomy and confirmed improvements in blood loss, transfusion requirements, morbidity, and length of stay without compromise of resection margins when employing a laparoscopic approach. Overall, 20% of the 450 hepatectomies were laparoscopic lobectomies. This proportion increased dramatically from 2006 to 2010, with nearly one fourth of all hepatectomies in this period being performed laparoscopically.

Intraoperative characteristics were compared using estimated blood loss, transfusion requirements, and operative times. There was significantly greater estimated blood loss in the open group (400 mL; range, 65 to 5000 mL) than in the laparoscopic group (150 mL; range, 20 to 1000 mL; $P < .0001$). The Pringle maneuver was also employed more frequently in the open group. Patients in the open group were 2.5 times more likely to receive a blood transfusion (95% confidence interval, 1.2 to 8.7). Blood loss and transfusion are important surrogate markers because they are independently associated with risk for postoperative complications. Operative duration averaged 160 minutes in the open hepatectomy group and 140 minutes in the laparoscopic group ($P = .009$).

Postoperative complications were more frequent in the open resection group (52% vs. 23%; $P = .001$); however, the grade of complication was not significantly different. Additionally, bile-specific complications were similar (8% open vs. 7% laparoscopic; $P = .2$). Mortality rates were 1% in the laparoscopic group and 3% in the open group. No instances of CO_2 embolization were detected during the laparoscopic procedures. Length of stay was also significantly reduced in the laparoscopic group (3 days; range, 1 to 13 days) compared with the open resection group (7 days; range, 2 to 57 days) ($P < .0001$).

Oncologic outcomes appear to be equivalent, with similar rate of R_0 resection and recurrence. The overall rate of negative margins was 97%, and there was no significant difference between groups ($P = .3$). The anatomic location of the tumors was similar. The median tumor size was 4 cm (range, 2 to 15 cm) in the laparoscopic group compared with 6.4 cm (range, 1 to 16 cm) in the open group.

Laparoscopic liver resection is a well-accepted approach for the appropriate indications. It will certainly continue to become more prevalent as surgeons become more comfortable with the techniques and as favorable results are reported. Incorporation of major hepatic resections into clinical practice should follow adequate training and familiarity initially with wedge resections and left lateral lobectomy to ensure acceptable results.

Suggested Reading

Abdalla EK, Vauthey JN, Ellis LM, et al: Radiofrequency ablation, and combined resection/ablation for colorectal liver metastases. *Ann Surg* 239:818–827, 2004.

Berber E, Pelley R, Siperstein AE: Predictors of survival after radiofrequency thermal ablation of colorectal cancer metastases to the liver: A prospective study. *J Clin Oncol* 23:1358–1364, 2005.

Brown RE, Bower MR, Martin RCG: Hepatic resection for colorectal liver metastasis. *Surg Clin North Am* 90:839–852, 2010.

Buell JF, Cherqui D, Geller DA, et al: The international position on laparoscopic liver surgery: The Louisville statement, 2008. *Ann Surg* 250:825–830, 2009.

Buell JF, Thomas MT, Rudich S, et al: Experience with more than 500 minimally invasive hepatic procedures. *Ann Surg* 248:475–486, 2008.

Cherqui D, Husson E, Hammoud R, et al: Laparoscopic liver resections: a feasibility study in 30 patients. *Ann Surg* 232:753–762, 2000.

Eisele RM, Neumann U, Neuhaus P, Schumacher G: Open surgical is superior to percutaneous access for radiofrequency ablation of hepatic metastases. *World J Surg* 33:804–811, 2009.

Gagner M, Rheault M, Dubuc J: Laparoscopic partial hepatectomy for liver tumor. *Surg Endosc* 6:97–98, 1992.

Kuvshinoff BW, Ota DM: Radiofrequency ablation of liver tumors: influence of technique and tumor size. *Surgery* 132:605–611, 2002.

Lortat-Jacob JL, Robert HG, Henry L: Un cas d'hepatectomie droit reglee. *Mem Acad Chirurg* 78:244–251, 1952.

Martin RCG, Scoggins CR, McMasters KM: Laparoscopic hepatic lobectomy: advantages of a minimally invasive approach. *J Am Coll Surg* 210:627–634, 2010.

McGahan JP, Browning PD, Brock JM, Tesluk H: Hepatic ablation using radiofrequency electrocautery. *Invest Radiol* 25:267–270, 1990.

Nguyen KT, Gamblin TC, Geller DA: World review of laparoscopic liver resection—2,804 patients. *Ann Surg* 250:831–841, 2009.

Pech M, Wieners G, Freund T, et al: MR-guided interstitial laser thermotherapy of colorectal liver metastases: Efficiency, safety and patient survival. *Eur J Med Res* 12:161–168, 2007.

Rossi S, Di Stasi M, Buscarini E, et al: Percutaneous radiofrequency interstitial thermal ablation in the treatment of small hepatocellular carcinoma. *Cancer J Sci Am* 1:73–81, 1995.

Scaife CL, Curley SA: Complication, local recurrence, and survival rates after radiofrequency ablation for hepatic malignancies. *Surg Oncol Clin N Am* 12:243–255, 2003.

Tanaka K, Shimada H, Nagano Y, et al: Outcome after hepatic resection versus combined resection and microwave ablation for multiple bilobar colorectal metastases to the liver. *Surgery* 139:263–273, 2006.

Vauthey JN, Chaoui A, Do KA, et al: Standardized measurement of the future liver remnant prior to extended liver resection: methodology and clinical associations. *Surgery* 127:512–519, 2000.

Vogl TJ, Straub R, Eichler K, et al: Malignant liver tumors treated with MR imaging-guided laser-induced thermotherapy: experience with complications in 899 patients (2,520 lesions). *Radiology* 225:367–377, 2002.

Vogl TJ, Straub R, Eichler K, et al: Colorectal carcinoma metastases in liver: Laser-induced interstitial thermotherapy—local tumor control rate and survival data. *Radiology* 230:450–458, 2004.

Wong SL, Mangu PB, Choti MA, et al: American Society of Clinical Oncology 2009 clinical evidence review on radiofrequency ablation of hepatic metastases from colorectal cancer. *J Clin Oncol* 28:493–508, 2010.

Pancreas and Spleen

BASIL J. AMMORI AND GEORGIOS D. AYIOMAMITIS

Laparoscopic Pancreatoduodenectomy

The videos associated with this chapter are listed in the Video Contents and can be found on the accompanying DVDs and *on Expertconsult.com.*

Recent advances in technology and surgical techniques have allowed a wide range of applications of minimally invasive surgery to be applied in patients with benign and malignant diseases of the pancreas. Whereas laparoscopic resection of the distal pancreas requires no anastomosis and therefore has gained worldwide acceptance (described in Chapter 23 of the *Atlas of Minimally Invasive Surgery*, 2009; see Suggested Readings at the end of this chapter), excision of cephalic lesions by minimal access techniques remains an underused approach because of its technical complexity and prolonged surgery.

Laparoscopic pancreatoduodenectomy (LPD) was first described in 1994. Since then, the procedure has been attempted in a relatively small number of patients worldwide with a high conversion rate. More recently, however, the worldwide experience with the totally laparoscopic approach to pancreatoduodenectomy has grown, and the procedure is being increasingly considered feasible and safe in the selected patient and in experienced hands.

OPERATIVE INDICATIONS

In a recent review of the world literature, cancer has been the indication for LPD in more than two thirds of patients, whereas cystic disease, neuroendocrine tumors, and chronic pancreatitis represent the remainder.

The complexity of resection and reconstruction and the prolonged duration of surgery mean that careful patient selection is paramount, especially early in the learning curve. Relative contraindications to LPD include patients with large tumors (>2 cm), potential vascular involvement, nondilated pancreatic or bile ducts, extension of tumor to the uncinate process that renders it in very close proximity to the superior mesenteric artery, acute pancreatitis, morbid obesity, and cardiorespiratory comorbidities. These patients are best offered open resection.

PREOPERATIVE EVALUATION, TESTING, AND PREPARATION

Patients with preoperative suspicion of vascular involvement may be further evaluated with endoscopic ultrasound (EUS) by an experienced gastroenterologist.

We prefer, whenever possible, to rely on magnetic resonance cholangiopancreatography to image the biliary tree and pancreatic duct to avoid preoperative biliary drainage unless jaundice has deepened (bilirubin >200 mmol/L or 11.7 mg/dL), because it has been shown to significantly increase the rate of postoperative complications and the need to resort to percutaneous transhepatic biliary drainage rather than endoscopic retrograde cholangiopancreatography. Insertion of a biliary stent induces inflammation and thickening of the bile duct and therefore increases operative difficulty. For similar reasons, chronic pancreatitis associated with a mass lesion within the head of the gland is best resected by open surgery.

Previous major abdominal surgery, especially within the upper abdomen (such as open cholecystectomy or laparotomy for peritonitis) is a relative contraindication to LPD. Certainly such adhesions could be divided laparoscopically, but to accomplish this the surgeon may need to either place ports in positions cumbersome for the LPD or place additional ports that could cause "crowding" and render surgery considerably more stressful. A decision could be made regarding whether such a patient is suitable for laparoscopic resection at the time of a staging laparoscopy.

The potential yield from a staging laparoscopy dictates that patients with suspected malignancy of the head of the pancreas or distal bile duct should undergo a staging laparoscopy before LPD, whereas patients with ampullary tumors and small duodenal tumors may proceed straight to resection. Laparoscopic ultrasonography may have a role to play in detecting small (<1 cm) hepatic lesions when suspected on preoperative imaging.

Surgeons contemplating LPD should have an established experience in open pancreatoduodenectomy and in advanced laparoscopic surgery, particularly in intracorporeal suturing.

PATIENT POSITIONING AND PLACEMENT OF TROCARS

All patients receive preoperative deep venous prophylaxis including thromboembolism-deterrent stockings and low-molecular-weight heparin (LMWH) unless epidural anesthesia is contemplated, in which case LMWH is administered after insertion of the epidural catheter and intravenous antibiotic prophylaxis. The surgery is carried out under general anesthesia, and

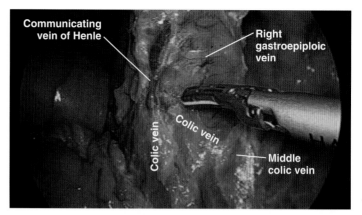

FIGURE 18-2 Communicating vein of Henle.

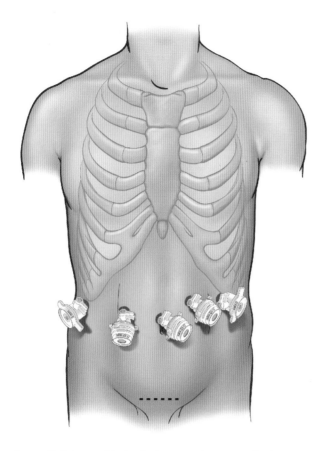

FIGURE 18-1 Port positioning for laparoscopic pancreatoduodenectomy.

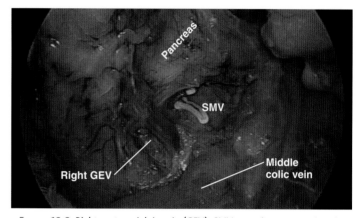

FIGURE 18-3 Right gastroepiploic vein (GEV). SMV, superior mesenteric vein.

patients receive epidural anesthesia selectively. The patient is placed in a flat Lloyd-Davies (French) position, with the surgeon standing between the patient's legs and the assistant on the patient's right or left according to the steps of the procedure. Most of the surgery is carried out with the patient in a 30-degree reverse Trendelenburg position to allow the colon and omentum to drop away from the upper abdomen. Surgery is most commonly conducted using a completely laparoscopic approach, although a recent review of the literature revealed that one fourth of the procedures were carried out using a hand-assist approach. The pneumoperitoneum is established and maintained at 12 to 15 mm Hg. The procedure may employ five trocars, as shown in Figure 18-1. A 30-degree laparoscope is employed routinely. The liver is retracted in a cephalad direction using an 80-mm angled Diamond-Flex retractor, which is fixed in position using a table clamp (Fast Clamp, Snowden-Pencer, San Diego, Calif.).

OPERATIVE TECHNIQUE

Resection

Most of the steps and principles of the resection and reconstruction of the LPD are the same as those in open surgery. After an exploratory laparoscopy, the gastrocolic omentum at the antrum and distal body of the stomach is divided with the ultrasonically activated scalpel (UAS), and the lesser sac is entered. With the posterior aspect of the antrum held and retracted upward by the assistant through the patient's leftmost lateral 5-mm port, any adhesions between the stomach and the anterior surface of the pancreas are divided. The transverse colon is then mobilized off the anterior surface of the pancreas and the second and third

portions of the duodenum; early in this process is the division of the communicating vein of Henle between the middle colic and right gastroepiploic veins (Fig. 18-2), which allows the transverse colon to fall away from the head of the pancreas and facilitates exposure of the superior mesenteric vein (SMV). Also, the right gastroepiploic vessels are encountered at the inferior border of the first part of the duodenum and their division (especially that of the vein, Fig. 18-3) enhances access to the SMV; the most superficial of these, the vein, is first dissected off its confluence with the SMV and divided between locking clips (Hem-o-lok, Weck Closure Systems, Research Triangle Park, N.C.). The artery that lies in a deeper position could be similarly clipped and divided if necessary. Identification of the SMV is facilitated by following the colic vein or the right gastroepiploic vein and by gentle mobilization of the inferior border of the body of the pancreas toward the neck, where the SMV can also be encountered. The anterior surface of the SMV is dissected and followed in a cephalad direction behind the neck of the pancreas to expose the confluence with the splenic vein and to further dissect the anterior surface of the portal vein and confirm resectability (Fig. 18-4).

If necessary, the hepatic flexure of the colon may be taken down to enhance exposure of the duodenum, although we have not found this step always necessary. The duodenum is extensively kocherized, exposing the inferior vena cava and left renal vein (Fig. 18-5) until the territory of the superior mesenteric artery (SMA) is reached, and separating the third and, if possible, the fourth parts of the duodenum from the transverse mesocolon until the infracolic compartment is reached (Fig. 18-6). In preparation for division of the antrum, the right gastroepiploic vessels are divided between locking clips along the inferior border of

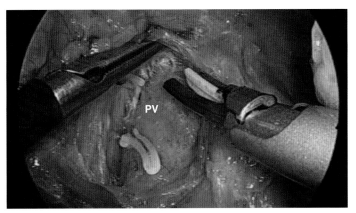

FIGURE 18-4 The portal vein (PV) and the superior mesenteric vein were dissected to confirm resectability.

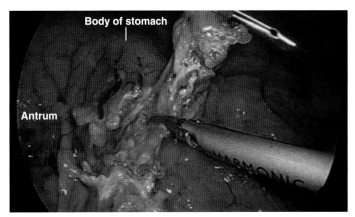

FIGURE 18-7 The right gastroepiploic vessels at the junction of the body and antrum of the stomach are clipped and divided.

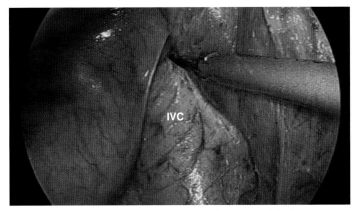

FIGURE 18-5 Kocherization of the duodenum and exposure of the inferior vena cava (IVC) and left renal vein.

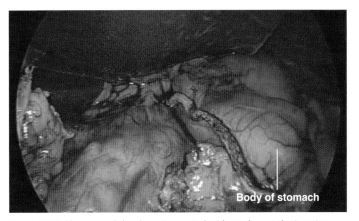

FIGURE 18-8 The stomach has been transected with staplers at the junction between its body and antrum.

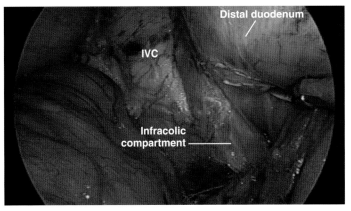

FIGURE 18-6 The distal duodenum was mobilized until the infracolic compartment was reached. IVC, inferior vena cava.

the junction between the antrum and body of the stomach (Fig. 18-7), and the vessels along the lesser curvature of the stomach in the region of the incisura and the lesser omentum are also divided with the UAS. The gastric antrum is then divided with endostaplers (Fig. 18-8) after ensuring that the nasogastric and nasojejunal tubes have been advanced no further than 50 cm. To avoid oozing from the staple line that could later obscure the operative field, we tend to oversew the distal staple line for hemostasis and to control the proximal staple line with the Harmonic scalpel (Ethicon Endo-Surgery, Cincinnati, Ohio), which will be incorporated in a suture line later when the gastrojejunostomy is constructed, and to wrap it with gauze. The body of the stomach

is then pushed into the left upper quadrant to facilitate exposure of the hepatic artery.

If a pylorus-preserving pancreatoduodenectomy is planned, the posterior aspect of the antrum and the duodenal bulb are mobilized off the pancreas. Care is taken to preserve the gastroepiploic arcade along the greater curvature of the stomach. The first part of the duodenum is then divided with an endostapler.

The peritoneum over the anterior surface of the hepatoduodenal ligament is then divided from left to right until its aspect over the upper border of the Calot triangle is also divided. With the assistant holding and retracting the antrum of the stomach caudally, dissection along the left border of the hepatoduodenal ligament allows for identification of the right gastric artery, which is then clipped and divided (Fig. 18-9). This allows the antrum of the stomach to fall away from the hepatoduodenal ligament and facilitates the dissection of the gastroduodenal artery. Dissection with the Harmonic scalpel then proceeds between the lower border of the common hepatic artery and the upper border of the body of the pancreas and duodenum. Group 8a (anterior hepatic) lymph nodes could be dissected off at this stage, mobilized off the common hepatic artery from left to right, and kept attached to the upper border of the head of the pancreas or removed separately for histologic analysis. Alternatively, this group of lymph nodes could be dissected before division of the neck of the pancreas (see the accompanying DVD as well as Expert Consult). This will lead to exposure of the gastroduodenal artery, which after meticulous dissection is mobilized (Fig. 18-10A), double-clipped, and divided with scissors (Fig. 18-10B). Holding the proximal stump of the gastroduodenal artery, the surgeon can mobilize the hepatic artery further in a cephalad direction. Division of the neurolymphatics in this region exposes the anterior surface of the portal vein and the left border of the common bile duct.

Attention is then diverted to dissection of the triangle of Calot, clipping and dividing the cystic artery, and mobilization of the gallbladder off its liver bed. The junction between the cystic duct and hepatic duct is dissected and identified, and, with the assistant retracting the gallbladder medially and anteriorly, the peritoneum along the right border of the hepatoduodenal ligament is divided with the UAS just behind the bile duct. This will facilitate mobilization of the posterior aspect of the common hepatic and bile ducts that will follow, which we find easier to do from a left-to-right direction. Care should be taken during this stage to avoid injury to the already exposed portal vein or one of its tributaries, especially in patients with prior biliary stenting. The common hepatic duct is suspended and lifted anteriorly with a thread and is divided transversely just proximal to its confluence with the cystic duct (Fig. 18-11); this could be accomplished with UAS if the duct is markedly dilated, with scissors if the duct is minimally dilated, or with a vascular endostapler if the duct is dilated and there is no biliary stent. The distal open end of the divided bile duct is oversewn with Vicryl (Ethicon, Somerville, N.J.) 3-0 suture, and a bulldog clamp is applied to the proximal end until the construction of the hepatico-jejunostomy.

Attention is then directed to division of the neurolymphatic channels along the right border of the hepatoduodenal ligament, ensuring that the lymph nodes encountered (group 12b) are dissected with the specimen. Care should be exercised to look for or exclude an aberrant right hepatic artery arising from the SMA

(even if careful study of preoperative images did not show one), which if encountered should be preserved to avoid ischemia to the hepatic duct and its consequences. The portal vein is thus exposed, and at this stage the uppermost tributary from the region of the head of the pancreas is clipped and divided.

The neck of the pancreas is then prepared for division. The tunnel behind the neck of the gland is completed, and a 3-0 Vicryl suture is placed into the inferior aspect of the pancreas and on either side of the intended point of neck division for hemostasis. A Vicryl 2-0 thread or a nylon tape is passed around the neck of the pancreas and grasped and lifted anteriorly by the assistant to facilitate transection of the neck of the pancreas (Fig. 18-12A). If the pancreatic duct is dilated (and we tend to preferentially select such patients whenever possible), the pancreas and duct are divided with the UAS (Fig. 18-12B); however, if the duct is not dilated, the middle third of the gland is best divided with sharp scissors to avoid sealing the pancreatic duct, which could occur if it were divided with the UAS.

Exposure of the infracolic compartment then proceeds after the greater omentum has been lifted off and placed in the supracolic compartment. The assistant holds upward the transverse mesocolon above the duodenojejunal flexure, and the proximal jejunum is then mobilized by dividing its peritoneal attachments along the right border of the inferior mesenteric vein and at the root of the transverse mesocolon. A window in the proximal jejunal mesentery is made, and the jejunum is divided with an endostapler about 5 cm distal to the duodenojejunal flexure (Fig. 18-13). The jejunal mesentery is divided with the UAS, with

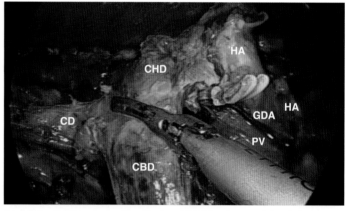

FIGURE 18-11 The common hepatic duct (CHD) has been mobilized; the gallbladder has been dissected off the liver bed and the cystic duct (CD) retracted laterally and caudally; and the CHD is divided with the ultrasonically activated scalpel. CBD, common bile duct; GDA, gastroduodenal artery; HA, hepatic artery; PV, portal vein.

FIGURE 18-9 The right gastric artery has been clipped and is to be divided.

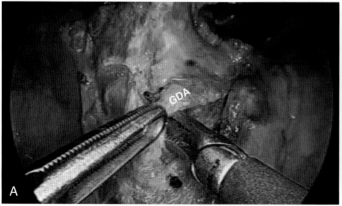

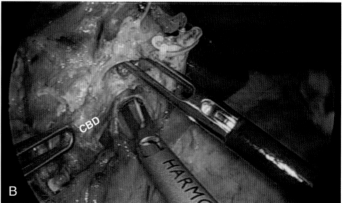

FIGURE 18-10 The gastroduodenal artery (GDA) has been dissected (A), clipped, and divided (B). CBD, common bile duct.

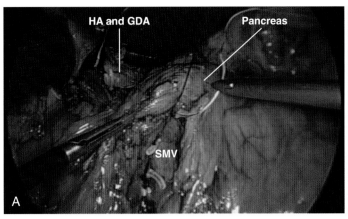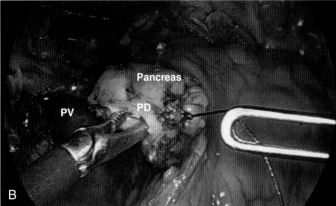

FIGURE 18-12 The neck of the pancreas was slung with a Vicryl thread **(A)** and was then divided with the ultrasonically activated scalpel **(B)**. HA, hepatic artery; GDA, gastroduodenal artery; PD, pancreatic duct; PV, portal vein; SMA, superior mesenteric artery.

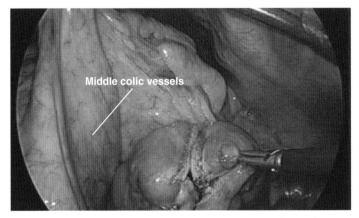

FIGURE 18-13 The proximal jejunum has been divided with a stapler.

or without the application of locking clips proximally on the vessels to be divided, and until the lower border of the pancreas is reached. The ligament of Treitz is divided along with any remaining attachments between the distal duodenum and the retroperitoneum. The mobilized and devascularized proximal jejunum is then delivered to the supracolic subhepatic space, and the greater omentum is returned to its resting position over the infracolic compartment.

The portal vein tributaries from the head of the pancreas (Fig. 18-14A) and the inferior pancreaticoduodenal vein (Fig. 18-14B) are very gently dissected, clipped, and divided. The posterior aspect of the portal vein is then peeled gently to the left off the uncinate process until a clear groove can be seen along the right border of the SMA; this groove is the target of the final stage of the resection. A further mobilization of the SMV and portal vein to the left will reveal the pulsating SMA. It is essential to optimize exposure for the mobilization of the uncinate process of the pancreas and for division of the SMA branches to the head and uncinate process. To facilitate this exposure, the divided antrum of the stomach, the gallbladder, and the devascularized jejunum are all placed in the right subhepatic space; the surgeon's left hand introduces a grasping forceps into the space between the head of the pancreas and the inferior vena cava (all adventitial attachments should have already been divided during kocherization of the duodenum) and lifts the head of the gland anteriorly, while the assistant retracts the SMV and portal vein to the left with a pledget, paying attention not to dislodge any clips off the portal vein tributaries.

The tissue to be divided along the parasuperior mesenteric artery groove described earlier can be viewed in three layers: the anterior and posterior layers containing neurolymphatic channels and supportive adventitial tissue, and the middle layer containing arterial branches that need to be secured. Dissection and division start at the caudal end of the groove and proceed in a cephalad direction. The anterior layer is first divided for about 1 cm using UAS, and any vessel is clipped and divided. The posterior layer containing neurolymphatics is also best clipped on the SMA side only (to minimize postoperative lymph leak) and divided with the UAS. This process is repeated as division progresses in a cephalad direction. The first substantial vessel to be encountered is the inferior pancreaticoduodenal artery (Fig. 18-15). Care should be taken at the start of this stage of pancreas-mesenteric division not to inadvertently divide the nearest major venous mesenteric tributary that joins the posteromedial border of the SMV because this could be pulled across to the right by too much traction on the pancreatic head. We have attempted to carry out the division along the para-SMA groove using a vascular stapler and were not pleased; bleeding had to be suture controlled. Moreover, one has to be very certain where the stapler is applied to avoid an injury to the SMA. The final resection view is shown in Figure 18-16.

The specimen is placed in a water-impervious bag (Fig. 18-17) that is then closed and parked in the left subphrenic space; the retrieval bag with the specimen is exteriorized through a separate Pfannenstiel incision at the end of the procedure.

The pneumoperitoneum could then be evacuated, if desired, for a 30-minute break to enable the patient and surgeon some physiologic recovery.

Reconstruction

The greater omentum is once again lifted up to the supracolic space, and the intestine is exposed. A stay suture is applied to the distal divided end of the jejunum to facilitate its handling. With the assistant holding upward the transverse colon or its mesentery close to the colon wall, a small window in the root of the transverse mesocolon to the right of the middle colic vessels is created. The divided jejunum is held by the stay suture and is delivered into the supracolic subhepatic space.

The pancreas is mobilized off the splenic vein for 1.5 to 2 cm to facilitate suturing of the posterior layer of the pancreatojejunal anastomosis. An end-to-side, single-layer, full-thickness, stented (Figs. 18-18 and 18-19) pancreatojejunostomy is constructed

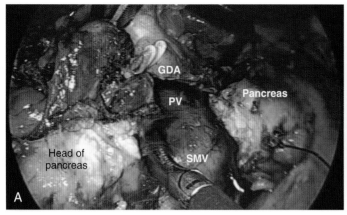 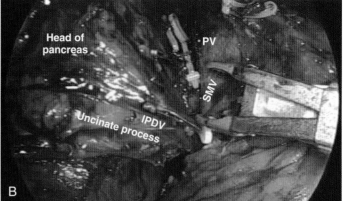

FIGURE 18-14 Dissection, clipping, and division of the venous tributaries from the pancreatic head to the portal vein (PV) and superior mesenteric vein (SMV) **(A)** as well as the inferior pancreaticoduodenal vein (IPDV) **(B)**. GDA, gastroduodenal artery.

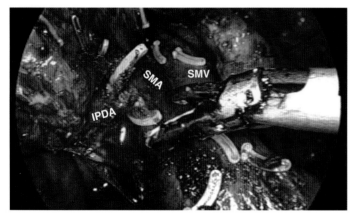 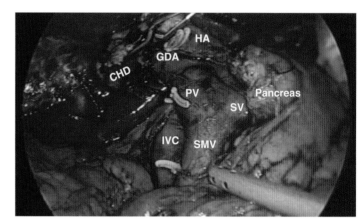

FIGURE 18-15 Dissection, clipping, and later division of the inferior pancreaticoduodenal artery (IPDA). SMA, superior mesenteric artery; SMV, superior mesenteric vein.

FIGURE 18-16 Final view at the end of the resection.

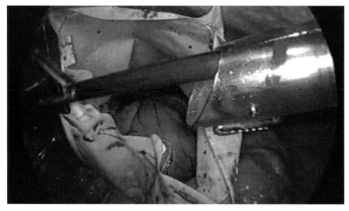 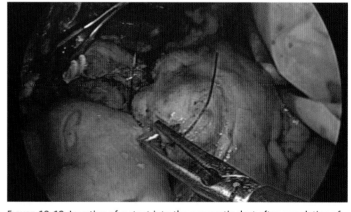

FIGURE 18-17 The resected specimen is placed in a water-impervious bag for retrieval through a Pfannenstiel incision at the end of surgery.

FIGURE 18-18 Insertion of a stent into the pancreatic duct after completion of the posterior layer of the end-to-side pancreatojejunostomy.

using 3-0 polydioxanone. This is the most challenging part of the reconstruction, and the ability to suture with both hands using forehand and backhand techniques is essential. Having tried interrupted and continuous suturing techniques, we now prefer the former; each suture is tied before the next is applied. The posterior layer is completed from the upper border of the pancreas to the lower border, and an internal stent 6 to 8 cm in length is then introduced into the pancreatic duct (see Fig. 18-18) and is not fixed. The anterior layer is completed leaving the last two or three sutures untied until they have been placed across the anastomosis. Care should be taken to ensure that each suture traverses the pancreatic duct and does not inadvertently catch its

opposite wall and obliterate the lumen. The completed view of the pancreatojejunostomy is shown in Figure 18-19. Some surgeons apply an end-to-end (fishmouth) technique to the pancreatojejunostomy, whereas others construct the pancreatic and biliary anastomoses through a small midline incision.

At a convenient point along the antimesenteric border of the jejunum and about 6 to 10 cm from the pancreatic anastomosis, the jejunum is opened longitudinally with the Harmonic scalpel for a distance slightly shorter than that of the width of the transacted bile duct. (The jejunal opening always stretches during suturing.) The bulldog is removed off the common hepatic duct, and an end-to-side choledochojejunostomy is fashioned using

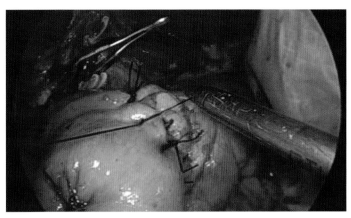

FIGURE 18-19 The completed end-to-side pancreatojejunal anastomosis that was fashioned with interrupted 3-0 PDS.

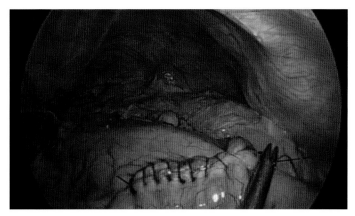

FIGURE 18-21 Hand-sutured end-to-side gastrojejunostomy using 3-0 Vicryl suture.

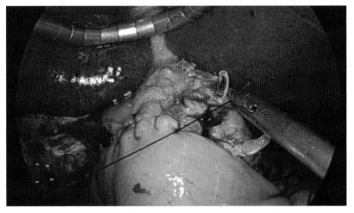

FIGURE 18-20 The completed end-to-side hepatojejunostomy that was fashioned with a continuous 4-0 Vicryl suture.

POSTOPERATIVE CARE

The patient is extubated at the conclusion of surgery and always transferred to the intensive care unit. Early mobilization is paramount, and jejunal feeding and oral fluids are commenced on the first postoperative day. The nasogastric tube could often be removed on the third postoperative day, and oral soft diet is commenced while the epidural analgesia is discontinued. More recently, we have been performing laparoscopic pancreatoduodenectomy without resorting to epidural anesthesia. The amylase concentration in the effluent fluid from the drains is measured on the third postoperative day in line with the International Study Group on Pancreatic Fistula guidelines, and the drains are removed if that concentration is low.

PROCEDURE-SPECIFIC COMPLICATIONS

Anastomotic leak from the choledochojejunal anastomosis requiring an open revision has been reported. Some surgeons advocate placement of a percutaneous T-tube catheter across the biliary-enteric anastomosis for drainage and postoperative radiologic assessment. Postoperative pancreatic fistula remains the most frequent specific major complication after pancreatic resection and is potentially life threatening, with associated increase in hospital stay and cost. Although LPD can be performed safely, the current mean rate of conversion to open surgery is just more than 10%.

RESULTS AND OUTCOME

To date, just fewer than 300 cases of LPD have been reported in the literature (Table 18-1). The technical difficulties of the operation and the lack of demonstrable benefit have led some to question the rationale of the minimally invasive approach for major pancreatic resections. Some early case series suggested that the hand-assisted approach to LPD shortened the operating time, although our recent review (see Table 18-1) showed that the totally laparoscopic approach was applied in two thirds of cases and the remainder performed by the robotic-assisted or the hand-assisted approach. Growth in experience with LPD is likely to lead to a reduction in operating time; Dulucq and associates reported a mean operative time of 287 minutes with 22 LPDs. Intraoperative blood loss during LPD compared favorably with that reported after open Whipple resection (338 vs. 740 to 1300 mL). A selection bias, however, may have contributed in favor of LPD.

one layer of continuous 4-0 Vicryl suture posteriorly. The anterior layer is completed either with a continuous 4-0 Vicryl suture if the duct is dilated (e.g., 8 mm or wider) (Fig. 18-20) or with interrupted sutures if it is not (described in Chapter 22 of the *Atlas of Minimally Invasive Surgery*, 2009; see Suggested Readings at the end of this chapter). The transverse colon mesenteric defect is then suture closed.

The jejunal loop is then traced in the infracolic compartment as it exits the mesocolon, and the length of the jejunum is measured to fashion an end-to-side antecolic gastrojejunostomy about 60 cm from the biliary anastomosis. The jejunum is suture-approximated to the stapled end of the stomach using a continuous 3-0 Vicryl suture that incorporates the staple line and takes seromuscular bites in the jejunal wall. The stomach and the jejunum are then opened with the UAS for about 5 cm, and a posterior inner layer is completed with continuous 3-0 Vicryl suture. The nasojejunal feeding tube is then located and advanced distally into the jejunum before completing the anterior layer of the gastrojejunostomy with a continuous 3-0 Vicryl suture in one layer (Fig. 18-21). Alternatively, a percutaneous feeding jejunostomy tube can be introduced into the jejunum distal to the gastrojejunostomy; it is secured to the jejunum with a pursestring 3-0 Vicryl suture and to the parietal peritoneum with interrupted sutures. Some surgeons, however, do not employ feeding tubes.

The abdomen is lavaged with warm normal saline, and two 20-French nonsuction drains are placed behind the biliary anastomosis from the right and in front of the biliary and pancreatic anastomoses from the left. A Pfannenstiel incision of about 6 cm is made, and the bag containing the resected specimen is removed; the incision is closed with polydioxanone.

Table 18-1 Summary of the Laparoscopic Pancreaticoduodenectomy Literature

Study	No. of Patients	Benign/ Malignant	Hand Assisted/Robotic Assisted/Totally Laparoscopic	Operative Time (min)*	Hospital Stay (days)*	Blood Lost (mL)*	Pancreatic Fistula: No. (%)	Postoperative Morbidity: No. (%)	Conversion to Open: No. (%)	No. of Lymph Nodes*	Follow-Up (month)*
Cuscieri (1994)	2	0/2	2/0/0								
Gagner & Pomp (1997)	10	2/8		510	22.7			2 (20)	4 (40)		
Staudacher et al (2005)	4	2/2	4/0/0	416	12	325	0	0	0	26	4.5
Kimura et al (2005)	1	0/1	1/0/0	300					0		
Mabrut et al (2005)	3	0/3	1/0/2	390	7	300	0				
Zheng et al (2006)	1	0/1			30	50					6
Dulucq et al (2006)	25	3/19	9/0/13	287	16.2	107		6 (27)	3 (12)	18	19
Lu et al (2006)	5	0/5	0/0/5	528		770	1 (20)	3 (60)	1 (20)		
Menon et al (2007)	1	0/1	0/0/1					0	0	17	12
Pugliese et al (2008)	19	1/12	7/0/6	482	18.5	180	3 (23)	7 (54)	6 (32)	11.6	32
Gumbs et al (2008)	3	3/0	0/0/3				1 (33)	1 (33)	1 (33)		20
Cai et al (2008)	1	0/1	0/0/1	510	14	800	0	0	0		23
Sa Cunha et al (2008)	2	/2	0/0/2	510	18.7	300	1 (50)	1 (50)	0		
Cho et al (2009)	1	1/0	0/0/1	450	14	200	0	0	0		
Palanivelu et al (2009)	75	3/72	0/0/75	357	8.2	74	5 (6.7)	20 (26.7)	0	14	60
Kuroki et al (2010)	9	5/4	0/0/9		19	642					
Kendrick et al (2010)	65	17/45	0/8/57	368	7	240	11 (16.9)	26 (40)	3	15	7.2
Guilianotti et al (2010)	60	15/45	0/60/0	421	22	394	19 (31.3)		11		
Ammori & Ayiomamitis (2010)	7	0/7	1/0/6	628.6	11.1	350	1 (14.3)	2 (28.6)	0	19.2	5
TOTALS	294	52/230	25/68/181	425.3	15.7	338	41 (17.7)	66 (30.3)	29 (10.4)	16.9	20.4

*Data shown represent mean.

The laparoscopic approach to pancreatoduodenectomy does not appear to shorten the postoperative hospital stay compared with what was reported from open series (an overall mean stay of 15.7 days), but appears to offer similar oncologic resection. The potential benefits of the laparoscopic approach to pancreatoduodenectomy may not be apparent during the immediate postoperative period; however, it is well established that patients return to normal activities faster and adjuvant chemotherapy may be initiated earlier. A randomized trial to compare LPD with open surgery will be extremely difficult to implement because the worldwide expertise in this complex procedure is very restricted. In addition, owing to the stringent selection criteria, the patients selected for LPD are likely to be a relatively small proportion of those requiring surgery.

The mean lymph node count in patients who underwent LPD for malignancy appears comparable to that reported by Western centers performing open pancreatoduodenectomy (16.9 vs. 16 to 17 nodes). The role of extended lymphadenectomy in patients undergoing pancreatoduodenectomy for periampullary cancer remains controversial. A meta-analysis of four randomized controlled trials that compared extended lymphadenectomy during pancreatoduodenectomy with standard resection showed greater morbidity with the former approach and no clear survival advantage. There are currently insufficient data to assess the adequacy of resection margins and long-term survival with LPD.

LPD requires an advanced degree of laparoscopic skills and should be performed in high-volume dedicated centers by surgeons who are experts in advanced laparoscopic surgery if optimal results are to be accomplished. Its feasibility and safety in such hands have been well demonstrated; it is now time to establish the evidence for the potential benefits of the laparoscopic approach in this setting and to confirm its long-term oncologic outcomes.

Suggested Readings

Ammori BJ: Pancreatic surgery in the laparoscopic era. *JOP* 4:187–192, 2003.

Ammori BJ, Ayiomamitis GD: Laparoscopic pancreaticoduodenectomy and distal pancreatectomy: A UK experience and a systematic review of the literature. *Surg Endosc* 25:2084–2099, 2011.

Bassi C, Dervenis C, Butturini G, et al: Postoperative pancreatic fistula: an international study group (ISGPF) definition. *Surgery* 138:8–13, 2005.

Bassi C, Molinari E, Malleo G, et al: Early versus late drain removal after standard pancreatic resections: Results of a prospective randomized trial. *Ann Surg* 252:207–124, 2010.

Bilimoria MM, Frantzides CT, Luu M, et al: Minimally invasive distal pancreatectomy. In Frantzides CT, Carlson MA, editors: *Atlas of Minimally Invasive Surgery*, Philadelphia, 2009, Saunders, pp 181–185.

Cai X, Wang Y, Yu H, et al: Completed laparoscopic pancreaticoduodenectomy. *Surg Laparosc Endosc Percutan Tech* 18(4):404–406, 2008.

Cho A, Yamamoto H, Nagata M, et al: A totally laparoscopic pylorus-preserving pancreaticoduodenectomy and reconstruction. *Surg Today* 39(4):359–362, 2009.

Cuschieri A: Laparoscopic surgery of the pancreas. *J R Coll Surg Edinb* 39:178–184, 1994.

Dulucq JL, Wintringer P, Mahajna A: Laparoscopic pancreaticoduodenectomy for benign and malignant diseases. *Surg Endosc* 20:1045–1050, 2006.

Dulucq JL, Wintringer P, Stabilini C, et al: Are major laparoscopic pancreatic resections worthwhile? A prospective study of 32 patients in a single institution. *Surg Endosc* 19:1028–1034, 2005.

Farnell MB, Aranha GV, Nimura Y, Michelassi F: The role of extended lymphadenectomy for adenocarcinoma of the head of the pancreas: Strength of the evidence. *J Gastrointest Surg* 12:651–656, 2008.

Gaghdadi S, Ammori BJ: Laparoscopic hepaticojejunostomy. In Frantzides CT, Carlson MA, editors: *Atlas of Minimally Invasive Surgery*, Philadelphia, 2009, Saunders, pp 169–177.

Gagner M, Pomp A: Laparoscopic pylorus-preserving pancreatoduodenectomy. *Surg Endosc* 8:408–410, 1994.

Gagner M, Pomp A: Laparoscopic pancreatic resection: Is it worthwhile? *J Gastrointest Surg* 1:20–25, 1997.

Giulianotti PC, Sbrana F, Bianco FM, et al: Robot-assisted laparoscopic pancreatic surgery: single-surgeon experience. *Surg Endosc* 24:1646–1657, 2010.

Gumbs AA, Gres P, Madureira FA, Gayet B: Laparoscopic vs. open resection of noninvasive intraductal pancreatic mucinous neoplasms. *J Gastrointest Surg* 12:707–712, 2008.

Kendrick ML, Cusati D: Total laparoscopic pancreaticoduodenectomy: Feasibility and outcome in an early experience. *Arch Surg* 145:19–23, 2010.

Kimura Y, Hirata K, Mukaiya M, et al: Hand-assisted laparoscopic pylorus-preserving pancreaticoduodenectomy for pancreas head disease. *Am J Surg* 189:734–737, 2005.

Kuroki T, Tajima Y, Kitasato A, et al: Pancreas-hanging maneuver in laparoscopic pancreaticoduodenectomy: A new technique for the safe resection of the pancreas head. *Surg Endosc* 24:1781–1783, 2010.

Lu B, Cai X, Lu W, et al: Laparoscopic pancreaticoduodenectomy to treat cancer of the ampulla of Vater. *JSLS* 10:97–100, 2006.

Mabrut JY, Fernandez-Cruz L, Azagra JS, et al: Laparoscopic pancreatic resection: results of a multicenter European study of 127 patients. *Surgery* 137:597–605, 2005.

Menon KV, Hayden JD, Prasad KR, Verbeke CS: Total laparoscopic pancreaticoduodenectomy and reconstruction for a cholangiocarcinoma of the bile duct. *J Laparoendosc Adv Surg Tech A* 17(6):775–780, 2007.

Palanivelu C, Rajan PS, Rangarajan M, et al: Evolution in techniques of laparoscopic pancreaticoduodenectomy: A decade long experience from a tertiary center. *J Hepatobiliary Pancreat Surg* 16:731–740, 2009.

Pugliese R, Scandroglio I, Sansonna F, et al: Laparoscopic pancreaticoduodenectomy: A retrospective review of 19 cases. *Surg Laparosc Endosc Percutan Tech* 18:13–18, 2008.

Sa Cunha A, Rault A, Beau C, et al: A single-institution prospective study of laparoscopic pancreatic resection. *Arch Surg* 143:289–295; discussion 295, 2008.

Staudacher C, Orsenigo E, Baccari P, et al: Laparoscopic assisted duodenopancreatectomy. *Surg Endosc* 19(3):352–356, 2005.

van der Gaag NA, Rauws EA, van Eijck CH, et al: Preoperative biliary drainage for cancer of the head of the pancreas. *N Engl J Med* 362:129–137, 2010.

Vollmer CM, Drebin JA, Middleton WD, et al: Utility of staging laparoscopy in subsets of peripancreatic and biliary malignancies. *Ann Surg* 235:1–7, 2002.

Zheng MH, Feng B, Lu AG, et al: Laparoscopic pancreaticoduodenectomy for ductal adenocarcinoma of common bile duct: A case report and literature review. *Med Sci Monit* 12:CS57–CS60, 2006.

BASIL J. AMMORI AND GEORGIOS D. AYIOMAMITIS

CHAPTER

19

Laparoscopic Cholecystojejunostomy

The videos associated with this chapter are listed in the Video Contents and can be found on the accompanying DVDs and on Expertconsult.com.

Obstructive jaundice is the most common presentation in patients with periampullary cancer (PAC), of whom 80% to 90% have unresectable disease and require palliative measures. PAC includes cancer of the head of pancreas, distal bile duct, ampulla or duodenum. These patients are generally debilitated and malnourished and have a median life expectancy of about 6 to 7 months for metastatic disease and 10 months for locally advanced nonmetastatic cancer. This should be taken into account when considering palliative measures to relieve jaundice, with emphasis placed on minimally invasive interventions. These interventions, however, should be expected to offer a high success rate in relieving the biliary obstruction with a durable result that lasts the patient's expected life. In the contemporary era of minimally invasive options, the place for open palliative biliary bypass with its antecedent morbidity has largely become extinct with the exception of the now less frequent scenario of the unexpectedly unresectable disease at laparotomy.

To date, more than 70 palliative laparoscopic biliary bypasses for PAC have been reported in the literature, with cholecystojejunostomy (CCJ) representing the large majority. This has been accomplished with high success rate in relieving jaundice in those selected patients and with minimal morbidity.

OPERATIVE INDICATIONS

At the outset, it is essential to establish that biliary bypass by CCJ is not an option in patients with benign distal biliary strictures because these patients are best managed by Roux-en-Y hepatojejunostomy (HJ) with or without resection of the underlying disease, such as in patients with chronic pancreatitis. This exclusion of benign disease relates to the fact that CCJ offers a shorter long-term patency compared with HJ.

A proposed algorithm for management of PAC that incorporates the applications of laparoscopic biliary and gastric bypass is outlined in Figure 19-1, and relevant aspects are discussed later.

Palliation of Obstructive Jaundice

Laparoscopic CCJ is therefore reserved primarily for patients with malignancy, and its primary role is for palliation of obstructive jaundice in patients with unresectable PAC. It is accepted that patients with obstructive jaundice and unresectable PAC cancer due to either metastatic or locally advanced disease are best treated by endoscopic insertion of a biliary stent whenever possible; the percutaneous transhepatic route is being reserved for failures of the endoscopic approach. Laparoscopic biliary bypass is a last resort in the uncommon instances of failure of the endoscopic and radiologic percutaneous approaches to biliary stent insertion.

Occasionally, the surgeon is faced with the diagnosis of inoperable disease at the time of staging laparoscopy. Consideration may be given to laparoscopic CCJ if the patient's biliary tree remains obstructed at the time of staging laparoscopy and the endoscopic approach to biliary drainage is not feasible because of gastric outlet obstruction (in which case, CCJ is combined with a gastrojejunostomy) or has failed.

Before Whipple Procedure

It is recognized that pre-resection biliary drainage using stents increases the risk for septic morbidity after resection and is therefore best avoided unless the patient is deeply jaundiced (e.g., bilirubin <11 to 14 mg/dL) or some delay is anticipated before resection with an inevitable further rise in bilirubin to above that threshold. An alternative to biliary stenting under those circumstances is to consider laparoscopic CCJ at the time of staging laparoscopy; this avoids the immediate and delayed risks for stent insertion and minimizes the number of interventions. Resection could be undertaken about 2 weeks later.

Prophylaxis

Patients with unresectable PAC who present with gastric outlet obstruction are usually managed by a palliative insertion of an expandable metal duodenal stent in the first instance. Failure of this endoscopic procedure is an indication to proceed to laparoscopic gastric bypass. If unresectability is due to a locally advanced rather than metastatic disease with its associated better prognosis, and if the patient has no distal biliary obstruction, then consideration should be given to a prophylactic CCJ. A typical example is in patients with uncinate process tumors that involve the superior mesenteric vessels as well as the distal duodenum, leading to duodenal obstruction. In the absence of metastases, future disease progression to involve the distal biliary tree is likely. A prophylactic CCJ at the time of gastrojejunostomy is a valid option and ensures a course of palliative

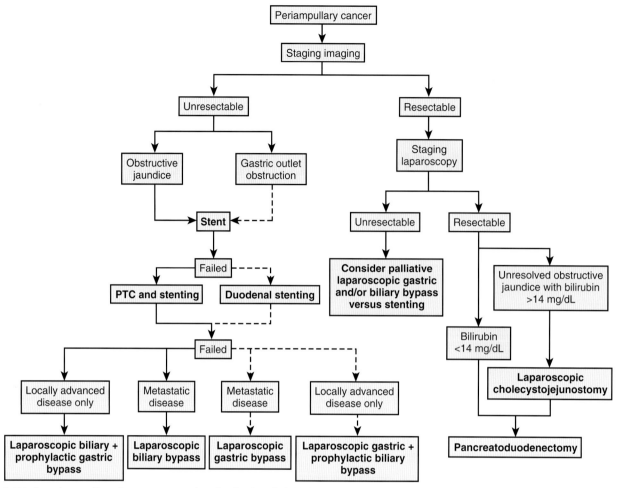

FIGURE 19-1 This flow chart outlines the management algorithm for the relief of biliary obstruction and/or gastric outlet obstruction in patients with periampullary cancer. *Stent* refers to duodenal and/or biliary stents, as appropriate. PTC, percutaneous transhepatic cholangiogram.

chemotherapy uninterrupted by a delayed onset of obstructive jaundice.

PREOPERATIVE EVALUATION, TESTING, AND PREPARATION

There are physical and safety conditions that ought to be considered before embarking on laparoscopic CCJ.

Physical Conditions

Clearly, a patent cystic duct is a prerequisite for CCJ to function. In addition, the point of insertion of the cystic duct into the bile duct should preferably be 1 cm or greater above the distal biliary stricture to achieve a durable biliary drainage for the duration of the patient's life expectancy, particularly in patients with locally advanced rather than metastatic disease who have a better survival outlook. To identify the biliary anatomy correctly, a magnetic resonance cholangiopancreatogram may be required. Alternatively, information could be obtained from staging computed tomography or from endoscopic retrograde cholangiopancreatography or percutaneous transhepatic cholangiography that has failed to achieve stenting (Fig. 19-2). If preoperative imaging information is not available or when in doubt, one could consider intraoperative transcholecystic cholangiography or laparoscopic ultrasound to delineate the anatomy of the cystic duct

insertion in relation to the stricture; however, we prefer to rely on preoperative imaging, thus avoiding extension of the duration of what is palliative surgery.

In the context of palliation, it is essential that the intraabdominal conditions not be hostile to the intended drainage procedure. The need to divide significant upper abdominal adhesions from previous major surgery, the presence of a bulky tumor that could preclude easy access to the gallbladder and hamper a tension-free anastomosis, the presence of ascites, or previous intestinal surgery with considerable adhesions render the option of CCJ unfavorable.

The presence of gallstones within the gallbladder is not a contraindication to CCJ because these can be evacuated at the time of surgery. However, the presence of gallstones in association with a diseased and contracted gallbladder is a contraindication to this procedure; this scenario is quite uncommon.

Safety Conditions

All the prerequisites for healing of an intestinal anastomosis should be respected. In particular, severely malnourished, edematous, and hypoalbuminemic patients have a higher risk for anastomotic leak and should not be offered surgical bypass under those circumstances.

Whether CCJ is carried out as a palliative procedure in patients with shortened life expectancy or as a pre-resection drainage procedure, it is essential that operative morbidity be kept to

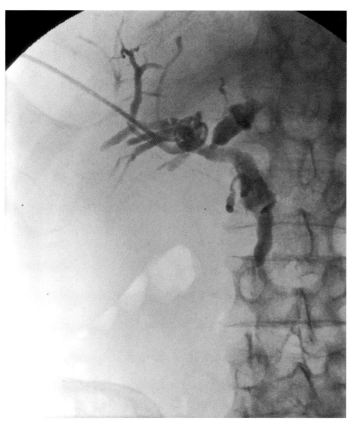

FIGURE 19-2 Preoperative percutaneous transhepatic cholangiogram in a patient with locally advanced pancreatic head cancer and a failed endoscopic retrograde pancreatography confirms a cystic duct insertion more than 1 cm above the stricture and, therefore, suitability for palliative laparoscopic cholecystojejunostomy if transcutaneous stenting fails.

the very minimum. Although the laparoscopic approach has its advantages as a minimally invasive procedure, it is equally important that the surgeon has established expertise in intestinal anastomoses and intracorporeal suturing.

PATIENT POSITIONING AND TROCAR PLACEMENT

Laparoscopic CCJ is carried out under general anesthesia with perioperative intravenous antibiotic coverage. The patient may be positioned supine with the surgeon and assistant standing to the left of the patient; alternatively, the patient may be placed in flat Lloyd-Davies position with the surgeon standing between the legs. Four ports are usually required, of which one employs a retractor against the liver to enhance exposure and access to the gallbladder. More recently, however, Tian and associates reported the first two cases of transumbilical single-incision laparoscopic CCJ demonstrating its feasibility, albeit at a rather prolonged operating time.

OPERATIVE TECHNIQUE

At laparoscopy, it is essential to establish that the gallbladder is distended in keeping with the preoperative imaging findings, rather than collapsed or contracted, and that there is no bulky disease that will preclude safe reach of jejunum to the gallbladder without tension. Any obvious tumor mass is biopsied if no prior histologic diagnosis has been obtained.

The omentum is lifted upward to expose the small intestine, and the duodenojejunal flexure is identified. A convenient loop of proximal jejunum is brought in an antecolic fashion to lie adjacent to the gallbladder. In cases of palliation, this could be about 50 cm from the duodenojejunal flexure, whereas in pre-resection CCJ, the loop is made about 75 cm long to allow for future reconstruction following pancreatoduodenectomy (Fig. 19-3). At the time of the subsequent pancreatoduodenectomy, 2 to 3 weeks after CCJ, the segment of jejunum at the CCJ may be resected en bloc with the gallbladder and the whole of the specimen, and the proximal jejunum is divided about 10 cm distal to the duodenojejunal flexure, leaving a free 60-cm loop of jejunum to be employed as a retrocolic Roux-en-Y loop for pancreatic and biliary reconstruction (see Fig. 19-3B).

In patients who require both a CCJ and a gastrojejunostomy, we prefer to construct the CCJ first and more distally before creating a gastrojejunostomy because the latter, if constructed first, could obscure the exposure for the CCJ.

The CCJ could be either sutured or staple-sutured. To fashion a fully sutured CCJ, an initial stitch is employed simply for the purpose of anchoring the jejunum to the gallbladder; it is continued over no more than 2 cm as a seromuscular posterior layer to the anastomosis-to-be. The jejunum is opened first in a longitudinal manner for about 1 cm using diathermy scissors or an ultrasonically activated scalpel, whereas the gallbladder is similarly opened; this minimizes the time that the gallbladder is kept open and therefore minimizes the contamination of the peritoneal cavity. If the gallbladder contained gallstones, these should be evacuated thoroughly to prevent future gallstone ileus or obstruction of the cystic duct or CCJ anastomosis. A continuous absorbable suture (e.g., Vicryl 3-0) is used to create a second posterior layer of the side-to-side CCJ and is continued to complete an anterior layer (Fig. 19-4). We do not find a second seromuscular anterior layer necessary for any gastrointestinal or pancreatobiliary anastomosis.

For a staple-sutured anastomosis, a single suture placed to anchor the jejunum to the body of the gallbladder is sufficient. A small enterotomy is made first and is followed by the creation of a similar opening in the gallbladder. Care should be exercised to suction spilled bile from the obstructed biliary tree to minimize contamination of the peritoneal cavity. A 35- to 45-mm vascular stapler is applied to create a side-to-side CCJ, and the common cholecystotomy-enterotomy is closed with a continuous absorbable suture.

The peritoneal cavity is copiously irrigated with warm saline to clear any bile contamination, and an abdominal nonsuction drain is selectively applied posterior to the anastomosis.

POSTOPERATIVE CARE

Oral fluids may be administered on the evening after surgery, and free fluids and liquid diet may be allowed the following day. We advise that patients adhere to a liquid diet for 7 days and then a soft diet for a further 7 days before resuming a normal solid diet. Prophylactic intravenous antibiotics may be continued for 24 hours after surgery. The abdominal drain is removed within 24 to 48 hours if there is no bile leakage.

Patients with unresectable PAC are then referred to the oncology services for consideration for palliative chemotherapy and possible entry into randomized controlled trials.

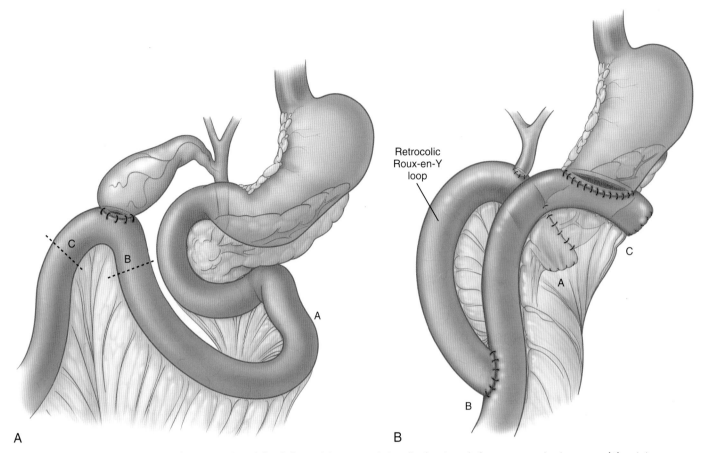

A

B

FIGURE 19-3 This diagram demonstrates the construction of the cholecystojejunostomy in jaundiced patients before pancreatoduodenectomy **(A)** and the subsequent classic resection (pancreatoduodenectomy with cholecystectomy and distal gastrectomy) and reconstruction **(B)**. The length of the afferent loop (A–B) is about 75 cm.

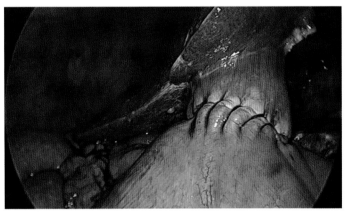

FIGURE 19-4 Operative image of the completed cholecystojejunal anastomosis.

RESULTS AND OUTCOME

The authors' experience with laparoscopic gastric and biliary bypass for PAC reported herein was associated with rapid postoperative recovery and short hospital stay. The addition of prophylactic gastric or biliary bypass neither prolongs the operating time significantly nor influences the duration of postoperative hospital stay but prevents future onset of obstructive symptoms. Pre-resection biliary bypass at the time of staging laparoscopy in deeply jaundiced patients with resectable pancreatic cancer appears safe and effective and does not preclude subsequent resection and reconstruction.

Palliation

The argument that CCJ is not a good biliary drainage procedure because of its poor long-term patency rates is true for patients with benign disease and expected extended survival but rather untrue in the context of palliation for unresectable periampullary carcinoma. This is because (1) there is a very small difference in patency rates between CCJ and HJ at 1-year follow-up and (2) only half the patients may be alive at that stage. In a retrospective cohort study of 1919 patients who had a surgical biliary bypass for pancreatic cancer, additional biliary interventions were required at 1, 2, and 5 years in 7.5%, 17.4%, and 26.0% of 945 patients initially treated with a CCJ compared with 2.9%, 11.0%, and 13.3% of 974 patients initially treated with an HJ. It is not practical to routinely apply laparoscopic HJ as a palliative biliary drainage procedure because it is technically more demanding, prolongs operating time and hospital stay, and carries higher morbidity. The authors reserve this procedure for the palliation of locally advanced PAC when endoscopic and percutaneous transhepatic approaches have failed and when the insertion of the cystic duct is within less than 1 cm from the upper end of the malignant distal biliary stricture. In a previous report, the authors applied laparoscopic CCJ to the large majority of their patients with advanced PAC (who either experienced failed biliary stenting or were found to have unresectable disease at staging laparoscopy) and encountered no recurrence of jaundice until the time of death in these selected patients. This experience contrasts with the findings by Tarnasky and colleagues, who evaluated ERCP images of 101 patients with malignant distal biliary obstruction and reported that a cystic duct insertion more than 1 cm above the stricture existed in only one third of the patients.

Several reports of laparoscopic CCJ, including the authors', have established the safety and effectiveness of this procedure in palliating obstructive jaundice in selected patients with an associated short hospital stay and low, if any, recurrence of jaundice before death. The advantage of long-term patency and fewer additional treatments with the surgical biliary bypass over plastic biliary stenting with an associated comparable mortality is well established from meta-analysis of several comparative studies. There is no doubt, however, that metal biliary stents, albeit more expensive, reduce the need for reintervention compared with plastic stents and may therefore offer an overall cost advantage. A randomized trial of metal biliary stents versus palliative surgical bypass reported comparable success rates in relieving jaundice and morbidity rates, with stenting being cheaper, although the surgery carried a far-reduced chance of long-term recurrence. For these reasons, we believe that metal biliary stenting should be considered as the first line of palliation in patients with locally advanced PAC, with surgery reserved for failures.

Prophylaxis

We have applied laparoscopic CCJ as a prophylactic procedure in patients who required palliative gastric bypass after failed attempts at endoscopic duodenal stenting, but only in patients with locally advanced rather than metastatic disease, who carry better prognosis. It is uncommon for patients to present with gastric outlet obstruction without obstructive jaundice; a typical example is that of an uncinate or distal duodenal tumor that causes duodenal obstruction and later progresses to obstruct the distal bile duct. The addition of a prophylactic laparoscopic biliary bypass to a therapeutic gastric bypass does not appear to increase operative morbidity or postoperative hospital stay, as the authors' data have shown. However, it is unnecessary to add a prophylactic bypass, biliary or gastric, in patients with metastatic disease because of their rather short life expectancy. Espat and colleagues found that 98% of 155 laparoscopically staged patients with unresectable histologically confirmed pancreatic adenocarcinoma, three fourths of whom had metastatic disease, did not require a subsequent surgical procedure to treat biliary or gastric obstruction.

Before Whipple Procedure

There is evidence to suggest that endoscopic biliary drainage before pancreatoduodenectomy is an ill advised, albeit common, practice. In a case-matched controlled study of pre-resection biliary drainage (89% underwent internal endoscopic biliary stenting) versus no drainage in 184 patients with pancreatic adenocarcinoma, drainage was associated with a stent-related complication rate of 23%, a greater likelihood of infected bile (82% vs. 7%), and a twofold increase in post-resection infectious complications. That said, endoscopic drainage does not appear to increase post-resection operative mortality, as a Cochrane review of two randomized trials with 125 patients undergoing pancreatoduodenectomy has found. On the other hand, it is worth noting that deep jaundice (serum bilirubin >10 mg/dL) may significantly increase the risk for intra-abdominal bleeding and operative time. For these reasons, it is our policy to avoid biliary drainage in the lightly jaundiced patient and to carry out

pre-resection laparoscopic CCJ at the time of staging laparoscopy in the deeply jaundiced patient (arbitrary figure of serum bilirubin ≥14 mg/dL) in whom endoscopic biliary stenting failed and in whom preoperative imaging has indicated that a CCJ is a valid option. We have found no incidences of implantation of cancer at the site of the CCJ anastomosis at the time of resection.

The data on laparoscopic CCJ indicate that it is a safe procedure with very low risk for anastomotic leak. It is essential, however, that this procedure be carried out by surgeons experienced in laparoscopic and hepatopancreatobiliary surgery in order to keep operative morbidity at a minimum in this vulnerable group of cancer patients.

In conclusion, laparoscopic cholecystojejunostomy has palliative as well as prophylactic applications in selected patients with unresectable periampullary carcinoma. In patients with resectable periampullary carcinoma, laparoscopic cholecystojejunostomy may play a role in pre-resection relief of deep obstructive jaundice. A careful evaluation of preoperative imaging is essential before embarking on palliative laparoscopic cholecystojejunostomy in order to ensure a cystic duct insertion of 1 cm or more above the stricture. Prophylactic bypass surgery does not prolong the operating time or hospital stay significantly, and it prevents future onset of obstructive symptoms.

Suggested Readings

Artifon EL, Sakai P, Cunha JE, et al: Surgery or endoscopy for palliation of biliary obstruction due to metastatic pancreatic cancer. Am J Gastroenterol 101:2031–2037, 2006.

Chekan EG, Clark L, Wu J, et al: Laparoscopic biliary and enteric bypass. Semin Surg Oncol 16:313–320, 1999.

Espat NJ, Brennan MF, Conlon KC: Patients with laparoscopically staged unresectable pancreatic adenocarcinoma do not require subsequent surgical biliary or gastric bypass. J Am Coll Surg 188:649–657, 1999.

Ghanem AM, Hamade AM, Sheen AJ, et al: Laparoscopic gastric and biliary bypass: a single-center cohort prospective study. J Laparoendosc Adv Surg Tech A 16:21–26, 2006.

Hamade AM, Al-Bahrani AZ, Owera AM, et al: Therapeutic, prophylactic, and pre-resection applications of laparoscopic gastric and biliary bypass for patients with periampullary malignancy. Surg Endosc 19:1333–1340, 2005.

Hodul P, Creech S, Pickleman J, Aranha GV: The effect of preoperative biliary stenting on postoperative complications after pancreaticoduodenectomy. Am J Surg 186:420–425, 2003.

Kuriansky J, Saenz A, Astudillo E, et al: Simultaneous laparoscopic biliary and retrocolic gastric bypass in patients with unresectable carcinoma of the pancreas. Surg Endosc 14:179–181, 2000.

Mezhir JJ, Brennan MF, Baser RE, et al: A matched case-control study of preoperative biliary drainage in patients with pancreatic adenocarcinoma: Routine drainage is not justified. J Gastrointest Surg 13:2163–2169, 2009.

Moss AC, Morris E, Leyden J, MacMathuna P: Malignant distal biliary obstruction: A systematic review and meta-analysis of endoscopic and surgical bypass results. Cancer Treat Rev 33:213–221, 2007.

Mumtaz K, Hamid S, Jafri W: Endoscopic retrograde cholangiopancreaticography with or without stenting in patients with pancreaticobiliary malignancy, prior to surgery. Cochrane Database Syst Rev 3:CD006001, 2007.

Rhodes M, Nathanson L, Fielding G: Laparoscopic biliary and gastric bypass: A useful adjunct in the treatment of carcinoma of the pancreas. Gut 36:778–780, 1995.

Schneider BP, Ganjoo KN, Seitz DE, et al: Phase II study of gemcitabine plus docetaxel in advanced pancreatic cancer: A Hoosier Oncology Group study. Oncology 65:218–223, 2003.

Shimi S, Banting S, Cuschieri A: Laparoscopy in the management of pancreatic cancer: Endoscopic cholecystojejunostomy for advanced disease. Br J Surg 79:317–319, 1992.

Srivastava S, Sikora SS, Kumar A, et al: Outcome following pancreaticoduodenectomy in patients undergoing preoperative biliary drainage. Dig Surg 18:381–387, 2001.

Shyr YM, Su CH, Wu CW, Lui WY: Prospective study of gastric outlet obstruction in unresectable periampullary adenocarcinoma. World J Surg 24:60–65, 2000.

Tarnasky PR, England RE, Lail LM, et al: Cystic duct patency in malignant obstructive jaundice: An ERCP-based study relevant to the role of laparoscopic cholecysto-jejunostomy. *Ann Surg* 221:265–271, 1995.

Taylor MC, McLeod RS, Langer B: Biliary stenting versus bypass surgery for the palliation of malignant distal bile duct obstruction: A meta-analysis. *Liver Transpl* 6:302–308, 2000.

Terwee CB, Nieveen Van Dijkum EJ, Gouma DJ, et al: Pooling of prognostic studies in cancer of the pancreatic head and periampullary region: The Triple-P study. Triple-P study group. *Eur J Surg* 166:706–712, 2000.

Tian Y, Wu SD, Chen YS, Chen CC: Transumbilical single-incision laparoscopic cholecystojejunostomy using conventional instruments: The first two cases. *J Gastrointest Surg* 14:1429–1433, 2010.

Urbach DR, Bell CM, Swanstrom LL, Hansen PD: Cohort study of surgical bypass to the gallbladder or bile duct for the palliation of jaundice due to pancreatic cancer. *Ann Surg* 237:86–93, 2003.

BASIL J. AMMORI AND GEORGIOS D. AYIOMAMITIS

Laparoscopic Management of Pancreatic Pseudocysts

20

The videos associated with this chapter are listed in the Video Contents and can be found on the accompanying DVDs and *on Expertconsult.com.*

A pancreatic pseudocyst (PP) is a collection of amylase-rich pancreatic fluid enclosed by a wall of fibrous granulation tissue without a true epithelial lining. In general, a peripancreatic fluid collection should be present for 5 to 6 weeks before the diagnosis of PP is considered. A collection that is present for less than this time is more accurately referred to as an acute peripancreatic fluid collection. An acute PP is defined as occurring after an episode of acute pancreatitis and complicates 2% to 10% of these patients with acute pancreatitis in whom the main pancreatic duct has been disrupted. A chronic PP is defined as occurring in association with chronic pancreatitis and arises in 10% to 30% of patients with this diagnosis. Pseudocysts also can complicate pancreatic trauma or ductal obstruction due to stricture or stone. The rate of spontaneous resolution of acute PPs has ranged from 30% to 85% in various reports.

Regarding the management of PP disease, it is essential to establish a diagnosis of pseudocyst while considering the possibility of a cystic neoplasm (see later). The management of PPs has evolved to include radiologic, endoscopic, and laparoscopic approaches. Endoscopic internal drainage of "acute" pseudocysts has been associated with low resolution rates; there also is a risk for secondary bacterial infection from inadequately débrided necrotic tissue within the pseudocyst cavity. Although endoscopic drainage techniques will continue to evolve, large persistent and symptomatic acute pseudocysts probably are best treated with an operative procedure.

Surgical treatment involves the creation of an internal communication between the PP and the gastrointestinal tract to allow the amylase-rich fluid within the PP to drain into the intestinal lumen. Open internal drainage consistently has produced good long-term results and therefore has been considered the treatment of choice. Open internal drainage most often was accomplished with a pseudocyst-gastrostomy or, if there was extensive infracolic extension, a Roux-en-Y pseudocyst-jejunostomy. These procedures now can be performed safely and effectively using laparoscopic techniques, and the literature contains a number of confirmatory series. Laparoscopic pseudocyst drainage adheres to the same principles as the open procedure, differing only in the nature of operative access.

OPERATIVE INDICATIONS

Because most PPs resolve spontaneously, internal drainage is reserved for pseudocysts that cause symptoms (e.g., abdominal pain and distention) or produce complications, such as gastric outlet obstruction, obstructive jaundice, abscess formation, pseudoaneurysm, gastrointestinal or intracystic bleeding, or pseudocyst rupture. In addition, PPs that are large (>6 cm), persistent (no regression after 6 weeks), or growing in size warrant intervention; if left untreated, these pseudocysts have a considerable complication risk.

If a PP patient fulfills the previously mentioned operative indications for internal drainage, then the surgeon should consider the following factors to determine the approach and timing of the laparoscopic intervention.

Availability of Endoscopic Drainage

If local expertise is available, a chronic PP can be drained endoscopically if (1) there is minimal necrotic debris in its cavity; (2) it has a retrogastric or juxtaduodenal location; and (3) the wall is less than 1 cm thick. Long-term resolution of a PP after stenting of the pancreatic duct is dependent on the presence of a communication between the duct and the PP and the subsequent absence of a stent-induced stricture in the proximal duct. The presence of necrotic debris within a PP (demonstrable on cross-sectional imaging or endoscopic ultrasound) may obstruct an endoscopically placed stent and predispose the cavity to infection. Endoscopic drainage of PP secondary to acute necrotizing pancreatitis has been associated with drainage failure (15%), other morbidity (13%), and recurrence (11%). With appropriate patient selection, success rates with endoscopic PP drainage can approach 100%.

Location of the PP

A retrogastric or juxtagastric PP can be drained by pseudocyst-gastrostomy. A PP that protrudes into the infracolic region may be drained in a dependent fashion using a pseudocyst-jejunostomy. A PP located in the tail of the pancreas may be managed by internal drainage or distal pancreatosplenectomy (open or laparoscopic).

Maturity of the Pseudocyst Wall

To create a stable anastomosis between the PP and the gastrointestinal tract, it is essential that a defined pseudocyst wall be demonstrable on a preoperative computed tomography (CT) scan. A PP wall with more than 1 cm thickness is a relative contraindication to endoscopic internal drainage; such a pseudocyst is best drained surgically.

Presence of Local Complications

An associated pseudoaneurysm should be embolized before surgical drainage of the PP. If gastric outlet or biliary obstruction is present, then PP drainage invariably will result in resolution of the obstruction. Percutaneous drainage by an interventional radiologist usually is reserved for the septic patient with an infected fluid collection because this procedure is associated with a considerable risk for pancreatocutaneous fistula and PP recurrence. If the patient has portal hypertension with varices, then surgical internal drainage may be safer, with a lower risk for bleeding, than endoscopic drainage.

Preoperative testing, evaluation, and preparation

Although cystic neoplasm of the pancreas is rare, this tumor can be mistaken for a PP. A history of acute pancreatitis suggests PP, but a pancreatic neoplasm also can precipitate an acute attack of pancreatitis. Radiologically documented development of a PP during the course of acute or chronic pancreatitis is somewhat reassuring. Weight loss, the lack of preexisting pancreatic disease (particularly in women), multilocularity or nodularity on imaging, a highly viscous cyst aspirate, and a markedly elevated carcinoembryonic antigen (>192 ng/mL) all make a cystic malignancy more likely.

The location, size, wall characteristics, and the presence of local complications (e.g., pseudoaneurysm) should be assessed with contrast-enhanced (intravenous and oral) CT. If the diagnosis is not clear after CT scanning, then additional information may be obtained with magnetic resonance imaging or endoscopic ultrasound (EUS). In addition to its high sensitivity (93% to 100%) and specificity (92% to 98%), the linear EUS probe can facilitate a cyst wall biopsy and cyst aspirate for tumor marker analysis.

Patient positioning and placement of trocars

All procedures are performed under general anesthesia, with broad-spectrum antibiotic coverage and prophylaxis against deep venous thrombosis. For laparoscopic pseudocyst-gastrostomy, the patient is placed in the French (lithotomy) position, with the surgeon standing between the legs, the first assistant and scrub nurse to either side, and the monitor over the patient's head. The surgeon's position for pseudocyst-jejunostomy may be on either side of the table or between the legs, depending on the PP location. The pneumoperitoneum is set at 12 mm Hg. A 10-mm port for the 30-degree laparoscope is placed one handbreadth away from the target (the PP-gastric or PP-jejunal anastomosis), and two or three 5- or 10-mm ports are placed on either side in order to achieve triangulation (Fig. 20-1). An additional 5-mm port may be placed laterally to retract the liver, spleen, and stomach if these organs impinge on the operative field.

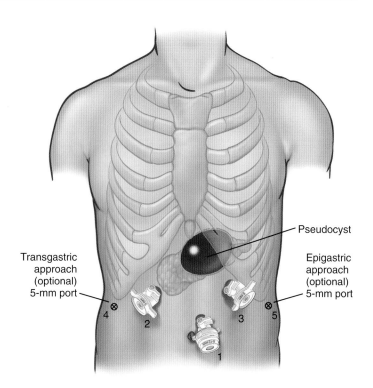

Figure 20-1 Placement of trocars. 1 = laparoscope (5-12 mm); 2, 3 = operating ports (5 mm); 4 = optional port for transgastric approach (5 mm); 5 = optional port for epigastric approach (5 mm).

Anatomic classification of pancreatic pseudocysts

The following section describes a surgically oriented approach to the classification of PP disease.

Large Retrogastric PP

This type is by far the most common and is readily visible and palpable on laparoscopy (Fig. 20-2). Internal drainage is readily achieved by the transgastric approach.

Small Retrogastric or Juxtagastric PP

This type is not readily visible or palpable on laparoscopy (Fig. 20-3). Although a small retrogastric PP can be located with the aid of laparoscopic ultrasound, transgastric drainage may be difficult because of the relatively small area of contact between the stomach and the pseudocyst wall. This type of PP is best managed through an exogastric (lesser sac) approach so that an ample-sized hand-sutured anastomosis may be performed. A juxtagastric PP may be contained within the splenic hilum or within the gastrohepatic ligament (Fig. 20-4); these also should be accessed with an exogastric approach, with division of the gastrocolic, lienogastric, or gastrohepatic ligaments and creation of a hand-sutured pseudocyst-gastrostomy.

Infracolic PP

This type protrudes through the mesocolon and into the infracolic compartment (Fig. 20-5) and thus is not amenable to dependent drainage with a pseudocyst-gastrostomy. In this case, a Roux-en-Y pseudocyst-jejunostomy should be performed.

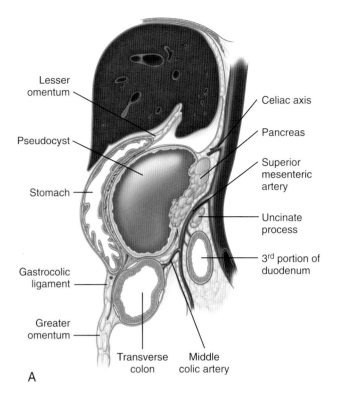

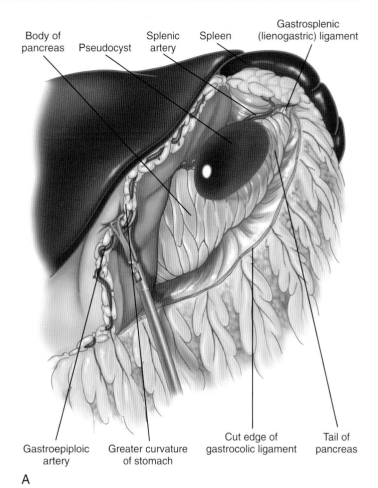

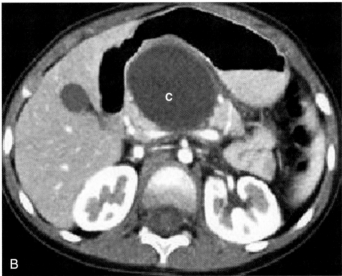

FIGURE 20-2 Large retrogastric pancreatic pseudocyst displacing the stomach. **A,** Sagittal schematic. **B,** Axial computed tomography image showing pseudocyst (c). This type of pseudocyst is visible and palpable at laparoscopy and can be drained through a transgastric approach (cystgastrostomy).

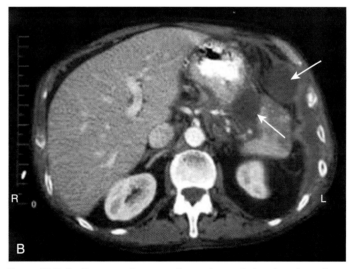

FIGURE 20-3 Small retrogastric pancreatic pseudocyst. **A,** Anterior schematic. **B,** Axial computed tomography image (*arrows* indicate pseudocysts). This type of pseudocyst is visible by division of the gastrocolic omentum (lesser sac approach) and can be drained with an exogastric approach (cystgastrostomy).

Small Juxtaduodenal PP

This type predominantly is located within the head of the pancreas (Fig. 20-6) and is associated with chronic pancreatitis. A small juxtaduodenal PP may be managed endoscopically using either EUS-guided aspiration and drainage or transpapillary pancreatic duct stenting. Failure to achieve lasting resolution by the endoscopic approach necessitates surgical drainage. The proximity of a juxtaduodenal PP to the medial wall of the second or third part of the duodenum makes pseudocyst-duodenostomy the best surgical option. Laparoscopic ultrasound often is essential to locate the pseudocyst if it is not visible after exposure of the pancreatic head.

OPERATIVE TECHNIQUE

Transgastric Approach

An anterior longitudinal gastrotomy of 7 to 8 cm is made using an ultrasonically activated scalpel (Ethicon Endo-Surgery, Cincinnati, Ohio) to provide access for *distal* internal drainage of the PP into the gastric lumen (Fig. 20-7). A needle is then introduced through the posterior gastric wall into the PP; this confirms its accessibility through the posterior gastric wall and

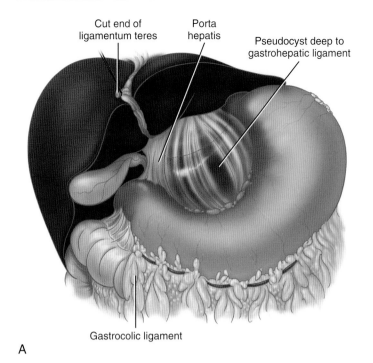

A

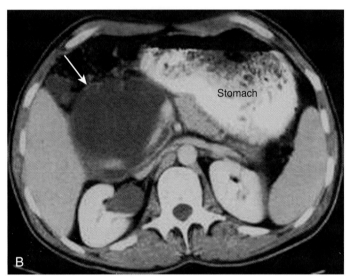

B

FIGURE 20-4 Juxtagastric pancreatic pseudocyst lying in the gastrohepatic ligament. **A,** Anterior schematic. **B,** Axial computed tomography image (*arrow* indicates pseudocyst). This type of pseudocyst can be drained with an exogastric approach through the lesser omentum (cystgastrostomy).

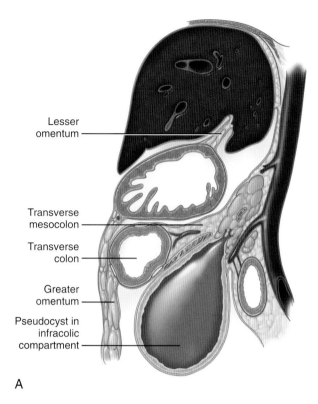

A

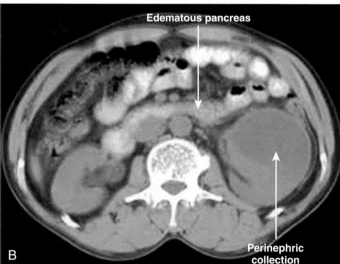

B

FIGURE 20-5 Large pancreatic pseudocyst extending into the infracolic compartment. **A,** Sagittal schematic. **B,** Axial computed tomography image. This type of pseudocyst can be drained with a Roux-en-Y cystojejunostomy.

provides fluid for amylase, cytology, and microbiology (Fig. 20-8). A 5-cm posterior gastrotomy extending into the PP lumen is created using the UAS, and any necrotic material is débrided (Fig. 20-9). The necrotic material is placed into a specimen bag (LapSac surgical tissue pouch, Cook Surgical, Bloomington, Ind.), which is removed at the end of the procedure (Fig. 20-10). Suturing of the pseudocyst-gastrostomy is necessary if the PP wall spontaneously detaches from the posterior gastric wall or if there is bleeding from the gastrotomy. (The latter particularly may be an issue in a patient with splenic or portal vein thrombosis and varices.) The anterior gastrotomy then is closed in one layer with a continuous 2-0 polyglactin suture (Vicryl, Ethicon, Somerville, N.J.; Fig. 20-11). Abdominal drains and nasogastric decompression of the stomach may be employed according to surgeon preference.

A modification of this approach is the intragastric approach, in which the ports are placed through the anterior gastric wall

after the initial laparoscopy. The procedure is then conducted within the gastric lumen. A modification of the anastomotic technique involves the use of a linear stapler to create the pseudocyst-gastrostomy. A stapled anastomosis may not be feasible, however, if the wall of the PP is too thick.

Exogastric Approach

The port placement for this approach is similar to the transgastric approach. For a small retrogastric PP or a small PP in the splenic hilum, the gastrocolic omentum is divided with the UAS. The PP then should be visible (Fig. 20-12) for fluid aspiration with an Endoneedle. A small PP in the gastrohepatic ligament is accessible after division of the ligament. Two adjacent 3- to 4-cm transverse openings are made, one into the stomach and the

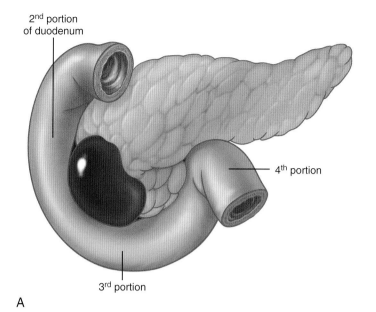

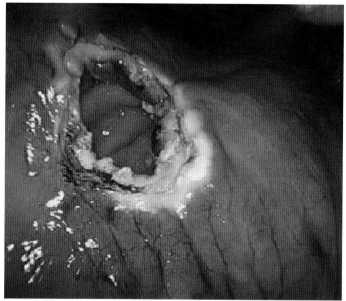

FIGURE 20-7 Longitudinal gastrotomy performed with the ultrasonic scalpel.

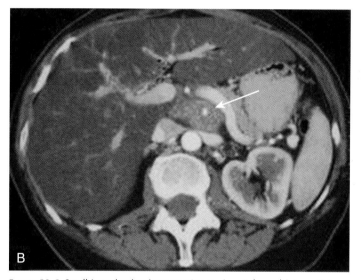

FIGURE 20-6 Small juxtaduodenal pancreatic pseudocyst *(arrow)* lying within the head of the pancreas. **A,** Anterior schematic. **B,** Axial computed tomography image. A cystoduodenostomy is performed if endoscopic drainage fails.

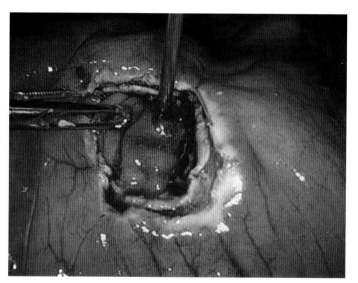

FIGURE 20-8 Needle sampling of pancreatic pseudocyst fluid for amylase, cytology, and microbiologic assays.

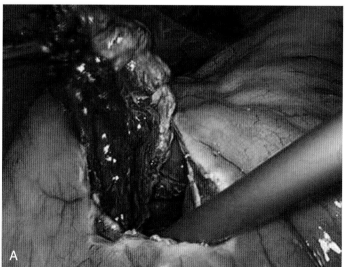

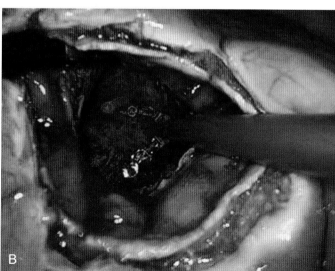

FIGURE 20-9 Débridement of necrotic tissue through the posterior gastrotomy.

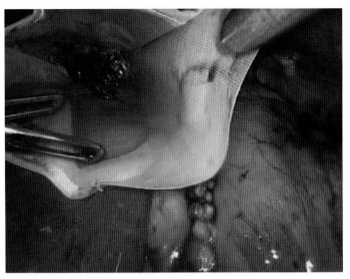

Figure 20-10 The necrotic pancreatic tissue is placed in a water-impervious bag, which is removed at the end of the operation.

other into the PP, close to the adhesion interface between the stomach and the PP (Fig. 20-13). The pseudocyst contents are evacuated, and the cavity is inspected (Fig. 20-14). A single-layer pseudocyst-gastrostomy then is constructed with a continuous 2-0 polyglactin suture (Fig. 20-15).

Pseudocyst-Jejunostomy Approach

Laparoscopic pseudocyst-jejunostomy is employed to drain a PP that protrudes into the infracolic compartment, an arrangement that renders dependent pseudocyst drainage into the stomach unlikely. Although a Roux-en-Y jejunal loop typically is employed for a pseudocyst-jejunostomy, some surgeons still apply a simple loop. We have adopted the former approach to minimize the potential consequences of a leak from the PP-jejunal anastomosis.

Inflammatory adhesions between the omentum and the PP wall are divided, and the omentum and transverse colon are

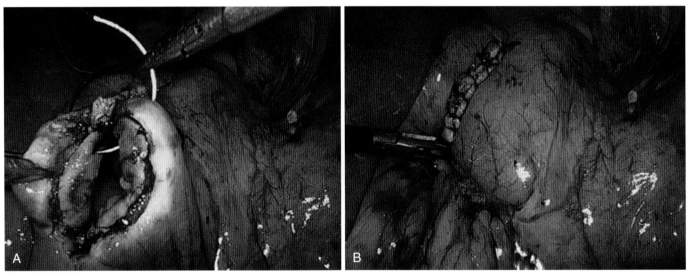

Figure 20-11 Closure of the anterior gastrotomy using a continuous suture in one layer.

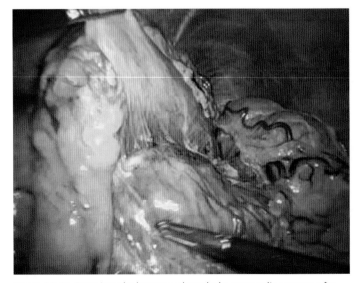

Figure 20-12 Entry into the lesser sac through the gastrocolic omentum for drainage of a small retrogastric pancreatic pseudocyst.

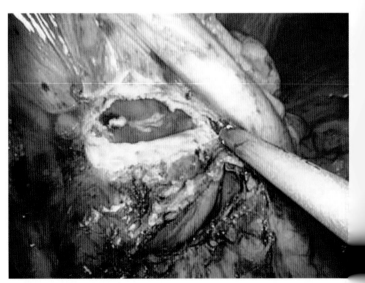

Figure 20-13 Two adjacent transverse openings are made, one into the stomach and the other into the pancreatic pseudocyst.

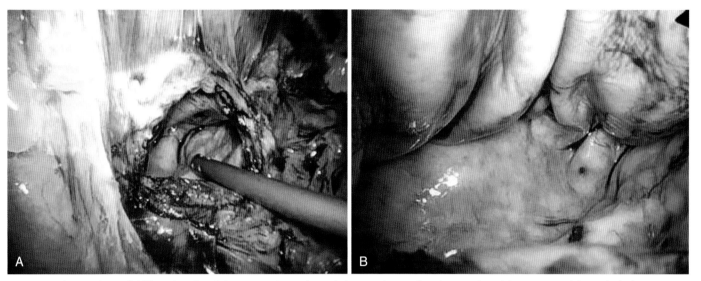

FIGURE 20-14 The pseudocyst fluid is aspirated, and the pancreatic pseudocyst is inspected to confirm absence of suspicious tumor nodules and whether a necrosectomy is needed.

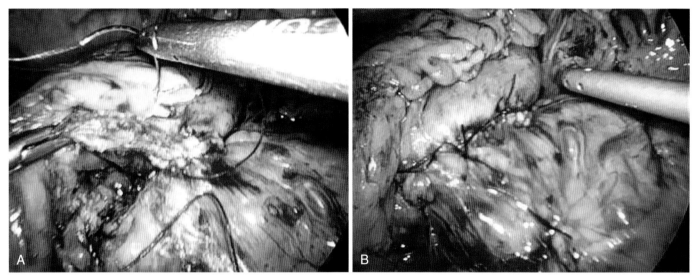

FIGURE 20-15 Side-to-side cystgastrostomy using continuous Vicryl 2-0 suture in one layer.

retracted superiorly by a triangular Diamond-Flex retractor (Surgical Innovations, Leeds, U.K.). The proximal jejunum is divided 50 to 75 cm from the duodenojejunal flexure with an endostapler, and a Roux loop 50 to 60 cm in length is constructed. A side-to-side jejunojejunal anastomosis is fashioned. (We prefer an intracorporeal single-layer hand-sutured anastomosis with continuous 2-0 polyglactin.) The mesenteric defect is then closed with sutures. The Roux loop is approximated to the PP wall with sutures. After needle sampling of the pseudocyst fluid, the PP is opened for about 3 to 4 cm, and its contents are débrided. The antimesenteric border at the end of the jejunal loop also is opened for 3 to 4 cm, and a side-to-side pseudocyst-jejunostomy is constructed with a single layer of continuous 2-0 polyglactin. Reinforcement with a second layer of interrupted sutures may be performed per the surgeon's discretion. Alternatively, the pseudocyst-jejunostomy can be constructed with endostaplers. Abdominal drains are not routinely employed.

POSTOPERATIVE CARE

Antibiotics are not continued after the operation. Oral fluids may be started as early as the evening of the operative day, depending on the clinical status. The abdominal drain and nasogastric tube, if employed, are removed on the first postoperative day. The patient may be discharged from the hospital when ambulatory and tolerating a liquid diet, which is continued for 10 days (allowing collapse of the PP and anastomotic healing) before solid food is resumed. Prophylactic proton pump inhibitors may be beneficial during the initial few weeks after pseudocyst-gastrostomy.

PROCEDURE-SPECIFIC COMPLICATIONS

- The main purpose of surgical treatment is to create a wide stoma between the PP and the gastrointestinal tract that provides dependent drainage. Failure to produce sufficient pseudocyst drainage may lead to PP recurrence. Recurrent PPs can be managed by further laparoscopic internal drainage following the same principles of primary surgical drainage.

- A pseudoaneurysm secondary to a PP can cause major hemorrhage, which can be difficult to control during an operation, whether open or laparoscopic. Ideally, a pseudoaneurysm should be identified on a preoperative CT scan or EUS and embolized in preparation for the operative procedure.

- Varices secondary to splenic or portal vein thrombosis or nonthrombotic portal hypertension may increase the risk for intraoperative bleeding, especially from a pseudocyst-gastrotomy. As described previously, a gastric anastomosis in this situation would benefit from suturing. The most likely source of postoperative gastrointestinal bleeding is the anastomosis. Although endoscopic control of this complication is possible, laparoscopic reexploration and suture hemostasis are recommended.

- Leak from a simple loop pseudocyst-jejunostomy, although rare, will require tube drainage (placed radiologically or at repeat laparoscopy), nasogastric decompression, somatostatin agonists, and parenteral nutrition. Drainage alone may be sufficient if a leak occurs in a Roux-en-Y pseudocyst-jejunostomy.

RESULTS AND OUTCOME

Internal drainage of a PP, particularly one arising from acute necrotizing pancreatitis, can be accomplished laparoscopically. An adequate stoma between the pseudocyst and the gastrointestinal tract that allows necrotic débridement and produces dependent drainage may be constructed. Failure to adequately débride pancreatic necrosis is a common cause of infectious complications and persistence of the PP after endoscopic transmural drainage. In the recent literature, laparoscopic drainage has been successful in achieving resolution of PP disease in more than 95% of cases, with very low morbidity and rapid recovery. At the senior author's institution, laparoscopic PP drainage has produced a 3.3% morbidity rate and a median hospital stay of 2 days, with a 6.7% recurrence rate at 15 months. Recurrence rates in open series, in which the follow-up times have been generally longer, have been about 15%.

Most PPs are large and retrogastric and thus are best drained by a transgastric approach. Smaller retrogastric or juxtagastric PPs are more efficiently drained using an exogastric approach through the lesser sac. Infracolic PPs cannot be dependently drained into the stomach and require a pseudocyst-jejunostomy. The rare instance of a persistent, symptomatic, but relatively small (<6 cm) PP within the head of the pancreas may be best drained into the adjacent duodenum, which could be accomplished laparoscopically.

In a series of 108 laparoscopically treated PPs, Palanivelu and coworkers employed transgastric pseudocyst-gastrostomy ($n = 90$), pseudocyst-jejunostomy ($n = 8$), and external drainage ($n = 8$); two patients required conversion to open pseudocyst-gastrostomy. Park and colleagues treated 29 PPs using laparoscopic intragastric ($n = 16$) or exogastric (lesser sac approach; $n = 9$) pseudocyst-gastrostomy, pseudocyst-jejunostomy ($n = 3$), and external drainage techniques ($n = 1$). One case was aborted because of extensive gastric varices. Minimally invasive PP drainage is highly effective, produces low morbidity and mortality, and has recovery and recurrence rates that compare favorably with open drainage.

Suggested Readings

Aljarabah M, Ammori BJ: Laparoscopic and endoscopic approaches for drainage of pancreatic pseudocysts: A systematic review of published series. *Surg Endosc* 11:1936–1944, 2007.

Behrns KE, Ben-David K: Surgical therapy of pancreatic pseudocysts. *J Gastrointest Surg* 12:2231–2239, 2008.

Bergman S, Melvin WS: Operative and nonoperative management of pancreatic pseudocysts. *Surg Clin North Am* 6:1447–1460, ix, 2007.

Bhattacharya D, Ammori BJ: Minimally invasive approaches to the management of pancreatic pseudocysts: Review of the literature. *Surg Laparosc Endosc Percutan Tech* 3:141–148, 2003.

Frantzides CT, Ludwig KA, Redlich PN: Laparoscopic management of a pancreatic pseudocyst. *J Laparoendosc Surg* 4:55–59, 1994.

Gumaste VV, Aron J: Pseudocyst management: Endoscopic drainage and other emerging techniques. *J Clin Gastroenterol* 44:326–331, 2010.

Hamza N, Ammori BJ: Laparoscopic drainage of pancreatic pseudocysts: A methodological approach. *J Gastrointest Surg* 14:148–155, 2010.

Lerch MM, Stier A, Wahnschaffe U, Mayerle J, et al: Pancreatic pseudocysts: Observation, endoscopic drainage, or resection? *Dtsch Arztebl Int* 106:614–621, 2009.

Owera AM, Ammori BJ: Laparoscopic endogastric and transgastric cystgastrostomy and pancreatic necrosectomy. *Hepatogastroenterology* 55:262–265, 2008.

Palanivelu C, Senthilkumar K, Madhankumar MV, et al: Management of pancreatic pseudocyst in the era of laparoscopic surgery: Experience from a tertiary centre. *Surg Endosc* 21:2262–2267, 2007.

Park AE, Heniford BT: Therapeutic laparoscopy of the pancreas. *Ann Surg* 236:149–158, 2002.

MARCO CASACCIA

Minimally Invasive Splenectomy for Massive Splenomegaly

The videos associated with this chapter are listed in the Video Contents and can be found on the accompanying DVDs and *on Expertconsult.com.*

The first reported laparoscopic splenectomy was done by Delaitre and Maignien and published in 1992. Minimally invasive splenectomy, more commonly called *laparoscopic splenectomy* (LS), is now a standard surgical option for splenic disease; some authors believe that LS is the treatment of choice. Reported advantages of laparoscopic over open splenectomy (without splenomegaly) include shorter hospital stay, less narcotic administration, faster recovery, and a quicker return to employment. Although the most common indication for LS has been idiopathic thrombocytopenic purpura, many other benign or malignant hematologic diseases can benefit from this procedure. In a multicenter study on LS from the Italian Registry of Laparoscopic Surgery of the Spleen (IRLSS), malignancy was the underlying diagnosis in 32.8% of 676 patients.

Massive splenomegaly, defined as an organ larger than 20 cm in greatest dimension, is associated with various malignancies; is frequently seen in older, more physiologically frail patients; and can be associated with coagulopathy, anemia, thrombocytopenia, and perisplenitis. These preconditions, along with the risk for intraoperative hemorrhage and specimen extraction difficulties, made LS in the setting of massive splenomegaly a difficult challenge during the early experience, and massive organ size was a contraindication for LS. Most studies comparing LS in normal and enlarged (nonmassive) spleens have shown that LS for splenomegaly is associated with longer operative times, increased blood loss, more perioperative complications, longer length of stay, and higher conversion rates than LS for normal-sized spleens. Despite these findings, the general consensus has been that LS in experienced hands is preferable to open splenectomy for nonmassive splenomegaly.

Ongoing improvement in instrumentation and accrued experience have increased the rate at which LS is being done for massive splenomegaly, and the massively enlarged spleen is now a relative issue in the consideration of LS. Although LS for massive splenomegaly should not be used by all surgeons, in the appropriate hands this procedure is feasible for spleens of almost any size.

OPERATIVE INDICATIONS

Benign splenic pathology seldom produces massive splenomegaly, with the exception of hemolytic anemia. Among malignancies, non-Hodgkin lymphoma (NHL) is by far the most common pathology associated with massive splenomegaly. Other associated malignancies include Hodgkin lymphoma (HL), idiopathic myelofibrosis, chronic lymphocytic leukemia, and hairy cell leukemia.

The patient with NHL may present with prominent retroperitoneal lymphadenopathy or hypersplenism without peripheral lymphadenopathy. Suspicious retroperitoneal lymphadenopathy is amenable to laparoscopic biopsy. The spleen is involved in 30% to 40% of patients with NHL. Treatment is directed at relieving the discomfort attributable to splenomegaly or preventing hematologic sequestration. Pancytopenia from the latter may prevent the administration of chemotherapy. Lymphoma confined to the spleen is rare (about 1% of NHL patients), but splenectomy may be curative. The patient with idiopathic myelofibrosis, chronic lymphocytic leukemia, or hairy cell leukemia may undergo splenectomy to treat symptomatic splenomegaly or hypersplenism, or both, similar to NHL.

In HL, the spleen typically is the first lymphoid basin that becomes involved below the diaphragm. The role of surgical staging has waned as imaging techniques and chemotherapy have improved, and staging is currently performed in about 5% of HL patients. A goal of noninvasive imaging in HL is to determine the presence of infradiaphragmatic disease. Staging laparoscopy, however, remains the most precise means of determining the presence and extent of abdominal involvement in patients with clinical Ann Arbor Stage I or II supradiaphragmatic HL; 20% to 35% of these patients have occult splenic or upper abdominal nodal involvement not detected by noninvasive imaging. An HL patient should be considered for staging laparoscopy (surface inspection, nodal sampling, liver biopsy) and splenectomy if the outcome of the procedure will influence subsequent therapy.

We consider most patients referred for elective splenectomy to be potential candidates for laparoscopic splenectomy. Contraindications to a minimally invasive approach include severe portal hypertension, uncorrectable coagulopathy, severe ascites, and most traumatic injuries. For a massive spleen that is less than 26 cm in greatest dimension, we proceed with LS in the absence of a contraindication. For a spleen that is larger than 26 cm in greatest dimension, we perform an open splenectomy through a left 14-cm subcostal incision. Similarly, other authors have suggested a cutoff dimension for laparoscopic splenectomy in the 27- to 30-cm range.

Hand-assisted laparoscopy or open splenectomy should be considered with extremely large spleens to avoid an intraoperative open conversion (per the guidelines of the European Association of Endoscopic Surgery), which is associated with an increased rate of postoperative morbidity. Other factors (e.g., morbid obesity, pancytopenia) may influence the surgeon to choose a more invasive approach. In the final analysis, the surgeon will have to judge whether to proceed with minimally invasive splenectomy for a massive spleen, a decision based on splenic size, relevant patient conditions, and the surgeon's own experience and expertise with the technique.

PREOPERATIVE EVALUATION, TESTING, AND PREPARATION

The preoperative evaluation for a splenectomy patient should include sonographic examination to establish spleen size. Splenomegaly is defined as a maximal splenic diameter greater than 15 cm; a maximal diameter greater than 20 cm is indicative of massive splenomegaly (specimen weight, obtained after splenectomy, is not helpful in deciding surgical approach). Thin-slice spiral computed tomography (CT) should be used if additional anatomic information is needed or if malignancy is suspected. In autoimmune or hemolytic disease, thin-slice spiral CT scan may detect accessory spleens. For patients with malignant hematologic diseases, CT scanning can reveal lymphadenopathy in the splenic hilum, perisplenic inflammation, or splenic infarction, all of which can increase the difficulty of the procedure. CT scanning with three-dimensional reconstruction can add helpful information on possible anomalous vascular supply to the spleen so that the surgeon can appropriately modify the dissection. Magnetic resonance imaging also is useful, but is not routinely needed.

If the patient has thrombocytopenia, then treatment with prednisone (1 mg/kg/day, beginning 5 to 7 days before surgery) is recommended to achieve a preoperative platelet count higher than 50×10^9/L. If the platelet count is not increased with prednisone, then intraoperative platelet transfusion may be performed after division of the splenic pedicle. If the patient has autoimmune thrombocytopenia (not a common cause of massive splenomegaly), then administration of immunoglobulin is recommended. If the patient has anemia, then preoperative transfusion to raise the hemoglobin to 10 g/dL is advisable. Vaccination against meningococcal, pneumococcal, and *Haemophilus influenzae* type B pathogens is performed at least 15 days before elective splenectomy. Antibiotic prophylaxis (e.g., cefazolin or clindamycin) is administered 30 minutes before skin incision.

If the patient has a massively enlarged spleen, then preoperative splenic artery embolization may decrease both splenic size and the risk for intraoperative hemorrhage. We do not, however, use routine preoperative embolization because no clear advantage has been shown with this approach. Preoperative splenic artery embolization has been associated with severe pain, pancreatitis, and other ischemic complications. Furthermore, if lymphoma is suspected, then preoperative embolization may result in splenic necrosis, thus increasing the difficulty of pathologic diagnosis.

PATIENT POSITIONING IN THE OPERATING SUITE

Laparoscopic splenectomy may be performed using a lateral decubitus, semi-decubitus, or supine approach, depending on surgeon preference, spleen size, patient characteristics, and the need for any concomitant procedures. The supine position provides access to the omental pouch, excellent visualization of the splenic hilum, and access to the rest of the abdomen if a concomitant procedure is planned. The decubitus position can facilitate bowel retraction away from the operative field, but full lateral decubitus alone is not recommended for a massive spleen because it will sag into the right upper quadrant, blocking the view of the hilum and making splenic manipulation extremely difficult. We prefer the semi-decubitus position for a massive spleen because the operating table can then be rotated to place the patient's body in the supine or decubitus position (or anywhere in between), depending on surgeon need at any given point in the procedure (Fig. 21-1A).

Using a bean bag, foam wedges, or other stabilizing device, the patient is positioned with the left side up at about a 45-degree angle (Fig. 21-1B). Cushions are place under the knees and ankles of both legs. The right arm is extended onto an arm board, and the left arm is elevated and secured in a flexed position over the patient's head. The patient is secured to the operating table with straps across the chest, hips, and legs to permit extreme rotation. The table is flexed to expand distance between the iliac crest and costal margin, and then reverse Trendelenburg tilt is applied (Fig. 21-1C). The monitors are placed on either side of the patient's head. The surgeon and the camera operator stand on the patient's right side, and the first assistant stands on the left, as shown in Figure 21-1B.

POSITIONING AND PLACEMENT OF TROCARS

Four ports are used, as shown in Figure 21-2. A 10-mm camera port is inserted at the umbilicus using the open technique. If the patient is large or tall, or if the splenomegaly is moderate, then this initial port may be placed superior to or to the left of the umbilicus, or both. Under laparoscopic guidance, a 5-mm port is placed in the subxiphoid area, a 10-mm port is placed variably under the costal margin along the midclavicular line, and a 10-mm port is placed in the left axillary line, halfway between the costal margin and the iliac crest. The surgeon should adjust port placement to accommodate organ size. In massive splenomegaly, the subcostal ports are positioned 4 cm below the medial and inferior tip of the spleen, parallel to the left costal margin, yet still allowing the instruments to reach the diaphragm. Occasionally the most lateral port cannot be placed below the spleen; in such a case, the port should be placed as low as possible. Infiltration with local anesthesia before insertion of each trocar helps reduce postoperative pain and confirms the precise location of each port.

OPERATIVE TECHNIQUE

A 30-degree angled 10-mm laparoscope is placed through port 1. Before initiating the splenectomy, an examination for liver and lymph node abnormalities and a search for accessory spleens is performed. The surgeon operates through ports 2 and 3 by means of an atraumatic grasper and a radiofrequency vessel sealer device (LigaSure Vessel Sealing System, Valleylab, Boulder, Colo.),

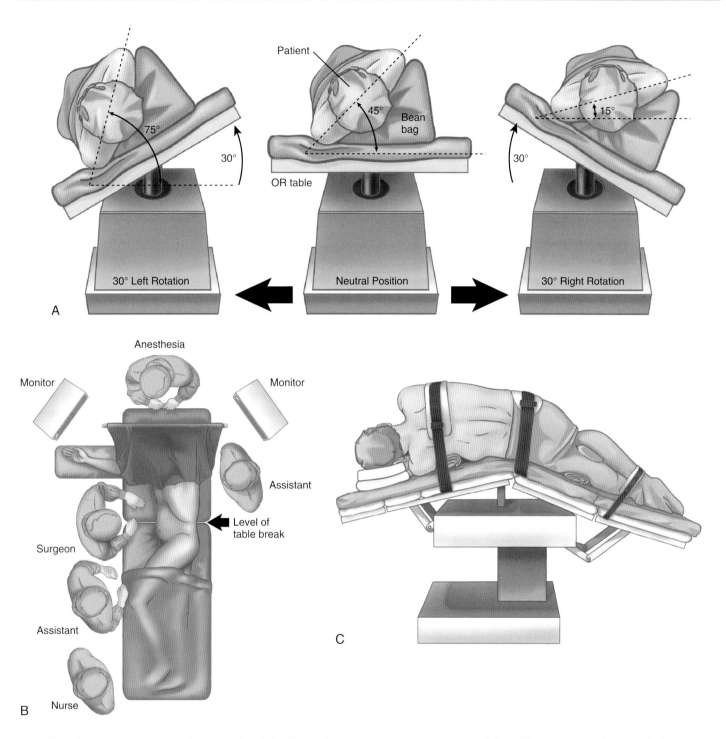

FIGURE 21-1 Operating room setup. **A,** Axial view of semi-decubitus position, demonstrating how a supine or full decubitus position may be obtained with extremes of operating table rotation. **B,** Overhead view of the left-side-up semi-decubitus position; *arrow* indicates level of table flex point. **C,** Side view of the same, showing expansion of the space between the costal margin and the iliac crest that was induced with table flexion.

and the first assistant uses port 4 for organ retraction and manipulation with a second atraumatic grasper.

Splenic Artery Ligation

The splenectomy begins with entry into the lesser sac through the gastrocolic ligament to obtain early ligation of the splenic artery. Although early splenic artery ligation may seem unnecessary and time-consuming in an uncomplicated splenectomy, this maneuver may decrease blood loss should unexpected hemorrhage occur during the hilar dissection of a massive spleen. The stomach is retracted superomedially with a grasper through port

2, and countertraction is placed on the spleen with a closed grasper (or other atraumatic retraction method) through port 4. The gastrocolic ligament is divided with the LigaSure device, and the lesser sac is entered. The pancreas is then identified and gently retracted inferoposteriorly. The pulsation of the tortuous splenic artery should be visible just superior to the pancreas. The visceral peritoneum overlying the splenic artery is opened with scissors. The artery is circumferentially dissected and then occluded (but not divided) with a clip or silk ligature (Fig. 21-3). We prefer to use ligature in case subsequent placement of a vascular stapler includes this control point so that the stapler action is not foiled.

Division of the Gastrosplenic Ligament and Short Gastric Vessels

After the gastrocolic ligament has been divided, the gastrosplenic ligament is placed on stretch by retraction of the stomach medially and the spleen laterally. If necessary, the assistant's grasper can be placed posterior to the gastrosplenic ligament, which can then be placed on stretch with anterolateral leverage of this grasper. The short gastric vessels subsequently are divided with the LigaSure device (Fig. 21-4), proceeding in the craniad direction. Division of the uppermost vessels can be quite difficult with a massive spleen; the gastric fundus and splenic upper pole can be in close contact, which hinders vessel exposure. Readjustment of traction-countertraction of the stomach and spleen can facilitate this exposure (Fig. 21-5). When using heat-generating dissection devices in this location, the surgeon should be vigilant to avoid thermal injuries to the gastric wall. In addition, the left crural bundle of the esophageal hiatus lies directly beneath the uppermost portion of the gastrosplenic ligament, so the surgeon should avoid catching the crural fibers during ligament transection.

Division of the Splenocolic Ligament

The patient is placed in a steep reverse-Trendelenburg position. The splenic flexure is partially mobilized by dividing the splenocolic ligament, the lower part of the phrenicocolic ligament, and the sustentaculum lienis (Figs. 21-6 and 21-7). The splenocolic ligament may be thin and avascular, covered by dense omentum, or hidden by the colon, which can be adherent to the splenic capsule. The sustentaculum lienis is another suspensory ligament that is in continuity with the splenocolic and phrenicocolic ligaments, and it provides support to the lower pole of the spleen. Exposure of these ligaments is obtained with gentle lifting of the spleen and gentle countertraction on the colon, and transection proceeds from medial to lateral using the LigaSure device. Care is taken around the inferior splenic pole because communicating vessels to the left gastroepiploic vein can be present in this location. A pedicle or stub of tissue is left on the spleen to provide a grasping point for subsequent manipulation.

Division of the Splenophrenic and Splenorenal Ligaments

We prefer to divide all of the suspensory splenic ligaments before performing the hilar dissection. If bleeding is encountered during

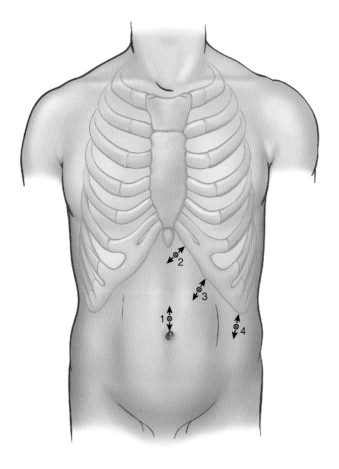

FIGURE 21-2 Port positions for a laparoscopic splenectomy involving massive splenomegaly. Placement is varied according to splenic size and patient body habitus.

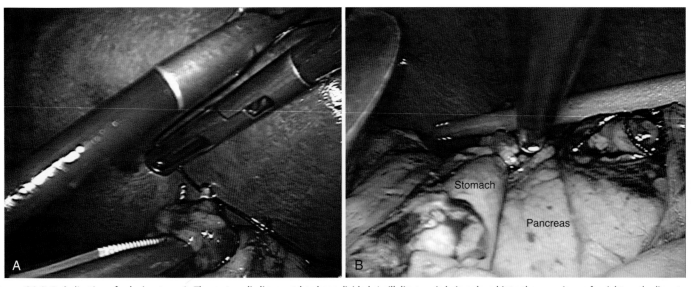

FIGURE 21-3 Early ligation of splenic artery. **A,** The gastrocolic ligament has been divided. A silk ligature is being placed into the open jaws of a right-angle dissector, which has dissected around the splenic artery. A closed grasper is retracting the spleen. **B,** The splenic artery, ligated in continuity, is seen superior to the pancreas. The stomach has been retracted medially, and the spleen has been retracted laterally with a suction-irrigator. Note that most of the spleen appears devascularized (*bluish color*), with the exception of the upper pole in the left of the photograph.

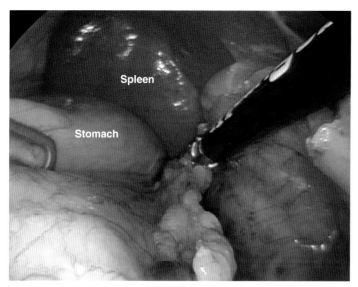

FIGURE 21-4 The gastrosplenic ligament, containing the short gastric vessels, is divided with the LigaSure device.

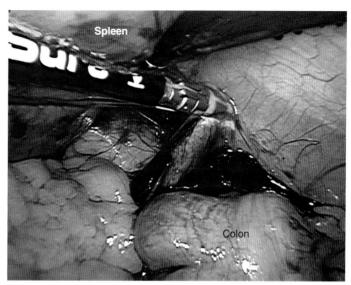

FIGURE 21-6 Division of the gastrocolic ligament with the LigaSure device. A grasper is lifting the inferior pole of the spleen.

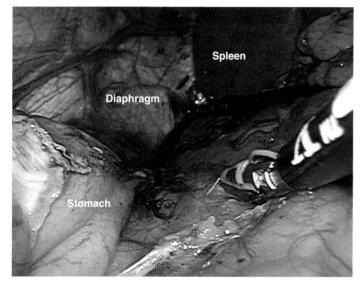

FIGURE 21-5 Division of the uppermost portion of the gastrosplenic ligament. The remaining short gastric vessel is shown, before its transection with the LigaSure device (approaching from the right in the photograph).

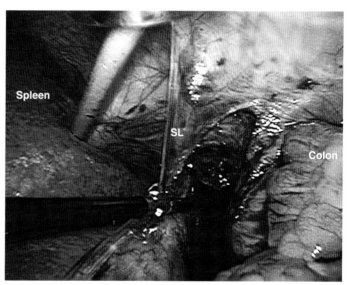

FIGURE 21-7 Division of the sustentaculum lienis (SL) with the LigaSure device.

hilar dissection, then control is easier to obtain if the spleen already has been mobilized. For division of the splenophrenic and splenorenal ligaments posterior to the spleen, the patient should be placed in full lateral decubitus position. Even with this positioning, it can be difficult to divide these ligaments around a massively enlarged spleen. If the patient has had radiation therapy, then these attachments can be particularly tough and fibrous.

Division of splenophrenic and splenorenal ligaments begins at the inferior pole and proceeds cephalad. A combination of hook electrocautery, the LigaSure device, and blunt dissection is used for this step. If exposure of the splenophrenic ligament is inadequate, then division of vessels to the inferior splenic pole may improve access to this ligament. Visualization of the splenophrenic ligament in the vicinity of the upper pole also can be difficult with a massive spleen because the organ blocks the camera view. It may be helpful at this point to swap the camera and operating ports (i.e., ports 3 and 4 in Fig. 21-2) to improve visualization of the upper pole. In addition, an atraumatic fan retractor should push the spleen inferomedially. After the

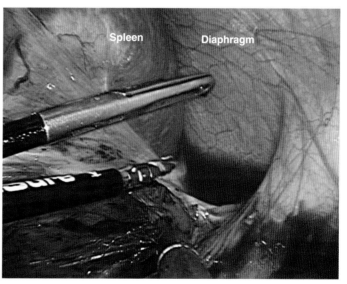

FIGURE 21-8 Division of the splenophrenic ligament at the superior pole with the LigaSure device.

posterior suspensory ligaments have been divided, the posterior dissection is joined to the anterior dissection by incising the phrenicocolic ligament back to the left crural bundle of the esophageal hiatus (Fig. 21-8). Excessive posterior dissection is avoided because the retropancreatic plane can be entered, which can set up a pancreatic tail injury.

Dissection of the Splenic Hilum

The table is rotated back to a semi-decubitus position. If the spleen at this point is not bluish in color (indicating ischemia), then it is likely that some arterial branches from the left gastro-epiploic artery remain to be divided, or the patient may have "distributed" hilar vasculature, such that the early ligation was not proximal enough to control all arterial branches. We prefer to transect any possible inferior pole arteries in order to thin out the splenic hilum as much as possible. One fortunate aspect of the massively enlarged spleen is that the hilar vessels become elongated, which make them easier to isolate.

Once the hilum has been adequately dissected, a linear vascular stapler is introduced through port 4. The upper and lower poles of the spleen are gently lifted using ports 2 and 3, exposing the hilum and pancreatic tail. The major splenic vessels are then divided with one or two cartridges (Fig. 21-9). The presence of malignant hilar lymphadenopathy increases the difficulty of the hilar dissection. All the macroscopically enlarged nodes should be harvested for disease staging. These nodes can be entwined with the hilar vessels, preventing application of a stapler across the hilum. In this case, a more proximal point of stapler transection should be used, taking care not to injure the pancreatic tail.

Extraction of the Spleen

For lymphoma, staging, or splenic malignancy, the spleen should be retrieved in toto. If careful pathologic analysis is not required, then the specimen may be morcellated inside a bag, avoiding spillage of specimen into the abdomen. Undetected spillage of splenic fragments may cause splenosis and recurrence of both benign and malignant disease. Spleens measuring up to 25 cm can be captured and extracted using a specimen bag such as the 15-mm Endo Catch II (Covidien, Norwalk, Conn.) (Fig. 21-10A). This instrument can be passed through one of the 10-mm port

sites after the port has been removed. If the surgeon intends to perform a minimally invasive splenectomy on an organ larger than 25 cm, then an appropriate-sized organ retrieval bag must be acquired before the operation.

Intra-abdominal insertion of a large organ retrieval bag is done by rolling the bag into a tube, grasping an end with a Kelly clamp, and gently dragging it into the abdomen through a 10-mm port site (number 4 in Fig. 21-2) with the port removed. The bag is unrolled inside the abdomen, the posterior lip of the open end is held toward port site 4, and downward countertraction is maintained on the closed end of the bag. With the patient in Trendelenburg position, the specimen is grasped by the hilum and dragged into the bag. Port site 4 is minimally enlarged, and the open end of the bag is delivered through this site. If the specimen does not need to be intact, then morcellation is performed using a ring forceps or similar instrument through port site 4. The bag is held tightly against the abdominal wall, the forceps is inserted into the open end of the bag, the specimen is morcellated, and individual fragments are pulled out of the bag. The process is monitored from inside the abdomen with the laparoscope to avoid small bowel injury or bag rupture.

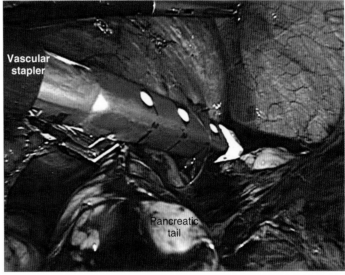

FIGURE 21-9 Division of the hilar vessels with the linear vascular stapler.

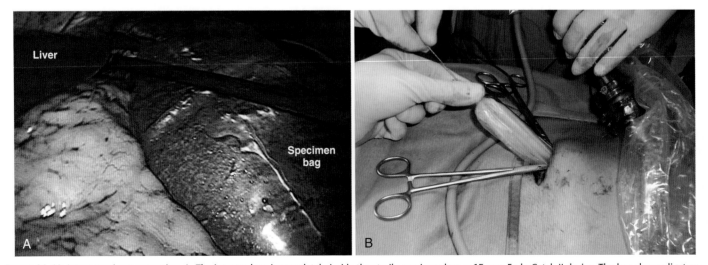

FIGURE 21-10 Intact specimen extraction. **A**, The intact spleen is completely inside the sterile specimen bag, a 15-mm Endo Catch II device. The bag closure ligature is controlled with a grasper. The spleen will be pushed into the pelvic area for extraction. **B**, Extraction of the intact spleen through a 5-cm Pfannenstiel incision.

If the spleen needs to be retrieved in toto, a subcostal incision connecting port sites 3 and 4 is made for bag extraction. Alternatively, a 5-cm Pfannenstiel incision may be employed (see Fig. 21-10B); this incision type has cosmetic advantages, and it may be less painful and result in fewer pulmonary complications than a subcostal incision. We prefer a Pfannenstiel incision for intact spleen retrieval.

After specimen extraction, the incision is closed temporarily with clamps, and the abdomen is reinsufflated. The operative site is irrigated and checked for hemostasis. We routinely place a closed-suction drain in the splenic fossa. The pneumoperitoneum is then evacuated, the fascia of all incisions 10 mm or greater is closed with 1-0 absorbable suture, and the skin is approximated with 4-0 intracuticular stitches.

POSTOPERATIVE CARE

The nasogastric tube is removed either in the recovery room or the next morning, depending on the duration and difficulty of the procedure. The urinary catheter usually is removed before the patient leaves the recovery room, and a dose of morphine chloridrate (10 mg by intramuscular injection) is given for analgesia. Further postoperative pain medication is given on an individual basis; most patients will not require additional narcotics. Acetaminophen is administered during the first night. Coanalgesia with a nonsteroidal anti-inflammatory drug (e.g., ketorolac tromethamine) may be added as necessary. The patient is given clear fluids on the morning after the operation; when clear fluids are well tolerated and there is no elevation of amylase and lipase, then the patient is allowed a full diet. The abdominal drain is withdrawn on postoperative day 1.

Intravenous amoxicillin (alternatively, erythromycin) is continued while the patient is hospitalized. The patient who is receiving intravenous cortisone is given oral steroids on postoperative day 1, overlapping with intravenous steroids; thereafter, steroid therapy is tapered. Perioperative anticoagulant prophylaxis is recommended for all patients (e.g., a low-molecular-weight heparin at 100 U/kg per day). If the patient has an associated coagulopathy or thrombocytopenia, then we usually administer it 6 to 12 hours after the operation, after ensuring that postoperative bleeding has not occurred.

We routinely perform a color Doppler ultrasonography on postoperative day 1 and before the patient's discharge to confirm portal and splenic vein patency before withdrawing anticoagulant prophylaxis. Further imaging studies are performed only in case of suspected postoperative complications. Platelet count is monitored for 3 to 6 months after splenectomy; if thrombocytosis develops, then antiplatelet therapy (e.g., acetylsalicylic acid) may be necessary.

PROCEDURE-SPECIFIC COMPLICATIONS

Possible pulmonary complications after splenectomy for a massive organ include left lower lobe atelectasis, pneumonia, and pleural effusion. Intraoperative hemorrhage usually is from laceration of the hilar or short gastric vessels, or the spleen itself, and is the main cause of open conversion. To minimize the hemorrhage risk, hemostatic scalpels that employ radiofrequency or bipolar energy are recommended. We prefer the 5-mm LigaSure device because of its small tip. When stapling the hilum, the stapler tip should be clear and free of tissue before it is closed; otherwise, hemorrhage from partial vessel transection might

result. Injury to the gastric fundus can occur during dissection of the upper splenic pole, where the interorgan distance is short. The fundus is relatively fixed in this region by the phrenoesophageal ligament, thus limiting gastric retraction.

Injury to the pancreatic tail can occur in up to 10% to 15% of cases involving massive spleens. This complication usually happens during the hilar stapling, especially if the pancreatic tail extends into the hilum. Blind application of the stapler should be avoided. An unrecognized pancreatic injury can produce hyperamylasemia, a peripancreatic fluid collection, a pancreatic abscess, amylase-rich drain fluid, and atypical postoperative pain. A routine check of serum amylase levels is done on postoperative day 1. Further studies for pancreatic injury should be guided by the patient's clinical condition.

Portal and splenic vein thrombosis is a potentially life-threatening complication that can occur months after surgery. Intestinal infarction and portal hypertension can result. Symptoms often are vague, including diffuse abdominal pain, nausea, fever, ileus, diarrhea, and decreased appetite. The reported rate of venous thrombosis ranges from 0.7% to 14%. Perioperative anticoagulant prophylaxis with a subcutaneous low-molecular-weight heparin should be performed for all patients. Risk factors for the development of this complication are the presence of myeloproliferative disorders associated with hypercoagulopathy, hemolytic anemia, hypersplenism, or hematologic malignancy. Patients at high risk for portal or splenic vein thrombosis should receive anticoagulant prophylaxis for 4 weeks. Diagnosis of this complication can be obtained with color Doppler ultrasonography or contrast-enhanced CT. After diagnosis of portosplenic thrombosis, intravenous heparin is begun immediately, with later transition to oral warfarin. Alternatively, therapeutic amounts of low-molecular-weight heparin also produce good results (90% recanalization if treated immediately).

The long-term risk for overwhelming postsplenectomy sepsis has been well documented and is highest within the first 2 years after splenectomy. One third of these infections, however, occur more than 5 years after splenectomy, so patients have a lifelong risk. Although the overall incidence of postsplenectomy sepsis is low (3.2%), the mortality rate is extremely high (40% to 50%). Infection mainly is from encapsulated organisms that normally are eliminated by the spleen. Preoperative vaccinations are administered as described earlier under Preoperative Evaluation, Testing, and Preparation. If the splenectomy was done nonelectively, then vaccinations should be given within the first month after the procedure.

RESULTS AND OUTCOME

Long-term outcome of the hematologic disease treated by LS has not been extensively studied. Reports on immune thrombocytopenic purpura have indicated that long-term results are similar after LS and open splenectomy. In cases of lymphoproliferative and myeloproliferative disease, the minimally invasive approach appears to have had a favorable effect on the postoperative morbidity and mortality rates. This positive effect is particularly relevant in these patients, who often need adjuvant chemotherapy or radiotherapy, or both. Large case series and nonrandomized comparative trials generally have reported better short-term outcomes after laparoscopic than open splenectomy.

A current interest has been the limit of splenic size that can be safely treated with a laparoscopic approach. The clinical guidelines of the European Association for Endoscopic Surgery have suggested that hand-assisted laparoscopic or open splenectomy should be considered for massive splenomegaly. A dimensional cutoff for the laparoscopic approach, however, has not been defined in the literature, as discussed earlier under Operative Indications. In general, operative time, blood loss, and conversion rate increase with splenic weight and size.

In a multivariate analysis of data from the Italian Registry of Laparoscopic Surgery of the Spleen (including 676 patients), hematologic malignancy and body mass index were independent risk factors for open conversion. The patient subgroup with hematologic malignancy, in particular, had a fourfold higher conversion rate compared with patients with benign disease (11.7% vs. 3.2%). Morbid obesity and hematologic malignancy are not, however, contraindications to LS. A mortality rate of 0.4% and a morbidity rate of 17.2% were reported from the IRLSS data. In the multivariate analysis, splenic size and open conversion were independent risk factors for postoperative complications; in converted patients, the morbidity rate was almost three times the rate in nonconverted patients.

The surgeon should always keep in mind this occurrence when assessing the feasibility of a laparoscopic approach to massive splenomegaly. It is not worth pushing the limits of this approach, considering that an additional incision for removal of the intact specimen for histopathologic evaluation is frequently required. Most authors agree that LS is an advanced laparoscopic procedure that, in the hands of an experienced surgeon, is a safe approach to splenectomy. They admit the existence of a learning curve, and many have reported that they have reached the limits of feasibility with the consequence of conversion mainly during the first laparoscopic approaches. Thus, we recommend mastering LS on smaller spleens before using the procedure to treat massive splenomegaly.

The available data are not adequate to impose specific limitations on the use of LS for massive splenomegaly. A prospective randomized trial (including a cost analysis) comparing laparoscopic and open splenectomy for massive splenomegaly would be optimum. Unfortunately, such a trial assuredly would be very difficult to accomplish in a proper fashion, considering the relatively low incidence of this clinical problem and the large number of technical details that would need to be controlled.

Suggested Readings

Casaccia M: Minimal-access open splenectomy. In Scott-Conner CEH, editor: *SAGES Manual of Strategic Decision Making: Case Studies in Minimal Access Surgery*, New York, 2008, Springer, pp 392–399.

Casaccia M, Torelli P, Cavaliere D, et al: Minimal-access splenectomy: A viable alternative to laparoscopic splenectomy in massive splenomegaly, *JSLS* 9:411–414, 2005.

Casaccia M, Torelli P, Pasa A, et al: Putative predictive parameters for the outcome of laparoscopic splenectomy: A multicenter analysis performed on the Italian Registry of Laparoscopic Surgery of the Spleen (IRLSS), *Ann Surg* 251:287–291, 2010.

Grahn SW, Alvarez J III, Kirkwood K: Trends in laparoscopic splenectomy for massive splenomegaly, *Arch Surg* 141:755–762, 2006.

Habermalz B, Sauerland S, Decker G, et al: Laparoscopic splenectomy: The clinical practice guidelines of the European Association for Endoscopic Surgery (EAES), *Surg Endosc* 22:821–848, 2008.

Kercher KW, Matthews BD, Walsh RM, et al: Laparoscopic splenectomy for massive splenomegaly, *Am J Surg* 183:192–196, 2002.

Owera A, Hamade AM, Bani Hani OI, et al: Laparoscopic versus open splenectomy for massive splenomegaly: A comparative study, *J Laparoendosc Adv Surg Tech A* 16:241–246, 2006.

Patel AG, Parker JE, Wallwork B, et al: Massive splenomegaly is associated with significant morbidity after laparoscopic splenectomy, *Ann Surg* 238:235–240, 2003.

Pomp A, Gagner M, Salky B, et al: Laparoscopic splenectomy: A selected retrospective review, *Surg Laparosc Endosc Percutan Tech* 15:139–143, 2005.

Torelli P, Cavaliere D, Casaccia M, et al: Laparoscopic splenectomy for hematological diseases, *Surg Endosc* 16:965–971, 2002.

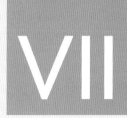

CONSTANTINE T. FRANTZIDES, MINH B. LUU, SCOTT N. WELLE, AND PAUL R. BALASH

Challenging Cases of Laparoscopic Enterectomy for Benign and Malignant Diseases of the Small Intestine

CHAPTER

22

The videos associated with this chapter are listed in the Video Contents and can be found on the accompanying DVDs and on Expertconsult.com.

Laparoscopic surgery for benign and malignant diseases of the small intestine has been well established. Resection of a small segment of bowel in an abdomen free of inflammation, bowel dilation, or adhesions is relatively straightforward, especially if laparoscopy-assisted techniques are used and part of the procedure is performed extracorporeally. We present two difficult scenarios in laparoscopic surgery as an update to our previous chapter, "Minimally Invasive Procedures on the Small Intestine," in the *Atlas of Minimally Invasive Surgery*, 2009 (see Suggested Readings at the end of this chapter). The first case involves the presence of inflammation, abscess, and a shortened mesentery due to Crohn's disease. A thickened and shortened mesentery creates a difficult and challenging scenario to safely dissect, mobilize, and resect the diseased part of the intestine. In addition, it precludes the use of laparoscopy-assisted techniques because the bowel segments cannot be exteriorized. Therefore, an intracorporeal anastomosis is required to avoid conversion to a laparotomy. The second scenario involves localization of small carcinoid tumors of the intestine. Localization of these lesions was aided by preoperative imaging; however, the ability to laparoscopically examine the small intestine is crucial. The application of laparoscopic surgery in these difficult cases should only be undertaken by surgeons with the appropriate experience and technical skills. We hope that the suggestions and techniques shown in this chapter and videos will help surgeons address these challenging cases laparoscopically.

OPERATIVE INDICATIONS

In general, the indications for laparoscopic enterectomy are the same as for open surgery. The initial management of Crohn's disease is medical and has evolved greatly in the past decade. Despite the development of new pharmaceuticals and immunomodulators, most patients with Crohn's disease require surgical intervention to treat the complications of a disease that currently has no cure. The common indications for surgery are complications of Crohn's disease (e.g., fistula, stenosis or obstruction, abscess), failure to improve with medical management, or the inability to tolerate long-term medical therapy. Inflammatory masses and abscesses with or without obstruction are infrequent complications of Crohn's disease but often require surgical intervention. Antibiotic therapy should be started, and large abscesses should be drained percutaneously (if safely accessible using CT or ultrasound).

The presence of masses in the small bowel is an indication for resection unless there is evidence of widespread metastatic disease. Imaging characteristics of benign versus malignant lesions are helpful, but the definitive diagnosis can only be made upon resection. Use of laparoscopic surgery to treat malignant lesions of the small bowel is based on an extrapolation of studies showing, from an oncologic standpoint, that laparoscopic surgery is as effective as open surgery.

PREOPERATIVE EVALUATION, TESTING, AND PREPARATION

Patients diagnosed with Crohn's disease should undergo evaluation of the entire gastrointestinal tract with small bowel series and endoscopies. Computed tomography (CT) is often used in lieu of small bowel series in the emergent setting to determine the presence of an abscess or a phlegmon. The patient's medical status should be optimized by correcting anemia, coagulopathy, dehydration, electrolyte imbalance, and malnutrition. In the absence of an obstruction, a mechanical bowel preparation should be performed to minimize the risk for peritonitis in the event of inadvertent perforation. Patients taking steroids should have a preoperative dose that is tapered postoperatively. Other immunosuppressive drugs can be discontinued before surgery, and their postoperative use is controversial. Postoperative use of infliximab is associated with an increase in morbidity.

Incidentally identified carcinoid tumors can be found during endoscopic or radiographic imaging performed for other purposes. When small bowel lesions suspicious for carcinoid tumors are seen on CT, the patient should be questioned for the presence of abdominal pain, nausea or vomiting, diarrhea, flushing, melena, or weight loss. Urinary 5-hydroxyindoleacetic acid and plasma chromogranin A levels are elevated in patients with carcinoid tumors but can also be elevated with certain foods, drugs, or other medical conditions. After diagnosis of a carcinoid tumor, indium-111 octreotide imaging (OctreoScan) can complement the CT scan in localizing other lesions but is not commonly used. CT scans should be reviewed with an experienced radiologist to assist in estimating the location of the small bowel mass. Capsule endoscopy can be used to complement CT findings to confirm the presence of small bowel masses. For small lesions, capsule endoscopy has a higher diagnostic yield than small bowel series and push enteroscopy. Until recently, small bowel endoscopy was very difficult and incomplete because of the length, redundancy, and complex turns of the small intestine. The development of double-balloon endoscopy has allowed for the examination of the entire small bowel. In general, per os or per anus, balloon endoscopy is able to examine one half to two thirds of the small intestine. Double-balloon endoscopy works by the use of a balloon on the endoscope and a balloon on the overtube. By alternating the gripping action (when inflated) of each of the balloons, this technique is able to provide forward advancement of the endoscope through the small bowel. When available, small bowel endoscopy can identify, mark (with ink), and biopsy small bowel lesions before resection.

Positioning and placement of trocars

The patient is placed in supine position with the arms tucked. Tucking the arms will allow the surgeon to stand by the patient's shoulder to view the lower abdomen and pelvis. The surgeon and camera assistant stand to the patient's left, and the first assistant stands to the patient's right. Four trocars are used and placed in a configuration similar to that for a right colectomy (see Chapter 11 in the *Atlas of Minimally Invasive Surgery*, 2009; see Suggested Readings at the end of this chapter). The initial trocar can be placed at the umbilicus or in the left subcostal position. Two ports are placed in the left upper and lower quadrants and one in the right mid to upper abdomen. The basic principles of trocar position and use should be followed: the camera port (umbilical) should be between the surgeon's left-hand (left lower quadrant) and right-hand (left upper quadrant) working ports. The retraction port (right abdomen) should be placed in a position that allows retraction of the terminal ileum and cecum without interfering with the surgeon's movements. This setup optimizes the dissection and manipulation of the distal small bowel and right colon. To evaluate the proximal small bowel, an additional trocar in the right lower quadrant may be necessary. The surgeon and camera assistant then switch to the patient's right and the first assistant to the left. Poor positioning of the trocars may be the main reason for conversion to open surgery.

Operative technique

Exposure

The right lower quadrant is exposed by placing the patient in slight Trendelenburg and left-tilt position. The omentum and transverse colon are retracted cephalad. This position allows for the examination of the right colon and distal ileum. The hand-over-hand technique is used to examine the small bowel from the terminal ileum toward the ligament of Treitz. To optimize the exposure of the proximal jejunum, the following changes are made: (1) The surgeon and camera operator now stand on the patient's right, and the first assistant stands on the patient's left. (2) The right upper quadrant port and right lower quadrant port become the surgeon's left-hand and right-hand working ports. (3) The first assistant can use the left upper port to retract the transverse colon cephalad to expose the ligament of Treitz. (4) The patient is placed in slight reverse-Trendelenburg with right-tilt position.

Dissection

The cecum is mobilized by dividing the lateral attachment or white line of Toldt. Blunt dissection is used to free the right colon

mesentery from the retroperitoneum. The inferior edge of the cecum and terminal ileum can be mobilized with the use of the Harmonic scalpel (Ethicon Endo-Surgery, Cincinnati, Ohio) or hook cautery. The right ureter is identified and confirmed by palpation and visualization of peristalsis. The use of a lighted ureteral stent will make the identification process easier. When a mesenteric abscess is encountered, it is probed bluntly and the purulent material aspirated (Figs. 22-1 and 22-2). Care is taken to avoid dissemination of pus throughout the abdomen, and irrigation should be kept to a minimum.

Small bowel mucosal lesions of 5 to 10 mm can be very difficult to identify laparoscopically. Preoperative imaging may aid in localizing the general vicinity of the lesions to the proximal, middle, or distal small intestine. Atraumatic graspers are used to manipulate the small intestine to allow close visualization of the bowel as well as instrument palpation. Because instrument palpation is not as sensitive as direct digital palpation, the use of other

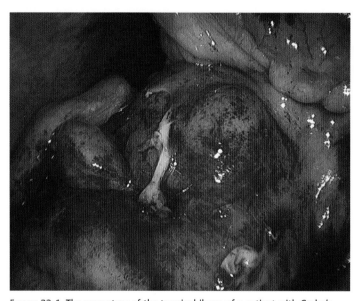

Figure 22-1 The mesentery of the terminal ileum of a patient with Crohn's disease is shown. This part of intestine appears inflamed, thickened, and shortened.

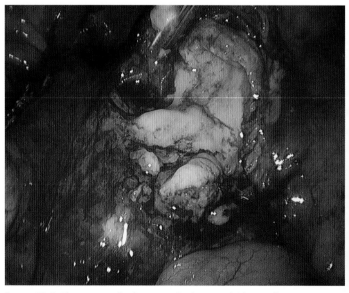

Figure 22-2 The mesenteric abscess cavity is opened. The purulent contents are carefully aspirated to prevent widespread spillage.

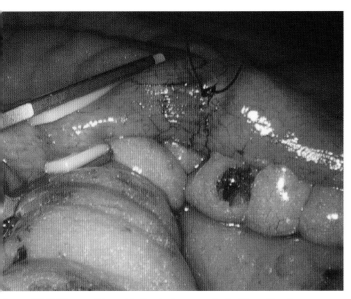

FIGURE 22-3 The small bowel lesion is shown marked with a silk suture. A slight increase in vascularity of the bowel wall is a clue to identifying the luminal mass.

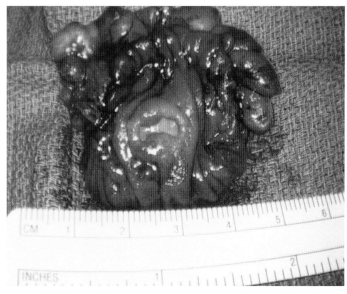

FIGURE 22-4 The small bowel specimen is opened showing a small (6 mm) intraluminal carcinoid tumor with a central mucosal ulceration.

signs and the preoperative localization are more essential. In the video of the small bowel carcinoid tumors included on the accompanying DVD (as well as on Expert Consult), a slight increase in the vascularity of the small bowel wall is a clue to the location of the tumor (Fig. 22-3). Multiple instrument manipulations are performed to confirm the presence of the small bowel lesion. A suture is placed to mark the location of the tumor, and the rest of the small bowel is examined. The second lesion, about 40 cm proximal to the first lesion, is identified in a similar fashion.

Resection

The proximal and distal bowel is divided using a linear stapler. The authors routinely use the white (2.5 mm) cartridge to divide the small bowel and the blue (3.5 mm) cartridge to divide the colon. The staple line should be inspected for bleeding and the staples examined to be sure that they are well formed. Beyond the manufacturer's instruction sheet, guidelines regarding selection of cartridge size are lacking. In general, large staples are used for thicker tissue to allow for adequate staple formation. Alternatively, selecting too large of a staple will increase the risk for staple line bleeding. A balance must be made to achieve an intact and hemostatic staple line. Cartridge compression of inflamed or thickened tissue before deployment of staples will also aid in forming the appropriate staple shape. This staple technology is currently part of a newer generation of linear staplers (see Chapter 43). Division of the normal mesentery can usually be accomplished with staples, clips, the Harmonic scalpel, or the LigaSure Vessel Sealing System (Valleylab, Boulder, Colo.). A thickened mesentery as a result of inflammation from Crohn's disease may present a real laparoscopic challenge for any ligating and dividing modality. Monopolar cautery or the Harmonic scalpel can be used to thin the mesentery and allow application of the linear stapler. Use of the LigaSure device may also prove to be inadequate because of the thickness of the mesenteric tissue. It is more likely that a green cartridge (4.8 mm) will be required to divide the thickened mesentery. Staple line bleeding should be expected when using larger staples and can be controlled with suture ligation.

Division of normal and nonthickened mesentery is relatively easy. The smallest staple size (2 mm or gray cartridge) should be used to achieve the best hemostasis. Minor bleeding of the mesentery staple line can be controlled using a Harmonic scalpel or suture ligation. The LigaSure device cannot be used for this purpose because of the presence of the staples that will prematurely inactivate the device.

The specimen is delivered from the abdomen using an Endo Catch bag (Covidien, Norwalk, Conn.). The bowel segment should be opened and examined to confirm the presence of the intraluminal mass (Fig. 22-4).

Reconstruction

After resection, bowel continuity is restored by creating a side-to-side anastomosis (Fig. 22-5) using a double-staple technique. The proximal and distal bowel segments are aligned using sutures so that the antimesenteric edges are in opposition. The sutures can be used to retract the bowel segments to be anastomosed so that they are in alignment with the trocar chosen for the introduction of the linear stapler. Enterotomies are created on the antimesenteric end of the staple line using the Harmonic scalpel and enlarged bluntly. After the enterotomy is made, the active blade of the Harmonic scalpel remains hot for several seconds, and care should be taken to avoid touching the active blade to the intestinal wall. Thermal injuries caused by the Harmonic scalpel may not be readily apparent; they often go unrecognized and can result in delayed intestinal perforation. A 60- × 3.5-mm cartridge and a 60- × 2.5-mm cartridge are used for large and small bowel anastomoses, respectively. Placement of the two jaws of the linear stapler into the bowel lumens through the enterotomies can be challenging. The placement of the larger jaw of the stapler first, the manipulation of stay sutures, and having a skilled first assistant can make the task easier. Before firing the stapler, ensure the bowel segments are appropriately aligned and that no other tissue is caught between the bowel segments. The bowel segments are gently stabilized with a grasper to prevent displacement, which is often seen with the advancement of the stapler cutting knife. The stapler is removed by opening the jaws slightly

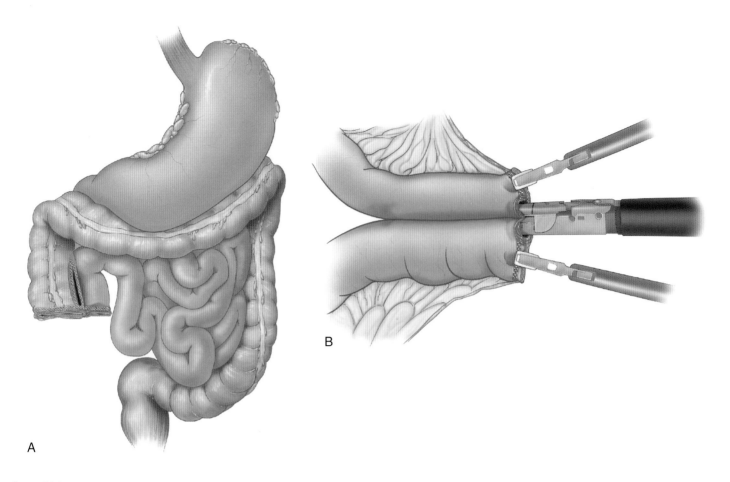

FIGURE 22-5 **A**, Diagrammatic representation of ileocolonic anastomosis following ileocecectomy for Crohn's disease. **B**, Diagrammatic depiction of intestinointestinal anastomosis.

and disengaging the bowel from the cartridge. Removing the stapler with the jaws wide open will result in a very large common enterotomy that will make closure more difficult. Failure to disengage the bowel from the cartridge will result in protrusion of the staple line through the common enterotomy and possibly disrupt the anastomosis. The staple line can be inspected for bleeding through the common enterotomy and closed by first reapproximating the bowel edges using sutures. Key to this step is incorporating the mucosa within the suture to ensure mucosa-to-mucosa approximation when the stapler is used. The staple lines should be inspected for integrity and hemostasis. Bleeding should be controlled with sutures or clips, and energy use should be avoided. The mesenteric defect is closed using a running silk suture to decrease the risk for an internal hernia. Needle bites should be superficial on the peritoneal surface of the mesentery to avoid bleeding that can result in a mesenteric hematoma, which may compromise the blood supply to the anastomosis.

POSTOPERATIVE CARE

Hospitalization averages 1 to 3 days, with the limiting factor for discharge being only the resolution of postoperative ileus. The amount of opioid use correlates with the duration of postoperative ileus. A postoperative nasogastric tube is not routinely used unless one was inserted preoperatively for bowel obstruction. No routine imaging is necessary unless there is a change in the expected postoperative course and clinical examination. Diet is restricted to clear liquids initially and advanced to a soft, low-residue diet.

MANAGEMENT OF PROCEDURE-SPECIFIC COMPLICATIONS

Complications of laparoscopic enterectomy include iatrogenic perforation of the gastrointestinal tract, anastomotic leak, intra-abdominal infection, and injury to the ureter. Unrecognized bowel injury may be secondary to trocar insertion or use of energy or direct manipulation. Laparoscopic access–related injuries can be avoided by the use of the optical trocar or open Hasson technique rather than the use of the Veress needle and subsequent blind insertion of a bladed trocar. In addition, the use of any energy source (electrocautery, Harmonic scalpel) should be judicious, and bowel manipulation should be performed with atraumatic instruments. Patients with intestinal perforation will develop signs and symptoms consistent with peritonitis; however, because of the early discharge after laparoscopic procedures, patients should be educated to keep a low threshold for consulting their surgeon if such symptoms develop.

Anastomotic disruptions can occur early or late. Early anastomotic leaks are usually the result of technical errors resulting in insecure anastomosis. These technical errors can be due to (1) stapler malfunction, (2) staple malformation secondary to thick tissue, (3) incomplete closure of a common enterotomy,

(4) tissue ischemia, and (5) tension at the anastomosis. Early leaks are usually the result of technical error because of gaps or disruption of the staple line. These technical errors can be due to staple malformation caused by using staples that are too small for the tissue thickness. When the tissue is too thick, malformation of the staple can occur, resulting in gaps. Incomplete closure of the common enterotomy can result in early leaks and can be prevented by the placement of alignment sutures. These sutures should incorporate the mucosa and the edges of the bowel wall and should be clearly seen above the staple cartridge. Leaks that occur after several days are the result of tissue ischemia. The anastomosis should be visualized for color changes that would indicate poor blood supply, and if these changes are present, the anastomosis should be revised. The anastomosis should also be checked for tension, and if tension is present, further mobilization of the intestine should be done until the anastomosis is tension free. We also routinely place a "crotch stitch" at the end of the staple line.

Injury to the right ureter can occur with ileocecectomy, and early identification of the ureter is crucial to injury prevention. The use of a lighted ureteral stent can ease and speed the process of identifying the ureter. If an injury to the ureter occurs and is recognized, a urologist should be consulted. Often, short-segment injuries can be primarily repaired in with single-layer, absorbable monofilament sutures over a stent. The area should also be drained.

RESULTS AND OUTCOMES

Ileocolic resection is the most commonly performed operation for Crohn's disease. Short-term outcomes are comparable to those after open surgery, with improved cosmesis, decreased pain, and shorter hospitalization. In the long term, about 30% of patients require a second operation. The risk for recurrent disease is higher in patients with multifocal disease and in those who smoke cigarettes. Laparoscopy theoretically will result in less adhesion formation and likely makes the second operation easier.

The small intestine represents the most common location of carcinoid tumors of the intestinal tract. Up to 20% of small bowel carcinoids are multifocal, and up to 30% can occur concurrently with other noncarcinoid tumors. The 5-year survival rate for small bowel carcinoids is about 70%. The rate of lymph node metastasis is more difficult to predict with small bowel carcinoids, and patients with lesions smaller than 1 cm can present with widely metastatic disease.

Suggested Readings

Alves A, Panis Y, Bouhnik Y, et al: Factors that predict conversion in 69 consecutive patients undergoing laparoscopic ileocecal resection for Crohn's disease: A prospective study, *Dis Colon Rectum* 48:2302–2308, 2005.

Appau KA, Fazio VW, Shen B, et al: Use of infliximab within 3 months of ileocolonic resection is associated with adverse postoperative outcomes in Crohn's patients, *J Gastrointest Surg* 12:1738–1744, 2008.

Avidan B, Sakhnini E, Lahat A, et al: Risk factors regarding the need for a second operation in patients with Crohn's disease, *Digestion* 72:248–253, 2005.

Fichera A, Michelassi F: Surgical treatment of Crohn's disease, *J Gastrointest Surg* 11:791–803, 2007.

Landry CS, Brock G, Scoggins C, et al: A proposed staging system for small bowel carcinoid tumors based on an analysis of 6,380 patients, *Am J Surg* 196:896–903, 2008.

Maartense S, Dunker MS, Slors FM, et al: Laparoscopic-assisted versus open ileocolic resection for Crohn's disease, *Ann Surg* 243:143–149, 2006.

Milsom JW, Hammerhofer KA, Bohm B, et al: Prospective, randomized trial comparing laparoscopic vs. conventional surgery for refractory ileocolic Crohn's disease, *Dis Colon Rectum* 44:1–8, 2001.

Modlin IM, Champaneria MC, Chan AK, et al: A three-decade analysis of 3,911 small intestinal neuroendocrine tumors: The rapid pace of no progress, *Am J Gastroenterol* 102:1464–1473, 2007.

Modlin IM, Lye KD, Kidd M: A 5-decade analysis of 13,715 carcinoid tumors, *Cancer* 97:934–959, 2003.

Simillis C, Purkayastha S, Yamamoto T, et al: A meta-analysis comparing conventional end-to-end anastomosis vs. other anastomotic configurations after resection in Crohn's disease, *Dis Colon Rectum* 50:1674–1687, 2007.

Sutton R, Doran HE, Williams EMI, et al: Surgery for midgut carcinoid, *Endocr Relat Cancer* 10:469–481, 2003.

Whelan G, Farmer RG, Fazio VW, et al: Recurrence after surgery in Crohn's disease, *Gastroenterology* 86:1826–1833, 1985.

Zeni TM, Bemelman WA, Frantzides CT: Minimally invasive procedures on the small intestine. In Frantzides CT, Carlson MA, editors: *Atlas of Minimally Invasive Surgery*, Philadelphia, 2009, Saunders, pp 97–101.

BORIS KIRSHTEIN

Laparoscopic Management of Acute Small Bowel Obstruction

23

The videos associated with this chapter are listed in the Video Contents and can be found on the accompanying DVDs and on Expertconsult.com.

Acute small bowel obstruction (SBO) is a common cause of emergency surgical admission and urgent surgical intervention. SBO most frequently results from postoperative adhesions, followed by primary hernia, metastatic malignancy, and inflammatory bowel disease. In an autopsy study of 752 cadavers, gross intra-abdominal adhesions were present in 67% and 28% of cadavers with and without previous laparotomy, respectively. The incidence of an adhesive SBO after open abdominal surgery, particularly following colorectal and pelvic surgery, is 12% to 17%. Despite advances in diagnosis and treatment, the operative intervention rate is 15% to 30%, and the perioperative mortality rate is 2% to 8%. The high incidence of postoperative adhesions resulted in more than 400,000 laparotomies for SBO in the United States in 1993, as reported in the National Inpatient Profile, at a total cost of $1.1 billion and an average hospital stay of 11 days.

Traditionally, exploratory laparotomy with open adhesiolysis has been the preferred treatment in patients requiring operative intervention. Laparotomy for treatment of SBO, however, may lead to additional adhesions, thereby increasing the risk for recurrent SBO. The cumulative recurrence rate of SBO after one open adhesiolysis for SBO has been reported as 7% at 1 year, 18% at 10 years, and 29% at 25 years. In patients with two episodes of SBO, recurrence rates were 17% at 1 year, 32% at 10 years, and 40% at 20 years; with three episodes of SBO, recurrence rates were 19% at 1 year and 40% at 20 years; and with four episodes of SBO, recurrence rates were 33% at 1 year and 60% at 10 years. There is ongoing research into prevention of postoperative adhesions; some of the more well-known devices that may inhibit adhesion formation include glycerol hyaluronate-carboxymethylcellulose (Seprafilm) and ferric hyaluronate gel (Intergel).

Laparoscopic adhesiolysis was first described by gynecologists for the treatment of chronic pelvic pain and infertility. This technique subsequently was used for diagnosis and treatment of chronic abdominal pain in adults and children. Laparoscopic adhesiolysis for SBO was first performed by Clotteau in 1990 and Bastug in 1991. The cumulative published experience since then has suggested that laparoscopic adhesiolysis for SBO may have the advantages of less postoperative pain, shorter recovery, shorter period of ileus, lower wound infection rate, lower incisional hernia rate, improved cosmesis, and decreased adhesion formation compared with open adhesiolysis. Purported disadvantages of laparoscopic adhesiolysis include limited visualization of the intra-abdominal space (from distended bowel loops) and the risk for bowel injury. Despite evidence from clinical series on laparoscopic management of SBO, laparoscopic adhesiolysis has yet to gain widespread acceptance.

OPERATIVE INDICATIONS

The main diagnostic challenges posed by SBO are to establish the underlining cause, identify any strangulation, and determine which patients can be managed nonoperatively. There is no single laboratory or radiographic parameter that will predict spontaneous resolution of SBO. Volume resuscitation, nasogastric suction, ongoing fluid maintenance, and close clinical observation are the cornerstones of nonoperative management of SBO. Gastric decompression provides symptomatic relief and decreases the need for intraoperative decompression. No definite advantage of using a long (intestinal) tube instead a conventional nasogastric tube has been observed. If the patient remains clinically stable, then a conservative approach can be tolerated almost indefinitely, as long as nutrition can be provided. Some clinicians will proceed to operative intervention if nonoperative management has not resolved the SBO after 48 to 72 hours. The maximal duration of nonoperative management for SBO is controversial; published reports have given cutoff periods ranging from 12 hours to 5 days.

As long as ischemia is not present, however, operative intervention for SBO can be delayed. The caveat to this guideline is that the presence of strangulation increases associated mortality to 30%. Thus, early diagnosis of strangulation in SBO is essential; yet, the detection of ischemia still is a function of clinical suspicion. Clinical symptoms and signs of bowel ischemia in SBO include severe abdominal pain, fever, tachycardia, peritoneal signs, leukocytosis (>18,000 white bloods cells/µL), metabolic acidosis, elevated lactate, and various computed tomography (CT) signs (see later); individually, none of these findings is neither sensitive nor specific for strangulation. The determination of whether a patient with an SBO has underlying bowel ischemia requires that the clinician integrate all the available data, including subjective complaints, physical examination, laboratory tests, and radiology.

Contraindications to laparoscopic adhesiolysis for SBO are listed in Table 23-1. These generally concern the severity or nature of the disease and the surgeon's ability to deal with these

Table 23-1 Contraindications to Laparoscopic Adhesiolysis

Absolute Contraindications	Relative Contraindications
Small bowel dilatation (>4 cm) on a plain abdominal film	Number of previous laparotomies >2
Peritonitis on physical examination	Multiple adhesions
Severe cardiovascular, respiratory, or hemostatic disease	
Hemodynamic instability	
Surgeon inexperience	

conditions. In general, an ideal candidate for minimally invasive release of SBO would (1) be hemodynamically stable; (2) not have generalized peritonitis; (3) have minimal small bowel dilatation; (4) not have a "frozen" abdomen (i.e., a peritoneal cavity obliterated with adhesions); and (5) not have multiple previous laparotomies. The risk for enterotomy (both recognized and delayed) appears to be higher in patients with multiple previous laparotomies. Successful completion of laparoscopic adhesiolysis for SBO would depend on patient selection as guided by Table 23-1.

PREOPERATIVE EVALUATION, TESTING, AND PREPARATION

Most patients with SBO present with abdominal pain, nausea and vomiting, constipation, and abdominal distention. The pain typically is intermittent and colicky in nature. Bowel sounds are often high pitched, increasing with the onset of cramping pain. Visible peristalsis or "laddering" of the small bowel may be observed in the patient with a thin abdominal wall. An obstruction in the proximal small bowel may present with nausea and vomiting without distention and constipation, whereas a more distal obstruction may present with abdominal distention and pain, with vomiting later in the course.

The plain abdominal radiograph (Fig. 23-1) remains the primary radiologic test performed in suspected SBO by virtue of low cost, wide availability, and utility. Identification of level of obstruction (small bowel vs. colon) on the plain film may be possible, although grossly distended small bowel can be mistaken for large bowel, and a colonic volvulus can be mistaken for small bowel. In addition, an obstructing colon cancer can cause an SBO in up to 15% of cases. On the other end of the spectrum, a normal abdominal radiograph does not exclude the diagnosis of SBO.

The oral ingestion of water-soluble contrast agents has become a common diagnostic and therapeutic procedure for SBO. Gastrografin (a mixture of sodium and meglumine diatrizoates) is a widely used contrast agent. Ingestion of this high-osmolarity substance draws water into the small bowel lumen, which is thought to decrease wall edema and stimulate motility. The therapeutic role of Gastrografin probably is limited to speeding resolution of an obstruction that would have resolved without an operation. Typically, 60 to 100 mL of Gastrografin is administered through the nasogastric tube after the diagnosis of SBO has been made and when there is no concern for strangulation or ischemia. Abdominal radiographs should be repeated 3 to 4 hours after Gastrografin administration (Fig. 23-2). If the contrast has reached the cecum and the patient is clinically well, then the patient may be started on liquids. The diet is advanced as tolerated, and early discharge should be possible. If the contrast does not reach the cecum within 24 hours, then surgical intervention may be required.

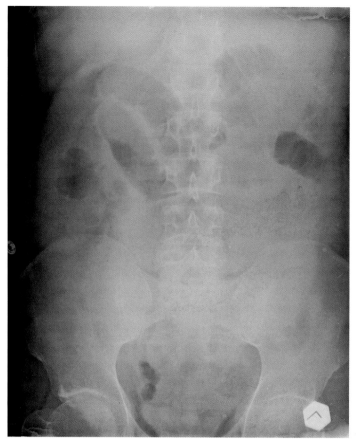

FIGURE 23-1 Supine abdominal radiograph in a patient with a small bowel obstruction.

If a diagnosis is not established with plain radiographs or a Gastrografin study, then ultrasound or CT, or both, may be used. CT scanning may detect the cause and site of the obstruction (Fig. 23-3) and may identify an underlying neoplasm. Slow passage of oral contrast, however, may hinder CT diagnosis of an obstruction. Administration of intravenous contrast can help identify thickened and ischemic bowel walls; signs of the latter include local mesenteric congestion, ascites, pneumatosis intestinalis, and reduced mural enhancement. The sensitivity of ultrasound in SBO detection has been reported to be 95% to 98% and may identify the level of obstruction in 70% to 81% of cases, which is better than plain radiographs (51% to 60%), but not as good as CT (93%). Ultrasound is particularly useful for the pregnant patient. Sonographic examination can be limited by obesity (secondary to a thick abdominal wall and intra-abdominal adipose) and distended gas-filled bowel loops. The use of magnetic resonance imaging in the diagnosis of SBO is an emerging application and is under study.

Before proceeding with adhesiolysis, the patient is fluid-resuscitated, and electrolyte abnormalities are corrected. A Foley catheter and nasogastric tube are inserted, and perioperative intravenous antibiotics are administered. Once operative intervention has been elected, opioid analgesia may be given as necessary.

PATIENT POSITIONING IN THE OPERATING SUITE

Patients are placed in supine position with both arms tucked. Nitrous oxide should not be used for anesthesia because this gas may exacerbate bowel dilation. After endotracheal intubation

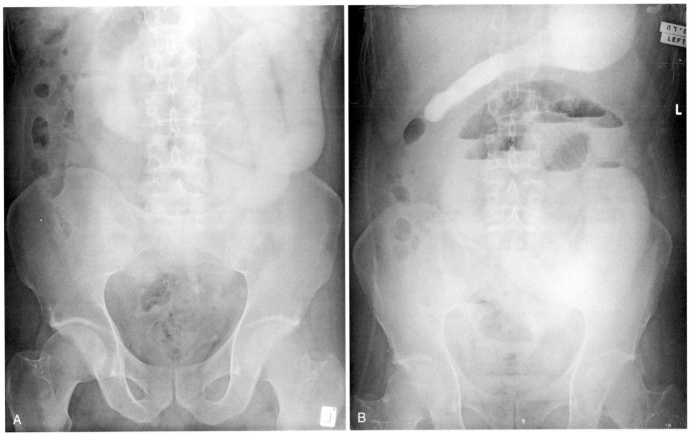

FIGURE 23-2 Gastrografin administration in a patient with a small bowel obstruction. **A,** Upright position, demonstrating contrast in the stomach and duodenum and dilated contrast-filled loops of the small bowel with air-fluid levels, but no distal filling. **B,** Supine position.

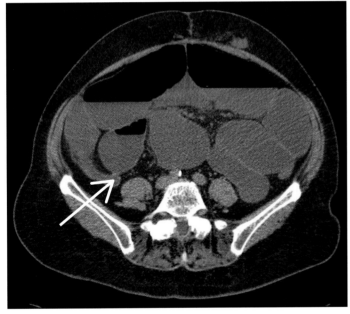

FIGURE 23-3 Computed tomography scan in a patient with a small bowel obstruction, demonstrating the point of obstruction. The *arrow* indicates a transition point between the dilated proximal small bowel and the collapsed distal small bowel.

under general anesthesia, the patient is secured to the operating table with straps, so that maximum tilt and rotation of the bed can be performed. A bean bag or a footboard may be used to help secure the patient in position. Lower extremity compression stockings or other compression device may be placed. Two video monitors are used, one on either side of the table. Initially,

the surgeon and the camera operator usually stand on the patient's left side, and the first assistant stands on the right side. An angled laparoscope is helpful to view around structures or adhesions.

POSITIONING AND PLACEMENT OF TROCARS

Bowel injury during peritoneal access for a minimally invasive adhesiolysis is a major risk of this procedure. The initial trocar should be placed away from existing scars in an attempt to avoid adhesions. The left upper quadrant is a common first-insertion site, particularly if the patient has a prior midline incision; adhesions may be the least troublesome in this location. Some investigators have recommended the use of CT or ultrasound to determine the best site for initial trocar insertion.

Multiple techniques exist to gain initial access to the peritoneal cavity, including the Hasson cannula (open technique), the Veress needle, and optical trocar insertion. It has remained controversial whether different access techniques yield different rates of bowel and vascular injuries, even in patients who have not had previous abdominal surgery. Insertion of a Hasson cannula remote from the umbilicus is performed with a muscle-sparing incision. An advantage of the open technique is the prompt identification of an access injury, if it occurs. The primary disadvantage of the open technique is extreme difficulty in the obese patient. If the Veress needle is used, then appropriate needle position should be verified with the saline drop test, and pressure should be monitored during subsequent insufflation.

Access with an optical trocar system involves placement of the laparoscope into the trocar, which allows the surgeon to visualize the abdominal wall layers during trocar insertion. Available optical-access trocar systems include the Visiport Optical Trocar (Covidien, Norwalk, Conn.), which uses a triggered spring-loaded blade that incrementally cuts through the abdominal layers; the Endopath Xcel Bladeless Trocar (Ethicon Endo-Surgery, Cincinnati, Ohio), which has a clear conical tip that is manually twisted back and forth to separate tissue; and the Kii Fios First Entry optical trocar (Applied Medical, Rancho Santa Margarita, Calif.), which has an aperture at its tip that allows gas insufflation once the tip has penetrated into the peritoneal cavity. Similar to the open technique, an optical trocar allows early identification of an insertion-related complication, yet has utility in obese patients.

After peritoneal access has been obtained, an adequate intra-abdominal space needs to be created to permit insertion of the remaining trocars. This usually requires lysis of some adhesions to the anterior abdominal wall, which may be done with finger dissection through the initial trocar site; the laparoscope also can be used to perform gentle blunt dissection. Insertion of a second trocar will allow sharp lysis of adhesions; insertion of a third trocar will add traction-countertraction capability to the sharp dissection. Three trocars (5 or 10 mm) generally are the minimum needed for a laparoscopic adhesiolysis. Electrocautery or ultrasonic dissection should be used sparingly to avoid a thermal bowel injury. If a loop of bowel is densely adhered to the anterior abdominal wall, then it may be safer to excise a small section of peritoneum or preperitoneal tissue in continuity with the loop instead of finding the precise plane between the peritoneum and bowel, a plane that likely is obliterated.

OPERATIVE TECHNIQUE

After establishment of pneumoperitoneum and an adequate operative space, a search for the transition zone between collapsed and distended bowel should be undertaken. A retrograde examination of the small bowel is begun at the cecum. Atraumatic graspers with nonlocking jaws can be used to run the decompressed distal small bowel. Resistance to retraction of the decompressed distal bowel may signify proximity of the transition zone. Manipulation of dilated proximal small bowel risks perforation and should be performed carefully, if it all. Grasping the mesentery or mesenteric fat to manipulate the proximal bowel decreases the likelihood of intestinal injury.

Simple adhesions may be lysed with cold scissors; as mentioned earlier, electrocautery, the ultrasonic scalpel, and other high-energy dissectors should be avoided, if possible. As the lysis of adhesion progresses, the surgeon may find that the initial trocar placement no longer provides a reasonable angle of attack. To improve this angle of attack, additional trocars can be placed, the initial trocars can be removed and repositioned, and the laparoscope can be rotated among the ports. Such rearrangement of operative ports can facilitate the dissection and identification of the transition point. In addition, the surgeon should take full advantage of operating table tilt and rotation to optimize the angle of attack and operative ergonomics.

Once the transition point of a simple obstruction has been identified and the adhesions involving this point have been cut, the adhesiolysis should be terminated. A complete dissection and adhesiolysis to the ligament of Treitz is unnecessary, prolongs the procedure, and increases the risk for a perforative complication, without adding any observable benefit to the operation. If the transition point cannot be found in simple obstruction, then we generally convert the procedure to a laparotomy.

After completion of the adhesiolysis, the areas of dissection should be inspected for bleeding or perforation. Small bleeding points may be controlled with clips, sutures, or careful electrocautery. Most serosal tears and enterotomies can be sutured laparoscopically. A minilaparotomy may be performed for bowel examination and repair under direct vision, if the situation warrants. After the final examination of the abdominal cavity, the abdomen is desufflated, completing the procedure.

If a released loop of bowel appears strangulated or ischemic, then it should be observed for return of color and peristalsis. If the loop is gangrenous or perforated, then resection and anastomosis are performed. If the patient is relatively thin, then this resection can be performed extracorporeally with conventional staplers through a small transverse incision. Otherwise, an intracorporeal resection with side-to-side anastomosis using endoscopic stapler-cutters is performed. If the viability of a bowel segment is not clear, then a second-look laparoscopy with possible resection may be performed in 24 to 36 hours.

Occasionally, unsuspected pathology is encountered, such as cancer, gallstone ileus, inflammatory bowel disease, or intussusception. The ability of the surgeon to identify an intraluminal mass may be enhanced with the use of laparoscopic ultrasound. If unsuspected and unknown pathology is encountered, then conversion to minilaparotomy or formal laparotomy may be necessary. If the patient has a preoperative diagnosis of malignant obstruction, such as from a colon cancer, then conversion of a nonelective procedure to an elective oncologic resection may be possible by inserting an endoscopic stent or with proximal diversion.

POSTOPERATIVE CARE

The nasogastric tube is left in place, and maintenance intravenous fluid is given until ileus has resolved. The diet then may be advanced as tolerated. The analgesic requirement after laparoscopic release of a simple obstruction should be minimal; the patient who requires excessive opioids may have a missed bowel injury.

MANAGEMENT OF PROCEDURE-SPECIFIC COMPLICATIONS

Procedure-specific complications to consider during and after a laparoscopic adhesiolysis include hemorrhage (including from solid organs), enterotomy, intra-abdominal abscess, bladder injury, or ureteral injury. The most common of these is enterotomy. There has been some suggestion that laparoscopic adhesiolysis for SBO leads to a higher rate of bowel injury than the open procedure. Inadvertent enterotomy appears to be more frequent in patients with a history of multiple previous laparotomies. The primary mechanism of inadvertent enterotomy is the adhesiolysis itself; less common mechanisms include perforation with the Veress needle or electrothermal injury. A recognized enterotomy typically can be repaired laparoscopically; extensive injury may necessitate an enterectomy. If an adhesiolysis-related enterotomy is recognized and repaired without subsequent sequelae, then some surgeons will not consider this a complication.

A patient with fever, tachycardia, hypotension, oliguria, or abdominal pain after laparoscopic adhesiolysis should be investigated or reexplored for a possible missed bowel injury. The

Table 23-2 Reported Results of Laparoscopic Adhesiolysis

Study	No. of Subjects	Surgery Time (min)	Conversion (%)	Bowel Injury (%)	Postoperative Complications (%)	Length of Stay (days)	Follow-Up (mo)	Reoperation (%)	Mortality (%)
Khaikin, 2007	31	75	32	NR	16	5.8	NR	NR	0
Kirshtein, 2005	65	40	28	4.6	6.4	4.2	24	NR	0
Borzellino, 2004	40	118	25	7.5	15	5	48	5	0
Chopra, 2003	34	138	32	4.6	39	7.3	NR	4.3	4.3
Levard, 2001	308	NR	41	8.4	47	4	1.6	4.5	2.2
Suter, 2000	83	NR	43	15.6	31	5.9	NR	9	2.4
Chosidow, 2000	134	72	16	3	5	5	NR	NR	0
Strickland, 1999	40	68	33	10	13	3.6	22	5	0
Léon, 1998	40	108	35	NR	NR	3	NR	17.5	0
Bailey, 1998	65	64	22	NR	NR	6.6	46	10.8	1.8
Navez, 1998	69	77	40	9	12	NR	NR	2.9	2.9
Ibrahim, 1996	33	NR	15	6.1	6	NR	NR	3	3
OVERALL RANGE	31-308	40-138	15-43	3-15.6	5-47	3-7.3	1.6-46	2.9-17.5	0-4.3

NR, not reported.

Table 23-3 Results of Laparoscopic Adhesiolysis for a Single Adhesive Band

Study	No. of Subjects	Patients with Single Band (%)	Successful Laparoscopic Adhesiolysis for Single Band (%)
Ibrahim, 1996	33	70	78
Léon, 1998	40	15	83
Strickland, 1999	40	30	75
Suter, 2000	83	42	68
Chosidow, 2000	134	31	NR
Levard, 2001	308	54	65
Lujan, 2005	61	41	84
TOTAL/MEAN (%)	699	40	76

NR, not reported.

Table 23-4 Comparison of Laparoscopic and Open Surgical Treatment of Small Bowel Obstruction

	Laparoscopic Adhesiolysis		Open Adhesiolysis	
	Wullstein (2003)	Khaikin (2007)	Wullstein (2003)	Khaikin (2007)
Operating time (min)	103	78	84	70
Postoperative hospital stay (days)	11.3	5	18.1	9
First bowel movement (days)	NR	3	NR	6
Oral intake (days)	5.1	NR	6.4	NR
Morbidity (%)	19	16	40.4	45
Recurrent bowel obstruction (%)	0-14.2	NR	0-4.6	NR

NR, not reported.

stable patient with mild symptoms can undergo CT scanning; the more symptomatic or unstable patient may be better managed with an immediate reoperation. The choice between laparoscopy or laparotomy for reoperation in this situation is surgeon dependent. It should be noted that unrecognized electrothermal intestinal injury may result in a delayed perforation, even occurring beyond the first postoperative week. The mortality rate from undetected bowel injury is 20% to 50%, which is far greater than with immediately recognized and repaired injury.

The frequency of conversions to laparotomy during laparoscopic adhesiolysis has been reported to range from 15% to 43%

(Table 23-2), although conversion by itself is not a complication. The most common cause for conversion has been dense and excessive adhesions; secondary causes include enterotomy and hemorrhage. To reduce the number of conversions, some surgeons use hand-assisted laparoscopy in select cases.

RESULTS AND OUTCOME

Recent literature has demonstrated that laparoscopic adhesiolysis for the treatment of SBO is safe, feasible, and reasonably effective in properly selected patients (see Table 23-1 for selection criteria). The perioperative mortality rate for this procedure has been 0% to 4.3% (see Table 23-2). The published success rate of laparoscopic adhesiolysis has ranged from 46% to 87%; cases in which a simple obstruction was secondary to a single adhesive band tend to have even better success rates (Table 23-3). The incidence of bowel injury has ranged from 3% to 15.7% (see Table 23-2). Laparoscopic adhesiolysis typically takes longer than the open procedure, but the length of stay and postoperative morbidity may be shorter with laparoscopic adhesiolysis, as suggested by uncontrolled data (Table 23-4). Conversion may increase the postoperative morbidity rate. The effect that laparoscopic adhesiolysis has on the rate of wound dehiscence and incisional hernia is not known for sure, but a logical assumption would be a decreased risk for wound complications, given the lack of a recent, large incision.

Suggested Readings

Bailey IS, Rhodes M, O'Rourke N, et al: Laparoscopic management of acute small bowel obstruction, *Br J Surg* 85:84–87, 1998.

Borzellino G, Tasselli S, Zerman G, et al: Laparoscopic approach to postoperative adhesive obstruction, *Surg Endosc* 18:686–690, 2004.

Burkill G, Bell J, Healy J: Small bowel obstruction: The role of computed tomography in its diagnosis and management with reference to other imaging modalities, *Eur Radiol* 11:1405–1422, 2001.

Chopra R, McVay C, Phillips E, Khalili TM: Laparoscopic lysis of adhesions, *Am Surg* 69:966–968, 2003.

Chosidow D, Johanet H, Montariol T, et al: Laparoscopy for acute small-bowel obstruction secondary to adhesions, *J Laparoendosc Adv Surg Tech A* 10:155–159, 2000.

Cirocchi R, Abraha I, Farinella E, et al: Laparoscopic versus open surgery in small bowel obstruction, *Cochrane Database Syst Rev* 2:CD007511, 2010.

Ghosheh B, Salameh JR: Laparoscopic approach to acute small bowel obstruction: Review of 1061 cases, *Surg Endosc* 21:1945–1949, 2007.

Ibrahim IM, Wolodiger F, Sussman B, et al: Laparoscopic management of acute small-bowel obstruction, *Surg Endosc* 10:1012–1014, 1996.

Khaikin M, Schneidereit N, Cera S, et al: Laparoscopic vs. open surgery for acute adhesive small-bowel obstruction: Patients' outcome and cost-effectiveness, *Surg Endosc* 21:742–746, 2007.

Kirshtein B, Roy-Shapira A, Lantsberg L, et al: Laparoscopic management of acute small bowel obstruction, *Surg Endosc* 19:464–467, 2005.

Léon EL, Metzger A, Tsiotos GG, et al: Laparoscopic management of small bowel obstruction: Indications and outcome, *J Gastrointest Surg* 2:132–140, 1998.

Levard H, Boudet MJ, Msika S, et al, for the French Association for Surgical Research: Laparoscopic treatment of acute small bowel obstruction: a multicentre retrospective study, *Aust N Z J Surg* 71:641–646, 2001.

Lujan HJ, Oren A, Plasencia G, et al: Laparoscopic management as the initial treatment of acute small bowel obstruction, *JSLS* 10:466–472, 2006.

Moran BJ: Adhesion-related small bowel obstruction, *Colorectal Dis* 9(Suppl 2): 39–44, 2007.

Nagle A, Ujiki M, Denham W, Murayama K: Laparoscopic adhesiolysis for small bowel obstruction, *Am J Surg* 187:464–470, 2004.

Navez B, Arimont JM, Guiot P: Laparoscopic approach in acute small bowel obstruction: A review of 68 patients, *Hepatogastroenterology* 45:2146–2150, 1998.

Strickland P, Lourie DJ, Suddleson EA, et al: Is laparoscopy safe and effective for treatment of acute small-bowel obstruction? *Surg Endosc* 13:695–698, 1999.

Suter M, Zermatten P, Halkic N, et al: Laparoscopic management of mechanical small bowel obstruction: Are there predictors of success or failure? *Surg Endosc* 14:478–483, 2000.

Szomstein S, Lo Menzo E, Simpfendorfer C, et al: Laparoscopic lysis of adhesions, *World J Surg* 30:535–540, 2006.

Wang Q, Hu ZQ, Wang WJ, et al: Laparoscopic management of recurrent adhesive small-bowel obstruction: Long-term follow-up, *Surg Today* 39:493–499, 2009.

Wullstein C, Gross E: Laparoscopic compared with conventional treatment of acute adhesive small bowel obstruction, *Br J Surg* 90:1147–1151, 2003.

Zerey M, Sechrist CW, Kercher KW, et al: The laparoscopic management of small-bowel obstruction, *Am J Surg* 194:882–887, 2007.

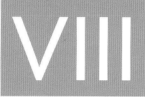

LINDA P. ZHANG, SCOTT Q. NGUYEN, AND CELIA M. DIVINO

Laparoscopic Reversal of the Hartmann Procedure

24

The videos associated with this chapter are listed in the Video Contents and can be found on the accompanying DVDs and *on Expertconsult.com.*

The Hartmann procedure was first performed by Henri Hartmann in 1921 for rectosigmoid cancer. He reported two patients with obstructing sigmoid carcinoma whom he treated with proximal colostomy, sigmoid resection, and closure of the rectal stump using an abdominal approach. The rationale for this procedure was a 38% mortality rate in patients undergoing an abdominoperineal resection for colorectal cancer during this period. Since that time, the Hartmann procedure has been used to treat various left-sided colonic diseases, such as perforated or obstructed tumors, ischemic colitis, traumatic colonic perforations, volvulus of the sigmoid colon, radiation injury, and complicated diverticular disease—the latter being the most common indication. The Hartmann procedure generally is considered the gold standard of treatment for benign sigmoid perforation. The procedure provides proximal diversion of the fecal stream and resection of the diseased portion of colon, but with no risk for anastomotic leak. It also allows time for the inflammation and intra-abdominal adhesions to improve or resolve before elective restoration of bowel continuity, which typically involves a several month wait.

Minimally invasive approaches have been applied to colostomy closure after a Hartmann procedure (i.e., Hartmann reversal) in an effort to decrease the morbidity and mortality associated with open colostomy closure. Early experiences with laparoscopically assisted Hartmann reversal were reported by Gorey and colleagues in 1993. The technical demands of this procedure have somewhat limited the widespread application of the laparoscopic Hartmann reversal. In addition, there really has not been a consensus on the optimal technique in performing a laparoscopic reversal. In this chapter, we describe our own technique and experience with laparoscopic reversal of the Hartmann procedure.

OPERATIVE INDICATIONS

There are risks associated with reversal of a Hartmann procedure. Morbidity rates for open Hartmann reversal can range from 30% to 40%, with anastomotic leak rates ranging from 0% to 15%. The perioperative mortality rate can be as high as 10%. Technical difficulty with dissection of the rectal stump secondary to dense adhesions, and the occasional need to perform a low anastomosis, can increase the risk for anastomotic failure. The use of various stapling devices since then has facilitated the performance of restorative procedures, particularly in the patient with a short rectal stump.

Studies have shown that patients with stomas score significantly lower on quality-of-life indexes than patients without stomas. Various medical and lifestyle issues associated with a stoma include skin rash, appliance leak, sexual dysfunction, parastomal hernia, and psychological distress. Even so, 40% to 45% of patients with a Hartmann procedure will never undergo reversal, usually because of medical comorbidity or social issues. Compared with open Hartmann reversal, the laparoscopic procedure offers the advantages of a smaller incision, shorter hospital stay, and less blood loss. These advantages may increase the candidate pool for colostomy closure, particularly in those who have multiple comorbidities.

The timing of a Hartmann reversal has been debated. In general, the patient who required a Hartmann procedure was a relatively sick individual whom the surgeon had deemed to have an unacceptable risk for primary anastomosis. It had been advocated to wait for about 6 months to allow patients to recuperate from the initial surgery and also to allow for the local inflammation and adhesions to diminish. More recent studies have suggested that operative difficulty appears to decrease after a waiting period as short as 15 weeks.

The laparoscopic approach can be limited by dense intra-abdominal adhesions, which can increase the difficulty of both abdominal access and mobilization of the rectal stump. This is especially true in the patient who had gross peritonitis from complicated diverticulitis. The open conversion rate for laparoscopic Hartmann reversal has ranged from 9% to 25%. In light of this, some surgeons have advocated hand-assisted laparoscopy for difficult cases to facilitate the dissection. Although there are no strict contraindications to performing laparoscopic Hartmann reversal, it is advisable that this procedure be performed by an experienced laparoscopic surgeon. It should be stressed that open conversion of a difficult laparoscopic Hartmann reversal is an acceptable outcome; such a conversion is not a complication in and of itself.

PREOPERATIVE EVALUATION, TESTING, AND PREPARATION

An evaluation of the patient's cardiac, pulmonary, and nutritional assessment should be performed. The patient with a poor nutritional status (e.g., preoperative serum albumin level < 3 g/dL) is at an increased risk for postoperative complications, such as anastomotic leak or fascial dehiscence. Because reversal of a Hartmann procedure is an elective operation, the patient with poor nutritional status should have the reversal postponed until the nutritional status can be optimized. Similarly, the patient with unstable cardiopulmonary disease should wait until his or her medical condition improves so that the procedure can be tolerated.

For the patient with diverticular disease, a barium enema can be performed to evaluate for any residual diverticular disease in the rectal stump. A colonoscopy through the stoma is performed to evaluate the proximal colon for any remaining diverticular disease or colon cancer. The patient who had a Hartmann procedure for colon cancer will require the standard preoperative malignancy evaluation, including a colonoscopy and a CT of the chest, abdomen, and pelvis. Neoadjuvant chemotherapy and radiation may be necessary depending on the results of the cancer staging.

It has been debatable whether preoperative mechanical bowel preparation of the remaining colon is necessary. Depending on the surgeon's preference, an oral cathartic solution or an ostomy enema can be administered to empty the colostomy proximally. Most surgeons have used an enema to evacuate the rectal stump. Patients should receive perioperative intravenous antibiotics, pneumatic sequential compression devices, and a Foley catheter. An orogastric tube may be necessary for better visualization of the upper abdomen and splenic flexure. Depending on the severity of the primary disease process and the degree of difficulty at the index procedure, ureteral stents can be placed to facilitate identification of the ureters.

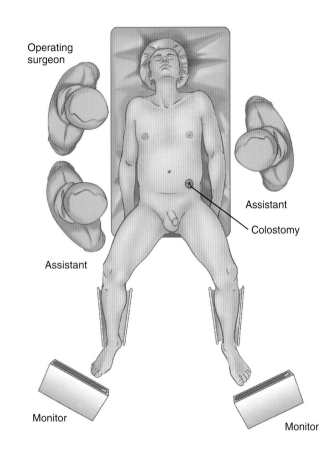

FIGURE 24-1 Low lithotomy position, with surgical team and monitor placement.

PATIENT POSITIONING IN THE OPERATING SUITE

The patient is placed in the low-lithotomy position. This allows for intraoperative endoscopy and placement of the end-to-end anastomotic stapling device. The legs are minimally flexed at the hip, which permits mobility of the laparoscopic instrumentation. The arms can be extended by their sides if the patient is obese. Alternatively, the arms can be tucked into the patient's sides to allow for maximal working room for the surgical team. All pressure points are padded, and the patient is secured on the table with a strap. One video monitor is placed on each side of the patient. For most of the procedure, the surgeon and first assistant stand on the right side of the table, and the second assistant stands on the left (Fig. 24-1).

POSITIONING AND PLACEMENT OF THE TROCARS

There are two accepted methods of gaining access into the abdomen (Fig. 24-2). Some surgeons advocate mobilizing the colostomy site and using the peristomal incision for a Hasson cannula. The abdomen is prepared and draped from the xiphoid to the pubis, and the stoma is left uncovered. The stoma site is excised, or an open cut-down technique can be used. The stoma is then mobilized, and the anvil of the circular stapling device is inserted into the lumen. A pursestring suture is placed to secure the anvil. The end of the left colon is then dropped into the abdomen. The fascia of the colostomy site is reapproximated using 0-0 polypropylene sutures, and the Hasson cannula is inserted between the sutures. The sutures are pulled tight to create an airtight seal around the cannula.

The second method of abdominal access involves initial port placement in the upper right or left abdomen, lateral to the rectus sheath. With this method, the stoma is either sewn closed with a 2-0 running silk suture or packed with gauze and covered with a sterile adhesive dressing. The abdomen is then prepared and draped from the xiphoid to the pubis. A Hasson cannula is inserted into the right or left upper abdomen, near the tip of the 11th rib lateral to the rectus sheath. This approach allows for safe access into the abdomen because there should be minimal adhesions in the upper quadrants. Lysis of adhesions thus can be done before mobilization of the colostomy.

Once the camera port is inserted, the peritoneal cavity is insufflated to 12 to 15 mm Hg, and visual inspection of the abdomen is performed. A 30-degree angled scope should be used to allow maximal visualization of the entire abdomen. Two to three additional trocars are placed under direct vision. The positions of these trocars are dependent on body habitus, length of abdominal cavity, and location of intra-abdominal adhesions. Generally, a 12-mm port is inserted in the right lower quadrant, where a stapling device can be used if the rectosigmoid stump requires further resection. Some surgeons prefer the camera port to be at the umbilicus. A 5-mm working trocar is inserted into the right upper quadrant. A third working port can be placed suprapubically or at the upper midline to aid with retraction.

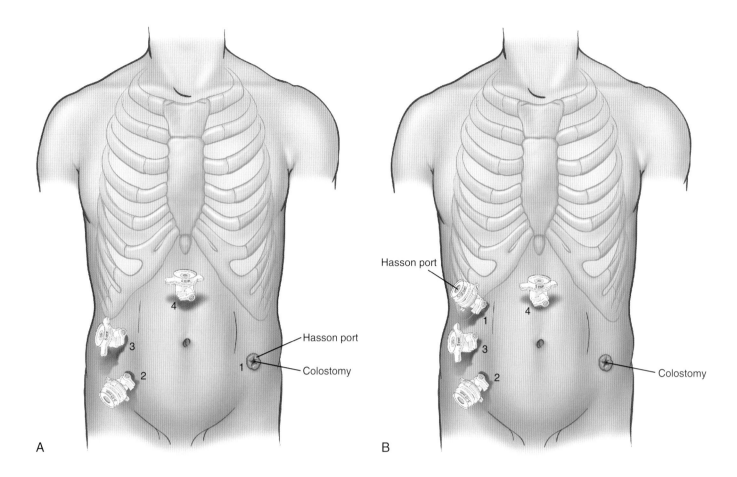

FIGURE 24-2 Port placement. **A,** Colostomy site used for Hasson cannula. **B,** Hasson cannula placed in right upper quadrant.

OPERATIVE TECHNIQUE

Lysis of Adhesions

Once access to the peritoneal cavity has been obtained, adhesiolysis will be necessary, especially at the midline and in the left lower quadrant. This can be achieved using dissection with Endo Shears (United States Surgical Corporation, Norwalk, Conn.), or with judicious application of electrocautery (to avoid thermal bowel injury). A bipolar vessel sealing device can be used for larger adhesions that may contain vessels. The lysis of adhesions is limited to the left side of the abdomen; adhesiolysis of other areas of the abdomen is unnecessary and should be avoided.

Identification and Dissection of the Rectal Stump

To identify the rectal stump, the patient is placed in the steep-Trendelenburg position with a rightward tilt. The small bowel is retracted to the right side of the abdomen. Some patients may have had a polypropylene suture placed on the rectal stump, or the stump may have been sutured to the anterior abdominal wall; these maneuvers facilitate the identification of the rectal stump. If there is no marking stitch, an EEA stapler or rectal dilator can be inserted transanally to aid in locating the rectal stump. Inability to locate the rectal stump is a common reason for conversion to laparotomy.

Once identified, the stump is dissected as needed. The bladder may be closely adherent to the rectum, and care must be taken

to avoid injuring the bladder (and vagina in women). Instillation of saline into the bladder with a three-way Foley catheter can aid in identifying the proper plane of dissection. The fat surrounding the end of the rectal stump is removed using Endo Shears (United States Surgical Corporation, Norwalk, Conn.) or a sealing device. If a long rectosigmoid stump with residual diverticulosis is present, then resection of the upper disease portion can be performed with a laparoscopic stapling device. A series of transanal dilator probes is then used to identify the widest circular stapler that the stump can accommodate.

Mobilization of the Colostomy

If the colostomy site was not used to access the abdominal cavity, then the colostomy site is mobilized at this time through a peristomal incision. The colostomy site is excised at the mucocutaneous junction circumferentially and mobilized down to the peritoneum. If necessary, the left colon containing residual diverticulosis may be brought out through the colostomy site and resected. The anvil of the circular stapling device is inserted into the lumen and secured with a 2-0 polypropylene pursestring suture. The end of the left colon, with the anvil in place, is dropped into the abdomen. The fascia at the colostomy site is closed using 0-0 polypropylene sutures. Alternatively, the site can be used as a working port by placing a balloon-tipped 10-mm trocar between the sutures and tightening them around the trocar.

Mobilization of the Splenic Flexure

The proximal colon should be mobilized to reach the rectal stump without tension. To accomplish this, the left colon and splenic flexure will need to be mobilized. Lateral attachments extending up to the splenic flexure are released along the line of Toldt. Care must be taken during this dissection, including visualization of the left ureter, because normal anatomy may be distorted after the index procedure. The splenic flexure is then mobilized. At this point, the proximal colon is brought down into the pelvis to determine whether a colorectal anastomosis can be performed without tension; additional mobilization is performed as necessary.

Anastomosis

The end-to-end stapling device is inserted transanally, with the head of the stapler positioned at the end of the rectal stump. The anvil within the end of the proximal colon is secured to the stapling device under direct laparoscopic visualization. The orientation of the left colon is checked to ensure that there is no mesenteric twisting. The bladder and vagina are retracted to avoid being caught in the staple line. The stapling device is closed and fired per the manufacturer's recommendations. After completion of the anastomosis, the cut tissue held within the stapler is inspected to confirm the presence of two complete "donuts." An air-leak test is then performed. The proximal left colon is occluded with a bowel grasper, the pelvis is filled with sterile saline, and a rigid sigmoidoscope (or bulb syringe) is inserted transanally to test the integrity of the staple line with air insufflation.

POSTOPERATIVE CARE

The patient can expect an average postoperative hospital stay of 3 to 4 days. Patient-controlled analgesia is used for pain control. No additional prophylactic antibiotics are needed. On the morning of postoperative day 1, the patient is placed on a clear liquid diet, encouraged to ambulate, and given deep venous thrombosis prophylaxis (subcutaneous heparin). The Foley catheter is removed. By postoperative day 2 or 3, the patient typically will have had flatus and can be advanced to a soft diet. When the patient is tolerating a soft diet, can ambulate, and has adequate analgesia with oral medication, then hospital discharge is possible, with a follow-up clinic visit in 1 to 2 weeks.

MANAGEMENT OF PROCEDURE-SPECIFIC COMPLICATIONS

The complications of laparoscopic Hartmann reversal are similar to those of open reversal and include wound infection, postoperative ileus, anastomotic leak, and intra-abdominal abscess. Most superficial wound infections after laparoscopic Hartmann reversal can be managed with antibiotics or by opening the wound, with closure by secondary intention. Because most of these infections occur at the previous colostomy site, it generally is recommended that the skin of the colostomy site be left open.

Postoperative ileus usually is less in laparoscopic Hartmann reversal compared with the open operation. The risk for anastomotic leak can be minimized by ensuring that there is no tension on the anastomosis and no twisting of the mesentery, and that the vascular supply to both ends is adequate. Various studies have shown a similar, if not decreased, rate of anastomotic leak in laparoscopic compared with open reversal. A typical anastomotic leak after a laparoscopic Hartmann reversal generally is small and contained within an intra-abdominal abscess. The patient should be made NPO and placed on antibiotics. Any intra-abdominal fluid collection should be assessed by interventional radiology for percutaneous drainage. Most small anastomotic leaks will resolve with this treatment. If the patient continues to be ill with fever, elevated white blood cell count, peritonitis, or an uncontained collection, then surgical intervention will be necessary. Unfortunately, such patients likely will need to have a colostomy reestablished.

RESULTS AND OUTCOME

A few hundred cases of laparoscopy-assisted Hartmann reversal have been published in case reports, single institution series, and multicenter series (i.e., retrospective data). When comparing laparoscopic with open Hartmann reversal, most studies have demonstrated less intraoperative blood loss, fewer abdominal wall hernias, decreased need for postoperative analgesia, and a shorter length of hospital stay (3 to 4 days vs. 5 to 8 days) with the minimally invasive approach. Not unexpectedly, the operative time has been equal or longer with laparoscopic reversal. This latter difference likely will decrease as surgeons become more proficient with this operation. The open conversion rate has ranged from 9% to 15%. Most studies did not find a difference in postoperative complication rates between open and laparoscopic groups. The long-term (>6 months) sequelae of abdominal wall hernia and reoperation were less with laparoscopic Hartmann reversal than with open reversal. These positive outcomes should result in an increased use of minimally invasive techniques for reversal of the Hartmann procedure.

Suggested Readings

Banerjee S, Leather AJ, Rennie JA, et al: Feasibility and morbidity of reversal of Hartmann's, *Colorectal Dis* 7:454–459, 2005.

Keck JO, Collopy BT, Ryan PJ, et al: Reversal of Hartmann's procedure: Effect of timing and technique on ease and safety, *Dis Colon Rectum* 37:243–248, 1994.

Khaikin M, Zmora O, Rosin D, et al: Laparoscopically assisted reversal of Hartmann's procedure, *Surg Endosc* 20:1883–1886, 2006.

Mazeh H, Greenstein AJ, Swedish K, et al: Laparoscopic and open reversal of Hartmann's procedure—a comparative retrospective analysis, *Surg Endosc* 23:496–502, 2009.

Rosen MJ, Cobb WS, Kercher KW, et al: Laparoscopic restoration of intestinal continuity after Hartmann's procedure, *Am J Surg* 189:670–674, 2005.

Rosen MJ, Cobb WS, Kercher KW, et al: Laparoscopic versus open colostomy reversal: A comparative analysis, *J Gastrointest Surg* 10:895–900, 2006.

Schmelzer TM, Mostafa G, Norton HJ, et al: Reversal of Hartmann's procedure: A high-risk operation? *Surgery* 142:598–606, 2007.

Siddiqui MR, Sajid MS, Baig MK, et al: Open *vs.* laparoscopic approach for reversal of Hartmann's procedure: A systematic review, *Colorectal Dis* 12:733–741, 2010.

Slawik S, Dixon AR: Laparoscopic reversal of Hartmann's rectosigmoidectomy, *Colorectal Dis* 10:81–83, 2008.

Sosa JL, Sleeman D, Puente I, et al: Laparoscopic-assisted colostomy closure after Hartmann's procedure, *Dis Colon Rectum* 37:149–152, 1994.

CONSTANTINE T. FRANTZIDES, SCOTT N. WELLE, AND TIMOTHY M. RUFF

Laparoscopic Colectomy for Diverticulitis

The videos associated with this chapter are listed in the Video Contents and can be found on the accompanying DVDs and *on Expertconsult.com.*

Colonic diverticular disease is common in Western society, occurring in about one third to two thirds of the population. It is hypothesized that a low-residue diet is a major causative factor. Age is another risk factor; diverticulosis is not uncommon in Americans in the fourth decade of life. Of patients with diverticulosis, as many as one fourth will develop diverticulitis.

The approach to the surgical management of diverticulitis depends greatly on the time of presentation. Many patients will present as a surgical emergency with the initial attack of diverticulitis. Historically, emergent surgery for diverticulitis was performed in either two or three stages. Since the 1980s, however, the practice of proximal diversion while leaving the diseased segment of colon behind (three-stage resection) has significantly decreased. Today, the Hartmann procedure is the most common two-stage operation. The initial stage of this operation is most commonly performed with the open approach; however, laparoscopic Hartmann procedure has been reported in the literature. More commonly, the second stage (i.e., Hartmann reversal) is performed laparoscopically. A single-stage approach to perforated diverticulitis has also been described. Additionally, with today's potent antimicrobial regimens, the treatment of contained perforated diverticulitis with intravenous antibiotics only has been accepted as an option.

OPERATIVE INDICATIONS

Elective colectomy for diverticulitis traditionally was reserved for the treatment of complications of the disease, such as recurrent attacks, perforation, abscess, fistula, stricture, or obstruction. Current recommendations are based on the clinical manifestations of the disease and the risk for recurrence and complications. It is advised that an elderly patient with a history of two episodes of diverticulitis or a younger patient (<50 years) with a history of one attack undergo an elective sigmoid colectomy to prevent a recurrent, more severe attack with the risks for complications. Both laparoscopic and open approaches for the elective treatment of diverticulitis have been described.

In this chapter, the technique for laparoscopic sigmoid colectomy with primary anastomosis in a complex case of diverticulitis is described. On the accompanying DVD (as well as on Expert Consult), we have included a video demonstrating the case of a patient with a history of multiple previous episodes of diverticulitis. The patient presented with a more severe recurrent

attack, failed conservative treatment with percutaneous drainage of an abscess and intravenous antibiotics, and developed a colovesical fistula. The incidence of fistulas in patients with diverticular disease, the most common cause of colovesical fistula, is accepted to be 2%, although some centers have reported higher percentages. Colovesical fistulas are more common in males. Women who present with colovesical fistulas are commonly older or have a history of hysterectomy. The diagnosis is made clinically and confirmed with cystoscopy. This acute case can be compared with the case described in Chapter 15 of the *Atlas of Minimally Invasive Surgery*, 2009 (see Suggested Readings at the end of this chapter), in which the patient was successfully treated with antibiotics and the inflammation subsided before resection.

PREOPERATIVE EVALUATION

The preoperative evaluation of a patient undergoing a colectomy for diverticulitis is determined by the timing of the patient's initial presentation.

When a patient presents with an acute attack of diverticulitis, a computed tomography (CT) scan to evaluate for perforation or abscess should be obtained. The patient is put on antibiotics covering aerobic and anaerobic bacteria. If an abscess is present, radiology-guided percutaneous drainage should be attempted. Patients with a microperforation may be managed conservatively with observation and antibiotics. If the inflammation improves with antibiotics, then the patient may undergo an elective resection.

The presence of a large perforation or diffuse peritonitis necessitates an urgent operation. Free colonic perforation secondary to diverticulitis is rare. Surgical management, whether open or laparoscopic, remains controversial.

If the patient presents with chronic diverticulitis, a barium enema to evaluate for stricture and fistula may be warranted in addition to a CT scan to evaluate for abscess and phlegmon.

For elective colectomy, a bowel preparation is recommended by most experts. The regimen consists of a traditional oral lavage with polyethylene glycol, followed by the administration of oral antibiotics (erythromycin and neomycin base) on the day before surgery. There is controversy surrounding the type of bowel preparation required and even whether bowel preparation is necessary. A single dose of a second-generation cephalosporin and

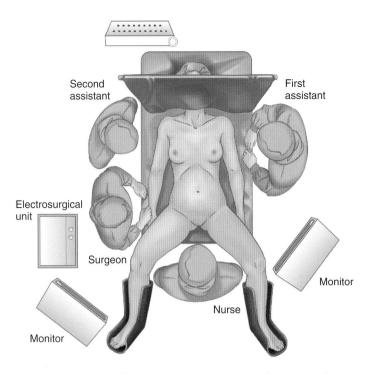

FIGURE 25-1 Patient positioning and operating room setup for laparoscopic sigmoid colectomy.

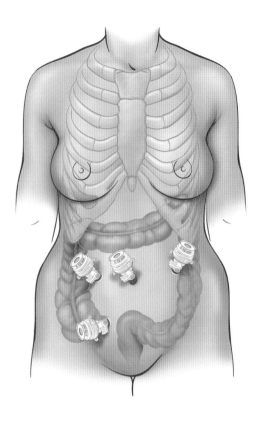

FIGURE 25-2 Trocar placement for laparoscopic sigmoid colectomy.

metronidazole is given intravenously 30 minutes before incision. Sequential compression devices are placed for the prevention of deep venous thrombosis. Foley catheter placement for bladder decompression is required.

PATIENT POSITIONING AND PORT PLACEMENT

For a laparoscopic sigmoidectomy, the patient is placed in the low lithotomy position with stirrups (Fig. 25-1). This positioning allows the end-to-end anastomotic (EEA) stapler to be used per the rectum. The left hip is elevated off the operating table by using a beanbag, viscoelastic cushion, or similar device. Placement of bilateral ureteral stents by a urologist, in particular infrared-illuminated stents (InfraVision, Stryker, San Jose, Calif.), is helpful in identifying the ureters when dealing with the phlegmon and inflammation of diverticulitis.

The surgeon stands on the patient's right, facing a monitor. The authors prefer to access the abdomen using the open Hasson technique inferior to the umbilicus. This incision can then be extended to remove the specimen. If the patient has had previous surgeries, it may be prudent to insert a bladeless optical trocar at a different site to access the abdomen. After the pneumoperitoneum is established, two additional 12-mm trocars are placed in the right abdomen, just inferior and superior to the level of the umbilicus (Fig. 25-2). The use of 12-mm trocars at all port positions allows for maximal instrument flexibility. The placement of additional trocars may be necessary depending on the extent of the operation and the complexity of dissection. There are no set rules for the perfect port positioning. The surgeon must carefully consider each trocar placement in relation to the dissection and also to the other trocars. The main reason for conversion to open is the malpositioning of the trocar sites.

OPERATIVE TECHNIQUE

The operating table is rotated to the patient's right, elevating the left side. This rotation, in addition to the patient's left hip already being elevated, will bring the patient close to the lateral decubitus position, facilitating mobilization of the sigmoid colon.

Mobilization of the sigmoid colon is often tedious and time-consuming because of the inflammation of diverticulitis. The colon is frequently densely adhered to the abdominal side wall. This mobilization can be accomplished bluntly with the use of a inflatable balloon retractor or sharply with scissors. One should be cautious using thermal energy during this dissection to avoid inadvertent injury to the bowel or underlying retroperitoneal structures. The proximal left colon is retracted medially, placing the colon under stretch using an atraumatic grasper. Sharp dissection is used to dissect the colon away from the lateral abdominal wall along the white line of Toldt with the use of hook electrocautery, scissors, or the ultrasonic scalpel. The bowel is then swept medially away from the side wall; again, the balloon retractor is useful for this portion of the procedure. The use of the illuminated stents is particularly helpful here to aid in identification of the ureter.

Depending on the extent of the diseased colon, the splenic flexure may need to be mobilized. For this portion of the procedure, the patient is placed in a steep reverse-Trendelenburg and right-tilted position so that the left side of the patient is elevated. This allows for the mobilization of the splenic flexure with sharp dissection while maintaining gentle traction on the colon.

During dissection in the pelvis, the patient is placed in steep Trendelenburg position. The small bowel may need to be retracted out of the pelvis with an inflatable balloon retractor. Once the

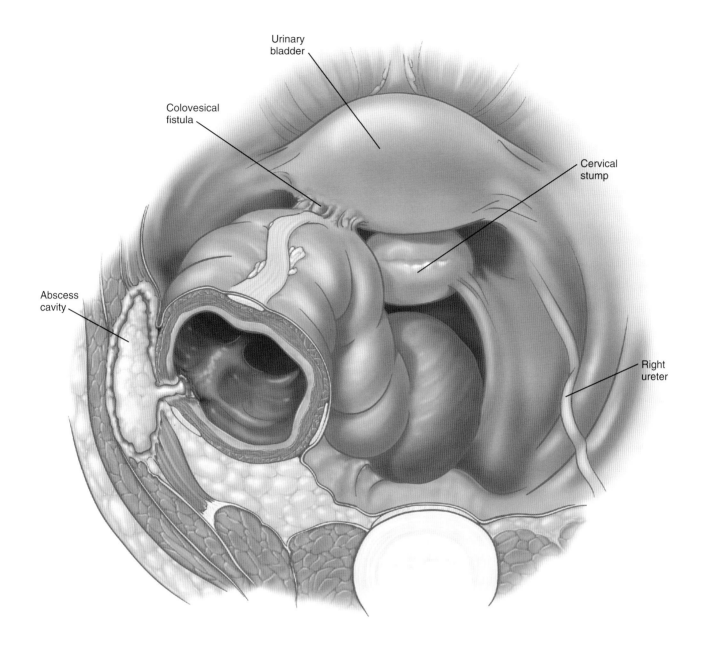

FIGURE 25-3 Pelvic anatomy. Note location of abscess cavity and colovesical fistula in a female patient with prior hysterectomy (see video on the accompanying DVD, as well as on Expert Consult).

colon is freed from its sidewall attachments, a combination of blunt and sharp dissection is used to sweep the colon and mesentery away from the underlying retroperitoneal structures. The presence of a phlegmon will require meticulous sharp dissection in the area of inflammation (Fig. 25-3). If an abscess cavity is encountered, it should be drained with caution to avoid peritoneal contamination. One should attempt to identify the ureter as it crosses the iliac artery near the external-internal bifurcation.

After the diseased colonic segment and mesentery are mobilized from the lateral abdominal wall, the main vascular trunk may be ligated without endangering the underlying ureter. The surgeon may score the peritoneum of the medial mesocolon, marking out a mesenteric wedge encompassing the segment to be resected. A small window is then bluntly created just underneath the mesenteric border of the colon at the distal point of transection. Using one or two loads of the linear articulating stapler, the colon is divided. Thickened tissue associated with diverticulitis will more likely than not require the use of the 4.8-mm (green) staple load. The mesentery is divided along the scored peritoneum to the point of proximal transection. The colon is divided proximally using the linear stapler-cutter. The resected colon and mesentery are placed in a polyethylene specimen bag. The proximal and distal staple lines are brought together to ensure the subsequent anastomosis will not be under tension. If not, further mobilization should be carried out. The umbilical trocar incision is extended, and the specimen is removed. The proximal end of colon is then delivered through this incision with the atraumatic grasper.

Alternatively, the surgeon may place the specimen into a camera bag after the distal transection before cutting the bowel proximally and then may deliver the bagged specimen through the enlarged umbilical incision. Before exteriorizing the colon with this technique, a marking stitch is placed at the margin of the devascularized colon. After the colon is delivered through the umbilical incision, it is divided proximally using the linear stapler-cutter. The colon is cleaned of mesenteric fat proximal to the staple line in preparation for the anvil of the EEA stapler. The staple line is excised, and the proximal colon is dilated with metal sizers in preparation for the head of the anvil. Generally speaking, a better functional result can be obtained by using the largest stapler diameter possible for the anastomosis. Typically, a 28-, 31-, or 34-mm diameter EEA stapler works well in this location. A pursestring suture is placed just underneath the staple line, either manually or with an automated pursestring applicator.

After sizing the proximal colon, the appropriate anvil is inserted, the pursestring suture is tightened, and the end of the colon is returned back into the abdomen. The incision is then closed, and pneumoperitoneum is reestablished. The EEA stapler is carefully maneuvered into the rectum; before insertion of the stapler, the rectum may need to be gently dilated. The surgeon should visualize the head of the stapler at the distal staple line of the rectal stump. The spike of the stapler should then be deployed directly through the center of the staple line; this will ensure better outcomes by avoiding the creation of parallel staple lines, which can lead to ischemia and perforation (Fig. 25-4A). The anvil is mated with the stapler, and the stapler is closed onto the anvil (Fig. 25-4B). The anastomosis is carefully checked for signs of tension and twisting before firing the stapler. Proper configuration of the staples is ensured by maintaining pressure on the firing levers of the staple gun for 10 seconds after firing. The stapler is reopened by rotating the Roticulator (Covidien, Norwalk, Conn.) three half-turns; the stapler is rotated gently 180 degrees and withdrawn from the rectum (Fig. 25-4C).

Several interrupted sutures can be placed to reinforce the EEA staple line.

Alternatively, if the surgeon feels that there is too much inflammation present to perform an anastomosis safely at this time, a colostomy may be created. After performing the distal resection, the specimen may be placed in a camera bag, and rather than delivering the colon through the umbilical port, it can be delivered through a suitable location in the left lower quadrant. Once delivered through the skin, the proximal resection can be performed and a colostomy matured in the usual fashion.

The presence of an abscess is considered by many surgeons a contraindication to performing a primary anastomosis. However, this is somewhat controversial. If the colon has been adequately prepared, there is no diffuse peritoneal contamination present, and a proper antibiotic coverage has been implemented, then a primary anastomosis can be safely performed, even in the presence an abscess. The case presented on the accompanying DVD (as well as on Expert Consult) is an example of this. The anastomosis is tested by immersing the staple line in saline and insufflating the rectum with air and methylene blue while clamping the bowel proximally. If a leak is present, then interrupted sutures are placed until the leak is sealed. Hemostasis is obtained and assured, the pelvis is irrigated and aspirated, the pneumoperitoneum is evacuated, and the port sites are closed to complete the operation.

POSTOPERATIVE CARE

Routine use of a nasogastric tube decompression is not necessary. A dose of ketorolac tromethamine is given in the operating room.

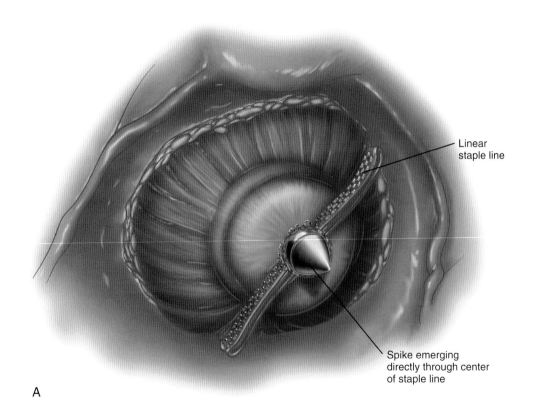

Linear staple line

Spike emerging directly through center of staple line

A

FIGURE 25-4 **A,** Piercing of the rectal stump with spike of the circular stapler.

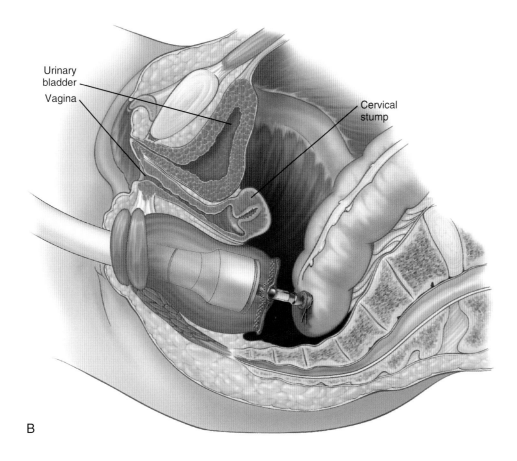

Urinary
bladder

Vagina

Cervical
stump

B

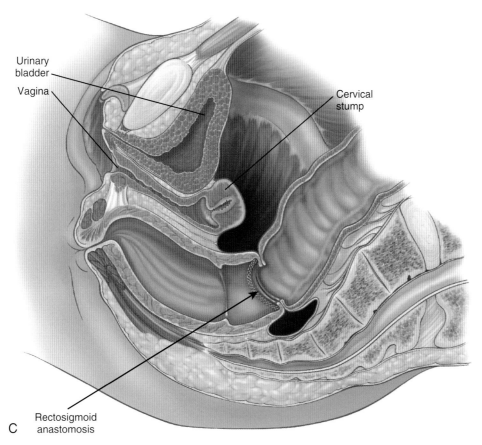

Urinary
bladder

Vagina

Cervical
stump

Rectosigmoid
anastomosis

C

FIGURE 25-4, cont'd   **B,** Mating of the anvil and head of the circular end-to-end anastomotic (EEA) stapler. **C,** Completed colorectal anastomosis.

Postoperative pain control is obtained with ketorolac and modest doses of oral opioids; intravenous opioids are avoided, and epidural or spinal anesthesia is not used because of known effects of prolonging postoperative ileus.

Early mobilization of the patient is important to quicken the return of bowel function. A clear liquid diet is started on postoperative day 1 and advanced to a low-residue diet when bowel function returns. The patient remains on this diet for several weeks before starting a regular diet. In the face of acute diverticulitis, the patient is continued on intravenous antibiotics while in the hospital and converted to oral antibiotics on discharge. Length of hospital stay is typically 2 to 4 days. On discharge, the patient is instructed to report fever, abdominal distention, pain, emesis, or wound drainage. The patient is followed up in the office at 1 week, 1 month, and 3 months.

PROCEDURE-SPECIFIC COMPLICATIONS

Primary intraoperative complications include bleeding and enterotomy. Hemorrhage can arise from splenic flexure mobilization, so the surgeon should use meticulous and gentle techniques around the spleen. Enterotomies can result from improper tissue handling with the graspers, and the use of 10-mm atraumatic graspers is encouraged. In the presence of dense adhesions and inflammation often seen with diverticulitis, an enterotomy should not necessarily be viewed as a complication because this event sometimes cannot be avoided. An enterotomy recognized intraoperatively can be closed primarily; if the injury is within several centimeters of one of the staple lines, then it may be more prudent to include the enterotomy with the specimen.

Postoperative complications include ileus, anastomotic stenosis, anastomotic leak, ureteral injury, and intra-abdominal abscess. Minimally invasive colectomy often produces some period of ileus, which may be prolonged if high doses of opioids are administered. Because the EEA circular stapler is used to perform the anastomosis in a sigmoid colectomy, this anastomosis is at an increased risk for stenosis compared with a side-to-side anastomosis. To minimize this risk, the largest possible EEA stapler should be used to perform the anastomosis. A leak in an end-to-end anastomosis is commonly due to technical error. The surgeon should ensure that the anastomosis is tension free, has good blood supply, is performed in the center of the rectal stump, encompasses the full thickness of the bowel wall, and passes an air leak test. We routinely reinforce the anastomosis with several interrupted sutures anteriorly. Leaks can still occur, however, despite following all recommended guidelines. A unique complication of the end-to-end anastomosis is twisting of the proximal bowel; the surgeon must carefully check alignment of the colon before firing the stapler. Another complication of a left colectomy is damage to the ureters. The use of lighted ureteral stents may

minimize the risk for injury; however, there is no replacement for meticulous dissection in the area of the ureter. If a ureteral injury is recognized, it may be prudent to obtain a urology consult to aid in the repair.

If the patient develops fever, pain, prolonged postoperative ileus, or an elevated white blood cell count, then the surgeon should investigate the cause with a contrasted CT scan of the abdomen. Early diagnosis of an anastomotic leak is preferable to a delayed diagnosis, which carries a higher morbidity rate. If a noncontained leak is discovered early, then prompt laparoscopy may be able to identify and repair the leak without the need for a colostomy. A delayed diagnosis may necessitate a laparotomy with a colostomy. If the patient develops a contained leak or intra-abdominal abscess, then this may be managed with percutaneous drainage, antibiotics, and close observation. These patients are at an increased risk for anastomotic stenosis or colocutaneous fistula; however, they often will not require a reoperation.

RESULTS AND OUTCOMES

Laparoscopic colectomy for complex diverticular disease can be a technically demanding procedure requiring advanced laparoscopic skills. In the hands of a qualified surgeon, however, the laparoscopic management of complex diverticulitis is feasible, achieves adequate resection, is safe, and has low overall morbidity. This approach offers the advantages of decreased pain, earlier return of bowel function, and shorter hospital stays compared with open surgery.

Suggested Readings

Agaba E, Zaidi R, Ramzy P, et al: Laparoscopic Hartmann's procedure: A viable option for treatment of acutely perforated diverticulitis. *Surg Endosc* 23:1483–1486, 2009.

Bruce CJ, Coller JA, Murray JJ, et al: Laparoscopic resection for diverticular disease. *Dis Colon Rectum* 39:S1–S6, 1996.

Frantzides C, Polymeneas G, Carlson M: Minimally invasive left colectomy. In Frantzides CT, Carlson MA, editors: *Atlas of Minimally Invasive Surgery*, Philadelphia, 2009, Saunders, pp 121–127.

Martel G, Bouchard A, Soto CM, et al: Laparoscopic colectomy for complex diverticular disease: A justifiable choice? *Surg Endosc* 24:2273–2280, 2010.

Richter S, Lindemann W, Kollmar O, et al: One-stage sigmoid colon resection for perforated sigmoid diverticulitis (Hinchey stages III-IV). *World J Surg* 30:1027–1032, 2006.

Siddiqui MR, Sajid MS, Khatri K, et al: Elective open versus laparoscopic sigmoid colectomy for diverticular disease: A meta-analysis with the Sigma trial. *World J Surg* 34:2883–2901, 2010.

Siddiqui MR, Sajid MS, Quereshi S, et al: Elective laparoscopic sigmoid resection for diverticular disease has fewer complications than conventional surgery: A meta-analysis. *Am J Surg* 200:144–161, 2010.

Vargas HD, Ramirez RT, Hoffman GC, et al: Defining the role of laparoscopic-assisted sigmoid colectomy for diverticulitis. *Dis Colon Rectum* 43:1726–1731, 2000.

MARK A. CARLSON

Minimally Invasive Low Anterior Resection with Total Mesorectal Excision for Malignancy

26

The videos associated with this chapter are listed in the Video Contents and can be found on the accompanying DVDs and *on Expertconsult.com.*

Current resective procedures for rectal cancer can have their origins traced to a radical pelvic extirpation described by Ernest Miles in the early 1900s, an operation now commonly known as the *abdominal-perineal resection* (APR). In Miles' original description of this operation, a cylinder of tissue was rapidly excavated from the pelvis (Fig. 26-1A), without preservation of neural structures. Five of his first 12 patients died, though none from hemorrhage. In addition, local recurrence was problematic in Miles' early experience with this technique. Nevertheless, the Miles procedure did represent an advance in rectal cancer surgery that, before this time, had been operated from a perineal approach.

With the advances in surgical science and technology in the 20th century, an interest in sphincter-preserving operations for rectal cancer evolved. The introduction of the circular surgical stapler in the late 1970s, which could create an end-to-end anastomosis with a single firing, facilitated the construction of a low rectal anastomosis. In addition, accumulated evidence indicated that the classic 5-cm distal tumor margin for rectal cancer was unnecessary; anastomotic recurrence was not observed to be an issue with a distal margin of 2 cm (or even less). Most patients undergoing operation for rectal cancer used to have an APR; the proportion gradually inverted, and now most patients have a transabdominal resection with anastomosis, without a permanent colostomy.

Although the rate of anastomotic reconstruction for rectal cancer resection has increased, the morbidity from these procedures, in terms of sexual and urinary dysfunction, has remained high. In the 1980s, Heald and colleagues demonstrated that sharp dissection of the mesorectum with preservation of known neural structures in the pelvis and intra-abdominal anastomosis (Fig. 26-1B) could produce excellent survival and recurrence rates without the associated morbidities. The procedure did require more time to perform than the cylindric resection shown in Figure 26-1A. The goal of Heald's procedure, however, was to remove all of the node-bearing mesorectum, without injuring important autonomic and sensory nerves. Heald's technique of total mesorectal excision (TME) has now become generally accepted among colorectal surgeons and is emphasized in this chapter.

Anterior resection of the rectum involves the removal of the mid to upper portion of the rectum in continuity with the lower sigmoid using a transabdominal approach (i.e., anterior, as opposed to a perineal resection), and typically reconstructed with a primary anastomosis. Addition of the "low" modifier generally indicates that the extent of resection is to the mid to lower rectum. In this chapter, the definition of low anterior resection (LAR) is the transabdominal removal of a continuous section of large bowel from the lower sigmoid to the mid to lower rectum, with a colorectal anastomosis.

OPERATIVE INDICATIONS

The primary indication for minimally invasive LAR with TME is localized, resectable adenocarcinoma of the rectum. In terms of the commonly used TNM classification system of the American Joint Committee on Cancer (AJCC), rectal tumors amenable to LAR with TME would include T1-3, N0-2 lesions or, generally speaking, stages I to III (Tables 26-1 and 26-2). It should be noted that in 2012, some guidelines (including the National Comprehensive Cancer Network) and experts still consider minimally invasive LAR for rectal cancer to be an experimental procedure, only to be performed within the confines of a clinical trial. As evident from the surgical literature, however, this procedure has been performed commonly (outside of trials) for rectal cancer in the Americas, Europe, and Asia since the mid-1990s. LAR for localized, resectable rectal cancer is intended to be curative; in some circumstances, however, palliative transabdominal resection for metastatic rectal cancer may be performed.

The resectability and the need for neoadjuvant therapy of a rectal cancer is dependent on the distance of the tumor from the anal sphincteric complex (Fig. 26-2) and the depth of tumor invasion (the T classification; see Table 26-1), and whether there are radiologically positive lymph nodes in the mesorectum (the N classification; see Table 26-1). Tumor location, depth of invasion, and nodal status are evaluated with computed tomography (CT), endorectal ultrasound (EUS), and/or magnetic resonance imaging (MRI), as discussed in the Preoperative Evaluation, Testing, and Preparation section.

A T1-2, N0 rectal cancer should undergo resection as primary therapy (Fig. 26-3). If the primary tumor is T1, N0, has a dimension of less than 3 cm, has favorable histopathology, and is within 8 cm of the anal verge (see Fig. 26-2), then local excision also may be acceptable treatment, particularly in the patient with increased operative risk or limited survival. Favorable histopathology has been defined as the absence of (1) perineural and lymphovascular invasion, (2) positive margins, and (3) poor differentiation. Recurrence appears to be higher after transanal compared with transabdominal resection of T1 lesions, and radiologically silent N1 disease may be missed by transanal excision of T1 tumors in up to two thirds of cases. As of 2012, the guidelines for transanal excision are in flux.

If selected, local excision may be accomplished with a conventional transanal approach or with transanal endoscopic microsurgery (TEM). Tumors located up to 20 cm from the anal verge have been resected with TEM in specialty centers. Of note, although TEM traditionally has been performed with a proprietary instrumental setup, it now appears that the technique can be reproduced using single-port instrumentation borrowed from laparoscopic surgery.

If the tumor is less than 5 cm from the anal verge, then abdominoperineal resection generally is recommended. This usually means that the tumor is within 1 cm of the sphincteric complex (see Fig. 26-2). Sphincter-preserving operations for tumors at or below this level are experimental and will not be covered in this chapter. Tumors that are more than 5 cm from the anal verge generally are amenable to LAR.

If the rectal cancer has been staged at T3-4 or N1-2, then the patient should undergo neoadjuvant chemoradiation (see Fig. 26-3). This treatment typically has involved continuous intravenous 5-fluorouracil along with 45 to 50 Gy (fractionated) of

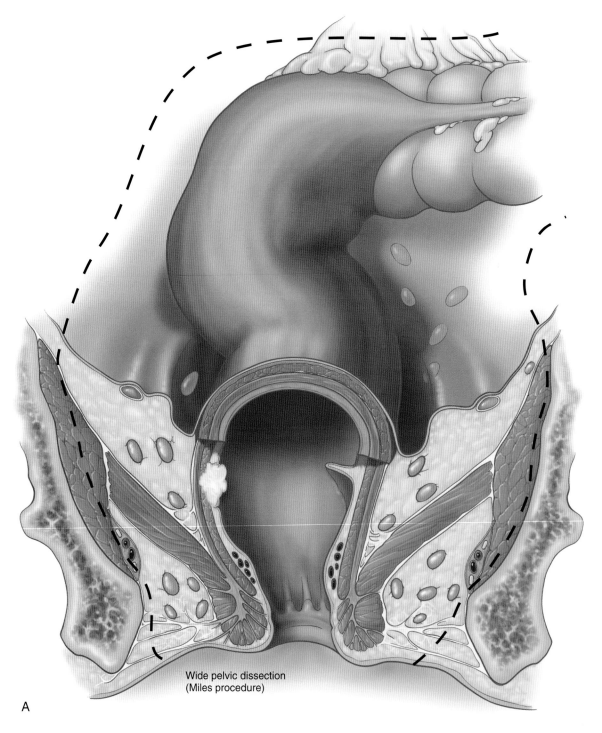

Wide pelvic dissection
(Miles procedure)

A

FIGURE 26-1 Extent of resection for rectal cancer. **A,** Traditional abdominoperineal resection (Miles procedure); coronal view.

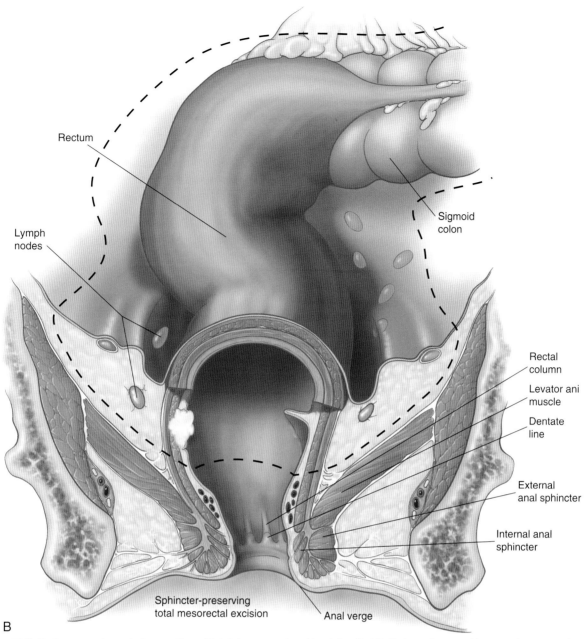

B

FIGURE 26-1, cont'd **B,** Contemporary low anterior resection with total mesorectal excision (after Heald). (Redrawn from Heald RJ: Rectal cancer in the 21st century—radical operations: Anterior resection and abdominoperineal excision. In *Mastery of Surgery*, ed 5, Philadelphia, 2006, Lippincott Williams & Wilkins, pp 1543–1444.)

Table 26-1 TNM Staging System for Colorectal Cancer

Primary Tumor (T)		Regional Lymph Nodes (N)		Distant Metastasis (M)	
TX	Primary tumor cannot be assessed	NX	Regional lymph nodes cannot be assessed	M0	No distant metastasis
T0	No evidence of primary tumor	N0	No regional lymph node metastasis	M1	Distant metastasis
Tis	Carcinoma in situ: intraepithelial or invasion of lamina propria	N1	Metastasis in 1-3 regional lymph nodes	M1a	Metastasis confined to one organ or site (e.g., liver, lung, ovary, nonregional node)
		N1a	Metastasis in one regional lymph node		
T1	Tumor invades submucosa	N1b	Metastasis in 2-3 regional lymph nodes	M1b	Metastases in more than one organ/site or the peritoneum
T2	Tumor invades muscularis propria	N1c	Tumor deposit(s) in the subserosa, mesentery, or nonperitonealized pericolic or perirectal tissues without regional nodal metastasis		
T3	Tumor invades through the muscularis propria into pericolorectal tissues				
T4a	Tumor penetrates to the surface of the visceral peritoneum	N2	Metastasis in 4 or more regional lymph nodes		
		N2a	Metastasis in 4-6 regional lymph nodes		
T4b	Tumor directly invades or is adherent to other organs or structures	N2b	Metastasis in 7 or more regional lymph nodes		

Used with the permission of the American Joint Committee on Cancer (AJCC), Chicago, Illinois. The original source for this material is the AJCC Cancer Staging Handbook, 7th edition (2010), published by Springer Science and Business Media LLC, www.springerlink.com.

Table 26-2 Anatomic Stages of the TNM System for Colorectal Cancer

Stage	T	N	M
0	Tis	N0	M0
I	T1	N0	M0
	T2	N0	M0
IIA	T3	N0	M0
IIB	T4a	N0	M0
IIC	T4b	N0	M0
IIIA	T1-T2	N1/N1c	M0
	T1	N2a	M0
IIIB	T3-T4a	N1/N1c	M0
	T2-T3	N2a	M0
	T1-T2	N2b	M0
IIIC	T4a	N2a	M0
	T3-T4a	N2b	M0
	T4b	N1-N2	M0
IVA	Any T	Any N	M1a
IVB	Any T	Any N	M1b

Used with the permission of the American Joint Committee on Cancer (AJCC), Chicago, Illinois. The original source for this material is the AJCC Cancer Staging Handbook, 7th edition (2010), published by Springer Science and Business Media LLC, www.springerlink.com.

pelvic radiation. This neoadjuvant chemoradiation requires about 6 weeks to complete. The transabdominal resection then should be performed 5 to 10 weeks after completion of the chemoradiation. A T1-2 tumor that is too close to the sphincter mechanism to permit a sphincter-preserving procedure also may undergo neoadjuvant chemoradiation in an attempt to make sphincter preservation possible, but the efficacy of this strategy is not clear.

A number of institutions have freely provided on the Internet their own guidelines for the management of rectal cancer. It would behoove the surgeon who operates on this disease to be familiar with a set of these guidelines.

Alternative Treatments

If the patient is medically unfit or otherwise refuses to undergo a major surgical procedure, then one or more of the following treatment alternatives may be considered: (1) primary chemoradiation with or without stenting (stenting is not effective in the lower rectum); (2) diverting colostomy for an obstructive lesion; (3) transanal excision; (4) TEM; or (5) transanal ablation with a variety of energy sources, including endocavitary radiation (as popularized by Jean Papillon in Lyon, France).

Contraindications

The contraindications to LAR for rectal cancer include (1) tumor invasion into the sphincteric complex; (2) tumor invasion into the pelvic sidewall, bladder (see later), or prostate (i.e., a T4b lesion); (3) tumor less than 2 cm from the sphincteric complex (see Fig. 26-2); (4) fecal incontinence; (5) unresectable M1 disease with minimal or no pelvic symptoms; and (6) medical contraindication to a major surgical procedure. A tumor that invades the sphincteric complex should be treated with an APR. As alluded to previously, there have been reports of LAR for tumors located less than 2 cm from the sphincteric complex, using an intersphincteric dissection (en bloc excision of the internal sphincter,

which can be performed robotically), with a coloanal anastomosis performed from the perineum. With preoperative chemoradiation, a high rectal cancer with bladder involvement may be resectable with an LAR and concomitant cystectomy.

A T4b lesion should undergo neoadjuvant chemoradiation in an attempt to reduce the T stage, perhaps making a resection feasible. A patient with rectal cancer who is not continent of stool should undergo an APR (with neoadjuvant therapy as indicated) so that the fecal stream is controlled with an end colostomy. If the patient has unresectable metastatic disease and an asymptomatic or minimally symptomatic primary rectal tumor, then it is reasonable not to undergo a major resection for the primary lesion but to proceed directly with chemotherapy. Simultaneous minimally invasive resection of a rectal adenocarcinoma and hepatic metastases may be feasible, but a description of this is beyond the scope of this chapter. Palliation of a symptomatic rectal cancer in the presence of unresectable metastatic disease should be individualized to each patient depending on functional status and life expectancy, but such treatment might include chemoradiation, proximal diversion, stenting, transanal ablation, or transabdominal resection.

Obesity (body mass index [BMI] >30) is a relative contraindication to a minimally invasive LAR. Although minimally invasive rectal resection has been shown to be feasible in obese patients, it probably would be best not to attempt minimally invasive LAR in a patient with a BMI greater than 30 early on in a surgeon's experience. In particular, centripetal obesity (i.e., excess adipose distributed in the abdomen), which is common in male patients, can increase the difficulty of dissection deep in the pelvis. The definition of *early experience* (the number of cases constituting the learning curve) for minimally invasive LAR is controversial and surgeon dependent but has been estimated to be in the range of the first 50 cases.

PREOPERATIVE EVALUATION, TESTING, AND PREPARATION

Ideally, all patients with rectal cancer should be discussed at a multidisciplinary tumor conference in both the preoperative and postoperative phase. Such a conference may include participation of medical oncology, surgical oncology, gastroenterology, radiation oncology, radiology, primary care, nursing, palliative care, and other specialties as needed. Evidence has been accumulating for a number of malignancies that patient outcome is improved if such discussions are performed routinely.

The patient with a rectal mass should undergo complete colonoscopy (including digital rectal examination and anoscopy) with biopsy of the mass. If the mass is located at the rectosigmoid junction, then tattooing the mass with dye (e.g., India ink) at the time of colonoscopy can facilitate the identification of the tumor in the event that the patient goes on to resection. If the biopsy confirms the presence of a rectal adenocarcinoma, then the patient also should undergo CT scanning of the chest, abdomen, and pelvis with oral, intravenous, and (ideally) rectal contrast. In addition, the patient should undergo an endoscopic ultrasound of the rectum to establish the depth of penetration (T stage) of the tumor and whether there is mesorectal adenopathy (N stage). In some centers, an MRI with an endorectal coil has been used to stage rectal tumors with impressive accuracy. A carcinoembryonic antigen (CEA) also is assayed on diagnosis of a rectal cancer. More elaborate tests for metastatic disease (e.g., positron

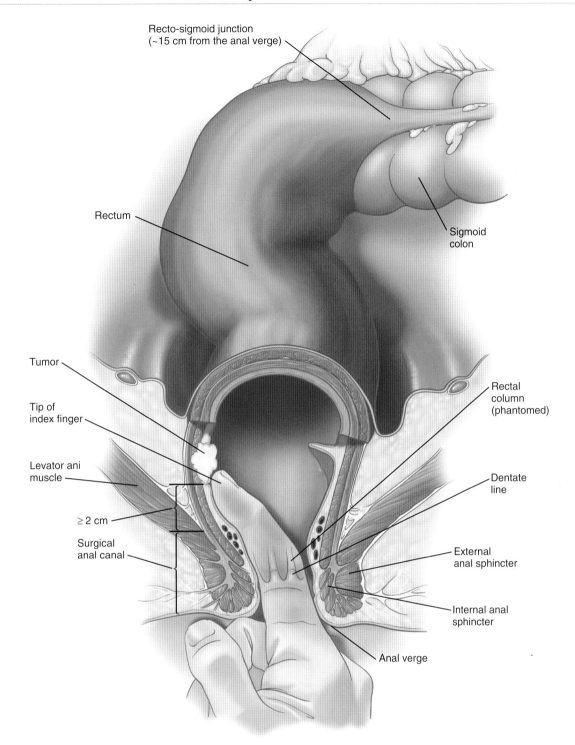

FIGURE 26-2 Digital determination of resectability (coronal view). The critical distance from the superior extent of the sphincteric complex to the tumor is measured using the examiner's finger as a ruler.

emission tomography [PET]-CT scanning) are not routinely indicated for rectal cancer.

If the patient with rectal cancer is a candidate for anterior resection of the rectum, then the surgeon should perform her or his own proctoscopy with digital rectal examination. Ideally, this should be done on a day before the actual resection. The surgeon should determine tumor diameter, fixation, circumferential location, and the distance of the tumor from the anal verge or sphincteric complex. Traditionally, the relevant distance has been that from the tumor to the anal verge, as measured with a proctoscope or a finger (see Fig. 26-2). As indicated earlier, the minimal distance (tumor to anal verge) for the safe performance of an LAR is about 5 cm. The precise location of the anal verge can vary

with sphincter contraction, introduction of an endoscope, and so forth, so the surgeon should be cautious when determining this distance in tumors of the lower rectum.

If the tumor is within reach of the surgeon's examining finger, then perhaps a more reliable (and relevant) distance to measure would be that between the sphincter mechanism and the tumor (see Fig. 26-2). This distance can be determined by sliding the index finger of the other hand into the anal canal to palpate the ring of the sphincteric complex while the tip of the examining finger is placed into the sulcus between the tumor and the rectal mucosa. Using the finger on the ring of the sphincteric complex, the surgeon touches the point on the examining finger where it crosses the sphincter, withdraws the fingers, and thereby can

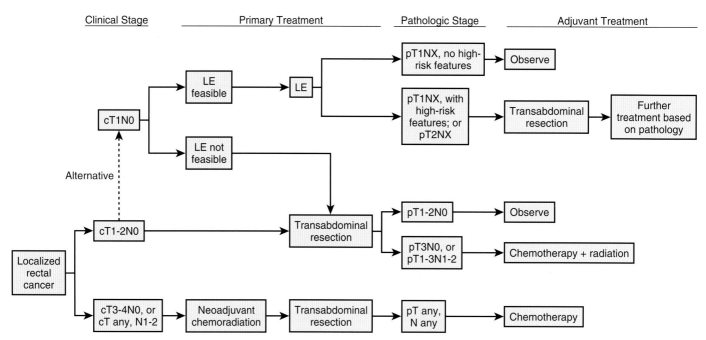

Clinical Stage   Primary Treatment   Pathologic Stage   Adjuvant Treatment

FIGURE 26-3 Algorithm for treatment of localized rectal cancer. See Table 26-1 for TNM staging definitions. LE, local excision. (© National Comprehensive Cancer Network, Inc. 2010, all rights reserved.)

obtain a direct measure of tumor-sphincter distance. Of note, it is easy to stretch the rectal mucosa and overestimate the tumor-sphincter distance, so the surgeon should not apply vigorous digital pressure. A minimum of 2 cm would be needed between the tumor sulcus proximally and the top of the sphincteric complex distally (i.e., not the anal verge) for the safe performance of an LAR. Of note, the critical distance of the tumor to the anal verge versus the sphincters obviously will not be the same, so the surgeon should use consistent terminology.

If the tumor has a clinical stage of T3 or N1-2, then neoadjuvant therapy should be given, as described previously. Although not required, it may be beneficial to restage the patient with CT or EUS after completion of the neoadjuvant therapy, before the resection. Documentation of disease progression after neoadjuvant therapy may alter the management, which can be discussed at the tumor conference. With regard to response to chemoradiation, an interesting scenario involves the patient who, after undergoing neoadjuvant therapy for rectal cancer as described previously, has a clinical complete response, that is, has no evidence of residual tumor. In 2012, most guidelines dictate that such a patient still should undergo transabdominal resection, followed by additional chemotherapy, even if pathologic examination of the specimen revealed no residual tumor (i.e., a pathologic complete response). Further investigation into this clinical situation might identify a subgroup of patients with rectal cancer who can be treated with primary chemoradiation, analogous to the management of anal canal cancer.

If a temporary ileostomy or permanent colostomy is planned, then an enterostomal therapist should see the patient before the operation. Regarding large bowel preparation, recent meta-analyses have claimed that mechanical bowel preparation is unnecessary and even detrimental to the patient. The landmark data from the 1970s, which demonstrated the efficacy of large bowel preparation in reducing postoperative infection, used a combination of oral antibiotics and mechanical bowel cleansing. Most studies of bowel preparation since then have focused on the effects of mechanical preparation and intravenous antibiotics, but not on oral antibiotics. It is from these studies that recent

meta-analyses have based their recommendation that mechanical bowel preparation should be omitted. Because oral antibiotics have been largely ignored in recent studies, the actual status of complete bowel preparation (oral antibiotics plus cathartics) with respect to minimally invasive colon resection in 2012 is controversial. The decision whether to perform a bowel preparation and which type to use is left to surgeon preference. For an LAR, it is reasonable to have the colon and rectum evacuated of solid stool to facilitate passage of endoscopes, staplers, and so forth.

PATIENT POSITIONING IN THE OPERATING SUITE

General endotracheal anesthesia is administered, and an orogastric tube and Foley catheter are inserted. A central venous catheter and arterial line are optional, depending on the patient's underlying comorbidities. Sequential compression devices are placed on both lower extremities, and the patient is placed in the low lithotomy position with both arms tucked (Fig. 26-4). The angle of thigh flexion should be less than 15 degrees to avoid interference with instrumentation during the splenic flexure mobilization. The buttocks should overhang the edge of the table to facilitate intraoperative sigmoidoscopy and transanal stapler insertion. The legs and feet are padded and strapped to the stirrups to secure the lower half of the patient during extremes of table maneuvering. The upper torso is secured to the operating table using two adjustable soft straps in an X configuration (see Fig. 26-4). The anesthesiologist should secure the head so that it will not roll during extremes of lateral tilt.

If the patient has an ample panniculus, then it may be helpful to place an additional soft strap underneath the panniculus at the level of the anterosuperior iliac spines (see Fig. 26-4) to prevent the patient from rolling off the table during lateral tilt. The Foley catheter is taped to the leg, away from the perineum. In men, the scrotum may need to be suspended away from the perineum with a single stay suture (or taped) to the medial thigh. Before the sterile preparation and draping, the operating table is placed through the

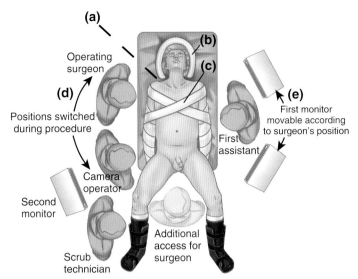

FIGURE 26-4 Overhead view of low lithotomy positioning for a minimally invasive low anterior resection. Position of monitor 1 is adjusted according to location of the dissection. No floor equipment should be present caudal to the *dotted line* (a). (b) Head support. (c) Chest straps. (d) Surgeon position. (e) Surgeon's monitor.

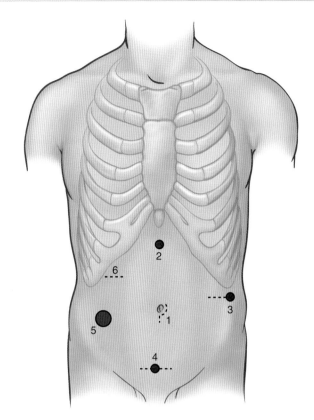

FIGURE 26-5 Positioning of ports and possible incisions for a minimally invasive low anterior resection. Options for incision use: 1 (periumbilical) = Hasson cannula, extraction; 3 = extraction, loop colostomy; 4 (Pfannenstiel) = stapler insertion, extraction; 5 = stapler insertion, 100p ileostomy; 6 = extraction, loop colostomy. Red = 5 mm port; blue = 12 mm port.

extremes of rotation and Trendelenburg position to ensure that the patient is immobilized and that surrounding equipment will not hinder table movement. In addition, the surgeon should make sure that a segment of left-sided bed rail is available for clamping of the post for a self-retaining retractor, either for the laparoscopic pelvic dissection or in case of open conversion.

If the patient's preoperative imaging indicated that the tumor or perineoplastic process was involving a ureter, or if there has been a history of pelvic inflammation, operation, or other event that may complicate the pelvic dissection, then the surgeon can consider placement of ureteral stents. In these situations, a stent can aid in the identification of the ureter and reduce the risk for ureteral injury. If a ureter is transected, then the presence of a stent can aid in identification of the ureteral lumen and subsequent repair. These stents are not without risk for urinary tract complications, so it would be reasonable to employ them selectively, in difficult cases.

After the patient has been positioned, a digital examination is performed to confirm location, size, and mobility of the tumor. A proctoscopy should not be performed at this point; otherwise, the colon will become distended and hamper the laparoscopic dissection. The patient's abdomen, lower chest, and flanks then are swabbed with an alcohol-based surgical preparation solution (e.g., ChloraPrep); the perineum is scrubbed with a solution of povidone-iodine and detergent (e.g., Betadine Surgical Scrub). The perineum and lower extremities are draped with separate sheets. The abdomen is draped so that the region from the pubis to the xiphoid, out to both flanks, is part of the sterile field. If the patient has a large panniculus with an underlying soft strap across the pelvis, then the prepared field may extend to the inferior extent of the panniculus.

The surgeon stands on the patient's right, the first assistant stands opposite to the surgeon, the camera operator stands on the right cephalad to the surgeon, and the scrub technician is positioned off the right leg (see Fig. 26-4). Two monitors are used, one on each side of the patient; the surgeon's monitor (on the patient's left) may need to be repositioned according to where the dissection occurs (e.g., cephalad for the splenic flexure mobilization, caudad for the mesorectal excision). The entire right side of the patient, from the head to the foot, should be free of

obstruction (e.g., intravenous poles, anesthesia machine, energy units) to allow the surgeon unencumbered movement.

POSITIONING AND PLACEMENT OF TROCARS

At a minimum, minimally invasive LAR requires access to both lower abdominal quadrants. If mobilization of the splenic flexure or fecal diversion is necessary, then three or all four quadrants will need to be accessible. In most patients, initial access may be obtained in the infraumbilical position with open insertion of a blunt 10-mm cannula (Hasson type), and this port subsequently will be used for the camera (Fig. 26-5). Alternatively, peritoneal access may be obtained with a Veress needle or with an optical trocar. If the position of the umbilicus has shifted inferiorly because of obesity, then it may be better to place the camera in the midline midway between the xiphoid process and the symphysis pubis. If there is an increased risk that the procedure may need to be converted to open (e.g., patient's BMI >35), then it would be prudent to use a vertically oriented incision for the camera port.

After the camera port has been inserted and the abdomen has been insufflated to 12 to 15 mm Hg, four additional ports (2 through 5) are placed in the diamond configuration, as shown in Figure 26-5. Although there is no absolute or constant arrangement for trocar placement, the positioning in Figure 26-5 is a general guideline that can be modified based on the patient's body habitus, previous surgical scars, and so forth. The diamond configuration allows reasonable access to all four quadrants of the abdomen.

Because the shape and anatomic relations of the abdominal wall can be distorted with distention, the actual insertion point for ports 2 through 5 should be determined by the surgeon only after the abdomen has been fully insufflated. If the abdominal wall is not excessively thick, then laparoscope transillumination should be used at each port site to identify and avoid laceration of abdominal wall vessels. The port size at positions 2, 3, and 4 in Figure 26-5 initially can be 5 mm, and then upsized to 12 mm later if necessary. The port at position 5 (superior to the right anterosuperior iliac spine) should be 12 mm to accommodate the endoscopic stapler-cutter, and should be positioned as lateral and inferior as possible to facilitate placement of the stapler across the distal rectum. Furthermore, if the surgeon encounters difficulty during the pelvic dissection, then she or he should not hesitate to place an additional port (typically in the right mid-abdomen) to improve pelvic retraction, instrument triangulation, and so forth.

OPERATIVE TECHNIQUE

Exploration

With the patient in a neutral position, the peritoneal surfaces, including the visible portions of the liver, are examined for tumor deposits or other disease. Any suspicious lesion is biopsied and sent for frozen section analysis. As the sensitivity of preoperative imaging has increased, it has become uncommon to discover metastatic disease at laparoscopy that was not suspected preoperatively. If a small solitary metastasis is found (e.g., a superficial liver nodule) and can be resected with minimal difficulty, then it would be reasonable to proceed with an oncologic resection (clearance of the primary tumor with nodes) and a metastasectomy. The patient's postoperative management can be discussed at a subsequent multidisciplinary tumor conference after all the pathologic data have been acquired. If multiple lesions or otherwise unresectable metastatic disease is found, then the decision to proceed with a palliative resection would depend on the symptoms caused by the primary tumor. For example, if a good-risk patient is suffering from anemia or pain, then a palliative resection (as opposed to a diverting colostomy) would be preferable. If the patient is being treated for tenesmus, then an APR likely will be needed. The acquisition of a good quality CT scan, however, should minimize the chance that a patient will come to operation with undiagnosed metastatic disease.

Proctoscopy

If the surgeon did not perform a proctoscopy on a prior date and the tumor cannot be localized on digital examination at the beginning of the anesthetic, then a rigid proctoscopy should be performed early on to establish the precise location of the rectal tumor. While the assistant compresses the distal sigmoid colon with a grasper, the surgeon can perform a proctoscopy with minimal insufflation to determine the distance between the tumor and the sphincter mechanism. It is important to prevent insufflation of the colon and small bowel during this step; otherwise, the laparoscopic working space will be compromised. If need be, the surgeon can mark the position of the tumor with India ink, or the assistant can place a marking stitch on the serosal surface of the anterior rectum.

Surgical Anatomy

Definitions and descriptions of pelvic anatomy are somewhat arbitrary and have been debated in the surgical and anatomic

literature for over 100 years. The following is an abbreviated synthesis of current opinions; this is not intended to be a final statement on the relevant pelvic anatomy. The *rectum* is about 12 to 15 cm long (see Fig. 26-2), depending on how the measurements are taken, and is arbitrarily divided into upper, middle, and lower thirds. The *rectosigmoid junction* is near the sacral promontory, typically an angled region of the large bowel where the epiploic appendices of the sigmoid colon become less prominent and where the longitudinal bands of the taenia coli diverge and coalesce, encircling the rectum. The anterolateral portion of the upper to mid rectum is covered with peritoneum, whereas the remainder is extraperitoneal. The peritoneum reflects off the mid rectum onto the bladder or the uterus, forming the *rectovesicular pouch* (in the male) or *rectouterine pouch* (in the female; sometimes known as the *pouch of Douglas*) or, simply, the *peritoneal reflection*.

The arterial blood supply to the rectum derives mainly from the *superior hemorrhoidal (rectal)* branches of the inferior mesenteric artery and, to a lesser extent, from the *middle* and *inferior hemorrhoidal* arteries, which derive from the internal iliac (hypogastric) arteries (Fig. 26-6). The middle hemorrhoidal vessels were described in older surgical literature to run in a structure called the *lateral ligament* (discussed under Operative Technique), but this arrangement has been questioned by numerous anatomic studies, and the presence of the middle hemorrhoidal vessels now is considered inconstant. Although the inferior (and middle) hemorrhoidal vessels are the primary supply to the anal canal, these vessels have an anastomotic network that can support a long rectal stump after ligation of the superior hemorrhoidal vessels.

Lymph from a tumor located below the pectinate (dentate) line (see Fig. 26-2) would drain primarily into the superficial inguinal nodes; a tumor above the pectinate line but still within the anal canal would drain primarily into the internal iliac nodes; and a tumor in the lower rectum would drain primarily into the mesorectal nodes (i.e., the inferior mesenteric basin) and internal iliac nodes. In light of this lymphatic anatomy, some surgeons, primarily from Japan, have advocated that an LAR for cancer should include an extended (also known as wide or lateral) lymphadenectomy, which encompasses the internal iliac nodes. Although there is a greater risk for urinary and sexual dysfunction with an extended lymphadenectomy, the Japanese results with this technique have been favorable. The majority view in Western countries, however, has favored removal of the lymph node basin associated with the mesorectum only (see Fig. 26-1B); this view has been supported with a meta-analysis. A rationale for not performing an extended lymphadenectomy, beyond the risk for autonomic nerve injury, is that once a rectal cancer has metastasized to the internal iliac nodes, the patient has a poor prognosis that is not affected by nodal clearance. The technique described in this chapter will clear nodes associated with the superior hemorrhoidal vessels only, and not an extended lymphadenectomy.

The *mesorectum* (Figs. 26-7 and 26-8; see Fig. 26-1B) is a bulk of fatty connective tissue that encases the rectum on its lateral and posterior aspect and contains blood vessels, lymphatic vessels and nodes, and nerves that supply the rectum. Anteriorly, the lower rectum may have a thin layer of mesorectum. The mesorectum is not a mesenteric structure per se because the former is not covered with peritoneum. The mesorectum is covered, however, by an investing fascial layer known as the *visceral endopelvic fascia* (alternatively, the *fascia propria* of the rectum). The apposing fascial layer on the pelvic wall is known as the *parietal endopelvic fascia*; posteriorly, covering the sacrum,

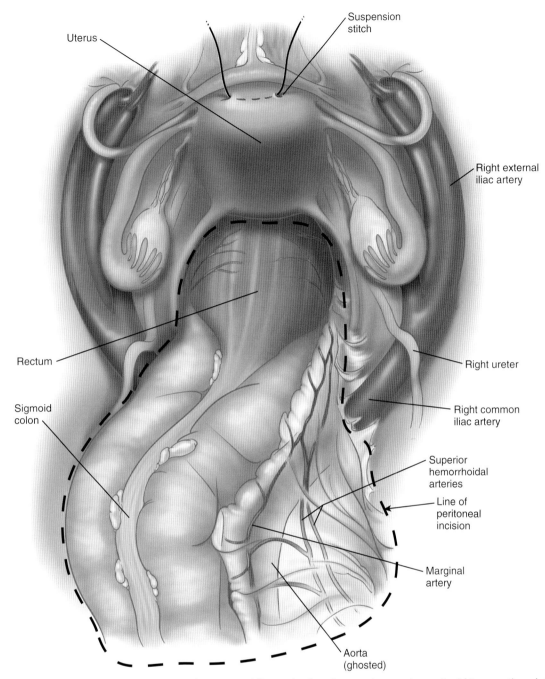

FIGURE 26-6 Peritoneal incision and the extent of vascular (mesosigmoidal) resection for a low anterior resection, as it might appear through the laparoscope.

this layer is known as the *presacral fascia*. The potential space between the visceral and parietal endopelvic fascia is the dissection plane for a TME, or the "holy plane" described by Heald. For the most part, this space only contains loose connective tissue that is amenable to sharp dissection.

In the posterior midline around the level of S4, the parietal and visceral endopelvic fascia fuse for a short distance to form the *rectosacral fascia* (see Fig. 26-7), sometimes known as *Waldeyer's fascia*. This fascial band should be transected sharply during a mesorectal dissection to avoid tearing of the presacral fascia and the underlying venous plexus. Distal to the rectosacral fascia, the parietal and visceral leaves of the endopelvic fascia separate again. Anterior to the lower rectum in the male, the seminal vesicles and the prostate are covered by *Denonvilliers' fascia* (see Figs. 26-7 and 26-8B); the equivalent structure in the female, covering the posterior vagina, is known as the *rectovaginal septum*. Whether or not Denonvilliers fascia should be

excised for oncological clearance during LAR is a matter of controversy; the risk of such an excision is that dissection anterior to this fascia (i.e., within the space containing the seminal vesicles and prostate) might injure nerves from the pelvic autonomic plexus.

The *anal verge* (see Fig. 26-2) represents the outer edge of the anal orifice, where the perianal skin angles sharply from the anal canal out to the perineum. The verge commonly is used by endoscopists as a point of reference to mark rectal tumors. The *anal sphincter* or *sphincteric complex* is a high-pressure zone within the anal canal that is formed by the tonic contraction of the *internal sphincter*, an autonomously controlled thickened portion of rectal circular muscle, and the somatic *external sphincter*, which is the continuation of the pelvic floor musculature (*levator ani* muscles) around the anal canal.

The *surgical anal canal* (see Fig. 26-2) is 4 to 5 cm in length, extending from the anal verge to the *anorectal ring*; the latter

225

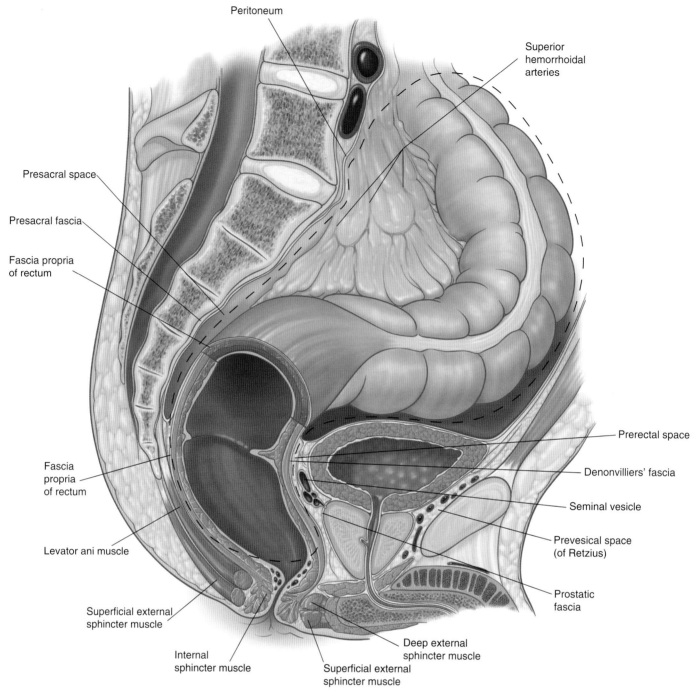

Peritoneum

Superior hemorrhoidal arteries

Presacral space

Presacral fascia

Fascia propria of rectum

Prerectal space

Denonvilliers' fascia

Seminal vesicle

Fascia propria of rectum

Prevesical space (of Retzius)

Levator ani muscle

Prostatic fascia

Superficial external sphincter muscle

Internal sphincter muscle

Deep external sphincter muscle

Superficial external sphincter muscle

FIGURE 26-7 Sagittal view of extent of mesorectal excision with relevant structures.

marks an angulation between the rectum and anal canal, just proximal to the sphincteric complex, and is where intraluminal pressure increases. The *pectinate* (or *dentate*) *line* within the anal canal divides it into proximal (upper two thirds) and distal (lower one third) segments. Below the pectinate line, the anal canal is lined with nonkeratinized squamous epithelium (without dermal appendages), which transitions into keratinized epithelium of the perianal skin (containing follicles and glands) around the level of the *intersphincteric groove* (the white line of Hilton in older literature), which is formed by the edges of the internal and external anal sphincters. The lining of the anal canal above the pectinate line is layered cuboidal epithelium (the *anal transition* or *cloacogenic zone*), which transitions into a single layer of columnar epithelium (i.e., rectal mucosa) near the distal *rectal columns* (or *columns of Morgagni*) in the region of the anorectal ring.

The relevant neuroanatomy for an LAR includes the *superior hypogastric plexus* (Fig. 26-9), which is located below the aortic bifurcation, generally in the plane between the parietal and visceral endopelvic fascia. This plexus is a center of sympathetic and sensory traffic to and from the pelvis. The right and left *hypogastric nerves* exit the plexus inferiorly and follow a course posterolateral to the mesorectum, about 1 to 2 cm medial to ureters. The hypogastric nerves can be adherent to the mesorectum and should be dissected carefully off this structure during the mesorectal dissection. Injury to a hypogastric nerve can affect emission function in the male and can also cause bladder dysfunction.

The hypogastric nerves intersect with the right and left *pelvic autonomic nerve plexus* (PANP, sometimes known as the *inferior hypogastric plexus*). The PANP is located on the pelvic sidewall at the level of S3-4 (see Fig. 26-9), directly in contact with the lateral mesorectum. In addition to the sympathetic input from the hypogastric nerve, the PANP receives parasympathetic input from the *pelvic splanchnic nerves* (also known as the *nervi erigentes*), which originate from the S2-4 sacral foramina. Branches from the PANP extend medially to the rectum, traveling through the "lateral ligament," whereas additional nerves from the PANP continue distally to support bladder and sexual function. To preserve the sexual and bladder functions of the PANP, these rectal branches should be transected flush with the surface of the visceral endopelvic fascia during an LAR, without violating the PANP.

Choice of a Dissection-Sealing Instrument

Similar to most minimally invasive abdominal procedures, hemostatic dissection for an LAR can be performed using a variety of instruments, including hook or scissors electrocautery, an ultrasonic scalpel, or a bipolar vessel sealing device. Both ultrasonic and bipolar vessel sealing instrumentation, developed for minimally invasive surgery during the 1990s and further refined in the 2000s, can seal and transect larger vessels such as the inferior mesenteric artery, although many surgeons still prefer to control vessels of this size with a vascular stapler load. Secondary to a lack of data demonstrating clear superiority of any one dissecting

and sealing instrument, the selection of this instrument largely remains an issue of personal preference for the surgeon. In this chapter, most of the dissection described is done with an ultrasonic scalpel.

Mobilization of the Splenic Flexure

Many patients undergoing an LAR for rectal cancer benefit from mobilization of the splenic flexure to facilitate construction of a low rectal anastomosis and to prevent excessive tension on the anastomotic staple line. If the patient has a redundant sigmoid colon or if a low rectal anastomosis is not anticipated, then it may be possible to bring the sigmoid colon (proximal to the left colic artery) down to the rectal stump, without mobilization of the splenic flexure, and to construct a tension-free colorectostomy. For the purpose of this chapter, it is assumed that the patient will require splenic flexure mobilization for safe performance of the anastomosis.

The patient is placed in reverse-Trendelenburg position with maximal lateral tilt to raise the left side. The descending colon is placed on gentle medial stretch with a laparoscopic Babcock grasper, and the peritoneal reflection of descending colon to the left sidewall (i.e., the white line of Toldt) is identified and incised parallel to the colon. The avascular plane between the descending colon and the sidewall is developed gently with blunt dissection.

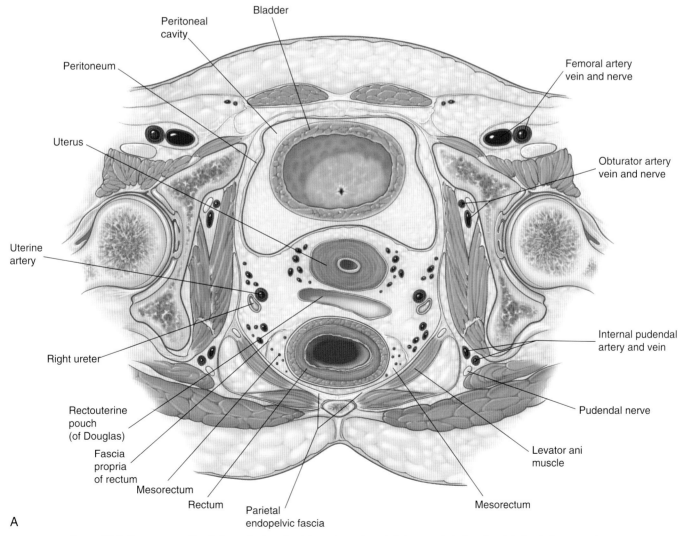

A

FIGURE 26-8 Transverse sectional views of relevant pelvic anatomy, from inferior aspect. **A,** Female pelvis, level of upper rectum.

Continued

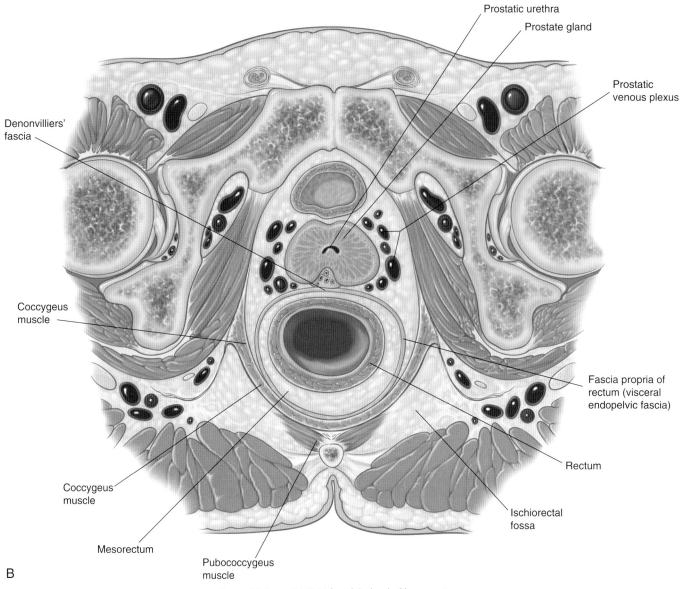

FIGURE 26-8, cont'd **B,** Male pelvis, level of lower rectum.

The incision in the peritoneal reflection is continued superiorly toward the splenic flexure of the colon. The avascular plane between the colon-mesocolon and sidewall is developed further as the incision in the peritoneal reflection is lengthened. As the splenic flexure is approached, the omentum from the transverse colon typically will limit this dissection.

The omentum then should be mobilized off of the transverse colon to facilitate transection of the splenocolic ligaments. The surgeon may find this easier to perform by standing between the patient's legs, with the monitor up by the patient's left shoulder (see Fig. 26-4). The omentum is retracted superiorly and anteriorly with the Babcock, and the plane between the posterior omental leaf and the transverse colon is entered sharply. The assistant can provide inferior stretch on the transverse colon to aid in this maneuver. If done properly, an avascular plane between the omentum superiorly and the transverse colon-mesocolon inferiorly will be entered, allowing the omentum to be mobilized from the latter without disruption its blood supply. The omentum should be mobilized off the distal half of the transverse colon. As the omentum is separated from the transverse mesocolon, the surgeon should be cautious not to injure the distal body of the pancreas, which lies at the posterior extent of this dissection.

After the omentum has been mobilized from the transverse colon, the splenic flexure is placed on gentle stretch with the Babcock grasper, the omentum is retracted superiorly, and the splenocolic ligament is transected. The dissection posterior to the colon and mesocolon should stay as close as possible to these structures to avoid dissecting posterior to the left kidney. During open mobilization of the splenic flexure, dissection behind the left kidney is avoided by palpating this organ; during a laparoscopic procedure, the location of the left kidney may be ascertained by periodically moving the left colon back and forth over the retroperitoneum and looking for a large immobile mass underneath. After the splenocolic ligament has been cut, the splenic flexure and proximal descending colon are mobilized as far as possible toward the midline.

Mobilization of the Sigmoid Colon

The patient is placed into Trendelenburg position with rightward lateral tilt (left side up), the surgeon moves back to the patient's right side, and the surgeon's monitor is moved down off the patient's left knee (see Fig. 26-2). With the sigmoid colon retracted medially, the line of Toldt is incised to the pelvic brim. The same

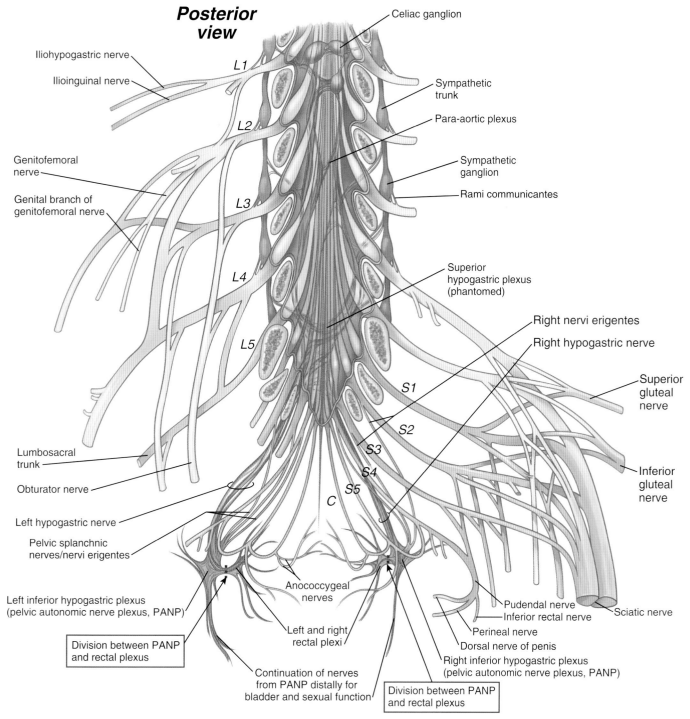

FIGURE 26-9 Relevant neural anatomy of the pelvis for a low anterior resection (coronal view, posterior aspect).

plane posterior to the mesocolon that was developed proximally is continued distally into the pelvis to mobilize the sigmoid colon to the midline. Typically, the first structure of importance encountered during this dissection is the left gonadal vein, which runs up from the internal inguinal ring along the lateral sidewall and empties into the left renal vein. This vein is not commonly involved with a rectal malignancy, so the vein should be preserved by maintaining the dissection anterior to it.

The left common iliac artery should become apparent during medial mobilization of the sigmoid colon. The surgeon can trace the path of this artery distally; at the point of the external-internal iliac bifurcation, the surgeon should be able to identify the left ureter (Fig. 26-10A). A gentle sweep, stroke, or squeeze with an instrument on the ureter should elicit a characteristic peristaltic

wave, providing positive identification of that structure. The left ureter should not be dissected free, but kept nestled in its surrounding connective tissue. As the dissection proceeds into the pelvis on the lateral side of the rectosigmoid colon, the surgeon should maintain constant awareness of the course of the left ureter because it will pass immediately lateral to the mesorectal dissection before entry into the bladder and can be prone to injury from the heat of a sealing device.

Transection of the Mesosigmoid and Lymphadenectomy

Some investigators (mostly from Japan) have suggested that an extended pelvic lymphadenectomy, variably consisting of high

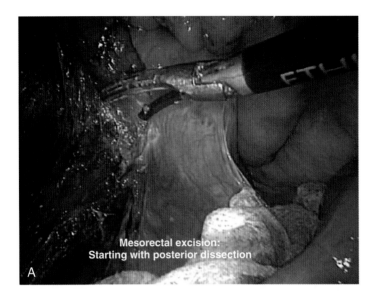

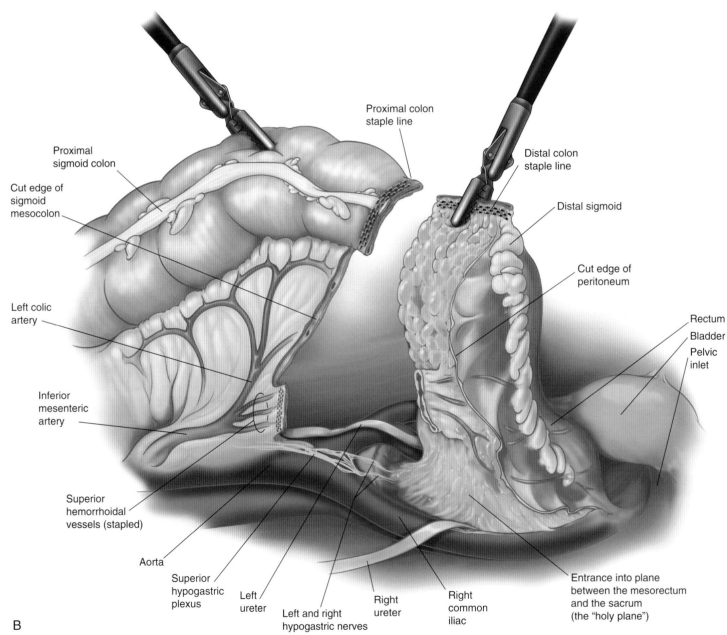

FIGURE 26-10 Entrance into the correct surgical plane at the beginning of the mesorectal excision. **A,** Photograph. **B,** Drawing.

ligation of the inferior mesenteric artery (IMA) combined with iliac and para-aortal nodal dissection, will decrease the risk for recurrence after LAR for rectal cancer. The advantage of an extended lymphadenectomy over a standard lymphadenectomy has not been demonstrated in a controlled trial, so most experts favor the performance of the latter, less extensive lymphadenectomy, including the mesorectum and distal mesosigmoid. In particular, the oncologic benefit of ligation of the IMA at its origin from the aorta has not been shown to be superior to an IMA ligation distal to the origin of the left colic artery. In the description in this chapter, the IMA will be transected distal to the origin of the left colic artery (see Fig. 26-6), primarily to preserve the proximal sigmoid colon for the colorectostomy. Alternatively, the surgeon can transect the IMA within 1 cm of the aorta, and then transect the inferior mesenteric vein just inferior to the pancreas.

With the patient in Trendelenburg position and some leftward lateral tilt, the sigmoid colon is elevated to place the inferior mesenteric vessels on stretch. The IMA and left colic artery branch should be visible as lines of tension within the mesocolon. The course of the left colic artery is followed out to the colon, and a point on the colon several centimeters distal to the left colic artery is marked with metal clips on the pericolic fat. A peritoneal incision is made on the medial side of the mesosigmoid, beginning at the metal clips, extending posteriorly to the level of the aorta, and staying inferior and parallel to the course of the left colic artery. Keeping the sigmoid colon retracted anteriorly and to the left, the medial peritoneal incision is continued inferiorly, below the aortic bifurcation and into the pelvis (see Fig. 26-6). The proximal rectum then is retracted anteriorly and to the left, and the peritoneal incision is continued along the groove where the peritoneum reflects off the mesorectum and onto the pelvic sidewall.

The sigmoid colon is elevated again, and the mesentery to the distal sigmoid within the previous peritoneal incision is transected with a vessel sealing device, beginning at the periphery. The marginal artery should be identified and sealed deliberately. As the mesenteric division proceeds centrally, the superior sigmoidal (hemorrhoidal) vessels (including branches of the IMA distal to left colic artery) will be encountered in a vascular pedicle (see Fig. 26-6). This pedicle should be isolated from the underlying aorta and pelvic brim with gentle blunt dissection; the aortic bifurcation should not be skeletonized because, otherwise, neural injury may occur. After a dissection window has been made beneath the mesenteric pedicle that contains the superior hemorrhoidal vessels, the pedicle may be transected with one or two vascular loads of a linear stapler-cutter. The course of the left ureter on the lateral side of the mesosigmoid should be checked before firing the stapler.

Mesorectal Dissection

With the mesentery to the distal sigmoid colon divided, the mesorectal dissection is begun on the posterior side. The patient is placed into maximal reverse-Trendelenburg position with neutral tilt. The rectosigmoid is elevated to place the mesorectum on anteroposterior stretch (see Fig. 26-10A). With gentle blunt dissection, a plane should become apparent between the sacral promontory and the mesorectal bulk (see Fig. 26-10A and B); this is the so-called holy plane of mesorectal excision described by Heald. This plane is developed around the posterior mesorectum while maintaining upward traction on the rectosigmoid. After the plane has been identified, the dissection can proceed with

a combination of sharp and blunt technique. No vascular structures of consequence should be encountered during the posterior mesorectal dissection.

Exposure of the posterior mesorectum will become limited as the dissection reaches the hollow of the sacrum. At this point, the dissection should move to the lateral and anterior locations. To enhance exposure of the rectouterine or rectovesicular space, a U-shaped suspension stitch can be placed in the uterus or lower bladder flap (see Fig. 26-6), brought out the abdominal wall superior to the pubis, and secured against the skin with a hemostat, thus lifting the uterus or bladder flap out of the line of sight. Alternatively, a Nathanson-type or fan-blade retractor can be placed against the uterus or bladder, with anterior lift provided by a self-retaining arm attached to a post on the bed rail.

The peritoneal incision previously made along the medial side of the mesorectum is continued distally, staying between the rectum and the right pelvic sidewall. As the surgeon descends deeper into the pelvis, all but the anterior portion of the rectum becomes retroperitoneal, until the rectum dives posterior to the uterus in the female or the bladder in the male (see Fig. 26-7). At the distal limit of the rectouterine or rectovesicular pouch, the medial peritoneal incision is carried anterior to the rectum and then across to the left pelvic sidewall, and the lateral and medial peritoneal incisions are connected (Fig. 26-11; see Fig. 26-6).

The mesorectal dissection of the distal rectum (i.e., below the level of the peritoneal reflection) can be accomplished by shifting the operative exposure among the posterior, anterior, and lateral approaches as needed so that the surgeon does not work "into a hole" by focusing exclusively on one side of the dissection. Retraction of the mesorectal bulk during these exposures should be done by grasping the epiploic appendices of the upper rectum or by pushing directly on the mesorectum with a broad-based laparoscopic retractor (e.g., fan-blade or balloon type), but not by grasping the mesorectum itself, which will tear easily and bleed. The anterior rectal wall also can be grasped for retraction, but the surgeon should avoid the region of the tumor if this is done.

During the lateral dissection of the mesorectum (both right and left sides), the surgeon may encounter bands of tissue running anterolaterally from the posterolateral mesorectum to the pelvic sidewall. In older texts, these tissue bands were described as the "lateral ligaments" that harbored the "middle rectal artery." More

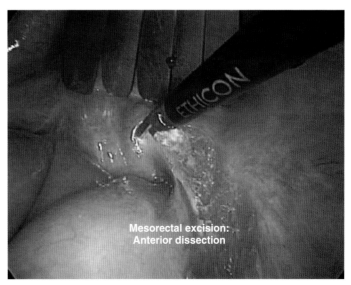

Mesorectal excision: Anterior dissection

FIGURE 26-11 Anterior peritoneal incision in the rectouterine or rectovesicular pouch.

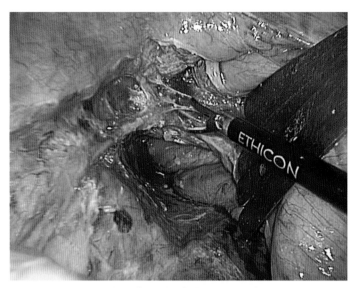

FIGURE 26-12 Division of the "lateral stalks" during a total mesorectal excision.

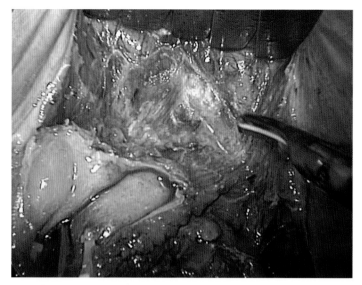

FIGURE 26-13 Dissection of Denonvilliers' fascia during the anterior portion of a total mesorectal excision.

recent cadaveric and clinical analyses have questioned whether the lateral ligament is a true anatomic structure, since there is only the occasional presence of a vessel requiring ligation in these tissue bands. In virtually all patients, the "lateral ligaments" simply are condensations of connective tissue that contain autonomic nerves to the rectum and inconsequential vessels. These tissue bands can be transected with impunity, such as with the ultrasonic scalpel (Fig. 26-12). The transection of the lateral bands should stay close to the mesorectum, however, to avoid injury to the ureter, which passes directly lateral in this region.

Below the level of the peritoneal reflection in the anterior dissection of the mesorectum, there is relatively little tissue that covers the lower anterior rectum. In this location, the surgeon will need to maintain the dissection plane close to the rectal wall. By maintaining downward traction on the anterior rectum and upward traction on the bladder, a plane containing fat and connective tissue between the anterior rectum and Denonvilliers' fascia can be identified (Fig. 26-13). This plane should be maintained all the way distally to the point of rectal transection. If possible, Denonvilliers' fascia should not be breached, but kept applied to the superior (patient) side of the dissection. If an anteriorly positioned tumor in the distal rectum has invaded through the rectal wall, then an en bloc excision of contiguous tissue (e.g., Denonvilliers' fascia, prostrate) should be attempted. Ideally, such a scenario would have been anticipated on a staging ultrasound or CT obtained after the neoadjuvant therapy so that the surgeon would be mentally prepared to perform a curative en bloc excision.

By continually switching among anterior, posterior, and lateral views, the distal dissection of the mesorectum can progress down to the pelvic floor, that is, to the levator ani complex. One potential problem the surgeon may encounter is difficulty with maintaining a uniform dissection plane 360 degrees around the mesorectum. This can be prevented by following the dissection plane from one operative field over to the next field and, as alluded to earlier, by avoiding prolonged dissection in one operative field; that is, the surgeon should not dissect himself or herself "into a hole." In the region of the transition between the rectum and the anal canal (just above the levators), the mesorectum will thin down and end. Posteriorly at this level, the mesorectum can turn into the rectal wall sharply (see Fig. 26-7), almost at a 90-degree angle, before the mesorectum abruptly terminates.

Distal Transection

A primary goal of the distal transection is to obtain an adequate distal tumor margin. During the past several decades, the minimal distal tumor margin recommended for an LAR for rectal cancer has decreased from about 5 cm to as low as 1 cm. Some authors have reported using a less than 1-cm distal margin with acceptable anastomotic recurrence rates in patients who completed neoadjuvant chemoradiation, but as of 2012, a tumor margin of less than 1 cm cannot be universally recommended. Before attempting the distal transection, the surgeon needs to know with confidence that the stapling device can be applied far enough distal to the tumor to ensure the minimal distal margin. If the surgeon cannot be certain about the location of the tumor during application of the stapling device, then the tumor site can be identified with a proctoscope and the level marked with a stitch on the anterior rectum.

The chosen site for transection should be cleaned of extraneous tissue around the rectal wall to allow maximal purchase of the staples. With the patient in maximal reverse-Trendelenburg and moderate leftward lateral tilt, a laparoscopic linear stapler-cutter with a 45-mm blue load (about 3.5-mm staple length) is inserted through the 12-mm port in the right lower quadrant. A 60-mm stapler load typically will be too long to fit within the pelvis at this level. Modern laparoscopic stapling devices can articulate the head 45 degrees with respect to the shaft; all of this angulation will be needed. The rectum is placed on cephalad stretch, and the open stapler is slowly worked across the chosen point of transection on the distal rectum (Fig. 26-14). The surgeon should ensure that the stapler is applied across the rectum as close to perpendicular as possible. This may require several rounds of (1) stapler reopening, (2) repositioning of the rectum within the stapler jaws, and (3) stapler reclosing before the optimal stapler angle is achieved. After stapler closure, the stapler is rotated back and forth to ensure that no sidewall tissue has been caught in the stapler jaws.

The tissue is compressed within the stapler jaws for 1 minute before firing the stapler. After the stapler has been fired, the tissue is compressed for an additional 15 to 20 seconds before opening the jaws and removing the stapler. If need be, a second load may be fired across the rectum to complete the transection. If more than two loads are required to complete the distal transection,

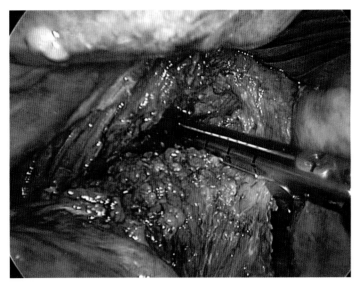

FIGURE 26-14 Division of the distal rectum with an endoscopic linear stapler-cutter.

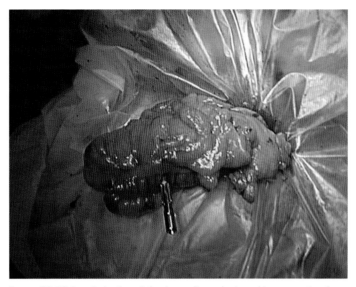

FIGURE 26-15 Exteriorization of the descending colonic end in preparation for the stapled colorectostomy. The specimen has been removed through the wound protector, and the anvil of the circular stapler has been inserted.

then the surgeon should consider that the distal transection was performed too obliquely across the rectum (as opposed to perpendicularly), which can compromise the distal tumor margin. An alternative method to perform the distal transection is to insert a nonarticulating, curved cutter stapler (e.g., Contour device, Ethicon Endo-Surgery, Cincinnati, Ohio) through a Pfannenstiel incision. This method is not always successful because of the angles that such a nonarticulating stapler will have to negotiate.

If the patient has a tumor located at the rectosigmoid junction, then the distal point of mesorectal excision need not be down to the level of the levator ani complex. With proximal rectal tumors, most authors and guidelines suggest that the level of rectal transection should be at least 5 cm distal to the most distal extent of the tumor. In such a case, the surgeon will need to cone down to the rectal wall just distal to where the 5-cm distal margin was identified. This path through the mesorectum will need to be cut with a vessel sealing device because the tissue will be heavily vascularized. Similar to the situation described previously, the rectum should be cleaned of all extraneous tissue at the level of transection before applying a stapler.

Proximal Transection and Specimen Extraction

There are numerous ways by which the proximal colonic transection and specimen removal can be performed; the choice depends on whether a defunctioning stoma will be employed, the degree of the patient's obesity and mesenteric mobility, and surgeon preference. A common technique is to complete the mesorectal dissection, the distal rectal transection, and ligation of the sigmoid vessels, and then to exteriorize the specimen, still attached to the descending colon, through a small incision (minilaparotomy). With the specimen extruded, the proximal colonic transection can be performed with a linear stapler-cutter, and the anvil of the circular stapler then can be inserted into the end of the descending colon in preparation for the anastomosis (Fig. 26-15).

If the surgeon intends to use a defunctioning stoma (see later discussion), then the surgical specimen can be extracted through the stomal incision. The stomal incision typically will be in the right lower quadrant (for a loop ileostomy) or in the right upper quadrant (for a transverse loop colostomy). In either case, the descending colon and rectum will need to be mobile enough so that the specimen can be exteriorized through a right-sided incision, at which point the proximal transection and anvil insertion can be performed. If the patient's anatomy will not permit this sequence of events, then an expedient option would be to make a transverse incision in the left lateral abdomen and to exteriorize the specimen there for transection and anvil insertion.

The typical incision for a diverting loop ostomy is positioned over the rectus abdominis muscle; see the full description for creating such an ostomy later. After a cruciate incision is made in the anterior rectus sheath and the rectus abdominis muscle is split vertically, a plastic wound protector (e.g., Alexis Wound Protector, Applied Medical, Rancho Santa Margarita, Calif.) is inserted (see Fig. 26-15) and specimen extraction proceeds, beginning with the staple line on the distal rectum. The incision in the rectus sheath can be extended laterally in a stepwise fashion until it is just big enough to allow passage of the specimen. The descending colon is extruded until the previously placed marking clips are visible. The proximal colonic transection then is performed with a linear stapler-cutter, and the specimen is passed off to a back table.

Before proceeding further, the surgeon should inspect the specimen for completeness of the mesorectal excision (i.e., the radial margin) and the length of the distal margin (Fig. 26-16). The mesorectal surface, particularly posteriorly, should be relatively smooth and without defects. Some have described the appearance of the surgical TME specimen as resembling a "baby's bottom" because there often is a shallow cleft in the posterior mesorectal surface. To assess the adequacy of the distal margin, the surgeon should not hesitate to open the specimen, which can be done by incising the anterior rectal wall in an axial direction, but avoiding a cut into the tumor. The surgeon should change gown and gloves after such an examination. If the tumor is within 2 cm of the distal staple line, then a frozen section of the distal margin should be obtained. If necessary, the distal tissue ring ("donut") that will be obtained from the circular stapler can be included in this examination. If the distal margin is positive, then conversion of the procedure to an abdominal perineal resection should be strongly considered.

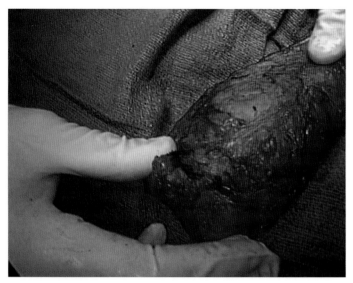

FIGURE 26-16 Inspection of the surgical specimen after extraction. Note intactness of mesorectum.

In preparation for the stapling of the colorectostomy, the end of the descending colon (about 1 cm) is cleaned of pericolic fat and other tissue so that the proximal staple line is clearly visible. Some patients will have diverticula in this region; if these become a problem, then it may be best to redo the colonic staple line several centimeters proximally. A pursestring suture then is placed about 5 mm from the end of the descending colon, either manually or with an automatic pursestring applicator (e.g., Purstring, Covidien, Norwalk, Conn.). The colonic staple line then is removed with a Mayo scissors, just distal to the pursestring (if an automatic pursestring device is used, the staple line is cut after the device has been applied). The region around the colonic end should be protected with laparotomy pads in case liquid stool is present. The end of the colon then is sized with dilators for the appropriate circular stapler, which, depending on the manufacturer, may be available in diameters of 25, 28, 29, 31, 33, and 34 mm.

Some authors advocate choosing a stapler that is one size greater than the largest dilator that the end of the descending colon can accommodate. For example, if the colonic end will only accept a 28-mm dilator, then a 31-mm stapler should be used. The rationale is that a larger anastomotic ring will be less susceptible to anastomotic stricture. This rationale should be balanced by the risk for splitting the wall of the descending colon by forcing an oversized anvil into the distal end. The surgeon will need to judge whether this risk is acceptable at each case, based mainly on the compliance of the colonic wall. If the colonic wall suffers a partial or full-thickness split, then it would be prudent to restaple the descending colon several centimeters proximally, and to start over. In most patients, it should be possible to use at least a 28- or 29-mm circular stapler.

After a stapler has been selected, the stapler anvil is inserted into the end of the descending colon and secured by tying the pursestring suture. At this point, additional pericolic fat may need to be trimmed from the region of the anvil so that extraneous tissue will not be incorporated into the circular staple line. The end of the descending colon with the anvil then is dropped back into the abdomen, the fascial incision is either closed (if it has been used just for specimen extraction) or towel-clipped (if the incision will be used for a loop ostomy), and the abdomen is reinsufflated.

If the surgeon does not intend to use a defunctioning stoma, then the specimen and descending colon may be exteriorized through an umbilical incision (e.g., an extension of the incision used for the Hasson cannula) or a low transverse incision (Pfannenstiel type), although this latter approach may have limited utility if the patient has a large pannus. Alternatively, the proximal colonic transection can be performed intracorporeally, with the specimen placed into a large polyethylene retrieval bag for removal through one of the above incisions. The colonic end then is brought out for anvil insertion, as described earlier. If the specimen is not overly bulky, then transanal extraction of the bagged specimen also is feasible. Use of this route would eliminate the need for a minilaparotomy but has technical issues that will not be discussed here.

The advantage of extruding an unbagged specimen through a small protected incision is that the extrusion can proceed from the stapled rectal end to the proximal end in a linear fashion (i.e., in "single file"), which should minimize the length of the minilaparotomy. If the specimen is placed within a bag, then the specimen can fold upon itself, increasing its transverse bulk and thereby increasing the length of the incision needed for specimen extrusion. Furthermore, there do not appear to be any oncologic issues with respect to extracting the specimen through a wound protector versus retrieval with a specimen bag. In this regard, the choice of extraction technique is influenced by surgeon preference.

Reconstruction with an End-to-End Colorectostomy

A number of reconstruction options have been described for LAR, including an intra-abdominal end-to-end colorectostomy with a circular stapler, a hand-sutured coloanal anastomosis performed from a perineal approach, an intra-abdominal robot-assisted intersphincteric coloanal anastomosis, and the construction of a colonic J pouch. This chapter describes reconstruction with the first technique, which involves an end-to-end anastomosis (EEA) between the descending colon and the distal rectum using a circular stapler. The following technique commonly is known as the double- or triple-stapling EEA technique, depending on how many of the stapling sequences are included in the name.

The rectal stump is irrigated with water or a diluted antiseptic-detergent (e.g., Betadine or Hibiclens). The anorectal ring is gently dilated with the insertion of four fingers; this is done to (1) facilitate transanal insertion of the circular stapler and (2) ease passage of the patient's first bowel movement. With the patient in steep-Trendelenburg position and no lateral tilt, the lubricated head of the circular stapler is inserted transanally. The progress of the stapler head toward the rectal staple line is monitored continually with the laparoscope. For a low rectal anastomosis, it typically is easiest to eject the spike of the stapler through or adjacent to the rectal staple line (Fig. 26-17). Ejection of the circular stapler spike through the anterior rectal wall, as may be done with an upper rectal anastomosis, usually is not possible during a low rectal anastomosis because of the proximity of the prostrate and bladder. Before ejecting the spike, the surgeon should visualize the impression of the stapler head against the end of the rectal stump, ensuring that the spike will be ejected through or adjacent to the staple line and parallel to the axis of the stump.

With the spike fully extended, the rectal wall over the head of the stapler is pressed down so that the rectal wall is flush with the head. If there is excessive fat or connective tissue over the

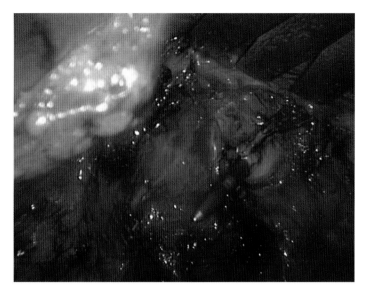

FIGURE 26-17 Ejection of the spike of the circular stapler adjacent to the staple line on the distal rectum.

impression of the stapler head that might impede the stapling process, then this tissue is excised at this time. The anvil of the stapler in the descending colon then is mated to the stapler spike, and the stapler is "closed," bringing the anvil in apposition to the stapler head. This closure should be monitored closely so that surrounding tissue does not get caught in the staple line. The typical circular stapling device has an indicator that will inform the surgeon when the device is completely closed. As discussed previously, the stapler is held in this compressed position for about 1 minute before it is fired. The stapler is fired, and the firing mechanism (handles of the stapler) are held compressed for another 30 seconds. The stapler then is "opened" partially (typically by unscrewing the closure mechanism by three half-turns), rotated gently 180 degrees to unseat the stapler head from the new staple line, and then slowly backed out of the anus, all under continual laparoscopic monitoring.

The stapler is opened on the back table, and the proximal and distal tissue rings ("donuts") are retrieved from inside the stapler mechanism. The rings are evaluated for their circular integrity; an incomplete ring should raise the suspicion of an incomplete anastomosis. If the integrity of the circular staple line is in question, then the surgeon can perform a gentle digital examination to palpate the anastomotic ring, or visualize it with a proctoscope. The distal ring should be sent for pathologic examination; this is particularly important if the distal tumor margin was close.

The course of the descending colon down to the anastomosis is inspected to confirm absence of both twisting and excessive tension. The colorectostomy then may undergo an air-pressure test. A proctoscope is inserted just inside the anus, with the end of the scope at the level of the sphincteric complex. Saline irrigation is squirted into the pelvis, just enough to submerge the anastomosis. The descending colon is compressed with a grasper at the pelvic brim, and air is insufflated with the proctoscope squeeze bulb until the distal colon is visibly distended. A persistent stream of bubbles signifies a leak.

If the pressure test detects a leak, then an attempt should be made to locate the leak and, if possible, oversew the area with laparoscopic suturing, taking bites of the descending colon serosa above and the rectal wall below. Of note, it would be quite difficult, if not impossible, to redo the anastomosis by stapling across the anorectum distal to the first transection. Such an

attempt likely would result in conversion of the procedure to an abdominoperineal resection. Most leaks from a properly executed colorectostomy with a circular stapler are small, so oversewing with proximal diversion should be adequate to allow the leak to heal. It would be prudent to divert any case in which a leak is detected, even if the leak is oversewn and the repeat pressure test demonstrates no bubbling. The surgeon should have a low threshold to protect any low rectal anastomosis with fecal diversion; therefore, if a problem arises with the pressure test, then all the more reason to divert.

Temporary Fecal Diversion

A long-standing surgical paradigm with respect to fecal diversion and LAR is that a protective ostomy will not prevent a leak but will, if a leak occurs, keep the patient from getting septic in the acute situation and permit the leak to heal over the long term. Controlled data has supported the use of a temporary defunctioning stoma in conjunction with LAR for cancer. The addition of a temporary stoma to the procedure, however, adds a new set of complication risks (e.g., stomal herniation, prolapse, wound sepsis) and also commits the patient to an additional closure procedure with all of its inherent risks; thus, temporary fecal diversion is not a benign addition to LAR.

Retrospective data from open surgery have indicated that the risk for anastomotic leak is elevated when the anastomosis is within 5 to 6 cm of the anal verge, so most authors have recommended routine fecal diversion for a low rectal anastomosis. Whether this strategy applies to minimally invasive LAR is not known for certain. Some have argued that an anastomosis constructed during a laparoscopic LAR will be less susceptible to leak compared with that in an open procedure, based on mostly vague or undefined physiologic patient benefits of minimally invasive surgery (in 2012, this argument is conjectural). On the other hand, there is evidence that TME may increase the risk for anastomotic leak. Therefore, the need for a temporary protective ostomy after minimally invasive LAR with TME remains controversial.

Because a temporary diverting ostomy does add risk for short-term and long-term morbidity and has well-known quality-of-life issues, safe avoidance of a stoma would be well received by surgeons and patients alike. Some surgeons believe that the optimal management plan is *not* to perform temporary diversion during minimally invasive LAR, and then to treat anyone who subsequently develops a leak with percutaneous drainage and antibiotics. The rationale here is that most leaks will be innocuous if diagnosed promptly, so a percutaneous drain in a fraction of patients would be much better than a colostomy bag in all patients. To some, this rationale is counter to established practice and decades of published experience. In 2012, whether the risk for morbidity from an anastomotic leak after a minimally invasive LAR is low enough to forgo routine diversion is unknown.

As described in this chapter, TME is performed with transection of the rectum close to the sphincteric complex followed by routine fecal diversion with a temporary defunctioning stoma, either a loop ileostomy or a loop transverse colostomy. The loop configuration is favored for temporary diversion because of the relative ease of reversing this stomal type. The advantages of an ileostomy include ease of construction and reversal, and perhaps improved quality of life compared with a colostomy; the disadvantages include well-described complications such as dehydration, electrolyte disturbances, and obstruction. Because a colostomy provides a more physiologic location to excrete stool, there is less risk for excessive fluid and electrolyte loss; in addition, because the transverse colon is more fixed in location than the ileum, there is less risk for volvulus, twisting, and so forth. The disadvantages of a colostomy include quality-of-life issues and the need for more dissection and mobilization. In addition, the larger fascial incision typically required for a loop colostomy may increase the risk for stomal herniation or prolapse.

To construct a temporary loop ileostomy, a loop of distal ileum is chosen with enough distance from the ileocecal valve to allow the loop to reach the anteromedial abdominal wall without tension or kinking. Tension on the ostomy can result in stomal retraction, so loop mobility is important. A disk of skin may be excised over the right rectus muscle at the level of the loop. The anterior rectus sheath is exposed with blunt dissection, and a cruciate incision is made in the sheath, large enough to accommodate the loop of ileum. The rectus muscle is separated in the direction of its fibers, taking care not to lacerate the inferior epigastric artery. The abdomen then is entered through the posterior layers, and the loop of ileum is brought up through the incision. The path through the abdominal wall may need digital dilation. Of note, the loop can be brought up directly from the peritoneal cavity (a "post"), or less commonly, the loop may be tunneled retroperitoneally, beginning near the cecum, up along the sidewall, and then out through the incision. This latter technique is intended to reduce the risk for prolapse, hernia, or mechanical obstruction associated with the post technique.

After the loop of ileum has been exteriorized, several anchoring sutures of 3-0 polyglactin can be placed from the serosal into the anterior rectus sheath. The ileum then is incised transversely for about two thirds of its circumference, and the edges of the ileum then are sewn to the skin with interrupted sutures of 3-0 polyglactin. These sutures should evert the ileum by taking, in sequence, full thickness of the cut ileal end, serosa 1 cm distal to the end, and then dermis. Eversion is needed to facilitate a seal to the ileostomy appliance, preventing effluent leakage and subsequent skin erosion. Some authors prefer a rod at the skin level to hold the loop in place, use minimal sutures on the ileostomy, and then remove the rod in 4 weeks.

If a colostomy is elected, then the transverse colon is preferable because the subcutaneous fat of the abdominal wall tends to be thinner in the medial upper abdomen compared with the lower quadrants. In addition, many patients will not have adequate length in the descending colon after an LAR to construct a left lower quadrant colostomy. The steps in construction of a transverse loop colostomy are similar to those of a loop ileostomy, except that the incisions and tract tend to be larger, and local mobilization of the colon may be needed to bring the transverse loop up through the rectal sheath so that there is no tension on the stoma.

Conclusion of the Procedure

The dissection areas are irrigated with saline, and as much fluid as possible is aspirated. Pelvic drainage is not routinely performed. Whether to use a drain in select patients (e.g., if the anastomosis is at risk) remains a perennial point of discussion. All incisions are infiltrated with a long-acting local anesthetic (e.g., bupivacaine), and the fascia of each port site larger than 5 mm is closed with suture. If the surgeon decides to perform an open conversion, then a long midline incision is made, incorporating the

infraumbilical and suprapubic port sites. If exposure of the splenic flexure is needed, then the midline incision can be extended to the xiphoid process. A midline incision generally is preferable to a transverse incision because the former can be extended to the symphysis pubis to enhance pelvic exposure.

POSTOPERATIVE CARE

Similar to most other surgical procedures, patient recovery after a minimally invasive LAR can be optimized (and expedited) with the use of a clinical pathway, which facilitates the standardization of postoperative care. The components of such a pathway are described in Table 26-3; this may be customized to surgeon preference or the local practice environment. The surgeon may need to modify the clinical pathway for a frail patient. Routine water-soluble contrast enema (to evaluate for leak) is not indicated. After discharge, the patient may be seen by the surgeon 1 and 6 weeks later. The patient with a temporary ileostomy may need additional patient education and intervention if high stomal output becomes an issue. The patient's operative findings and surgical pathology should be discussed at the multidisciplinary tumor conference so that final treatment and surveillance recommendations can be made.

MANAGEMENT OF PROCEDURE-SPECIFIC COMPLICATIONS

The main procedure-specific complication of LAR (whether open or laparoscopic) is anastomotic leak. Complications of temporary stomas, alluded to earlier, will not be detailed here. The primary risk factor for an anastomotic leak is a low rectal anastomosis, that is, if the anastomosis is within 5 to 6 cm of the anal verge. Secondary risk factors may include technical issues with the anastomosis, surgeon inexperience, tumor diameter, tobacco use, diabetes mellitus, prolonged operative time, pelvic drainage, and (possibly) preoperative neoadjuvant therapy. The prevention of anastomotic leak is primarily the responsibility of the surgeon, that is, proper decision making and operative execution. The weight of published data, as previously mentioned, supports the use of a temporary defunctioning stoma when a low rectal anastomosis is contemplated.

A leak may manifest in the first several days to several weeks after the procedure, but most commonly after 7 to 10 days. Symptoms may be minimal to life-threatening and may include fever, tachycardia, abdominal pain, and ileus. If a stable patient develops one or more of these symptoms, then an abdominal CT scan with intravenous and oral contrast can be obtained. If the anastomotic ring is located in the upper rectum, then careful installation of rectal contrast may be possible. If the stable patient has evidence of a leak (usually a pelvic fluid collection), then this should be drained percutaneously with CT guidance. The patient is given intravenous antibiotics and is maintained NPO until the clinical signs resolve. For the patient with a defunctioning stoma, this typically is all the intervention that is needed. For the stable patient without a defunctioning stoma, a longer period of observation and NPO status likely will be needed (with parenteral nutrition as indicated) until the leak resolves. If such a patient does not progress, then operative intervention will be needed, as described below.

If the patient becomes unstable or has generalized peritonitis, then immediate operative intervention is needed. The patient is

Table 26-3 Example Postoperative Clinical Pathway for a Minimally Invasive Low Anterior Resection

Postoperative Day	Activity	Fluids and Diet	Analgesia	Other
0	Patient in chair for 2 hr; ambulate in evening	Clear liquids	Acetaminophen and/or NSAID*; oral opioid for breakthrough pain	
1	Ambulate four times per day	Discontinue intravenous fluids; regular diet	Acetaminophen and/or NSAID[†]; oral opioid for breakthrough pain	
2	Ambulate four times per day	Regular diet	Acetaminophen and/or NSAID[†]; oral opioid for breakthrough pain	Stomal nurse visit; remove Foley catheter
3	Ambulate four times per day	Regular diet	Acetaminophen and/or NSAID[†]	Discharge

*If the patient undergoes open conversion, place a thoracic (T8-9) epidural catheter, and infuse continuously with bupivacaine for 48 hr.
[†]Nonsteroidal anti-inflammatory drug.

resuscitated and given intravenous antibiotics. The patient is placed in the low lithotomy position, and the abdomen is explored through a midline laparotomy. Contaminated fluid is washed out. Identification and assessment of the leak can be facilitated with a digital examination or proctoscopy (hence the need for perineal access). If possible, the anastomotic leak is oversewn, closed-suction drains are placed into the pelvis, and a proximal defunctioning stoma is created. If the anastomosis has to be taken down for the creation of an end colostomy, then the patient most likely will be left with a permanent stoma.

RESULTS AND OUTCOME

As discussed previously, some still consider minimally invasive LAR to be an experimental procedure that should not be performed outside the confines of a controlled trial. The reality is that this procedure is being performed outside of controlled trials, although the vast majority of LARs currently (as of 2012) still are performed with open technique. The major scientific question that still needs to be answered in this respect is whether the long-term oncologic outcome of minimally invasive LAR is as good as after the open procedure. A definitive answer probably will require another 10 years. The short- to mid-term data that have accrued so far suggest that the oncologic outcomes have *not* differed between the open and laparoscopic approaches.

A wealth of published data demonstrate that minimally invasive resection of colon cancer (above the peritoneal reflection) has multiple short-term advantages over open resection, including less blood loss, less pain, shorter ileus, better pulmonary function, shorter hospital stay, and improved quality of life in the first 30 days. This is offset by longer operative time with the laparoscopic approach and the fact that this approach cannot be applied to all patients. Review of large databases has suggested that perioperative morbidity is less with laparoscopic than open colon resection; a 2011 meta-analysis of randomized controlled trials of laparoscopic versus open colorectal resection, however, found a higher rate of intraoperative complications (including hollow viscus injury) in the laparoscopic group. This nonconcordance of retrospective versus controlled data is a reminder of how these two sources of information can produce different answers to the same clinical question.

The data comparing minimally invasive to open rectal resection are not as abundant as with colon resection, but so far similar conclusions as described previously appear to be valid. Moreover, collective review of the published data has not identified differences in circumferential margin acquisition, nodal clearance, anastomotic leak rate, overall morbidity, mortality, and short-term disease-free survival or overall survival in

laparoscopic versus open LAR with TME for rectal cancer. Specifically, data from uncontrolled or retrospective series or short-term trials have documented a mortality rate from laparoscopic LAR in the range of 0% to 3%. The anastomotic leak rate has been in the range of 5% to 15%. The published rate of open conversion has varied widely, from nearly 0% to more than 30%. It should be emphasized that all these data were derived from expert centers that operate on relatively large numbers of patients with rectal cancer, so these observations likely represent a best-case scenario. The question of open versus laparoscopic LAR with TME is under active study, and a number of controlled trials on this subject are in progress.

In well-trained hands, it appears that minimally invasive LAR with TME can be performed with short-term equivalency to the open procedure, with possible short-term benefits from the laparoscopic approach. If the long-term oncologic outcome actually is observed to be better with the laparoscopic approach, then gradual migration to this approach would be desirable. If it is assumed that the long-term oncologic outcomes are equivalent, however, then the movement of the surgical community to perform laparoscopic LAR in preference to open LAR may become more of a philosophical issue. That is, will the technical difficulty of accomplishing the minimally invasive dissection justify any short-term benefits? Will patient advocacy groups favor the minimally invasive approach?

For most surgeons who already perform laparoscopic LAR, the answers to the above questions probably would be "yes." Other surgeons might argue that oncologic clearance and neural preservation are the primary considerations in this procedure, so an argument over incision length would not be relevant. Interestingly, the relative absence of controlled data demonstrating the superiority of the minimally invasive approach did not prevent the mass migration of surgeons to laparoscopic cholecystectomy and Nissen fundoplication during the 1990s. In these nononcologic scenarios, the laparoscopic approach was embraced because of quicker patient recovery, improved cosmesis, and (perhaps) a decreased risk for perioperative morbidity.

As implied above, the paradigm shift in surgical preference for the minimally invasive approach for some procedures has not required multi-institutional controlled trials. As the benefits of laparoscopic surgery become more difficult to ferret out (especially with major oncologic resections), however, the randomized controlled trial appears to have more relevance. Unfortunately, for reasons beyond the scope of this discussion, a well-designed and well-executed randomized controlled trial is getting more difficult to accomplish. In any event, the debate of open versus laparoscopic LAR likely will continue for years to come.

ACKNOWLEDGMENTS

I would like to express my gratitude to Drs. Jon S. Thompson and Edibaldo Silva for their critical reading of this manuscript.

Suggested Readings

Baik SH, Gincherman M, Mutch MG, et al: Laparoscopic vs open resection for patients with rectal cancer: Comparison of perioperative outcomes and long-term survival, *Dis Colon Rectum* 54:6–14, 2011.

Chand M, Heald RJ: Laparoscopic rectal cancer surgery, *Br J Surg* 98:166–167, 2011.

Fry DE: Colon preparation and surgical site infection, *Am J Surg* 202:225–232, 2011.

Georgiou P, Tan E, Gouvas N, Antoniou A, et al: Extended lymphadenectomy versus conventional surgery for rectal cancer: A meta-analysis, *Lancet Oncol* 10:1053–1062, 2009.

Heald RJ, Ryall RD: Recurrence and survival after total mesorectal excision for rectal cancer, *Lancet* 1:1479–1482, 1986.

Kang SB, Park JW, Jeong SY, et al: Open versus laparoscopic surgery for mid or low rectal cancer after neoadjuvant chemoradiotherapy (COREAN trial): Short-term outcomes of an open-label randomised controlled trial, *Lancet Oncol* 11:637–645, 2010.

Kapiteijn E, Marijnen CA, Nagtegaal ID, et al: Preoperative radiotherapy combined with total mesorectal excision for resectable rectal cancer, *N Engl J Med* 345:638–646, 2001.

King PM, Blazeby JM, Ewings P, et al: Randomized clinical trial comparing laparoscopic and open surgery for colorectal cancer within an enhanced recovery programme, *Br J Surg* 93:300–308, 2006.

Laurent C, Leblanc F, Wutrich P, et al: Laparoscopic versus open surgery for rectal cancer: Long-term oncologic results, *Ann Surg* 250:54–61, 2009.

Lindsey I, Guy RJ, Warren BF, Mortensen NJ: Anatomy of Denonvilliers' fascia and pelvic nerves, impotence, and implications for the colorectal surgeon, *Br J Surg* 87:1288–1299, 2000.

Lujan J, Valero G, Hernandez Q, et al: Randomized clinical trial comparing laparoscopic and open surgery in patients with rectal cancer, *Br J Surg* 96:982–989, 2009.

Miles WE: A method of performing abdominoperineal excision for carcinoma of the rectum and of the terminal portion of the pelvic colon, *Lancet* 2:1812–1814, 1908.

National Comprehensive Cancer Network. NCCN Clinical Practice Guidelines in Oncology (NCCN Guidelines): Rectal Cancer. Version 4.2011 (February 25, 2011). Accessed June 13, 2011, from http://www.nccn.org.

Ohtani H, Tamamori Y, Azuma T, et al: A meta-analysis of the short- and long-term results of randomized controlled trials that compared laparoscopy-assisted and conventional open surgery for rectal cancer, *J Gastrointestinal Surg* 15:1375–1385, 2011.

Prins H, Lacy A: Minimally low anterior resection and abdominal perineal resection. In Frantzides CT, Carlson MA, editors: *Atlas of Minimally Invasive Surgery*, Philadelphia, 2009, Saunders.

Sammour T, Kahokehr A, Srinivasa S, et al: Laparoscopic colorectal surgery is associated with a higher intraoperative complication rate than open surgery, *Ann Surg* 253:35–43, 2011.

Takahashi T, Ueno M, Azekura K, Ohta H: Lateral ligament: Its anatomy and clinical importance, *Semin Surg Oncol* 19:386–395, 2000.

Tan WS, Tang CL, Shi L, Eu KW: Meta-analysis of defunctioning stomas in low anterior resection for rectal cancer, *Br J Surg* 96:462–472, 2009.

Tjandra JJ, Kilkenny JW, Buie WD, et al: Practice parameters for the management of rectal cancer (revised), *Dis Colon Rectum* 48:411–423, 2005.

George S. Ferzli, Michael F. Timoney, and Sean Rim

Lateral Decubitus Approach to Minimally Invasive Low Anterior Resection

27

The videos associated with this chapter are listed in the Video Contents and can be found on the accompanying DVDs and *on Expertconsult.com.*

The questions and controversies that have surrounded the minimally invasive low anterior resection for rectal cancer have, to a large extent, been answered or refuted. These issues involve the learning curve, patient safety, cost, operative time, and whether it is possible to perform an oncologically sound resection with a laparoscopic approach. Recent data have suggested that the number of laparoscopic low anterior resections a surgeon needs to perform to obtain reasonable technical proficiency is in the range of 15 to 80. Studies on perioperative outcome have shown that laparoscopic low anterior resection has acceptable (perhaps improved) morbidity and mortality compared with the open procedure.

Pathologic specimen analysis and short-term follow-up so far have demonstrated that minimally invasive rectal resection is oncologically sound; long-term survival and recurrence data currently are accruing. Objections concerning the potential for port-site metastasis in laparoscopic colorectal resection have not been borne out. Laparoscopic colorectal resection has been associated with increased operative time and equipment costs compared with open resection. On the other hand, the former approach has been associated with an earlier return of bowel function, an earlier return to work, decreased pain scores and pain medication requirements, and a shorter length of stay.

The traditional approach to the laparoscopic low anterior resection has been with the patient supine, typically in a modified lithotomy position. The technical obstacles to this approach included difficulty in dissection of the transverse colon and the splenocolic ligament. On the other hand, the lateral approach in the decubitus position provides excellent visualization of the transverse and left colon and allows improved access to the splenic flexure. This permits easy mobilization of the colon without requiring excessive traction, while minimizing the number of ports needed. A low rectal dissection can be performed, and the colorectal anastomosis is constructed with a traditional end-to-end stapler technique.

OPERATIVE INDICATIONS

The lateral decubitus approach to low anterior resection can be used for a patient undergoing minimally invasive colorectal resection for benign diseases such as diverticulitis. It also is suitable for high-grade dysplasia and invasive colorectal cancer that is amenable to curative resection, before or after chemoradiation.

If a patient with rectal cancer is being considered for a low anterior resection, then the tumor location has to allow a 2-cm distal margin in the specimen for pathologic clearance. In addition, a rectal stump of 1 to 2 cm should be maintained to preserve anorectal function. The patient should have good anorectal function before resection.

PREOPERATIVE EVALUATION, TESTING, AND PREPARATION

The preoperative management of patients undergoing laparoscopic low anterior resection varies according to the surgical indication. Candidates must be medically fit to undergo general anesthesia, possibly prolonged, and must be able to withstand the physiologic challenges that pneumoperitoneum imposes. The following testing and preparation can be applied to any patient having this procedure, except that endoscopic ultrasound (EUS) and magnetic resonance imaging (MRI) usually are reserved for the patient with rectal cancer.

Digital Rectal Examination and Rigid Proctoscopy

Digital rectal examination and rigid proctoscopy are performed to determine the distance of a cancerous lesion from the anal verge, the size and texture of the lesion, and whether the lesion is fixed to adjacent structures. The distance from the anal verge and fixation are particularly important in the clinical determination of lesion resectability, the likelihood of performing a safe anastomosis, and the possible need for neoadjuvant chemoradiation.

Colonoscopy

Colonoscopy is mandatory to evaluate the entire bowel for extent of disease, as well as synchronous lesions. If full colonoscopy is not feasible, contrast enema and computed tomography (CT) colonography are reasonable alternatives.

Tattoo

A lesion that is not palpable on digital examination should be tattooed during colonoscopy to help identify it laparoscopically.

Computed Tomography

CT of the abdomen and pelvis is useful for determining the extent of local disease and evaluating the entire abdomen for metastasis, for example, to the liver or peritoneal surface.

Endorectal Ultrasound and Magnetic Resonance Imaging

Depending on the surgeon's preference or the hospital's protocol, EUS and MRI are useful in the staging of rectal cancer. Both modalities have high sensitivity for the detection of local extension into the rectum or pelvis, thus determining the need for neoadjuvant chemoradiation.

Mechanical Bowel Preparation

Recent meta-analyses of the colorectal literature have discouraged the use of mechanical bowel preparation (MBP) before colon surgery. Nevertheless, a randomized, multicenter trial in 2010 of patients undergoing rectal resection with or without MBP demonstrated improvement in infectious and overall morbidity in patients with MBP, although there was no difference in the rate of anastomotic leak.

PATIENT POSITIONING IN THE OPERATING SUITE

The patient is placed in the right lateral decubitus position (Fig. 27-1). The right leg is flexed 30 degrees at the hip, and the left leg is extended with a pillow placed between the knees. The buttocks are positioned toward the edge of the table. Sequential compression devices are placed on both legs, and the patient is taped securely to the table. The right arm is extended over an arm board, and the left arm is positioned over a pillow on a Mayo stand. An axillary roll is placed under the right axilla. The arms are properly cushioned and supported to avoid a perioperative neurapraxia. The table is flexed and the kidney rest may be raised, extending the left flank and maximizing the working space. The operative field is prepared and draped to allow exposure from the left nipple down to the pubic symphysis, and from the umbilicus to the posterior axillary line. The anus must be accessible under the drapes so as to place the EEA device, as if performing a colonoscopy. Two video monitors are required—one at the head of the table to the patient's left, the other at the foot of the table.

POSITIONING AND PLACEMENT OF TROCARS

Laparoscopic low anterior and rectal resection in the right lateral decubitus position requires three trocars, with the option of a fourth (Fig. 27-2). A 10-mm trocar is inserted in the left midclavicular line, 2 to 3 cm above the level of the umbilicus. This serves as the optical port. A 5-mm trocar is inserted in the left subcostal region at the level of the anterior axillary line. This serves as the working port, through which the retraction and dissection instruments are placed. It can be converted to a 10-mm port if needed later in the operation. A 5-mm trocar is inserted under the left 11th rib at the level of the midaxillary line. This is used for the retraction and dissection instruments. If a fourth port is needed, it may be placed in the suprapubic region. A 10-mm 30-degree laparoscope is used for the procedure.

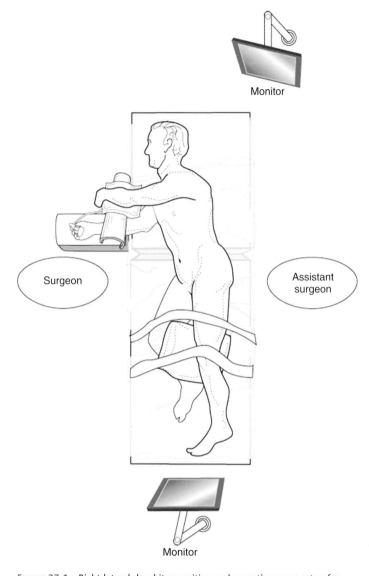

FIGURE 27-1   Right lateral decubitus position and operating room setup for a minimally invasive low anterior resection. (© Anne Erickson, CMI.)

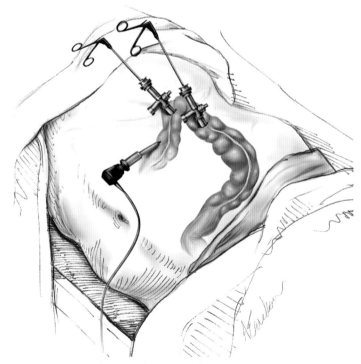

FIGURE 27-2   Port placement for a minimally invasive low anterior resection in the right lateral decubitus position. (© Anne Erickson, CMI.)

OPERATIVE TECHNIQUE

Mobilization of the colon and rectum is performed in two stages. The colon is mobilized in the first stage. This is best performed with the surgeon standing on the right side of the table and facing the upper monitor. The patient is placed in a 30-degree reverse-Trendelenburg position. This allows gravity to aid in the retraction of the colon, which facilitates the dissection of the splenic flexure and identification of the left ureter. Most of the planes are avascular, and dissection can be safely performed with an ultrasonic or bipolar dissector, or with electrocautery (hook or scissors).

The operation is begun by retracting the greater curvature of the stomach anteriorly to enter the lesser sac. The left hand retracts the mid-curvature, and the thin avascular layer of omentum that connects the stomach to the transverse colon (also known as the gastrocolic ligament) is entered bluntly or with an energy source. Care should be taken to ensure that the dissection does not extend into the mesocolon, which could cause bleeding or colonic ischemia. Depending on the transparency of the tissue, the division of the gastrocolic ligament proceeds toward the splenic flexure with electrocautery or with a dissecting-sealing device.

The advantage of the lateral decubitus approach becomes apparent during the dissection of the splenic flexure. As the colon is retracted inferiorly and medially with the right hand, the splenocolic ligament is transected (Fig. 27-3). This may best be performed using a sealing device because this ligament may contain small vessels. The flexure should fall away naturally from its attachments. The white line of Toldt then can be opened inferiorly toward the sigmoid colon. Careful attention to the planes of dissection must be maintained to avoid entering the lateral attachment of Gerota fascia, which would medialize the left kidney and reduce exposure of the operative field.

The second stage of mobilization involves dissection of the sigmoid colon and the rectum. This may be achieved with the surgeon standing on the left side of the table, facing the lower monitor. The patient is placed in a 30-degree Trendelenburg position. The small bowel is displaced with the aid of gravity out of the pelvis and is kept superiorly and to the patient's right. The white line of Toldt is incised further using electrocautery, and the avascular plane is entered to dissect the descending colon and sigmoid away from the sidewall (Fig. 27-4).

Care must be exercised to identify the ureter because its inadvertent injury is one of the major pitfalls of this operation. The ureter is identified as it courses along the psoas fascia. It is positioned medial to the gonadal vessel and crosses over the common iliac as it travels toward the trigone of the bladder. A gentle pinch of the ureter with an atraumatic grasper will generate ureteral peristalsis, confirming its identification.

As the peritoneal reflection in the pelvis is approached, it is incised along its anterior border 180 degrees, over the surface of the rectum. When dissection approaches the right side, great care must again be taken to identify the right ureter. Indeed, constant awareness of the ureters is essential throughout the remainder of the operation. The dissection of the rectum proceeds along the presacral fascia, using a combination of blunt dissection and an energy device.

At this point, a fourth 5-mm suprapubic trocar may be placed to aid in the anterior and lateral retraction of the rectum. Most of the posterior dissection of the rectum is avascular, but the median sacral artery (a direct branch of the aorta) will require ligation to avoid potentially heavy bleeding. The lateral suspensory ligaments of the rectum are avascular and can be dissected bluntly or with the aid of an energy device. An irradiated pelvis can present technical challenges to the operating surgeon. In the early postradiation period, perirectal tissue can be friable, leading to bleeding. Later on, irradiated tissue can become tough and woody, making the dissection difficult.

After the rectal mobilization, the vascular supply to the distal colon is ligated. The inferior mesenteric artery, just distal to the

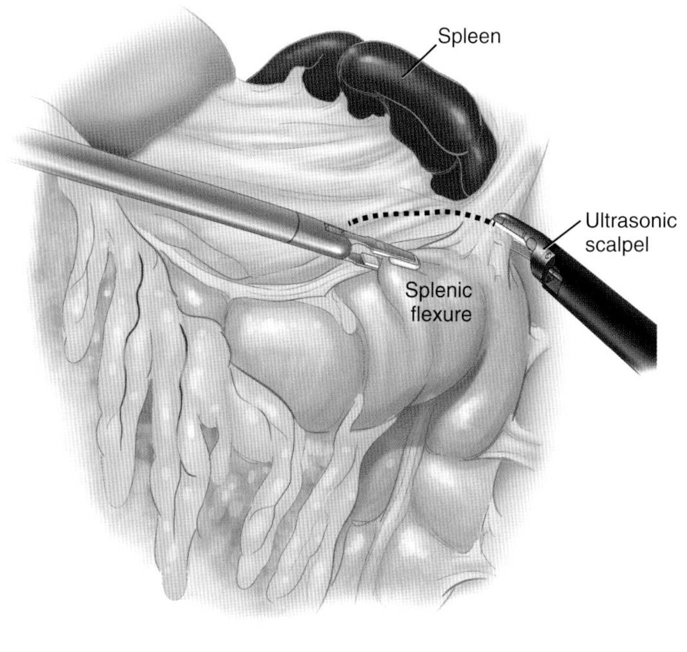

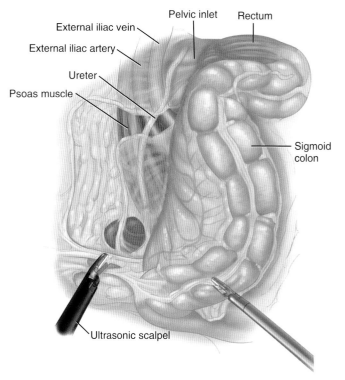

FIGURE 27-3   Transection of the splenocolic ligament.

FIGURE 27-4   Mobilization of the sigmoid colon. Inferior is at the top of the drawing.

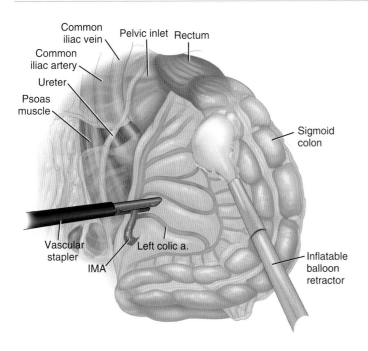
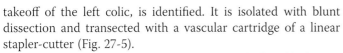

FIGURE 27-5   Ligation of the inferior mesenteric artery, distal to the left colic artery. Inferior is at the top of the drawing.

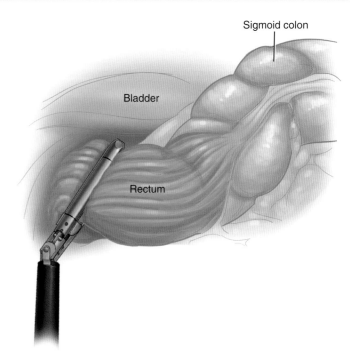

FIGURE 27-6   Transection of the distal rectal margin with the roticulating endo-GIA stapler. Inferior is at the top of the drawing.

takeoff of the left colic, is identified. It is isolated with blunt dissection and transected with a vascular cartridge of a linear stapler-cutter (Fig. 27-5).

The distal end point of dissection is the end of visible disease in a case of diverticulitis, or 2 cm beyond the lesion in colorectal carcinoma. When the distal end point of dissection has been reached, the surgeon inserts a finger into the rectum to identify the levators and to ensure that the dissection has proceeded beyond the lesion and not below the dentate line.

The proximal and distal borders of resection now should be determined. In the case of colorectal carcinoma, the lesion should have been identified by palpation or tattoo marking, or both. The distal resection margin of diverticular disease typically is at the peritoneal reflection. In the severe case of diverticulitis, however, that margin may extend lower into the pelvis. The proximal boundary of resection for diverticular disease is a section of colon that is not involved with inflammation, which can be determined after the bowel has been extracorporealized.

A 60-mm roticulating endo-GIA stapler is used to transect the distal margin (Fig. 27-6). This often can be achieved with a single firing of the stapler. If the rectum or perirectal tissue is too wide or thick, then multiple stapler applications may be needed. A limiting factor to stapling of the distal margin may be the male narrow pelvis. In this situation, two or three firings of a 45-mm endo-GIA stapler may be required to work across the distal margin. If multiple applications of the endo-GIA stapler are required, then the staple line must follow along the "crotch" (vertex) of the prior stapler application to avoid crossing the prior staple line. Such crossing could lead to stapler misfire or to is-chemic "tongues" of rectum that might result in anastomotic leakage.

With the distal rectum transected, the proximal rectosigmoid can be extracorporealized. The incision for the low lateral port is extended to 5 cm. A wound protector is placed in this incision to avoid infection and the possibility of seeding the incision with cancer. The descending colon and rectum (containing the speci-men) are exteriorized through this incision. After the proximal

colonic transection is performed with a linear stapler-cutter, the anvil of an appropriately sized EEA stapling device is inserted in the proximal bowel and tied in place with a pursestring suture around the anvil. The surgeon may use a disposable or reusable pursestring device or may opt to hand-sew a pursestring on the colonic end. The bowel (with the anvil in place) is returned to the abdominal cavity to perform the anastomosis in the pelvis.

Alternatively, the proximal resection can be performed intra-abdominally. The specimen is placed in an endoscopic specimen bag and brought out through the wound. This avoids specimen contact with the wound and obviates the need for a wound protector.

The colorectal anastomosis is performed in the usual manner. The extraction wound is closed, and the abdominal cavity rein-sufflated. The EEA stapler is inserted into the anus and advanced toward the proximal rectal stump. When the circular end is seen at the staple line, gentle traction is applied to the rectal stump, and the spike is twisted through this tissue. The descending colon then is juxtaposed to the rectum by grasping the hollow cylinder of the anvil and inserting the EEA spike into it (Fig. 27-7). The stapler is closed and fired, creating the colorectal anastomosis. The stapler "donuts" then are inspected for continuity, and the staple line is inspected with the rigid proctoscope for bleeding and for any discontinuity.

The anastomosis is tested for leakage by flooding the pelvis with water, compressing the colon proximal to the site, and instilling air into the rectum with the proctoscope. Bubbles ema-nating from the region of the anastomosis indicate a leak. A second leak test then may be performed by instilling an iodine solution into the rectum with a bulb syringe. A leak is indicated by billowing of the dark iodine solution through the clear fluid in the pelvis. The management of an anastomotic leak identified in the operating room depends on the clinical scenario and the surgeon's level of expertise. The options for such a leak include resection and redo of the anastomosis; reinforcement of

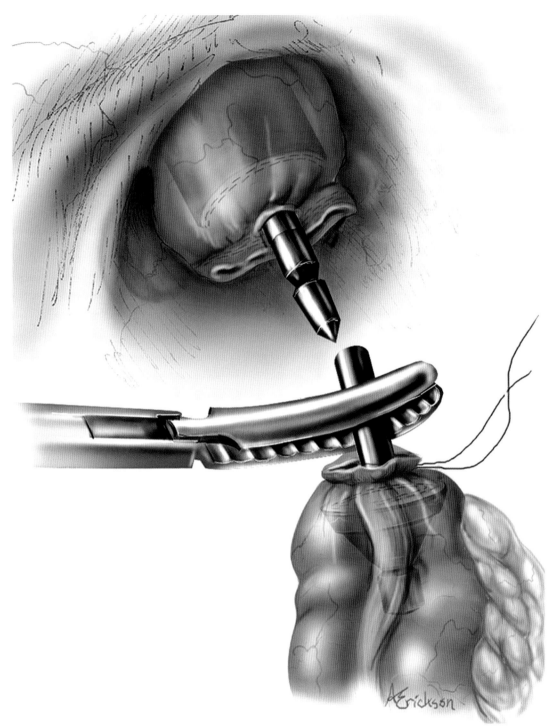

FIGURE 27-7   Connection of the EEA stapler anvil in the proximal colon with the spike of the EEA stapler penetrating through the rectal stump. (© Anne Erickson, CMI.)

the identified area of leak with intracorporeal sutures; diverting ileostomy; or closed-suction drainage. After the anastomosis has been performed, the irrigant is aspirated, hemostasis is confirmed, and the wounds are closed.

In about 20% of low colorectal anastomoses, there is insufficient length of descending colon to perform a tension-free anastomosis (Fig. 27-8). In such a case, it may be necessary to ligate and transect the inferior mesenteric vein (IMV) to provide full mobilization of the descending colon for a tension-free anastomosis. This maneuver adds a significant amount of time to the operation. Some authors, however, recommend routine IMV ligation to ensure familiarity with the anatomy and methodology for cases in which it is absolutely necessary. This is a technically

difficult maneuver and, if not performed correctly, may compromise the blood supply to the proximal anastomosis.

Ligation and transection of the IMV may be routinely performed before takedown of the splenic flexure or as needed when there is an insufficient length of descending colon. The transverse colon is retracted superiorly, and the small bowel is allowed to fall to the patient's right. The IMV should be visible at the root of the mesocolon as it ascends toward the pancreas and the splenic vein. Sharp dissection of the attachments of the fourth portion of the duodenum (i.e., the ligament of Treitz) is performed. Use of electrocautery should be minimal here to avoid duodenal injury. The vein is retracted anteriorly with the left hand, and sharp dissection is continued under it with the right

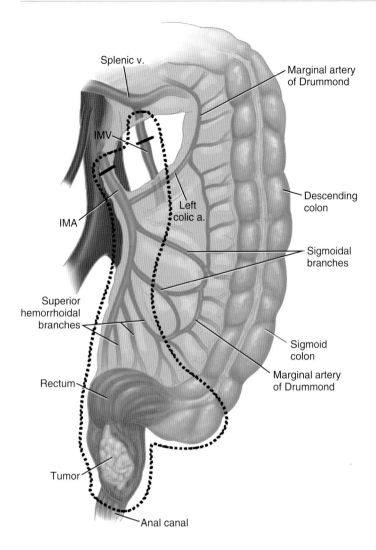

FIGURE 27-8   High ligation of the internal mesenteric artery and vein (IMA/IMV) during low anterior resection for malignancy. Superior is at the top of the drawing. Note the intact marginal artery, which is important in this scenario for perfusion of the colonic side of the anastomosis.

hand to mobilize the vein circumferentially. The IMV then may be doubly clipped and divided or divided with a sealing device. The mesocolon to the left of the IMV is divided to the border of Gerota fascia. The descending colon should now have greater mobility, allowing for a tension-free anastomosis.

POSTOPERATIVE CARE

We have adopted a "fast-track" clinical pathway for most of our colorectal surgery patients. They are required to sit in a chair or to walk on the same day as surgery. In an effort to avoid ileus, narcotic medication is avoided, and unless there is a contraindication, the patient is given intravenous or oral nonsteroidal anti-inflammatory drugs (NSAIDs) for pain. The patient is given clear liquids on the day of surgery or on postoperative day 1. The diet then is advanced to full liquids or regular, as tolerated. Routine postoperative laboratory tests are monitored on day 1. The urinary catheter is removed within the first 24 to 48 hours. Closed-suction drainage in the pelvis has not been shown to prevent infection, and we avoid its routine use. Patients are maintained on perioperative prophylactic antibiotics for 24 hours from anesthesia end time, and discharged on day 2 or 3.

MANAGEMENT OF PROCEDURE-SPECIFIC COMPLICATIONS

Bladder and sexual dysfunction are well-known complications of low anterior resection. Although the rate of bladder dysfunction is roughly equal between open and laparoscopic procedures, the rate of severe erectile dysfunction is almost twice as high for laparoscopic rectal surgery as for open (41% versus 23%, respectively).

The acceptable rate of clinically relevant anastomotic leakage is 3% to 6%, but some reported rates are as high as 30%. Patient-specific risk factors include malnutrition, steroid use, tobacco or alcohol use, cardiovascular disease, ASA score, and diverticulitis. Intraoperative risk factors include low anastomosis, poor anastomotic blood supply, prolonged operating room time, bowel obstruction, male gender, obesity, perioperative blood transfusion, and intraoperative septic conditions not conducive to primary anastomosis. It is unclear whether radiation is a risk for anastomotic leak. If a patient has been placed on preoperative bevacizumab (monoclonal antibody to vascular endothelial growth factor), then it is advisable to wait 60 days before surgery to minimize the risk for an anastomotic leak. The mortality rate of anastomotic leakage ranges from 0% to 30%. Although many leaks may occur in the hospital during the immediate postoperative period, a leak still may occur at home, after the patient has been discharged in apparent good condition.

RESULTS AND OUTCOME

We determined that our learning curve for optimal performance of the previously described technique was 38 cases. Our rate of conversion was 3% in the beginning and has decreased toward 0% with experience. Our morbidity and mortality rates were very low. Operative times decreased steadily each year in our series. The mean operative time for our entire study period was 125 minutes; in the fourth year, the mean operative time had decreased to 108 minutes. We have found that this technique is ideal for the patient who presents the surgeon with a technical challenge, such as from obesity, prior surgery, or ventral hernia (Fig. 27-9). Although this technique originally was designed for the patients with low, left-sided lesions, we have found that it is also applicable to those with lesions of the splenic flexure and proximal descending colon.

In 2007, we published results from our initial series of 100 patients who underwent colon resection with the medial to lateral approach. We have found that the number of procedures ("learning curve") to the optimal performance of a laparoscopic colon resection with this technique was 38. The average length of stay was 4 days for the entire series. Our rate of conversion was 3% in the beginning and decreased toward 0% with experience. Our rate of morbidity in the late group was 12% and included surgical site infection ($n = 2$), incisional hernia ($n = 1$), dehiscence ($n = 1$), acute renal failure ($n = 1$), anastomotic leak ($n = 1$), and cardiac arrest ($n = 1$). There was one death from cardiac disease in the late group, for a mortality rate of 2%. Operative times decreased steadily each year in our series. By our fourth year, the mean operative time was 108 minutes. The overall mean operative time for our entire study period was 125 minutes.

The advantages of the laparoscopic approach to colon resection are becoming increasingly apparent in the surgical literature.

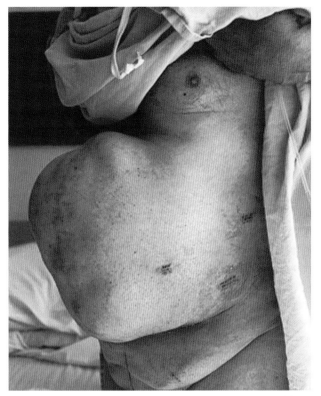

FIGURE 27-9   Patient with a preoperative massive ventral hernia with loss of domain who underwent a successful minimally invasive low anterior resection (LAR) in the right lateral decubitus position (photograph taken after LAR).

Recent data from the National Surgical Quality Improvement Program (NSQIP) database have demonstrated that, despite longer operative time, laparoscopic colectomy confers a significant improvement in the rate of surgical site infection (SSI) compared with open colectomy (9.5% laparoscopic vs. 16.1% open, $P < .001$). Another recent study from Massachusetts General Hospital demonstrated a significantly lower rate of anastomotic leak with laparoscopic compared with open sigmoid resection for

diverticular disease. A recent review of the Nationwide Inpatient Sample database (NIS, from the Healthcare Cost and Utilization Project, HCUP) demonstrated that the use of laparoscopy in colon resection was an independent predictor of a decreased mortality rate with respect to open colectomy.

In our practice, we have found that the technique of a lateral decubitus approach to laparoscopic low anterior resection is ideal for patients who present the surgeon with technical challenges. These include obese patients, those who have had prior surgery, and those with ventral hernia. Although this technique was designed and originally described for patients with low, left-sided lesions, we have found that it also is applicable to lesions of the splenic flexure and proximal descending colon.

Suggested Readings

Abraham NS, Young JM, Solomon MJ: Meta-analysis of short-term outcomes after laparoscopic resection for colorectal cancer, *Br J Surg* 91:1111–1124, 2004.

Bretagnol F, Panis Y, Rullier E, et al, for the French Research Group of Rectal Cancer Surgery (GRECCAR): Rectal cancer surgery with or without bowel preparation: The French GRECCAR III multicenter single-blinded randomized trial, *Ann Surg* 252:863–868, 2010.

Ferzli GS, Fingerhut A: Trocar placement for laparoscopic abdominal procedures: A simple standardized method, *J Am Coll Surg* 198:163–173, 2004.

Guller U, Jain N, Hervey S, et al: Laparoscopic vs. open colectomy: Outcomes comparison based on large nationwide databases, *Arch Surg* 138:1179–1186, 2003.

Jayne DG, Brown JM, Thorpe, H, et al: Bladder and sexual function following resection for rectal cancer in a randomized clinical trial of laparoscopic versus open technique, *Br J Surg* 92:1124–1132, 2005.

Kim J, Edwards E, Bowne W, et al: Medial-to-lateral laparoscopic colon resection: A view beyond the learning curve, *Surg Endosc* 21:1503–1507, 2007.

Kingham TP, Pachter HL: Colonic anastomotic leak: Risk factors, diagnosis, and treatment, *J Am Coll Surg* 208:269–278, 2009.

Murray A, Lourenco T, de Verteuil R, et al: Clinical effectiveness and cost-effectiveness of laparoscopic surgery for colorectal cancer: Systematic reviews and economic evaluation, *Health Technol Assess* 10:1–141, 2006.

Murray B, Huerta S, Dineen S, Anthony T: Surgical site infection in colorectal surgery: A review of the non-pharmacologic tools of prevention, *J Am Coll Surg* 211:812–822, 2010.

Nelson H, Sargent D, Wieand HS, et al, for the Clinical Outcomes of Surgical Therapy Study Group: A comparison of laparoscopically assisted and open colectomy for colon cancer, *N Engl J Med* 350:2050–2059, 2004.

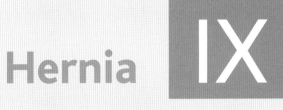

MICHAEL J. ROSEN

Minimally Invasive Ventral Hernia Repair with Endoscopic Separation of Components

The videos associated with this chapter are listed in the Video Contents and can be found on the accompanying DVDs and on Expertconsult.com.

A ventral incisional hernia is a protrusion of viscera through a previous abdominal incision into the subcutaneous tissue; the hernia contents typically are enveloped in a serous sac in continuity with the peritoneum. Because 11% to 20% of laparotomies result in an incisional hernia, incisional herniorrhaphy is one of the most common general surgical procedures, with more than 250,000 cases annually in the United States. Although the full economic burden of abdominal wall reconstruction is unknown, informal industry estimates have suggested that related health care costs amount to $2.5 to $3 billion per year.

An understanding of the objectives of ventral hernia repair can provide insight into the ideal technique and strategy for this procedure. A defect in the ventral abdominal wall predisposes patients to incarceration of the bowel and mesentery, which can lead to obstruction, strangulation, and perforation. In addition to these life-threatening complications, a ventral hernia can cause paradoxical movement of the abdominal contents during respiration, which can compromise pulmonary function (a particular problem in the patient with underlying lung disease). Complaints of back and abdominal pain due to the absence of the abdominal wall musculature also are common with ventral hernia. All of these scenarios can have a negative effect on quality of life, decrease functional activity, and produce long-term disability. Given the wide spectrum of patients suffering from abdominal wall defects and the range of defect anatomy, a tailored approach for each hernia would be prudent.

One of the foremost goals of ventral hernia repair is the prevention of intestinal herniation. Although primary suture repair of the defect could accomplish this goal, this technique was associated with an unacceptably high recurrence rate in all but the smallest of hernias. The introduction of prosthetic mesh dramatically reduced the recurrence rate after incisional hernia repair. Prosthetic mesh can be placed using a variety of techniques; no single technique has been able to provide an acceptable solution in every patient.

Laparoscopic ventral hernia repair was first reported in 1993 and generally was accepted as an approach to ventral hernia repair. In a typical laparoscopic incisional hernia repair, a large prosthetic mesh is placed in the retromuscular and intraperitoneal position. A possible advantage of the laparoscopic approach has been the avoidance of extensive soft tissue dissection; overall, the rate of wound complications and mesh infections has been less with laparoscopic compared with open repair. Although

placement of a large, retromuscular mesh to bridge a wide defect can prevent bowel herniation, use of this technique will not produce a functional, dynamic abdominal wall. In the active and thin patient, some form of a bulge or paradoxical motion can persist after repair and may result in patient dissatisfaction. In our practice, we have reserved the typical laparoscopic incisional hernia repair (with a large retromuscular and intraperitoneal mesh) for the obese or elderly patient. A slight bulge often is imperceptible by such a patient and thus of little consequence; furthermore, the risk for wound complications in this scenario usually outweighs other issues.

In 1990, Ramirez and others described a method of hernia repair in which the lateral abdominal wall musculature was separated to provide a tension-free fascial advancement for the repair; this technique was termed *components separation.* This repair method has undergone several modifications but essentially involves entrance into the lateral abdominal muscular compartment. This typically has been accomplished with large lipocutaneous flaps, incision of the external oblique fascia lateral to the linea semilunaris, and separation of the external and internal oblique muscles. As such, this technique essentially has been a major abdominal wall reconstruction. Problematic wound morbidity has been associated with components separation and has limited its widespread acceptance. Recent modifications, however, have enabled this procedure to be performed with endoscopic access to the lateral abdominal wall while achieving similar myofascial advancement.

Several investigators have begun evaluating the combination of (1) an endoscopic components separation with (2) a laparoscopic repair using a retromuscular and intraperitoneal mesh. Using the laparoscopic technique, the defect can be closed and prosthetic mesh placed to reinforce the repair. This minimally invasive functional abdominal wall reconstruction might offer the ideal physiologic reconstruction of the abdominal wall. This chapter focuses on the technical details of an endoscopic components separation with midline fascial reapproximation and reinforcement with a large subfascial mesh.

OPERATIVE INDICATIONS

An ideal abdominal wall reconstruction for a midline incisional hernia would provide a minimally invasive technique to release the external oblique muscles, enable laparoscopic adhesiolysis, reapproximate the midline, and reinforce the repair with permanent prosthetic material. Ideally, such a reconstruction would be performed without creation of the large lipocutaneous tissue flaps. Our approach is to perform an endoscopic components separation combined with a laparoscopic mesh herniorrhaphy that includes restoration of the linea alba, as described later.

Patient factors that favor a laparoscopic ventral hernia repair include a smaller defect region, lack of severe adhesions, a history of previous prosthetic infection, and a high risk for wound morbidity (e.g., secondary to obesity, advanced age, immunosuppression, or diabetes). Factors that support an open approach include known severe adhesions, a defect that extends to the bony confines of the abdomen (e.g., iliac crest, costal margin), and the need for formal abdominal wall reconstruction. The latter need is common in patients who do manual labor or are young, thin, active, and athletic, particularly if the defect is more than 10 cm wide.

Obese patients should be counseled to lose weight before ventral hernia repair. The morbidly obese patient may be given the option to lose weight by dieting or to undergo a bariatric procedure before definitive repair of the abdominal wall. Cessation of smoking is mandatory for all patients because smoking has been associated with an increased risk for wound complications and repair failure. A patient with a large pannus, skin ulcerations, or an extensive scar may be better served with a panniculectomy or scar revision as part of an open procedure.

The ideal candidate for minimally invasive ventral hernia repair with endoscopic components separation and midline reapproximation is a thin, active patient with an 8- to 10-cm wide defect, without an extensive midline scar, who desires a functional abdominal wall. An active patient who has undergone a previous laparoscopic incisional hernia repair may develop bulge at the repair site that represents flexing of the prosthesis where it bridges the defect. If the patient is dissatisfied with this result, then components separation may be an option for revision. If the patient has a hernial defect 12 cm or more in transverse dimension or has an abdominal wall that has been scarred with multiple stomas, drains, or infections, then midline approximation of the linea alba may not be possible, and other repair options should be considered.

PREOPERATIVE EVALUATION, TESTING, AND PREPARATION

Determination of the width and rostral and caudal extent of the hernia defect is important, as is determining other associated defects, such as "Swiss-cheese" defects (multiple small defects along a midline incision, associated with the sawing action of suture loops) or lateral defects associated with prior stomas. A preoperative abdominal pelvic computed tomography (CT) scan is routine for this determination. In addition, it is important to determine by CT whether there is loss of various layers of the abdominal wall. If a stoma is present, then its exact location within the rectus or the lateral abdominal wall can be ascertained. We no longer perform preoperative bowel preparation because it can produce bowel distention, making adhesiolysis more difficult.

The patient should be counseled before the procedure that transfascial fixation sutures will be placed to secure the mesh and medialize the rectus muscle, so there may be a degree of postoperative discomfort. Placement of an epidural catheter for postoperative pain management can be considered. Hospital stay for several days typically will be required. Managing a patient's expectations for an immediate flat abdomen is important; although the hernia sac is not excised, it usually becomes obliterated after the defect has been closed. A postoperative seroma still is possible.

PATIENT POSITIONING IN THE OPERATING SUITE

Prophylactic antibiotics are administered, and a Foley catheter and an oral gastric tube are inserted. The patient is positioned supine on the operating table with the arms extended, not tucked. When performing an endoscopic components separation, the lateral trocar must be placed in the posterior axillary line, which may not be possible if the arms are adducted. The patient is prepared widely to permit lateral trocar placement. Two laparoscopic towers are placed, one on either side of the patient's head.

POSITIONING AND PLACEMENT OF TROCARS

The costal margins and inguinal ligaments are identified and marked. The linea semilunaris, representing the lateral edge of the rectus muscle, is typically 8 to 10 cm from the midline (or edge of the defect); this landmark also is drawn bilaterally on the patient's abdomen. Placement of a port medial to the linea semilunaris (i.e., through the rectus muscle) will make the endoscopic separation difficult and might result in an open conversion. To insure port placement, we place the initial port (10 mm) just inferior to the 11th rib (Fig. 28-1). In general, the second port (5 mm) is placed in the posterior axillary line, 4 fingerbreadths inferior to the initial port. After the inferior release is completed, the third 5-mm port is placed within the release region, medial to the upper port. This port should be placed in a line with the cephalad transection of the external oblique muscle as it is taken over the costal margin.

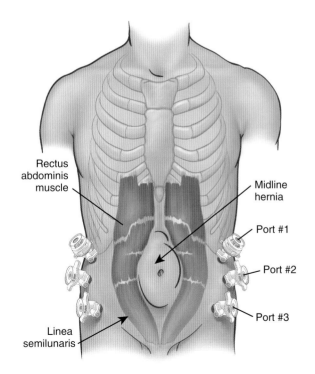

Rectus abdominis muscle

Midline hernia

Port #1

Port #2

Port #3

Linea semilunaris

FIGURE 28-1 Port positions for an endoscopic separation of components.

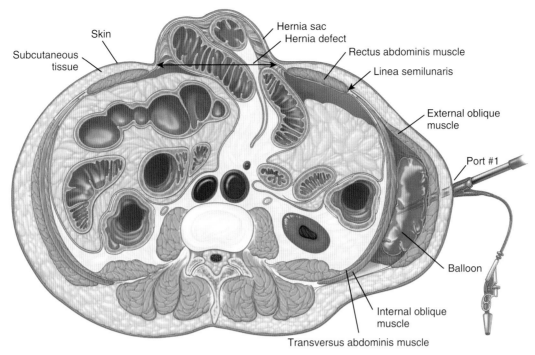

FIGURE 28-2 Creation of the space between the external and internal oblique muscles. Cross-sectional view from the feet.

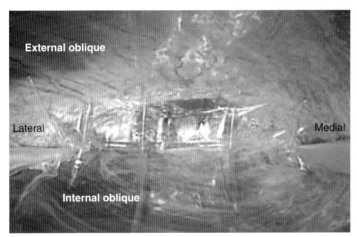

FIGURE 28-3 Endoscopic view into the inflated balloon, which is dissecting the space shown in Figure 28-2. View is caudal.

OPERATIVE TECHNIQUE

The bilateral endoscopic components separation is performed first. Performing this maneuver first prevents the potential problem of air leak into the abdomen, which can occur if the ports initially are placed into the peritoneal cavity. At the site chosen for port 1 (see Fig. 28-1), the external oblique fascia is localized with Kocher clamps through a 1-cm incision, incised sharply, and spread in the direction of its fibers. The internal oblique muscle with its filmy anterior fascia is identified, and the avascular plane between the external and internal oblique fascia is developed with narrow retractors.

A bilateral laparoscopic inguinal hernia balloon dissector (Covidien, Norwalk, Conn.) is passed into the space between the external and internal obliques and advanced caudally down to the inguinal ligament (Fig. 28-2). The balloon should meet little or no resistance because it is traversing an avascular plane. Inflation of the balloon separates the external oblique muscle from the underlying internal oblique muscle. This maneuver is performed under direct visualization from within the balloon to confirm the appropriate orientation of the respective muscle fibers (Fig. 28-3).

After inflation, the balloon dissector is removed, and a 30-mL balloon-tipped port is inserted through port site 1. Carbon dioxide insufflation to 10 to 12 mm Hg will allow adequate visualization yet should prevent subcutaneous emphysema. The tip of the camera can be used to complete the posterior lateral dissection bluntly. A 5-mm port (number 2 in Fig. 28-1) then is placed as far laterally as possible to provide the best angle to incise the external oblique fascia. Using scissors and cautery, the external oblique fascia is transected 2 cm lateral to the linea semilunaris in a caudal direction down to the inguinal ligament (Figs. 28-4 and 28-5); this also is known as the *fascial release*. Too medial an incision, crossing over the linea semilunaris, will result in a full-thickness defect and a lateral hernia. Such a defect would be difficult to repair, and would require a different operative approach. Maintenance of a 2-cm margin lateral to the linea semilunaris during the fascial release will prevent this complication.

After the fascia is released caudally, another 5-mm port (number 3 in Fig. 28-1) is placed through the area of the fascial release, medial to the initial camera port, to provide visualization of the rostral fascial transection. The camera then is repositioned in the posterior axillary line (port 2), and the scissors are placed in the inferior port. Transection of the external oblique fascia in the rostral direction is continued to a point 3- to 5-cm superior to the costal margin (Fig. 28-6). Meticulous hemostasis should be maintained during this maneuver because the bleeding from external oblique muscle trauma can occur in this region.

An identical components separation is performed on the contralateral side. After completion of bilateral components separation, the trocars for the laparoscopic intraperitoneal hernia repair are placed into the abdominal cavity. The port sites used for the endoscopic components separation may be reused to place the intra-abdominal trocars. All adhesions of the intra-abdominal contents to the posterior surface of the entire anterior abdominal wall are divided so that no attachments remain between the viscera and abdominal wall (Fig. 28-7). The transverse and longitudinal dimensions of the hernia defect are measured using spinal needles and a 15-cm ruler placed within the peritoneal cavity.

The fascial defect is reapproximated before mesh application. We typically do not excise the hernia sac or remove the peritoneum from the fascia, but this is an option. A small stab wound in the skin is made at the superior end of the hernia, and one end of a 1-0 polypropylene suture is dragged through the skin and fascial edge of the hernia defect with a suture passer (Fig. 28-8). The suture end is held within the abdomen with a laparoscopic grasper. The suture passer then is reinserted through the same skin incision and through the contralateral fascial edge. The suture end then is grasped with the passer and dragged out of the abdomen, making a loop to approximate the defect (Fig. 28-9).

Using the same general technique, these fascial approximation sutures also can be placed in a figure-of-eight fashion.

A series of these interrupted sutures are placed every 2 to 3 cm over the length of the hernia defect to create a secure musculofascial approximation. The insufflation pressure is

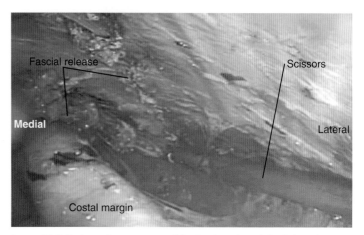

FIGURE 28-6 Endoscopic appearance of fascia, viewed cranially. Release is performed superior to the costal margin.

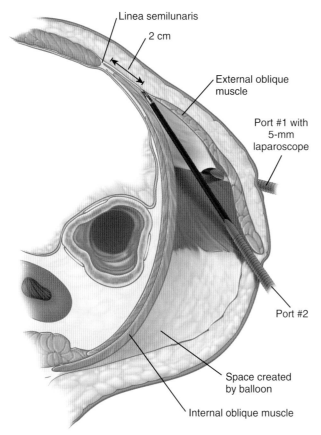

FIGURE 28-4 Fascial release. The scissors are transecting the external oblique fascia 2 cm lateral to the linea semilunaris.

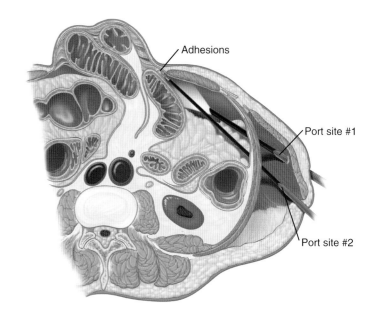

FIGURE 28-7 Laparoscopic adhesiolysis in preparation for the mesh placement.

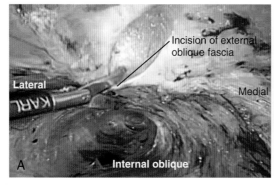
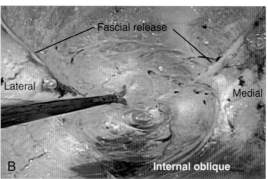

FIGURE 28-5 A, Endoscopic appearance of initial portion of fascial release described in Figure 28-4; caudal view. B, Endoscopic appearance after extensive incision, showing wide degree of fascial release.

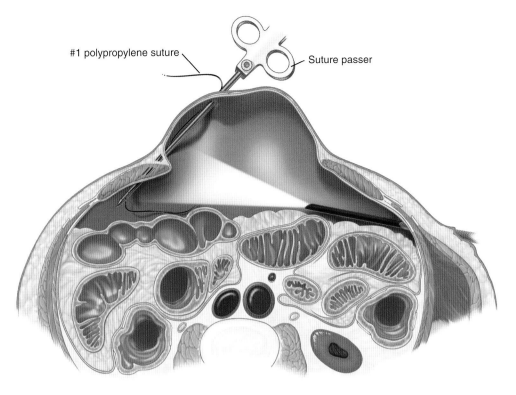

FIGURE 28-8 Placement of the suture into the peritoneal cavity for reapproximation of the midline fascia.

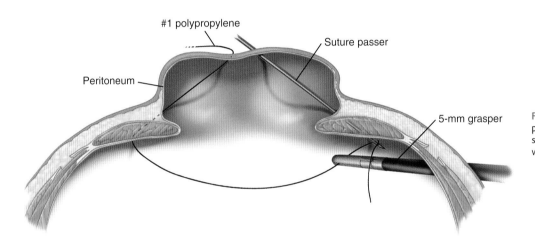

FIGURE 28-9 Suture placed in Figure 28-8 is pulled back out of the abdomen with the suture passer, completing a closure loop that will help pull the midline together.

decreased, and the sutures are tied with the knots below the skin on the fascia (Fig. 28-10). If the skin incisions are too large or the skin over the hernia is very thin, then these sites may leak insufflated CO_2. An occlusive dressing placed over these holes can address this issue. Because these sutures typically are placed under a fair amount of tension, the repair may become disrupted with prosthetic reinforcement. Therefore, a hernia mesh is prepared with dimensions based on the original defect measurements plus at least 4 cm of overlap. We believe it is important to use the original defect dimensions for the mesh to reduce the risk for recurrence. Downsizing the mesh for a closed defect, which might be done to reduce overlap and simplify fixation, is not advisable at this time. We typically use a nonresorbable synthetic mesh covered with an adhesion barrier, for which there are a number of commercially available options. This prosthesis is placed intraperitoneally in the underlay position and secured with transfascial sutures (Fig. 28-11). After placement of these transfascial sutures, a laparoscopic tacker is used to seal the mesh periphery (to prevent bowel from insinuating between the mesh and peritoneum) and flatten the mesh against the abdominal wall.

POSTOPERATIVE CARE

After a complex abdominal wall reconstruction, the patient typically is kept NPO until passage of flatus to minimize the risk for abdominal distention and retching, which are events that could lead to an early recurrence. Two postoperative doses of antibiotics are given. The patient is encouraged to ambulate the morning after surgery and is asked to wear an abdominal binder for at least 6 weeks.

MANAGEMENT OF PROCEDURE-SPECIFIC COMPLICATIONS

Loss of Intra-abdominal Working Space

After laparoscopic closure of the midline defect, the intra-abdominal working space will be diminished. With larger defects, reapproximation of the midline can bisect the abdomen into two separate spaces, which would make subsequent mesh placement very difficult. For this reason, we typically limit the components

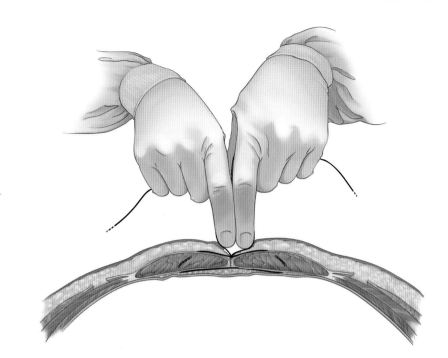

FIGURE 28-10 Tying of sutures for the midline reapproximation.

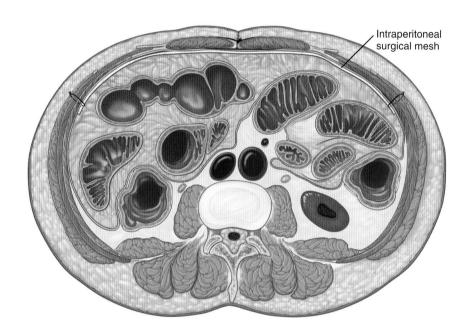

Intraperitoneal
surgical mesh

FIGURE 28-11 Placement of the reinforcing
intraperitoneal mesh using the sublay technique
with tacks and transfascial sutures.

separation procedure with laparoscopic mesh placement to the
defect that is less than 12 cm in width.

Postoperative Pain

These procedures typically result in more postoperative pain
than a standard laparoscopic ventral hernia repair because of the
additional transfascial sutures and the tension on the midline
fascial closure. Managing initial patient expectations for this discomfort in the early postoperative period is critical. Patients with
chronic pain at transfascial fixation sutures can be managed with
local injections or removal of the offending suture.

Seroma

Laparoscopic ventral hernia repair with intraperitoneal mesh
placement produces a seroma in virtually all patients. The patient

should be counseled not to expect a flat abdomen in the immediate postoperative period, nor to be concerned with an initial
bulge of a seroma. With the fascial closure technique, however,
the hernia sac usually is obliterated, and seroma rarely is a
problem that requires intervention.

Skin

Transfascial sutures placed in the midline or through a prior scar
can result in dimpling of the skin. Meticulous attention to appropriate release of the dermis from the transfascial sutures can
eliminate this problem. A patient with a large scar from a wound
that healed by secondary intention may not be the ideal candidate
for this procedure as described in this chapter because the scar is
not revised, and some patients will be unhappy with the cosmetic
result. Therefore, in our practice, the patient with a large midline
scar typically is offered an open repair with scar revision.

Hematoma

Hematomas can occur at the site of the muscle release during the components separation. The external oblique is at the greatest risk for postoperative bleeding as it extends over the costal margin, where the muscle usually is thicker. We have used either an ultrasonic scalpel (e.g., Harmonic scalpel, Ethicon Endo-Surgery, Cincinnati, Ohio) or a vessel-sealing device (e.g., LigaSure Vessel Sealing System, Valleylab, Boulder, Colo.) to obtain hemostasis in this region.

RESULTS AND OUTCOME

Endoscopic components separation has provided another minimally invasive approach to the reconstruction of complex midline hernia in the patient who desires a functional abdominal wall. In the treatment of these challenging defects, wound morbidity with endoscopic components separation has been substantially reduced and approaches the rates obtained with standard laparoscopic ventral hernia repair. To date, there is only one small series with short-term follow-up that describes the complete minimally invasive procedure (endoscopic components separation combined with laparoscopic midline closure and intraperitoneal mesh reinforcement), but the results are encouraging.

When attempting to determine the ideal approach to ventral hernia repair, it is important to consider the complexity of the patient, the size of the hernia defect, and the presence of contamination in each study. Each of these factors can dramatically affect the outcome and morbidity of abdominal wall reconstruction. Despite the heterogeneous nature of ventral hernia, we believe that the following reconstructive concepts may be applied: (1) prosthetic mesh should be applied with the sublay technique, as opposed to the onlay or inlay technique; (2) the mesh should have wide lateral overlap with respect to the defect to maximize surface ingrowth and support from the sublay positioning; (3) the rectus musculature should be reapproximated whenever possible; and (4) every step should be taken to minimize wound- and mesh-related morbidity.

Suggested Readings

Bachman SL, Ramaswamy A, Ramshaw BJ: Early results of midline hernia repair using a minimally invasive component separation technique, *Am Surg* 75:572–577, 2009.

Harth KC, Rosen MJ: Endoscopic versus open component separation in complex abdominal wall reconstruction, *Am J Surg* 199:342–347, 2010.

Malik K, Bowers SP, Smith CD, et al: A case series of laparoscopic components separation and rectus medialization with laparoscopic ventral hernia repair, *J Laparoendosc Adv Surg Tech A* 19:607–610, 2009.

Jin J, Rosen MJ: Laparoscopic versus open ventral hernia repair, *Surg Clin North Am* 88:1083–1100, 2008.

Ramirez OM, Ruas E, Dellon AL: "Components separation" method for closure of abdominal wall defects: An anatomic and clinical study, *Plast Reconstr Surg* 86:519–526, 1990.

Rosen MJ, Fatima J, Sarr MG: Repair of abdominal wall hernias with restoration of abdominal wall function, *J Gastrointest Surg* 14:175–185, 2010.

Rosen MJ, Jin J, McGee MF, et al: Laparoscopic component separation in the single-stage treatment of infected abdominal wall prosthetic removal, *Hernia* 11:435–440, 2007.

Rosen MJ, Williams C, Jin J, et al: Laparoscopic versus open-component separation: A comparative analysis in a porcine model, *Am J Surg* 194:385–389, 2007.

CONSTANTINE T. FRANTZIDES, SCOTT N. WELLE, AND TIMOTHY M. RUFF

Laparoscopic Repair of Complex Scrotal Hernia

29

The videos associated with this chapter are listed in the Video Contents and can be found on the accompanying DVDs and on Expertconsult.com.

The repair of complex scrotal hernias presents a unique challenge for the general surgeon. Use of the preperitoneal space offers several advantages during repair. The tissue planes are often relatively clean, the anatomy is easily appreciated, and the mesh may be placed posterior to the defect, which offers a mechanical advantage over anterior placement. The laparoscopic approach is able to fully utilize these advantages. The laparoscopic transabdominal preperitoneal (TAPP) approach to complex scrotal hernia repair also offers the advantages of being able to inspect bowel viability and to reduce the hernia contents and sac under direct visualization. Some controversy surrounds laparoscopic repair of these complex hernias. Discussion of this controversy is beyond the scope of this chapter; we believe that the laparoscopic TAPP repair is a safe, effective therapeutic option for complex scrotal hernias.

OPERATIVE INDICATIONS

Traditionally, the presence of an inguinal hernia was an indication for surgery in a patient able to tolerate anesthesia, regardless of whether the patient was symptomatic. The patient who presents with a large complex scrotal hernia, however, will probably have symptoms, for example, pain or intermittent bowel obstruction. These types of hernias also have an increased likelihood leading to life-threatening complications. Consequently, although repair of these hernias is still elective, surgical repair should be considered sooner rather than later. We prefer the laparoscopic TAPP approach for such hernias. Contraindications for a TAPP repair include the inability to tolerate a general anesthetic, the presence of infection, and moderate coagulopathy. Previous lower abdominal surgery may be considered a relative contraindication for a TAPP laparoscopic repair.

PATIENT PREOPERATIVE EVALUATION, PREPARATION, AND POSITIONING

The preoperative TAPP patient should undergo the required evaluation for general anesthesia. Aspirin and other nonsteroidal anti-inflammatory medications should be stopped 1 week before surgery. Shaving of the groin area should be done immediately before surgery. All patients should receive a single dose of first-generation cephalosporin, or equivalent antibiotic, to cover skin flora before incision in accordance with accepted guidelines.

The patient is placed in the supine position with both arms tucked. For large incarcerated scrotal hernias, placement of a Foley catheter is generally recommended. The video monitor is placed at the foot of the bed. The surgeon may stand on the same side as the hernia or the opposite side of the bed depending on preference. The assistant and camera operator stand on the side opposite of the surgeon.

TROCAR PLACEMENT

We prefer to access the abdomen using the open Hasson technique. A curvilinear incision is made inferior to the umbilicus, a 10-mm trocar is placed and the pneumoperitoneum is established. Two additional 10-mm trocars are then placed lateral to the rectus abdominis muscle at the same level as the infraumbilical port (Fig. 29-1).

OPERATIVE TECHNIQUE

The patient is placed in Trendelenburg position to allow displacement of the small intestine and omentum from the lower abdomen, and the hernia defect is identified (Fig. 29-2). Using gentle traction, the hernia contents are reduced. External pressure on the scrotum may be used to facilitate the reduction. With large incarcerated scrotal hernias, the bowel can often become very adherent to the cord structures and sac. Care must be taken to avoid iatrogenic injury to the bowel wall and cord structures during reduction. Reduction of the sac should be attempted without performing intestinal adhesiolysis because the lysis of these adhesions only increases the chance for bowel injury. After the bowel is returned to the abdomen, the hernia sac is evaginated into the abdominal cavity with steady pressure elevating the peritoneum away from the anterior abdominal wall. This maneuver can be facilitated by inserting a grasper into the inguinal defect and grabbing the end of the hernia sac. With large hernias, the sac can be very adherent to the cord, making reduction difficult. If unable to fully reduce the sac, at this point it is better to open the peritoneum and complete the mobilization and reduction from the preperitoneal space. The peritoneum is opened above the inguinal ring using hook electrocautery from the median umbilical ligament to a point about 10 cm laterally.

The inferior epigastric vessels are identified and preserved as they come up from the internal inguinal ring and course along the anterior abdominal wall (Fig. 29-3). The avascular plane between the peritoneum and underlying transversalis fascia is then bluntly dissected with a palpation probe or similar device, opening the preperitoneal space. Medially, the dissection is carried out until the Cooper ligament overlying the superior pubic ramus is clearly exposed. Often, a small blood vessel originating from the obturator artery is identified overlying Cooper ligament, and care must be taken to avoid injury to this vessel during dissection of the preperitoneal space or while anchoring the mesh in place.

Attention is then turned to dissecting the remaining hernia sac free from the spermatic cord. A combination of traction-countertraction pulling along the cord is used to reduce the sac.

Sharp dissection may also be used with care to avoid damaging the cord structures. Complete reduction of the hernia sac is important to minimize the probability of recurrence.

Once the sac is reduced, the space beneath the spermatic cord structures is developed that is necessary to allow the mesh to be placed around the cord in a keyhole fashion. Because of the proximity of the external iliac vessels, extreme caution needs to be taken when dissecting in this location. The spermatic cord is elevated, and with blunt dissection, a window underneath the cord is easily developed.

After the hernia sac has been completely reduced and the spermatic cord clearly delineated, attention is turned to the lateral dissection. When developing the lateral preperitoneal space, most of the adipose tissue can be left on the muscle layer,

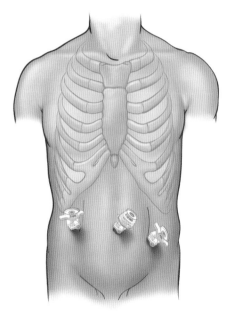

FIGURE 29-1 Trocar placement for laparoscopic scrotal hernia repair.

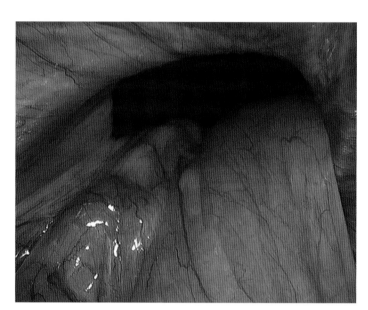

FIGURE 29-2 Laparoscopic view of large left scrotal hernia with incarcerated sigmoid colon.

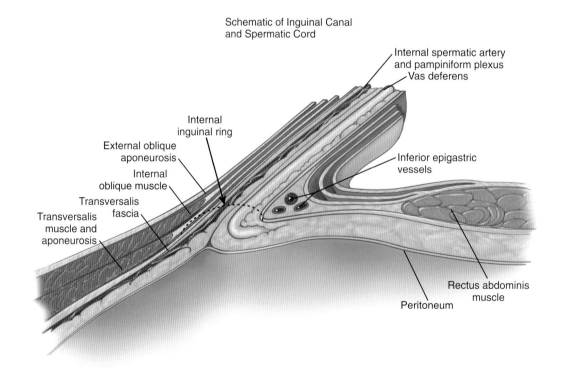

Schematic of Inguinal Canal
and Spermatic Cord

Internal spermatic artery
and pampiniform plexus
Vas deferens

Internal
inguinal ring

External oblique
aponeurosis

Internal
oblique muscle

Transversalis
fascia

Transversalis
muscle and
aponeurosis

Inferior epigastric
vessels

Rectus abdominis
muscle

Peritoneum

FIGURE 29-3 Schematic drawing of inguinal anatomy.

minimizing the risk for injury to the nerves crossing in this region. With large scrotal hernias, often the genital branch of the genitofemoral nerve separates from the spermatic cord, increasing the chance for injury. After this lateral dissection is completed, the surgeon should have a clear view of the pubic tubercle, Cooper ligament, internal inguinal ring, all hernia defects, the spermatic cord, the inferior epigastric vessels, and the arch of the transversalis aponeurosis. If all of these structures are clearly seen, the surgeon is ready for placement of the mesh.

The size of the defect is measured from the pubic tubercle to 3 cm lateral to the edge of the fascial defect to allow ample coverage of the hernia defect by the mesh. An instrument with a known dimension (e.g., the open jaws of a grasper) may be used to accurately measure the operative field laparoscopically. A number of prefabricated mesh products are available; however, we prefer to use a sheet of polypropylene mesh cut to the calculated size with a keyhole fashioned to surround the cord structures. The mesh is rolled around a 5-mm instrument and placed into the abdomen through a 10-mm trocar.

After the mesh has been inserted and unfurled, it is positioned around the spermatic cord by passing a grasper underneath the cord and dragging the inferior wing of the keyhole through the window. A marking stitch placed into the upper outer corner of the inferior wing may be used to facilitate this positioning. Care must be taken to ensure that the mesh does not become twisted or folded as it is brought underneath the cord. The mesh is flattened against the myopectineal orifice, ensuring that the inguinal floor, femoral triangle, and internal ring are all well covered by the mesh before fixation. If unable to obtain this coverage, then further dissection or repositioning of the mesh may be required.

Mesh fixation during laparoscopic inguinal hernia repair is controversial. The firing of tacks or staples from a posterior approach into the anterior abdominal wall has been implicated in causing chronic abdominal pain, presumably from nerve entrapment. Although fixation of mesh would appear to prevent slippage or migration of the mesh without subsequent recurrence, there are reports of favorable results without mesh fixation and also with fixation using other means such as glues. We prefer an intermediate approach, using judicious staple placement for mesh fixation.

Multiple different staplers and tackers are available for mesh fixation; we prefer to use a multifire straight hernia stapler (Endopath EMS, Ethicon Endo-Surgery, Cincinnati, Ohio). The ability to partially deploy the staple and then engage the mesh with one arm of the staple while the other arm bites into the tissue is a major advantage of the use of this stapler. This is in contrast to the helical tacker, which requires a full firing before ejection of the tack. Additionally, the force required for firing the straight stapler is considerably less than a helical tacker. Consequently, control over the depth of penetration using the straight stapler is better than with a helical tacker. The mesh should be secured medially to the pubic tubercle and the medial portion of Cooper ligament. Superiorly, staples may be placed along the edge of the mesh into the transversalis aponeurosis, medial to the inferior epigastric vessels. The inferior and superior wings of the keyhole should be approximated (Fig. 29-4). The mesh should be closed around the cord such that a 5-mm instrument can be slid easily alongside the cord.

During mesh fixation, the surgeon needs to be cognizant of the structures underlying the mesh. No staples should be placed inferior to Cooper ligament into the area inferomedially containing the iliac vessels (triangle of doom) or in the area inferolaterally containing the genitofemoral, femoral, and lateral femoral cutaneous nerves (triangle of pain). Additionally, one needs to be aware of the force used to secure the staples to the abdominal wall as injury to nerves and vessels anterior to the inguinal floor can occur if the force is too great.

On completion of the mesh fixation, the field is checked for hemostasis, and the peritoneal flap is closed to cover the mesh. Staples or sutures may be used to secure the flap over the mesh. Decreasing the pneumoperitoneum pressure before closing the flap may facilitate this closure. No portion of the mesh should be visible after the flap is reapproximated. All 10-mm port sites are closed, and the pneumoperitoneum is evacuated. The surgeon should then ensure that both testicles are present in the scrotum because during reduction of the hernia a testicle may be pulled into the inguinal canal. If the patient has developed a massive pneumoscrotum, then decompression can be accomplished with the use of an 18-gauge angiocatheter.

POSTOPERATIVE CARE

One dose of ketorolac can be administered in the operating room. The patient can usually be discharged home the same day with oral opioid for pain control. Lifting restrictions (no greater than 10 to 15 pounds) should be encouraged for at least 4 to 6 weeks. The patient should be evaluated postoperatively at 1 week, 1 month, and 3 months.

PROCEDURE-SPECIFIC COMPLICATIONS

Complications specific for the TAPP repair of large scrotal hernias include bladder injury, epigastric vessel laceration, spermatic cord injury or constriction, scrotal seroma or hematoma, and chronic groin pain and neuropathy. The risk for bladder injury can be minimized by maintaining bladder decompression. If the bladder is injured, then a urology consult may be considered to assist with the repair. In this scenario, the avoidance of permanent mesh placement should be considered. Epigastric vessel laceration typically is the result of trocar insertion. Transillumination of the abdominal wall with the laparoscope before placing the lateral trocars can minimize this risk. A bleeding inferior epigastric vessel can be suture-ligated with the aid of a laparoscopic needle passer. Injury to the spermatic cord can be avoided by careful dissection in the vicinity of the cord and by ensuring the mesh keyhole has not been closed too tightly around the cord structures. If the spermatic artery is injured, the testicle will likely undergo acute necrosis or atrophy. After the reduction of large hernias, the scrotum becomes a large empty potential space. Seromas are a common complication after scrotal hernia repairs. Scrotal hematomas are also common. Hematomas can result from excessive blunt dissection resulting in tearing of small capillary vessels of the cremasteric muscle fibers or an underlying coagulopathy. Both seromas and hematomas can usually be managed nonoperatively with rest, scrotal elevation, and ice as needed. The surgeon needs to resist the temptation of draining these fluid collections because doing so may introduce bacteria, infecting the collection and contaminating the mesh. Postherniorrhaphy chronic groin pain and neuropathies are the result of nerve injury or entrapment occurring during dissection or mesh fixation. The published incidence of nerve injury is 2% to 4%. The most commonly injured nerves are the femoral branch of the genitofemoral nerve, resulting in pain in the groin, scrotum, and upper thigh, loss of the cremasteric reflex, and ejaculatory

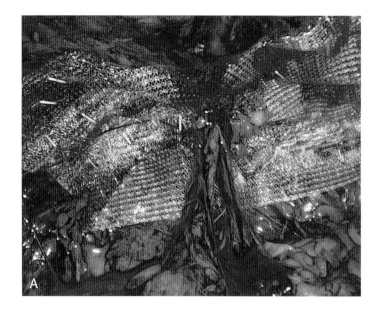

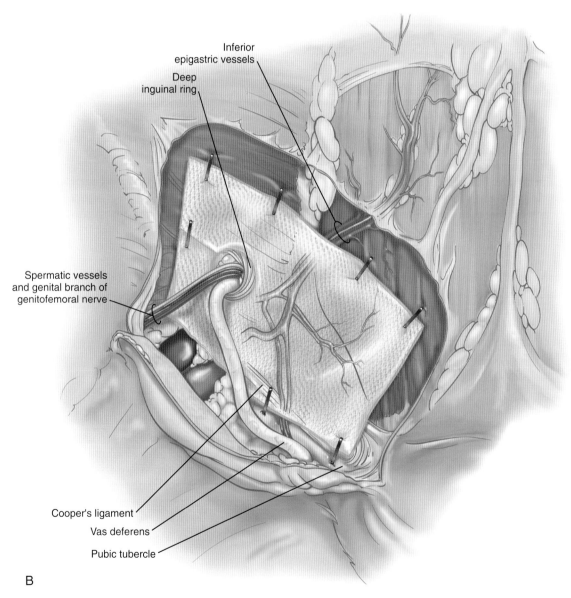

Figure 29-4 Placement of polypropylene mesh with a cut keyhole for laparoscopic scrotal hernia repair. **A,** Laparoscopic view. **B,** Schematic drawing.

dysfunction; and the lateral femoral cutaneous nerve, resulting in pain in the groin anterior and medial thigh. Less commonly, the ilioinguinal and iliohypogastric nerves can be injured if excessive force is used during the firing of the fixation device. The risk for chronic groin pain can be minimized by judicious mesh fixation as described earlier. The treatment of posthernior-rhaphy pain has variable success but is beyond the scope of this chapter.

RESULTS AND OUTCOMES

The adoption of laparoscopic inguinal hernia repair into the mainstream has been met with some resistance. Older papers reported that laparoscopic repairs resulted in a faster return to work and less chronic pain and numbness than open surgery. The laparoscopic repair, however, also resulted in longer operating times and higher complication rates. Other papers also reported higher recurrence rates with the laparoscopic repair. More recent reports, however, demonstrate the laparoscopic repair to be comparable to traditional repair for elective, reducible inguinal hernias. Of still some controversy is the laparoscopic repair of large incarcerated or strangulated scrotal hernias because of anticipated problems and complications in dissecting the extended hernia sac. Our unpublished results demonstrate the TAPP repair to be safe, effective, and durable in these types of hernias. Several smaller reports confirm that the TAPP repair of incarcerated scrotal hernias are not associated with higher complication or recurrence rates compared with the open repair and demonstrate an effective therapeutic option.

Suggested Readings

Deeba S, Purkayastha S, Paraskevas P, et al: Laparoscopic approach to incarcerated and strangulated inguinal hernias. *JSLS* 13:327–331, 2009.

Ferzli GS, Kiel T: The role of the endoscopic extraperitoneal approach in large inguinal scrotal hernias. *Surg Endosc* 11:299–302, 1997.

Frantzides C, Zografakis J, Carlson M: Laparoscopic transabdominal preperitoneal inguinal hernia repair. In Frantzides CT, Carlson MA, editors: *Atlas of Minimally Invasive Surgery*, Philadelphia, 2009, Saunders, pp 215–220.

Lantis JC 2nd, Schwaitzberg SD: Tack entrapment of the ilioinguinal nerve during laparoscopic hernia repair. *J Laparoendosc Adv Surg Tech A* 9:285–289, 1999.

Legnani GL, Rasini M, Pastori S, Sarli D: Laparoscopic trans-peritoneal hernioplasty (TAPP) for the acute management of strangulated inguino-crural hernias: A report of nine cases. *Hernia* 12:185–188, 2008.

Leibl BJ, Schmedt CG, Kraft K, et al: Laparoscopic transperitoneal hernia repair of incarcerated hernias: Is it feasible? Results of a prospective study. *Surg Endosc* 15:1179–1183, 2001.

Leibl BJ, Schmedt CG, Kraft K, et al: Scrotal hernias: A contraindication for an endoscopic procedure? Results of a single-institution experience in transabdominal preperitoneal repair. *Surg Endosc* 14:289–292, 2000.

McCormack K, Scott NW, Go PM, et al: Laparoscopic techniques versus open techniques for inguinal hernia repair. *Cochrane Database Syst Rev* 1CD001785, 2003.

Rosenberger RJ, Loeweneck H, Meyer G: The cutaneous nerves encountered during laparoscopic repair of inguinal hernia: New anatomical findings for the surgeon. *Surg Endosc* 14:731–735, 2000.

Seid AS, Amos E: Entrapment neuropathy in laparoscopic herniorrhaphy. *Surg Endosc* 8:1050–1053, 1994.

Stark E, Oestreich K, Wendl K, et al: Nerve irritation after laparoscopic hernia repair. *Surg Endosc* 13:878–881, 1999.

Laparoscopic Mesh Repair of Parastomal Hernia

CONSTANTINE T. FRANTZIDES, JACOB E. ROBERTS, SCOTT N. WELLE, AND TALLAL M. ZENI

30

The videos associated with this chapter are listed in the Video Contents and can be found on the accompanying DVDs and on Expertconsult.com.

The incidence of parastomal hernias after ileostomy and colostomy can be extremely high, 36% and 48%, respectively. Most occurrences are seen within the first 2 years after creation of the stoma. Several randomized trials have demonstrated the superiority of laparoscopic ventral hernia repair over the open approach; in contrast, although parastomal hernia is an incisional type of hernia, there is no consensus on the best method for this herniorrhaphy. The options for the surgical management of parastomal hernia include primary fascial repair, stomal relocation, and placement of varying types and shapes of mesh.

Traditional open parastomal hernia repair appears to have unacceptable rates of complications and hernia recurrence. Primary fascial repair has a recurrence rate of 46% to 76% at the ostomy site. Although stomal relocation results in a lower rate of hernia recurrence at the previous ostomy site than primary repair, it can be associated with an incisional hernia at the laparotomy site and a parastomal hernia at the new stoma site.

Over the past few years, several authors have reported their experience with laparoscopic parastomal hernia repair. Recently, laparoscopic parastomal hernia repair with synthetic mesh has also been described. The technique may result in lower rates of hernia recurrence; it appears to be safe, and the incidence of mesh erosion is low, although further studies are required. Advantages over the open techniques include avoidance of stoma relocation, reduction in postoperative pain, and decreased wound complications and other complications inherent to laparotomy.

OPERATIVE INDICATIONS

Asymptomatic patients may be managed conservatively; however, as many as 30% will require a surgical correction. The primary indication is the same as for other incisional hernias: pain, obstruction, bowel incarceration or strangulation, and persistent symptoms (i.e., difficulty with ostomy appliances, leakage, or skin maceration). Because there is a significant risk for recurrence, the symptoms must be substantial so that benefits outweigh the risks.

In this chapter, our technique is illustrated in the case of a permanent ileostomy parastomal hernia. The patient had undergone a laparoscopic total proctocolectomy with end ileostomy for ulcerative colitis 15 years earlier, performed by the senior author (CTF). The patient was experiencing intermittent bowel obstructions, with abdominal pain interfering with his everyday life. Our operative technique incorporates those principles applied in laparoscopic ventral hernia repair as well as in paraesophageal hernia repair with mesh, as described in the *Atlas of Minimally Invasive Surgery,* 2009 (see Suggested Readings at the end of this chapter).

PREOPERATIVE EVALUATION

Patients should undergo the necessary medical evaluation to determine fitness for general anesthesia. The history and physical examination should focus on all previous operations, and if possible all medical records should be obtained. The location, size, and extent of the parastomal hernia should be well documented, in addition to any incisional hernias present, to formulate an operative plan. It is imperative to obtain a computed tomography scan on all patients to determine size, location, and presence of any undiagnosed hernias. A standard bowel prep consisting of polyethylene glycol and oral antibiotics would be a prudent practice. This is justified by the potential risks for inadvertent enterotomy secondary to laparoscopic enterolysis often necessary during these operations.

PATIENT POSITIONING AND PLACEMENT OF TROCARS

The patient is placed supine on the table with both arms secured at the patient's side. Appropriate safety measures including belts or straps are placed to secure the patient for needed rotational changes. A urinary bladder catheter is placed for decompression to avoid inadvertent injury to the bladder.

The surgeon and assistant typically stand on the side opposite the hernia, facing the monitor. There is no consensus in the literature regarding establishment of pneumoperitoneum in patients with a stomal hernia or ventral hernia. Instead of using the blind insertion of the Veress needle in a previously operated abdomen, it would be advisable to use an optical bladeless trocar well away from the previous surgical site to gain access into the abdominal cavity. Another option includes the use of an open Hasson technique. Two additional 10-mm trocars are usually placed on the contralateral side of the hernia. Extra trocars may be placed as needed.

OPERATIVE TECHNIQUE

The operating table may be manipulated to change the patient's position to aid with the exposure and ease of surgical maneuvering. The use of a 30-degree laparoscope allows for better visualization of the anterior abdominal wall and the parastomal hernia (Fig. 30-1). Initially, the entire abdominal wall should be freed of all adhesions. This clearing of the abdominal wall allows for the identification of any associated midline incisional hernias in addition to the parastomal hernia. Adhesiolysis should be carried out with scissors rather than using an energy source. Thermal injury to the intestine with an energy source, such as the Harmonic scalpel (Ethicon Endo-Surgery, Cincinnati, Ohio) or electrocautery, can result in a full-thickness injury to the bowel that may not be seen initially.

Midline incisional hernias encountered after adhesiolysis may be repaired at the time of parastomal hernia repair (see the *Atlas of Minimally Invasive Surgery*, 2009 [see Suggested Readings at the end of this chapter]).

In the repair of parastomal hernias, the hernia contents are reduced using gentle traction with atraumatic graspers; the fascial defect is repaired with interrupted nonabsorbable sutures (Fig. 30-2). Because of the acute angles created by the location of the stoma on the abdominal wall, suturing with laparoscopic needle drivers and a free needle in this location can be challenging. Consequently, the use of the Endo Stitch (Covidien, Norwalk, Conn.) in this situation could be advantageous. In addition, extracorporeal knot-tying techniques ensure better formation of knots when tying tissue under tension. After the defect is closed, the bowel is anchored to the fascia with interrupted nonabsorbable sutures. The repair is then reinforced, with mesh acting as a buttress. A sheet of PTFE mesh (DualMesh, W. L. Gore and Associates, Flagstaff, Ariz.) is measured and fashioned into a horseshoe shape. The mesh is rolled up and passed through a trocar into the abdomen. Contact between mesh and skin should be avoided, and gloves should be changed before contact with the mesh. The mesh is placed around the ostomy site and secured to the anterior abdominal wall with a 10-mm hernia stapler (Endopath EMS, Ethicon Endo-Surgery, Cincinnati, Ohio). It is important to allow a 5-mm space between the mesh and the bowel, which may result in improved mesh ingrowth away from the bowel, thus reducing migration and subsequent erosion. Use of external counterpressure against the abdominal wall when firing the hernia stapler is imperative to ensure adequate fixation. The mesh is secured circumferentially to complete the repair (Fig. 30-3).

POSTOPERATIVE CARE

Early ambulation and use of the incentive spirometer are strongly encouraged after surgery. A clear liquid diet can be initiated after surgery and advanced as tolerated. A 1- to 2-day hospitalization is usually necessary. The patient should be educated to recognize symptoms consistent with a perforation (e.g., tachycardia, fever, increasing abdominal pain, persistent nausea, or failure to progress) and instructed to maintain a low threshold for contacting the surgeon. Patients should be followed up in 7 to 10 days after surgery to ensure good progression. It is important that the

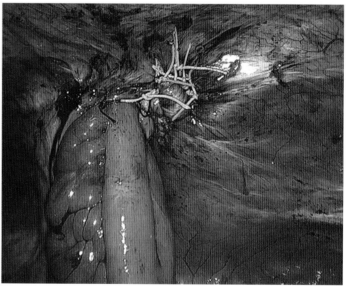

FIGURE 30-2 Laparoscopic repair of parastomal hernia with interrupted nonabsorbable sutures.

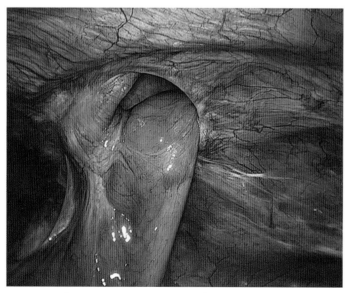

FIGURE 30-1 Laparoscopic view of parastomal hernia.

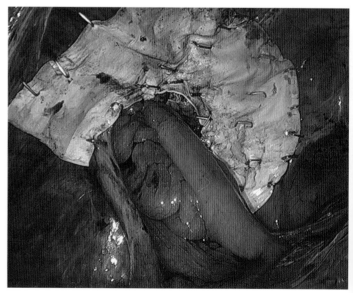

FIGURE 30-3 Mesh reinforcement of parastomal hernia repair.

patient avoid lifting anything greater than 10 to 15 pounds or any strenuous activity for 6 to 8 weeks after surgery.

PROCEDURE-SPECIFIC COMPLICATIONS

Complications associated with the laparoscopic repair of parastomal hernia include enterotomy, bowel obstruction, and mesh erosion. The occurrence and identification of an enterotomy at the time of surgery creates a logistical problem. In a prepped bowel, the enterotomy may be able to be laparoscopically repaired without gross spillage of enteric contents; thus, the use of synthetic mesh would not be precluded. However, if there is gross spillage of enteric contents, then the hernia repair should be performed with a biologic mesh, or the repair should be deferred to a later operation.

Missed intestinal injury after hernia repair is the most feared complication and can occur even in the hands of the most experienced of surgeons. Invariably under such circumstances, reoperation with removal of the mesh is imperative.

Bowel obstruction after parastomal hernia repair can occur with bowel herniating over the mesh, through the mesh keyhole, or from adhesions; if suspected, a computed tomography scan will often delineate it, and the complication can subsequently be managed accordingly.

RESULTS AND OUTCOMES

Several randomized trials have demonstrated the superiority of laparoscopic ventral hernia repair over the open approach. There is no consensus, however, on what is the best approach for the repair of parastomal hernias. Several authors have reported their experience with laparoscopic parastomal hernia repair; these studies include small numbers of patients and limited follow-up, allowing little room for establishing guidelines.

Within these reports, no one surgical technique dominates. There are many variations described: mesh type (synthetic vs. biologic), mesh modification (slit vs. nonslit), and techniques (keyhole vs. sling [Sugarbaker] vs. primary repair vs. stomal relocation). One consistency, however, is that the use of mesh for parastomal hernia repair results in fewer hernia recurrences. The technique for repair and mesh placement remains controversial. Recently, two of the larger studies report that keyhole techniques are associated with higher recurrence rates than the sling, or the modified Sugarbaker, technique. However, in these reports, the keyhole-type procedures were performed without fascial defect closure and without anchoring the bowel to the fascia, as we describe. In our small unpublished series of six patients using the previously described technique, no recurrences have been reported at a mean follow-up of 4 years, with no short- or long-term complications. These results are encouraging, although larger patient numbers and long-term follow-up assessment for this type of repair are still needed.

Suggested Readings

Craft RO, Huguet KL, McLemore EC, et al: Laparoscopic parastomal hernia repair, *Hernia* 12:137–140, 2008.

Frantzides CT, Carlson MA, Zografakis JG: Laparoscopic ventral hernia repair. In Frantzides CT, Carlson MA, editors: *Atlas of Minimally Invasive Surgery*. Philadelphia, 2009, Saunders, pp 221–226.

Frantzides CT, Granderath FA, Granderath UM, Carlson MA: Laparoscopic hiatal herniorrhaphy. In Frantzides CT, Carlson MA, editors: *Atlas of Minimally Invasive Surgery*. Philadelphia, 2009, Saunders, pp 31–40.

García-Vallejo L, Concheiro P, Mena E, et al: Parastomal hernia repair: Laparoscopic ventral hernia meshplasty with stoma relocation. The current state and a clinical case presentation, *Hernia* 15:85–91, 2010.

Hansson BM, Bleichrodt RP, de Hingh IH: Laparoscopic parastomal hernia repair using a keyhole technique results in a high recurrence rate, *Surg Endosc* 23:1456–1459, 2009.

Hiranyakas A, Ho YH: Laparoscopic parastomal hernia repair, *Dis Colon Rectum* 53:1334–1336, 2010.

Jani K: Laparoscopic paracolostomy hernia repair: A retrospective case series at a tertiary care center, *Surg Laparosc Endosc Percutan Tech* 20:395–398, 2010.

Lo Menzo E, Martinez JM, Spector SA, et al: Use of biologic mesh for a complicated paracolostomy hernia, *Am J Surg* 196:715–719, 2008.

McLemore EC, Harold KL, Efron JE, et al: Parastomal hernia: Short-term outcome after laparoscopic and conventional repairs, *Surg Innov* 14:199–204, 2007.

Muysoms EE, Hauters PJ, Van Nieuwenhove Y, et al: Laparoscopic repair of parastomal hernias: A multi-centre retrospective review and shift in technique, *Acta Chir Belg* 108:400–404, 2008.

Urinary System and Adrenal Glands

WOONG KYU HAN AND SEUNG CHOUL YANG

Video-Assisted Minilaparotomy Surgery for Living Donor Nephrectomy

Video-assisted minilaparotomy surgery (VAMS) is a hybrid of laparoscopic and open surgical techniques. A VAMS procedure typically is performed through a minilaparotomy, with a laparoscope and internal retractors placed through stab incisions. VAMS does not require pneumoperitoneum or gas insufflation; instead, the abdominal wall is lifted with internal retractors to provide a working space. Visualization of the operative field during VAMS may be obtained with both direct viewing and the laparoscope. Conventional instrumentation from both open and laparoscopic surgery may be employed in a VAMS procedure; instruments modified specifically for VAMS also may be used. The VAMS approach is particularly well suited for extraction of an intact solid organ through a minimal incision, such as with VAMS living donor nephrectomy, the topic of this chapter. The operative field in our description of VAMS living donor nephrectomy actually is the retroperitoneal space. Although we acknowledge that the use of the term *minilaparotomy* may not be entirely accurate in this circumstance (i.e., the peritoneal cavity is not entered), we still will employ the VAMS terminology for the sake of consistency.

OPERATION INDICATIONS

VAMS living donor nephrectomy is indicated for the removal of an intact kidney with ureter from a living organ donor for transplantation into a suitable recipient with end-stage renal disease. Donors should undergo proper medical and psychosocial evaluation preoperatively per the routine of the transplantation unit. The decision to permit voluntary donation of a kidney is made after a determination that there is no complicating mental dysfunction. The donor should be healthy and free of major medical problems, such as unstable coronary anatomy, heart failure, arrhythmia, valvular disease, coagulation disorders, thromboembolic disorders, and chronic lung disease (Table 31-1). Other contraindications to donor nephrectomy include age younger than 18 years, impaired renal function, renal disease, hypertension, diabetes mellitus, body mass index (BMI) more than 35, and pregnancy. Relative contraindications include microscopic hematuria, stone disease, and an abnormal kidney. In general, a history of multiple previous abdominal procedures is not a contraindication for VAMS donor nephrectomy because a retroperitoneal approach is used.

PREOPERATIVE EVALUATION, TESTING, AND PREPARATION

Each donor should undergo routine screening, including a medical history, physical examination, BMI determination, ABO blood typing, general biochemistry panel, hematology panel, pathogen antigen and antibody panels, 24-hour urine collection (for creatinine clearance, urinalysis, protein quantification, and culture), electrocardiogram, chest radiograph, and pregnancy testing. A donor BMI higher than 35 is a relative contraindication to donor nephrectomy, because of increased risk for postoperative donor morbidity. The glomerular filtration rate (GFR) should be 80 mL/minute or higher, or 2 standard deviations above the normal range based on age, sex, and body surface area. Donors with hypertension (blood pressure >140/90 mm Hg, as measured with ambulatory blood pressure monitoring) generally are excluded. Donors with diabetes (as defined in Table 31-1) also are excluded.

If asymptomatic microscopic hematuria (>3 red blood cells per high-power field) is diagnosed, then urine cytology and full urologic examination should be performed to eliminate the possibility of malignancy or stone disease. Renal biopsy is performed if there is a concern for glomerular pathology; if this is negative, then donation still may be considered. Candidates with more than 250 mg protein in a 24-hour urine collection are excluded. A candidate with a prior history of malignancy (especially melanoma or hematologic, renal cell, testicular, choriocarcinoma, bronchial, or breast cancer) typically is excluded from living kidney donation.

An asymptomatic candidate with a history of a single stone, no abnormal urine analysis findings (hypercalciuria, hyperuricemia, cystinuria, hyperoxaluria, or metabolic acidosis), and no evidence of nephrocalcinosis or multiple stones on computed tomography (CT) scan may be accepted for donation. An asymptomatic candidate with an existing single stone smaller than 1.5 cm in diameter, or a stone that can be removed intraoperatively, may be accepted for donation. On the other hand, candidates with bilateral stone disease, nephrocalcinosis, or recurrent stones should be excluded.

After the donor undergoes psychological and medical screening, donor-recipient compatibility is determined. A donor with ABO incompatibility and crossmatch positivity with the recipient traditionally has been excluded from donation; however, select

Table 31-1   Contraindications for Donor Nephrectomy, for the Donor

Absolute Exclusion Criteria

Age <18
Glomerular filtration rate <80 mL/min, or 2 standard deviations below
    normal based on age, sex, and body surface area
Hypertension: blood pressure >140/90 mm Hg
Diabetes: history of diabetes or random blood glucose levels ≥200 mg/dL,
    fasting blood glucose levels ≥126 mg/dL, or 2-hr glucose levels
    ≥200 mg/dL in an oral glucose tolerance test
Proteinuria: protein levels >250 mg/24 hr
High risk for perioperative morbidity and mortality, including presence of
    renal disease, cardiovascular disease, or pulmonary disease
Transmissible disease (HIV, hepatitis)
Psychiatric problems
Pregnancy

Relative Exclusion Criteria

Asymptomatic microscopic hematuria >3 red cells/high-power field
Obesity: body mass index >35 kg/m²
Nephrolithiasis, single stone
Multiple medical comorbidities
History of malignancy

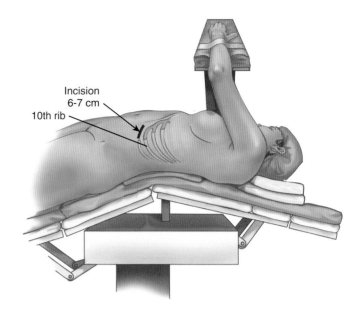

FIGURE 31-1 The semilateral position for VAMS donor nephrectomy.

mismatches of this type have been transplanted recently. The candidate with a transmissible disease such as HIV, hepatitis, cytomegalovirus (CMV) infection, or syphilis also is excluded.

CT scanning is performed routinely to delineate the renal vascular anatomy. Renal scintigraphy is performed routinely to rule out urinary obstruction and to determine right versus left renal function. The left kidney generally is chosen for donation, because of the longer length of the vessels on the left. The right kidney may be used, however, if the left kidney has one or more of the following: multiple renal vessels; a relative function of more than 10% below normal; or a duplicated ureter.

PATIENT POSITIONING IN THE OPERATION SUITE

The patient is placed in the semilateral position on the operating table, as shown in Figure 31-1. The torso is positioned with the level of the kidney over the central point of bed flexion. The ipsilateral arm is fixed on an arm board, which is positioned between the upper neck and the head. A cushioning roll (viscoelastic polymer gel) is placed under the axilla. A rolled sheet is placed under the back of the patient to stabilize the torso. The contralateral leg is bent slightly, the ipsilateral leg is stretched, and a cushion is placed between the legs. The operating table then is flexed about 30 degrees at the level of the kidney. On completion of positioning, the ipsilateral shoulder will be rotated up and the hips will remain flat with respect to the table. The table flexure will have expanded the operative area between the costal margin and the iliac crest. A Foley catheter is placed. All wires, tubes, and lines are routed along the top of the operating table, near the edge. If these objects are left to fall directly off the table, then they will hinder subsequent installation of the retractors.

POSITIONING AND PLACEMENT OF TROCARS

The operative space in our description of VAMS donor nephrectomy is the retroperitoneal space. In general, the operative space in a VAMS procedure is established with (1) a piercing

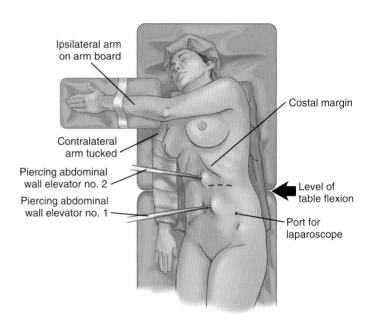

FIGURE 31-2 Basic retraction procedure for VAMS donor nephrectomy.

abdominal wall elevator, (2) a piercing peritoneal (visceral) retractor, and (3) blades from an external self-retaining retractor system. The piercing abdominal wall elevator, as its name implies, enters the operative space through a separate stab incision and provides lift to the abdominal wall (Fig. 31-2). Because the operative space will be open to the atmosphere through the minilaparotomy incision, lift from abdominal wall elevator will expand this space. As described in detail later, the head of the piercing peritoneal retractor is inserted into the operative space through the minilaparotomy incision, positioned against the anteromedial abdominal wall, and held in place with an arm that pierces through the abdominal wall and is clamped to the external system.

The external self-retaining retractor system we employ is a Thompson type (Thompson Surgical Instruments, Traverse City, Mich.), specifically developed for VAMS donor nephrectomy.

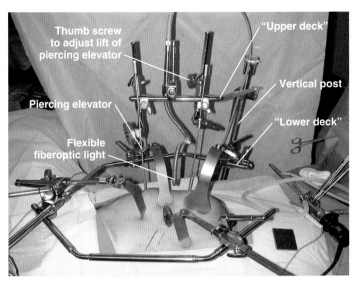

FIGURE 31-3 Setup for the external self-retaining retractor system for VAMS donor nephrectomy. Patient's right side is up, with the head to the left.

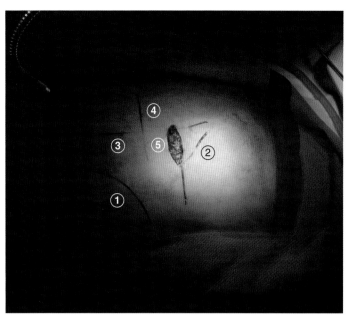

FIGURE 31-5 Skin incision for VAMS donor nephrectomy. Patient's left side is up, with the head to the right. (1) Iliac crest; (2) costal margin (10th rib); (3) lateral margin of rectus abdominis; (4) umbilical level; (5) skin incision.

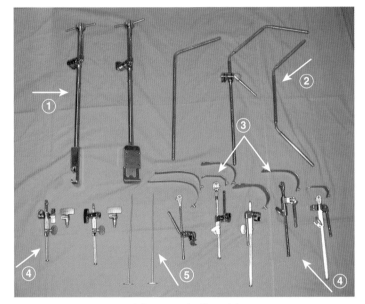

FIGURE 31-4 Components of the external self-retaining retractor system: (1) two rail clamps; (2) three types of horizontal crossbars; (3) an assortment of surgical blades; (4) various clip-on and sliding handles; and (5) a pair of piercing abdominal wall elevators.

(Fig. 31-3 shows system setup; system components are shown in Fig. 31-4). This device can provide both horizontal and vertical traction simultaneously by means of its "double-decker" configuration (see Fig. 31-3). A major advantage of this configuration is that the donor nephrectomy can be performed without the need for a retracting assistant.

A 6- to 7-cm transverse skin incision is made 2 fingerbreadths superior to the level of the umbilicus, beginning at the lateral border of the rectus abdominis and extending laterally to the costal margin (Fig. 31-5; see Fig. 31-2). The subcutaneous fat is dissected off of the abdominal wall fascia, including the anterior rectus sheath. The lateral half of the rectus sheath is incised transversely (Fig. 31-6), and this incision is carried laterally through the fascia enveloping the external oblique muscle. The muscle layers are split in the direction of their fibers, and the rectus is retracted medially to expose the peritoneum, which is not violated.

The inferior half of the incision is elevated with a hand-held Richardson retractor, and the underlying peritoneum is swept away from the abdominal wall. When an adequate space has been created, the Richardson is replaced with the Mayo (Balfour) blade of the Thompson retractor; the blade is connected to a horizontal bar, which in turn is affixed to a vertical post, which is clamped to a bed rail on the side contralateral to the operation, about level with the groin (Fig. 31-7). The Mayo blade will provide upward traction so that the operative field may be prepared. The peritoneum and the abdominal wall then are further separated with a sponge stick to develop the retroperitoneal space.

After the retroperitoneal space has been developed, a 10-mm (or 5-mm) trocar is placed about 7 cm inferior to the minilaparotomy in the anterior axillary line, just superior to the iliac crest (Fig. 31-8; see Fig. 31-2). A 10-mm (or 5-mm) laparoscope is inserted through this port. A piercing abdominal wall elevator then is passed through the abdominal wall from inside the operative space, exiting about 4 cm medial and inferior to the minilaparotomy (Fig. 31-9; see Fig. 31-2). The "T" end of the elevator is positioned against the inner abdominal wall, and the externalized arm of the elevator then is clamped to the horizontal bar of the Thompson retractor. The Mayo blade that was positioned earlier is removed, and the horizontal bar then is adjusted to its maximal height (about 30 cm above the table) on the vertical post; this horizontal bar will constitute the "upper deck" of the external retractor system (Fig. 31-10; see Fig. 31-3). The lift provided on the anterolateral abdominal wall by the piercing elevator can be adjusted with a thumb screw on the device that attaches the elevator to the horizontal bar (see Fig. 31-3).

The hand-held Richardson retractor is used to elevate the upper half of the incision, and the retroperitoneal space is developed superiorly with a sponge stick. A second piercing abdominal wall elevator is placed about 10 cm superior to the first elevator, in the same vertical line (see Fig. 31-2). The second elevator also is attached to the upper horizontal bar (see Figs. 31-3 and 31-10), and lift is adjusted as needed with the thumb screw.

A second vertical post is placed, this time ipsilateral to the operative side, about 5 cm inferior to the level of the axilla (see

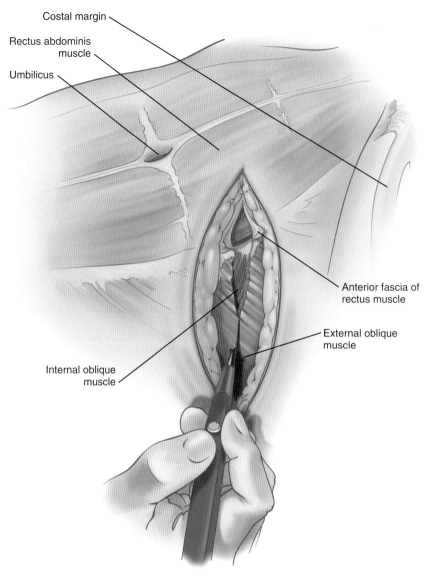

Costal margin

Rectus abdominis muscle

Umbilicus

Anterior fascia of rectus muscle

External oblique muscle

Internal oblique muscle

FIGURE 31-6 Incision of fascial layers for the minilaparotomy of VAMS donor nephrectomy.

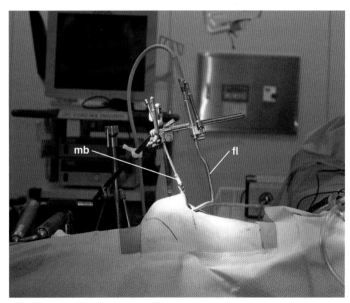

FIGURE 31-7 Mayo blade (mb) of the Thompson retractor elevating the inferior portion of the incision, allowing development of the retroperitoneal space. Patient's left side is up, with the head to the right. fl, Adjustable fiberoptic light.

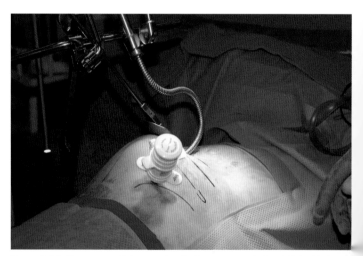

FIGURE 31-8 Placement of the port for the laparoscope. Patient's left side is up, with the head to the right.

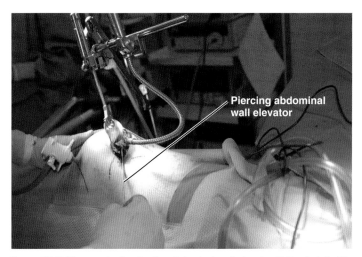

FIGURE 31-9 Placement of a piercing abdominal wall elevator. Patient's left side is up, with the head to the right.

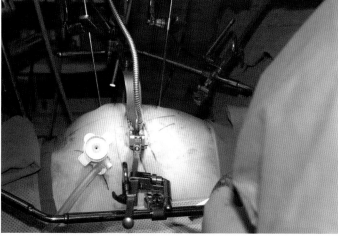

FIGURE 31-11 Retraction of the operative space using blades placed on the lower deck of the external system. Patient's left side is up, with the head to the right.

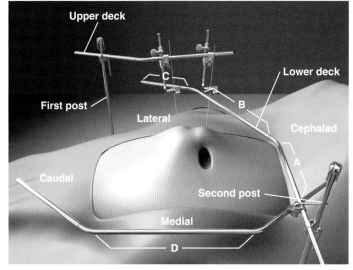

FIGURE 31-10 Graphic of the external retractor system, demonstrating the double-decker configuration and the two vertical posts. Patient's left side is up, with the head to the right.

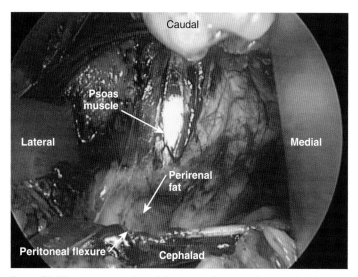

FIGURE 31-12 Laparoscopic view of the retroperitoneum after creating the operative space for left VAMS donor nephrectomy. An Army-Navy retractor is seen at the lower left of the photograph, further mobilizing the peritoneal sac.

Fig. 31-10). Horizontal bar no. 2 is affixed to this second post and extends over the anterior side of the patient; horizontal bar no. 3 is affixed to bar no. 2 and extends over the posterior side of the patient (see Figs. 31-4 and 31-10). Horizontal bars no. 2 and no. 3 constitute the lower deck of the external retractor system. A large Harrington (heart-shaped) blade is installed on section C of the lower deck (see Fig. 31-10), and a narrow blade is placed on section D, so that traction and counter-traction can be maintained on the operative space (Fig. 31-11). The peritoneal sac is swept medially; the Harrington blade is used to keep the peritoneal sac out of the operative field (Fig. 31-12). An Army-Navy retractor may be used to facilitate this dissection, as guided by laparoscopic visualization (see Fig. 31-12). The final operative setup of the retraction system is depicted in Figure 31-13.

OPERATIVE TECHNIQUE

The following description is for a left donor nephrectomy. The ureter is identified with gentle blunt dissection running along the medial surface of the psoas muscle (Fig. 31-14). Using gentle lateral traction on the ureter, this structure is dissected down to the bifurcation of the iliac artery, using judicious application of

electrocautery. The ureter should not be skeletonized, but rather mobilized with the surrounding fat and small vessels intact. After the ureter has been mobilized, the lower pole of the kidney is released from medial adhesions (Fig. 31-15). The medial border of the kidney is separated from the peritoneal sac until the hilum is reached. The kidney then is retracted medially with a retractor blade on its lateral side, and the lateral attachments of the kidney to the spleen and abdominal wall are cut.

The gonadal vein is encircled with a right-angle clamp and then ligated (Fig. 31-16). Tributaries to the renal vein are divided with ties on the specimen side and locking clips on the donor side. The hilum of the kidney is lifted gently with a retractor blade to expose the lumbar vein on the underside of the renal vein. The lumbar vein is isolated and ligated (Fig. 31-17). The renal vein is dissected medially until the adrenal vein is identified on the superior surface; the adrenal vein then is ligated (Fig. 31-18). The left renal vein is dissected circumferentially, cleaning off the adjacent connective tissue and fat. The left renal artery then is identified and mobilized to its juncture with the aorta.

After the major hilar vessels have been dissected, the left ureter is divided above two titanium endoclips placed on the donor side (Fig. 31-19). The left renal artery then is transected

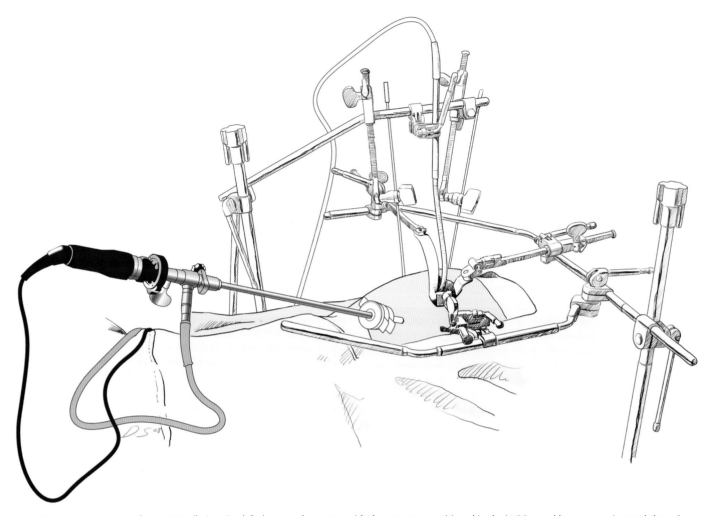

FIGURE 31-13 Operative setup for a minimally invasive left donor nephrectomy, with the retractors positioned in the incision and laparoscope inserted through its port.

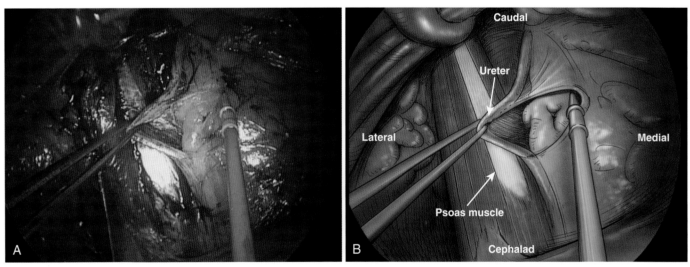

FIGURE 31-14 Dissection of the ureter for left VAMS donor nephrectomy.

between titanium clips (Fig. 31-20), and the stump on the donor side is oversewn with continuous 5-0 polypropylene suture. The left renal vein is ligated with an extra-large Hem-o-lok clip (Weck Pilling, Research Triangle Park, NC) and transected (Fig. 31-21); the donor stump of the renal vein also is oversewn with continuous 5-0 polypropylene suture. During a right donor nephrectomy, Satinsky vascular clamps may be used to control the renal vein to facilitate its transection.

After the renal vessels have been cut, the kidney is extracted in a lap sac. If the size of the kidney is larger than the incision, then the retractor blades are removed so that the minilaparotomy incision may be slightly enlarged. After the specimen has been removed, the operative field is inspected for hemostasis. The camera port then is removed, and a closed-suction drain is placed through this port site. An anatomic, layered closure of the minilaparotomy incision then is performed.

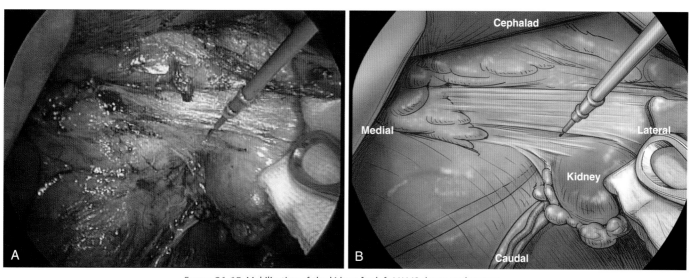

FIGURE 31-15 Mobilization of the kidney for left VAMS donor nephrectomy.

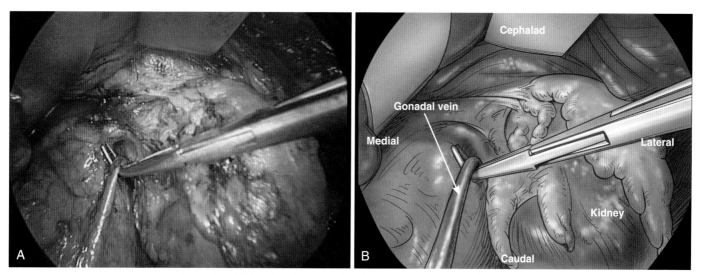

FIGURE 31-16 Dissection of the gonadal vein for left VAMS donor nephrectomy.

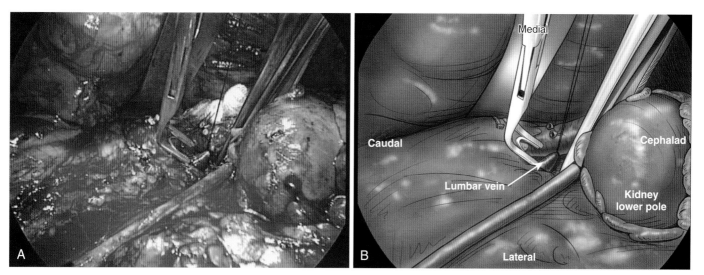

FIGURE 31-17 Dissection of the lumbar vein for left VAMS donor nephrectomy.

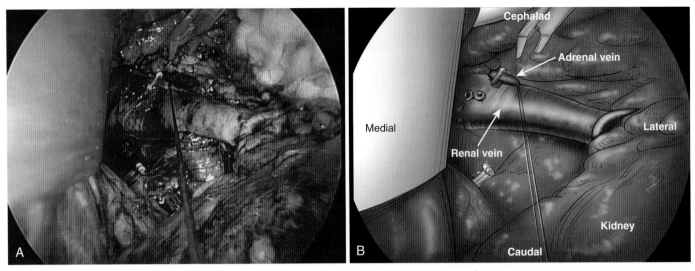

FIGURE 31-18 Dissection of the adrenal vein for left VAMS donor nephrectomy.

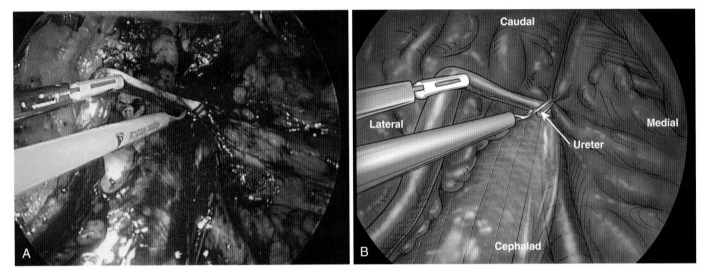

FIGURE 31-19 Transection of the ureter for left VAMS donor nephrectomy.

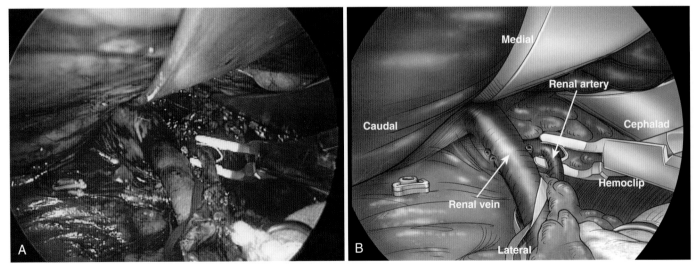

FIGURE 31-20 Ligation of the renal artery for left VAMS donor nephrectomy.

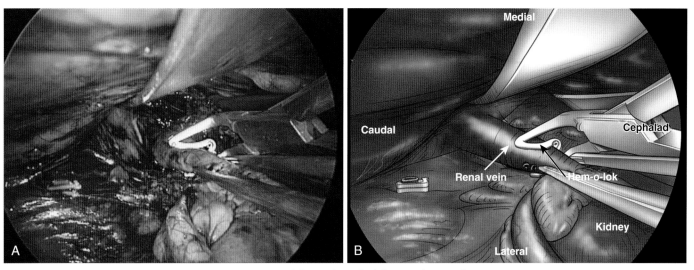

FIGURE 31-21 Ligation of the renal vein for left VAMS donor nephrectomy.

POSTOPERATIVE CARE

After surgery, early ambulation is encouraged. Urine output is maintained with intravenous hydration. Complete blood counts and serum chemistries are monitored. The bladder catheter generally is removed on postoperative day 1. The closed-suction drain is removed 2 to 3 days after surgery, and the patient typically is discharged 3 to 5 days after surgery. Follow-up visits are scheduled at 1, 3, and 6 months and annually after the operation. Testing at these visits includes urinalysis, complete blood count, and broad chemistry panel. An abdominal sonogram to image the remaining kidney is obtained annually.

MANAGEMENT OF PROCEDURE-SPECIFIC COMPLICATIONS

Excessive retraction on the minilaparotomy may predispose the patient to wound dehiscence, which has a 1.5% incidence in this procedure. To minimize the risk for this complication, strong retraction on the wound edge is used only when necessary, as during the hilar dissection. Lymphocele is a rare complication (0.1% incidence) of the retroperitoneal approach. To minimize the risk for this complication, lymphatics should be coagulated or ligated thoroughly during the procedure. If drainage of lymphatic fluid persists in the postoperative period, then the drain is maintained and the patient is placed on a low-fat diet. If this dietary manipulation does not resolve the leak, then the patient is placed on a medium-chain triglyceride diet (or nothing per os), and total parenteral nutrition is instituted. Any fluid collection not adequately drained by the closed-suction drain placed at the operation should undergo percutaneous drainage by an interventional radiologist.

RESULTS AND OUTCOME

Between 2003 and 2010, 720 VAMS living donor nephrectomies (120 right and 600 left) were performed at the Yonsei Severance Hospital. The mean age was 39 ± 11 years. Right-sided donor nephrectomy was done because of vascular anomalies, relatively poor renal function, or nephrolithiasis on the left side. Eighty and 45 patients had multiple renal arteries and veins, respectively.

Three patients had duplicated ureters that were implanted with a common channel. The mean operative time was 189 minutes (range, 60 to 380 minutes), and the mean warm ischemia time was 197 seconds (range, 0.5 to 15 minutes; minus the 15-minute outlier, the range was 30 to 270 seconds). With the donor patients placed on a modification of diet in renal disease (MDRD), the preoperative GFR (normalized to a body surface area of 1.7 m^2) was 92 ± 15 mL/minute; the GFR at 1 year while still on the MDRD was 64 ± 10 mL/minute.

The intraoperative complication rate was 3.8% ($n = 27$), including renal artery branch laceration, laceration of the junction of the gonadal or lumbar vein with the renal vein, and failure of lumbar vein ligation slip ($n = 3$ each). Five patients had an estimated blood loss of more than 500 mL or required blood transfusion, including one case of renal vein laceration. There was no open conversion, and there was no injury to bowel, liver, spleen, or other adjacent organ. The reported rate of intraoperative complications for other forms of living donor nephrectomy has been 4.6% to 4.9%.

Our postoperative complication rate after VAMS living donor nephrectomy ($n = 40$, or 5.6%) was lower than after other types of living donor nephrectomy, according to a 2009 meta-analysis of laparoscopic and open procedures (10.9% and 10.8%, respectively). Wound dehiscence ($n = 11$, 1.5%) was the most frequent postoperative complication; however, secondary wound closure was not needed in any patient. A blood transfusion was given in nine patients (1.4%) for presumed postoperative bleeding; however, no patient underwent reoperation for bleeding. Other complications in our series included wound site pain ($n = 5$), urinary retention ($n = 4$), and paresthesia of the scrotum and thigh ($n = 2$), which were all managed nonoperatively. Massive lymphorrhea (>500 mL/day) occurred in three patients and was treated with prolonged drainage and, in one patient, with readmission and insertion of a pigtail catheter. In one patient, partial slippage of the renal artery clip was detected on a CT scan, and this patient underwent reoperation. Complications exceeding grade IIIb (Clavien-Dindo classification) did not occur in our series.

Regarding kidney recipient outcomes in our experience, the postoperative 1-year MDRD GFR was 54.8 ± 23.7 mL/minute. Delayed graft function occurred in seven patients (1.0%). There was one recipient who had a vascular complication, and the ureteral complication rate was 1.1% (8 patients). This latter rate was lower than that reported for either open or laparoscopic living donor nephrectomy. The 1-year and 5-year graft survival rate was 98.6 and 98.2%, respectively. Twenty-one grafts were lost during the entire study period; the most frequent cause of graft loss was patient death (with a functioning graft kidney, $n = 8$) and then acute rejection ($n = 7$). A primary nonfunctioning kidney occurred in one recipient.

ACKNOWLEDGMENTS

We would like to thank Dr. Kyung Hwa Choi and D. S. Jang for their support with medical illustrations.

Suggested Readings

Antcliffe D, Nanidis TG, Darzi AW, et al: A meta-analysis of mini open versus standard open and laparoscopic living donor nephrectomy, *Transplant Int* 22:463–474, 2009.

Choi KH, Yang SC, Lee SR, et al: Standardized video-assisted retroperitoneal mini-laparotomy surgery for 615 living donor nephrectomies, *Transpl Int* 24:973–983, 2011.

Han WK, Lee HY, Jeon HG, et al: Quality of life comparison between open and retroperitoneal video-assisted minilaparotomy surgery for kidney donors, *Transpl Proc* 42:1479–1483, 2010.

Kim S, Huh K, Kwon K, et al: Kidney transplantation in Yonsei University from 1979-2003, *Clin Transpl* 183–192, 2003.

Kim SI, Rha KH, Lee JH, et al: Favorable outcomes among recipients of living-donor nephrectomy using video-assisted minilaparotomy, *Transplantation* 77:1725, 2004.

Lee YS, Jeon HG, Lee SR, et al: The feasibility of solo-surgeon living donor nephrectomy: Initial experience using video-assisted minilaparotomy surgery, *Surg Endosc* 24:2755–2759, 2010.

Yang SC: Video-assisted minilaparotomy surgery (VAMS)-live donor nephrectomy: 239 cases, *Yonsei Med J* 45:1149–1154, 2004.

Yang SC, Ko WJ, Byun YJ, Rha KHO: Retroperitoneoscopy assisted live donor nephrectomy: The Yonsei experience, *J Urol* 165:1099–1102, 2001.

Yang SC, Park DS, Lee DH, et al: Retroperitoneal endoscopic live donor nephrectomy: Report of 3 cases, *J Urol* 153:1884–1886, 1995.

Yang SC, Rha KH, Kim YS, et al: Retroperitoneoscopy-assisted living donor nephrectomy: 109 cases, *Transpl Proc* 33:1104–1105, 2001.

Quoc-Dien Trinh, Jesse D. Sammon, and Kevin C. Zorn

Laparoscopic Partial Nephrectomy

CHAPTER

32

The videos associated with this chapter are listed in the Video Contents and can be found on the accompanying DVDs and *on Expertconsult.com.*

Relative to radical nephrectomy (RN), nephron-sparing surgery with partial nephrectomy (PN) has been demonstrated to provide equivalent oncologic control, improved renal function, a lower risk for cardiovascular disease, and improved overall survival. Techniques developed for obligatory PN (solitary kidney, renal insufficiency, synchronous tumors, genetic predisposition) have also been used in the setting of a healthy contralateral renal unit. As a consequence, RN is no longer an acceptable option when a PN is indicated and is technically feasible. Moreover, wide dissemination of surgical techniques and continued improvement in instrumentation have made PN the preferred approach for small masses of the kidney.

More recently, laparoscopic partial nephrectomy (LPN) has been shown to have functional and oncologic outcomes comparable to those of open surgery. LPN is technically more demanding to perform, and it has been shown to have a steep learning curve. In this chapter, we describe our transperitoneal technique for LPN and discuss strategies for the prevention and management of complications.

OPERATIVE INDICATIONS

The indications for partial nephrectomy include bilateral tumors or a mass in the presence of renal insufficiency or in a solitary functioning kidney. In addition, the indications for PN now include the patient with a normal contralateral kidney. The indications for LPN have broadened to include more challenging cases, such as tumors larger than 4 cm, multiple tumors, hilar tumors, and completely endophytic masses.

Contraindications for LPN are similar to those for open PN, including active peritonitis, coagulopathy, bowel obstruction, and severe cardiopulmonary disease. Renal anatomic anomalies, such as horseshoe or ectopic kidney, do not preclude the laparoscopic approach, provided that adequate preoperative imaging has been obtained to delineate renal vascular supply. Relative contraindications are related to the surgeon's experience and comfort level. A history of previous abdominal or ipsilateral kidney surgery may be considered a relative contraindication. A retroperitoneal approach may be preferable in such a case to avoid intra-abdominal adhesions.

Obesity had been considered a relative contraindication to LPN. Initial access in obese patients (body mass index [BMI] >30 kg/m^2) can be difficult, resulting in a higher likelihood of abdominal wall vessel injury and subcutaneous dissection. Longer trocars and bariatric laparoscopic instrumentation should be available. Skin-to-peritoneum distance can be calculated from abdominal imaging. Port placement and entry angle to the subcutaneous tissue should allow for instrument triangulation and freedom of movement. With adequate operative experience, LPN in obese patients may be attempted. The Cleveland Clinic experience with obese patients (BMI >30 kg/m^2) has suggested that LPN is technically feasible in this patient group. Specifically, when compared with a cohort of open PN controls, obese patients undergoing LPN experienced reduced blood loss and analgesic requirement, quicker return of bowel function, reduced hospital stay, and shorter convalescence; operative times and complication were similar. Comparing obese and nonobese subjects undergoing LPN, other authors have reported longer operative times and increased blood loss with the obese group, but with similar complication and conversion rates and recovery period. Overall, an obese patient appears to have a comparable outcome to that of a nonobese patient when undergoing LPN by an experienced surgeon. We recommend that initial operative experience with LPN should be obtained with nonobese patients to minimize the risk for complications and open conversion.

Although PN remains the standard of care for small renal masses, ablative techniques have demonstrated acceptable oncologic outcomes in series with short-term follow-up, and represent viable alternatives to PN. Preliminary studies appear to have favored cryoablation rather than radiofrequency ablation, but this may change with additional data. Interestingly, observational series (i.e., no resection or ablation) have shown that very few patients demonstrate disease progression while on active surveillance. Some have suggested that delayed intervention may be a viable management strategy.

PREOPERATIVE EVALUATION, TESTING, AND PREPARATION

As part of the preoperative workup, all patients should have a complete history and physical examination, with particular attention to prior abdominal surgical history. During the assessment, the patient's body habitus, location of previous surgical incisions, and presence of skeletal deformities should be noted. Each of these factors can influence the choice of laparoscopic approach, patient positioning, and port placement. The informed consent discussion should include the risk for bleeding, injury to peritoneal contents, and the possibility of open conversion, which occurs in about 5% of LPN procedures.

Preoperative laboratory studies include a complete blood count, serum chemistries, coagulation panel, urinalysis, and urine culture. Chest radiograph and electrocardiogram also are obtained. Additional pulmonary function studies and cardiac workup are ordered as needed. Clinical suspicion of advanced disease or metastasis should entail additional imaging, such as a chest computed tomography (CT), head CT, and bone scan. A type and screen is obtained, and two units of packed red blood cells are crossmatched. Anticoagulants and platelet inhibitors should be stopped 5 to 7 days before surgery.

Candidates for LPN should undergo a staging workup with CT or magnetic resonance imaging (MRI). An abdominopelvic CT scan, with and without intravenous contrast and with a 10-minute delayed phase and coronal and sagittal reconstructions, is our imaging modality of choice. This study provides an excellent depiction of perirenal anatomy, including the location and number of renal vessels, as well as the location of the ureter. A CT scan is helpful in detecting the presence of aberrant renal vessels, which are known to occur in 25% to 40% of kidneys. If an accessory vessel is suspected but not well defined on CT, some surgeons recommend that an angiogram (CT, MRI, or conventional) should be performed to rule out the presence of vascular variants.

CT also allows the surgeon to assess the relationship of the kidney (position and rotation) to adjacent structures and to obtain an accurate estimate of the amount of perirenal fat present. In patients with a history of atherosclerosis, one should carefully examine the noncontrasted images of the CT scan to identify renal artery wall calcifications. If mural calcification is present, particularly at the ostium, the renal artery should be dissected and clipped at a point where the vessel is free of atherosclerotic disease. Vessel fracture during clip application can cause severe arterial hemorrhage. Imaging also can be used to calculate the RENAL (*r*adius of tumor; *e*xophytic/endophytic properties, *n*earness of tumor to the collecting system; *a*nterior/posterior descriptor; *l*ocation relative to the polar line) Nephrometry Score (RNS), a standardized classification system that quantifies the salient anatomy of renal masses. In patients undergoing LPN, a higher RNS is associated with an increased estimated blood loss, warm ischemia time, and length of hospital stay.

Gadolinium-enhanced MRI also is a suitable consideration for patients with renal impairment or contrast allergy. Finally, if there are concerns regarding the residual renal function, a MAG-3 (mercaptoacetyl triglycine, chelated to technetium-99m) nuclear scan with differential function may be useful.

Preoperative bowel preparation rarely is needed, and depends on the anticipated difficulty of the case. In our experience, if the kidney is not involved with an inflammatory process, then the patient is placed on a clear liquid diet the day before surgery and the bowel preparation omitted. Another option is a limited bowel preparation protocol consisting of a clear liquid diet and a bottle of magnesium citrate the day before surgery. If significant difficulty with dissection is expected, then the patient should undergo a full mechanical bowel preparation along with antibiotics the day before surgery. All patients should be given a parenteral antibiotic, usually a first-generation cephalosporin, in the preoperative holding area. Subcutaneous heparin and pneumatic compression stocking are administered before anesthesia induction.

An orogastric tube and Foley catheter also are inserted before patient positioning.

PATIENT POSITIONING IN THE OPERATING SUITE

The patient is placed in a modified lateral decubitus position using an underlying beanbag, with the thorax rotated back slightly at 30 degrees (Fig. 32-1). The lower hand is padded and placed on an armrest. The lower leg is flexed at the knee 90 degrees, and the upper leg is left extended. Pillows are placed between the legs for adequate support. Padding is placed under the lower ankle to relieve pressure in this area. An axillary roll then is placed 5 cm caudal to the axilla to protect the brachial plexus from a stretch injury. Additional padding is placed under the lower elbow to prevent ulnar nerve compression. The beanbag then is placed on vacuum to secure the final position. The umbilicus and spine should be visible to ensure adequate exposure in the rare need for an emergent open conversion. Surgical towels are placed over the skin at the hip and knee levels, and 3-inch silk tape is wrapped circumferentially at these levels to completely secure the patient to the table. Finally, an armrest is fastened to the table and secured to support the padded ipsilateral arm. Careful attention to final position and pressure padding is essential because bed rotation during surgery is often required to optimize exposure and assist with gravity bowel retraction. Care is taken not to obstruct any intravenous line.

POSITIONING AND PLACEMENT OF TROCARS

Transperitoneal access is our preferred approach to LPN, given the larger working space, familiar landmarks, greater versatility of instrument angles, and improved ease of suturing that this approach affords. The important anatomic landmarks for initial access are the subcostal margin, the umbilicus, and the rectus abdominis muscle. Standard port placements for right- and left-sided procedures are summarized in Figures 32-2 and 32-3 (four ports for left and five for right), respectively.

In patients with previous abdominal surgery, the initial entry site should be well away from scars and prior surgical fields. We favor the use of a 12-cm, 14-gauge Veress needle to insufflate the abdomen. Initial access is obtained at the level of the umbilicus, about 8 to 10 cm lateral to the midline. A greater distance should be used in an obese patient in whom the abdominal pannus falls with gravity. The surgeon should confirm correct placement by first applying gentle suction through the needle using a 10-mL syringe to ensure that no bowel contents or blood is aspirated. Saline should then be injected and aspirated; on release of the syringe, the fluid meniscus should drop secondary to the negative intra-abdominal pressure. Failure to gain access should prompt an open approach with the Hasson technique.

Once the Veress needle is in proper position, insufflation then is initiated with CO_2 to raise the intra-abdominal pressure to 20 mm Hg. The surgeon should examine and percuss the abdomen periodically during insufflation to confirm proper Veress placement and ensure that no significant subcutaneous emphysema is developing. When the appropriate intra-abdominal pressure is achieved, the needle is removed. An Optiview trocar (Ethicon, Cincinnati, Ohio) then is placed under camera guidance.

All remaining ports are placed in a subcostal configuration under direct visual guidance using a 5-mm, 0-degree laparoscope

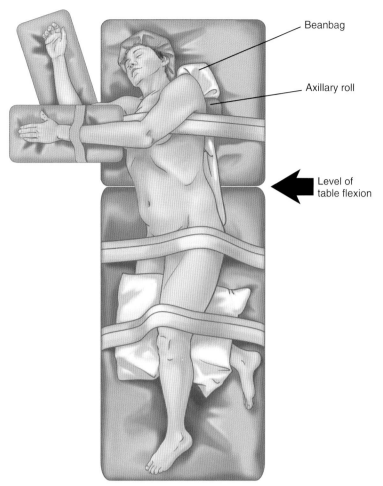

FIGURE 32-1 Patient positioning for a laparoscopic partial nephrectomy.

(see Figs. 32-2 and 32-3). We have developed a generalized approach for renal surgery in which nearly identical trocar configurations are used for both extirpative and reconstructive procedures. Adaptation of a standard approach simplifies surgical planning and facilitates transferring of laparoscopic techniques to the trainee. The entry sites of the trocars are marked after the abdomen has been insufflated.

We routinely place two 5-mm trocars through the pararectus line so that all ports are distanced at least 7 to 8 cm from one another. A lateral trocar is placed along the midaxillary line, halfway between the anterosuperior iliac spine and the costal margin. For a right-sided procedure, another 5-mm port is placed in the midline, 2 to 5 cm below the xiphoid process, to assist with liver retraction. Throughout the procedure, additional 5-mm ports can be placed as needed. This standard configuration can be varied according to individual patient anatomy and tumor location.

OPERATIVE TECHNIQUE

Bowel Mobilization

The colon is mobilized medially by incising along the line of Toldt to expose the kidney (Fig. 32-4). A relatively avascular plane between the posterior mesocolon and Gerota fascia is developed using both sharp and blunt dissection. To facilitate surgical instrumentation, we currently use the EnSeal TRIO (Ethicon) for dissection. The device allows for controlled, smoke-free tissue

and vessel sealing. The instrument also can be used as a scissors for cold cutting of adhesions near bowel structures, or as a blunt dissector. During right-sided LPN, the liver is retracted anteriorly and cephalad to expose the upper renal pole. The liver is held in position using a 5-mm Alice grasper in the subxiphoid port. During left-sided LPN, the spleen, splenic flexure, and pancreas are reflected medially.

Hilar Dissection

The ureter and gonadal vein packet are dissected en bloc and lifted anterolaterally off the psoas muscle toward the renal hilum. Extended dissection is used to locate the renal vein and to visualize its entire anterior surface. The renal vein can be identified by tracing the gonadal vein proximally to its insertion in the renal vein on the left side, or to its insertion in the inferior vena cava just caudal to the hilum on the right side. The renal artery usually is posterior to the renal vein. The vessels are circumferentially dissected in preparation for clamping (Fig. 32-5). To minimize iatrogenic vascular injury, some authors have advocated that the renal artery and vein not be completely skeletonized during this dissection.

Tumor Identification

The Gerota fascia is opened from a medial to lateral direction to expose the tumor and a sufficient amount of normal parenchyma. Dissection of the perirenal fat allows for increased kidney

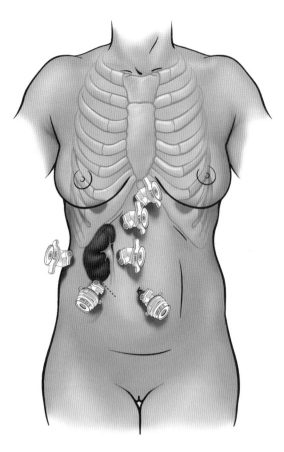

FIGURE 32-2 Port placement technique for right-sided laparoscopic partial nephrectomy.

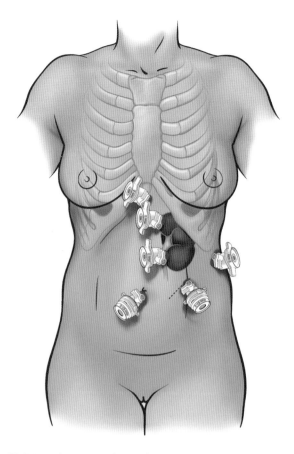

FIGURE 32-3 Port placement technique for left-sided laparoscopic partial nephrectomy.

FIGURE 32-4 The colon is mobilized medially by incising along the line of Toldt to expose the kidney.

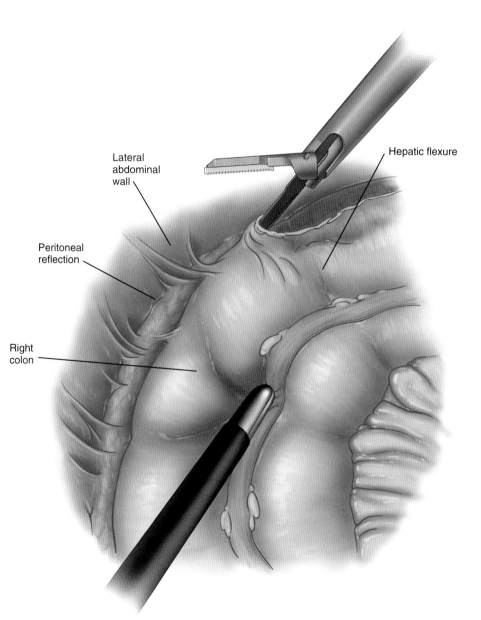

Lateral abdominal wall

Hepatic flexure

Peritoneal reflection

Right colon

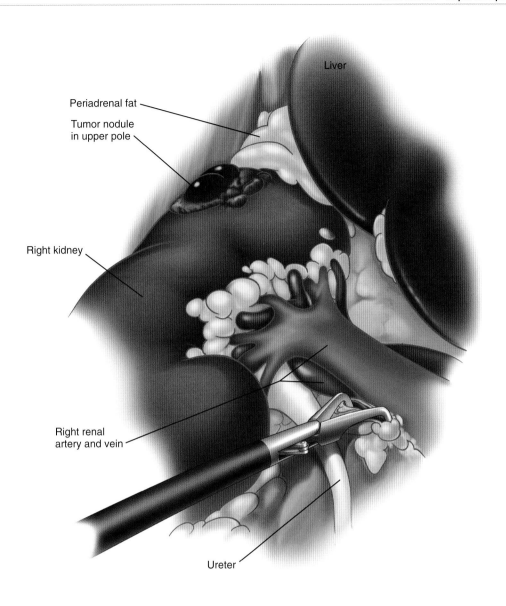

Liver

Periadrenal fat

Tumor nodule in upper pole

Right kidney

Right renal artery and vein

Ureter

FIGURE 32-5 The hilar vessels are skeletonized in preparation for renal clamping.

mobility, enhanced visualization of satellite tumors, use of intraoperative ultrasonography, and improved versatility of tumor resection and suturing angles. Intraoperative ultrasound can be used to obtain more accurate information on the location, depth, and extent of the tumor to ensure an oncologic resection with negative margins. These considerations are especially important in the context of hilar and endophytic masses. The margins of resection are scored with cautery after their demarcations with the ultrasound probe.

Hilar Clamping

Before clamping, all necessary sutures and instruments are made available to ensure that resection and renorrhaphy are performed efficiently during warm ischemia. Intravenous mannitol may be administered before clamping to facilitate osmotic diuresis, which is believed to promote renal protection. Hilar clamping can be performed using either laparoscopic bulldog clamps or a Satinsky clamp. If bulldog clamps are used, the renal artery is clamped first, followed by the vein (Fig. 32-6). Alternatively, a laparoscopic Satinsky clamp, inserted through the 12-mm

suprapubic port, is placed across the hilum. For select tumors, resection may be performed with exclusive renal artery clamping or without any hilar clamping. For endophytic, larger, or centrally placed tumors, both the renal artery and vein should be clamped.

We prefer to use bulldog clamps rather than a Satinsky clamp. The laparoscopic Satinsky requires a 12-mm port and limits mobilization of the kidney during tumor excision and renorrhaphy. Moreover, we prefer placing two bulldog clamps on the artery to ensure complete occlusion and a single clamp on the vein to prevent back bleeding. Before hilar clamping, one or two 3-0 barbed polyglyconate sutures (V-Loc, Covidien, Mansfield, Mass.) are anchored to the capsule 1 cm away from the excision line. This deep layer suture is anchored before warm ischemia so that the surgeon has control on the position of the kidney, which facilitates a fast and efficient tumor excision and renorrhaphy.

Tumor Excision

With the hilar vessels clamped, sharp and cold excision of the tumor is carried out with an adequate margin of normal parenchyma (Fig. 32-7). The preserved perirenal fat that is attached to

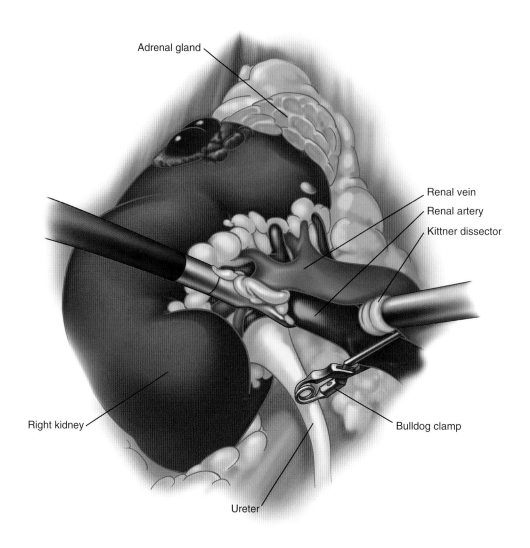

Adrenal gland

Renal vein

Renal artery

Kittner dissector

Right kidney

Bulldog clamp

Ureter

FIGURE 32-6 Clamping of the renal artery using a bulldog clamp.

the tumor is grasped and placed on counter-traction to elevate the tumor away from the tumor bed. The assistant uses suction to ensure visualization and to provide counter-traction. To guide the tumor resection, the surgeon needs to systematically integrate information from the CT, intraoperative ultrasound (if performed), and laparoscopic visualization. After resection, the tumor-containing specimen is placed aside for later retrieval.

Renal Reconstruction

Renorrhaphy is performed in two layers. The initial deep renorrhaphy layer closes the collecting system and major transected vessels. This is performed quickly with the self-retaining V-Loc barbed suture in a running fashion. Throws of the deep renorrhaphy layer are placed about 1 cm apart; the number and placement of the suture throws are determined by size of the defect, the depth of tumor invasion, and the extent of involvement of the collecting system and segmental vessels. Suturing the bed of the PN defect minimizes the chance for arteriovenous fistula or the development of an aberrant communication between the vessels and collecting system (Fig. 32-8). If necessary, an additional suture can be placed on a large parenchymal blood vessel.

The second renorrhaphy layer is performed using 0-0 polyglactin sutures (Vicryl, Ethicon, Somerville, NJ) placed about 1 cm apart along the renorrhaphy margin. All sutures are anchored with a knot and a Hem-o-lok clip (Weck Pilling, Research Triangle Park, NC) and are secured in a compressive guillotine fashion using the sliding clip technique. Sutures should be placed between 0.5 and 1 cm from the edge of the renorrhaphy to allow sufficient purchase of tissue and to minimize the chance of a capsular tear. For particularly large defects, oxidized cellulose bolsters (Surgicel, Johnson & Johnson, New Brunswick, NJ) may be positioned under the suture loops of the outer renorrhaphy layer; use of these bolsters is based on surgeon preference. A biologic hemostatic agent also can be layered directly on the PN bed underneath the bolster. There are a number of tissue sealants available: gelatin matrix thrombin sealant (Floseal, Baxter, Deerfield, Ill.), fibrin glue (Tisseel, Baxter), polyethylene glycol hydrogel (Coseal, Baxter), and cyanoacrylate glue (Dermabond, Ethicon, Cincinnati, Ohio). After tightening the Hem-o-lok clips, additional throws may be placed in a running or mattress fashion. The parenchymal renorrhaphy typically requires three to five sutures, depending on the length of the renorrhaphy margin (Fig. 32-9).

Removal of Hilar Clamps

After completion of the renorrhaphy, the hilar clamps are removed. Intravenous administration of mannitol can be repeated 2 to 3 minutes before hilar unclamping, but there is no clear

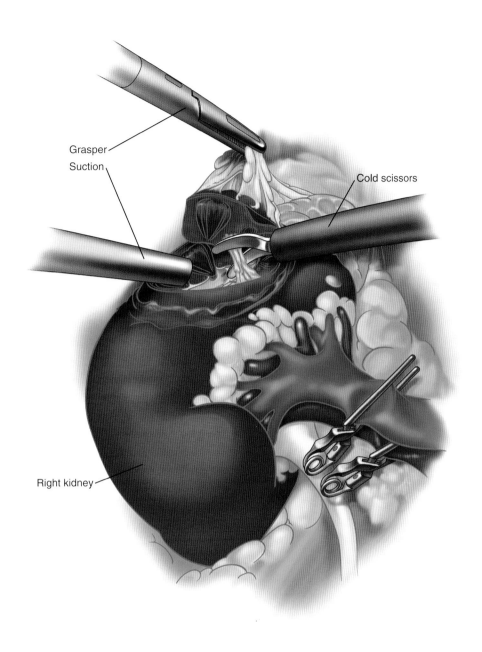

Grasper
Suction
Cold scissors
Right kidney

FIGURE 32-7 Tumor excision using cold scissors.

evidence to support this maneuver. If bulldog clamps were used, then the venous clamp is removed first, followed by the arterial clamp. Otherwise, the Satinsky clamp is unclamped and kept in an adjacent space while hemostasis is confirmed. If gentle oozing is present, a laparoscopic sponge can be used to apply direct pressure, and the Hem-o-lok clips can be further tightened. Once hemostasis is confirmed, the clamp is carefully removed under direct vision, and the warm ischemia time is noted. Hemostasis always should be rechecked after slight desufflation of the pneumoperitoneum, before removal of the laparoscopic trocars.

Specimen Retrieval

Depending on tumor size, a 10- or 15-mm Endo Catch (Covidien, Norwalk, Conn.) bag is used for specimen extraction. After placing a Jackson-Pratt drain, one of the port sites is extended, and the specimen is withdrawn. The fascia and skin then are

closed. Before completing the procedure, it is important for the surgeon to inspect the specimen and confirm grossly negative margins.

POSTOPERATIVE CARE

Serial hemoglobin levels are followed in the recovery room and postoperative period. Intravenous fluids, analgesics, and thromboprophylaxis are administered as per institution protocol. On the morning after surgery, the Foley catheter is removed, ambulation is permitted, and clear liquids are started. If the drainage output is minimum, then the drain may be removed on postoperative day 2. If the drainage output is more than 150 mL per 24 hours, then a creatinine level is obtained on the drainage fluid. The drain can be removed if the creatinine is at serum level. The length of stay typically is 2 days at our institution. After discharge, the patient is advised to restrict physical activity for 2

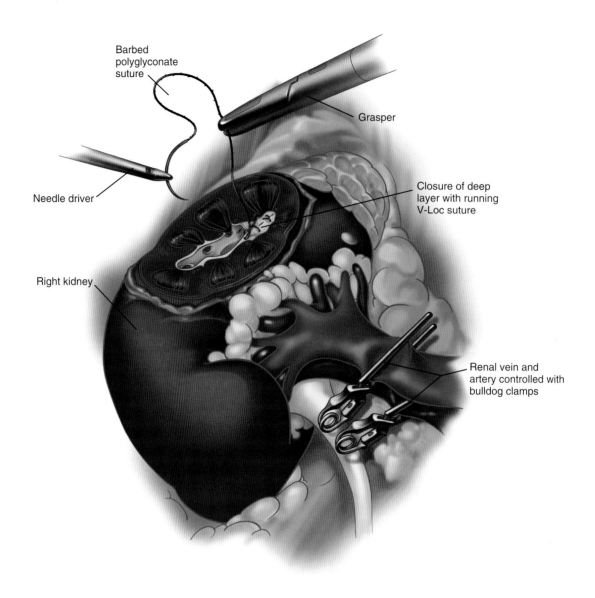

Barbed
polyglyconate
suture

Grasper

Needle driver

Closure of deep
layer with running
V-Loc suture

Right kidney

Renal vein and
artery controlled with
bulldog clamps

FIGURE 32-8 Deep layer closure technique performed with barbed polyglyconate suture in a running fashion.

to 3 weeks to minimize the risk for dehiscence of the renorrhaphy. The initial follow-up at 4 weeks includes a physical examination, complete blood count, and serum creatinine level.

MANAGEMENT OF PROCEDURE-SPECIFIC COMPLICATIONS

Hemorrhage

A serious vascular injury may occur during dissection of the renal hilum. Meticulous dissection and good exposure can help prevent intraoperative hemorrhage. Gentle application and removal of the vascular clamps are key to avoiding vascular wall damage. We prefer detachable bulldog clamps, which avoid inadvertent tugging that may occur with the use of the laparoscopic Satinsky clamp. Use of the bulldog clamps also frees an additional port for the duration of the warm ischemia time. Should venous bleeding be encountered, it usually can be controlled by direct pressure with a sponge or instrument while the insufflation pressure is increased. Small bleeding vessels can be cauterized or clipped, but sutured repair may be indicated for larger vascular injuries.

Renal parenchymal bleeding during hilar clamping may occur because of insufficient arterial occlusion or unrecognized accessory vessels. Attention to preoperative imaging should minimize this occurrence. An inadequate renorrhaphy may result in bleeding after the hilum is unclamped. Pneumoperitoneum may be increased transiently (20 to 25 mm Hg) and direct compression applied while the sliding renorrhaphy clips are retightened. The bipolar instrument and a short 3-0 Vicryl suture with an end-loaded LapraTy clip (Ethicon, Cincinnati, Ohio) also can be used to help control vascular bleeding. As discussed previously, a contingency plan should always be in place should uncontrolled bleeding take place. Failure to adequately control unexpected bleeding laparoscopically necessitates open conversion; the appropriate surgical trays should be open and accessible.

A symptomatic decrease in serial hemoglobin, accompanied by fluctuations in vital signs or urine output, usually indicates postoperative hemorrhage. Transfusions and close monitoring of vital signs are usually sufficient to manage postoperative bleeding. Late postoperative hemorrhage may result from a pseudoaneurysm or arteriovenous fistula and usually presents as gross hematuria. It is important to suspect a vascular complication

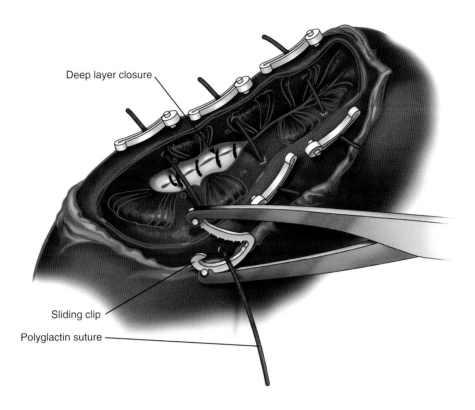

FIGURE 32-9 Parenchymal layer closure, sliding Hem-o-lok clip technique, performed with polyglactin sutures spaced 1 cm apart.

when a patient presents with postoperative hematuria. This type of hemorrhage may require renal angiography and angioembolization. Surgical exploration (and completion nephrectomy) is the next step if angioembolization fails to control bleeding.

Bowel Injury

Unrecognized bowel injury is a potential complication of any abdominal procedure and may occur from port or instrument insertion as well as from cautery. A bowel injury that is recognized at the time of surgery should be immediately repaired, and general surgery should be consulted as needed. When the bowel injury is not recognized intraoperatively, postoperative signs and symptoms include nonspecific gastrointestinal symptoms, anorexia, low-grade fever, and an abnormal white blood cell count. The patient can deteriorate rapidly if the injury is not promptly recognized and managed. A CT scan with oral and intravenous contrast may help identify an injury and visualize intra-abdominal fluid collections. If an injury is diagnosed in the postoperative period, then open exploration usually is required to evacuate bowel spillage and perform the necessary repair. With the use of Enseal and other advanced energy devices, the threat of inadvertent bowel injury due to electrical arcing appears to have decreased.

Urine Leak and Urinoma

If there is evidence of a postoperative urine leak (e.g., elevated drain creatinine levels, high drain output), then the drain should be left in place and the urine output monitored. CT urography should be considered for persistent leakage or symptoms to assess for a urinoma and to ascertain the position of the drain relative to the collection. The position of the drain may need to be changed or a percutaneous drain placed if there is an undrained collection. Serial imaging may be used to monitor the resolution of a urinoma. Retrograde placement of a ureteral stent should be considered if there is persistent high-volume drainage or evidence of distal obstruction on the CT urogram.

Other Procedure-Specific Complications

Insufflation complications include subcutaneous emphysema and gas embolism. Leaking trocar sites or incorrectly positioned trocars can allow CO_2 to travel under the skin and into the mediastinum, resulting in potentially life-threatening pneumomediastinum or pneumothorax. Other complications include nerve injury, chronic pain syndrome, and orchialgia. Several authors have reported cases of chronic pain syndrome or nerve injury after LPN that presented as a constant burning discomfort in the ipsilateral flank, requiring narcotics and pain clinic consultation. Ipsilateral orchialgia has been described to occur in up to 10% of patients after laparoscopic kidney surgery.

RESULTS AND OUTCOME

A brief description of complication rates associated with LPN at centers of excellence is shown in Table 32-1. Gill and colleagues recently compared the outcomes of 1800 consecutive open PN (OPN) and LPN at three large referral centers. They showed that LPN was associated with shorter operative time, decreased operative blood loss, and shorter length of stay. The likelihood of intraoperative complications was comparable

Table 32-1 Complication Rates of Laparoscopic Partial Nephrectomy Performed at Centers of Excellence

First Author	No. of Subjects	Mean Tumor Size (cm)	Mean Operative Time	Mean Ischemia Time	Overall Complications (%)	Medical Complications (%)	Hemorrhage (%)	Urine Leak (%)	Wound Infections, Sepsis (%)	Renal Failure (%)
Ramani	200	2.9	199	28.7	33.0	12.0	10.0	4.5	3.0	2.0
Simmons	200	3.0	226	34.7	19.0	9.0	5.5	2.0	1.0	0.5
Wright	49	2.3	267	32.7	14.3	8.2	2.0	4.1	N/R	N/R
Venkatesh	123	2.6	204	28.0	20.6	8.1	2.4	10.6	N/R	N/R
Schiff	66	2.2	144	18.2	9.0	3.0	1.5	3.0	N/R	N/R
Link	217	2.6	186	27.6	12.4	6.9	1.8	1.4	1.4	0.9
Bollens	39	2.3	120	9.0	30.7	20.5	2.5	7.7	N/R	N/R
Lifshitz	184	2.5	220	31.0	13.0	4.9	N/R	N/R	N/R	N/R
Abukora	78	2.1	186	31.5	29.5	12.8	7.7	6.4	N/R	N/R
Porpiglia	90	3.1	116	27.1	24.4	12.2	7.8	4.4	N/R	N/R
Pierorazio	102	N/R	193	18.0	N/R	N/R	N/R	N/R	N/R	N/R

N/R: not reported.

between the two groups. Conversely, LPN was associated with longer ischemia time and more postoperative complications. Renal functional outcomes were similar 3 months after OPN and LPN. Three-year cancer-specific survival rates for patients with a single cT1 N0 M0 renal cell carcinoma were 99.3% and 99.2% after LPN and OPN, respectively. Similarly, Porpiglia and associates performed an analysis of the available literature and reached similar conclusions. Specifically, intermediate oncologic and functional outcomes of LPN are similar to those of OPN. Conversely, ischemia time is longer after LPN, and a steeper learning curve is necessary to reach satisfactory complication rates. The authors concluded that optimal patient selection is needed for the novice laparoscopic surgeon to ensure high-quality patient care.

Suggested Readings

Abukora F, Nambirajan T, Albqami N, et al: Laparoscopic nephron sparing surgery: Evolution in a decade, *Eur Urol* 47:488–493; discussion 493, 2005.

Bollens R, Rosenblatt A, Espinoza BP, et al: Laparoscopic partial nephrectomy with "on-demand" clamping reduces warm ischemia time, *Eur Urol* 52:804–809, 2007.

Fazeli-Matin S, Gill IS, Hsu TH, et al: Laparoscopic renal and adrenal surgery in obese patients: Comparison to open surgery, *J Urol* 162:665–669, 1999.

Gill IS, Kavoussi LR, Lane BR, et al: Comparison of 1,800 laparoscopic and open partial nephrectomies for single renal tumors, *J Urol* 178:41–46, 2007.

Lifshitz DA, Shikanov S, Jeldres C, et al: Laparoscopic partial nephrectomy: Predictors of prolonged warm ischemia, *J Urol* 182:860–865, 2009.

Lifshitz DA, Shikanov SA, Deklaj T, et al: Laparoscopic partial nephrectomy: A single-center evolving experience, *Urology* 75:282–287, 2010.

Link RE, Bhayani SB, Allaf ME, et al: Exploring the learning curve, pathological outcomes and perioperative morbidity of laparoscopic partial nephrectomy performed for renal mass, *J Urol* 173:1690–1694, 2005.

Pierorazio PM, Patel HD, Feng T, et al: Robotic-assisted versus traditional laparoscopic partial nephrectomy: Comparison of outcomes and evaluation of learning curve, *Urology* 78:813–819, 2011.

Porpiglia F, Volpe A, Billia M, et al: Assessment of risk factors for complications of laparoscopic partial nephrectomy, *Eur Urol* 53:590–596, 2008.

Porpiglia F, Volpe A, Billia M, Scarpa RM: Laparoscopic versus open partial nephrectomy: Analysis of the current literature, *Eur Urol* 53:732–742; discussion 742–743, 2008.

Ramani AP, Desai MM, Steinberg AP, et al: Complications of laparoscopic partial nephrectomy in 200 cases, *J Urol* 173:42–47, 2005.

Schiff JD, Palese M, Vaughan ED Jr, et al: Laparoscopic vs open partial nephrectomy in consecutive patients: The Cornell experience, *BJU Int* 96:811–814, 2005.

Simmons MN, Gill IS: Decreased complications of contemporary laparoscopic partial nephrectomy: Use of a standardized reporting system, *J Urol* 177:2067–2073; discussion 2073, 2007.

Spaliviero M, Gill IS: Laparoscopic partial nephrectomy, *BJU Int* 99:1313–1328, 2007.

Trinh QD, Saad F, Lattouf JB: The current management of small renal masses, *Curr Opin Support Palliat Care* 3:180–185, 2009.

Van Poppel H, Becker F, Cadeddu JA, et al: Treatment of localised renal cell carcinoma, *Eur Urol* 60:662–672, 2011.

Venkatesh R, Weld K, Ames CD, et al: Laparoscopic partial nephrectomy for renal masses: Effect of tumor location, *Urology* 67:1169–1174; discussion 1174, 2006.

Volpe A, Cadeddu JA, Cestari A, et al: Contemporary management of small renal masses, *Eur Urol* 60:501–515, 2011.

Wright JL, Porter JR: Laparoscopic partial nephrectomy: Comparison of transperitoneal and retroperitoneal approaches, *J Urol* 174:841–845, 2005.

CHAD A. LAGRANGE

Minimally Invasive Radical Prostatectomy

The videos associated with this chapter are listed in the Video Contents and can be found on the accompanying DVDs and *on Expertconsult.com.*

Minimally invasive radical prostatectomy (MIRP) encompasses both laparoscopic radical prostatectomy (LRP) and robot-assisted radical prostatectomy (RARP). The first LRP was described by Scheussler in 1993. Subsequently, Binder described the first RARP in 2000. It is estimated that most radical prostatectomies performed in the United States during 2011 will be done with robotic assistance and that RARP is the most common robotic surgery performed worldwide.

In general, MIRP offers several advantages over other forms of radical prostatectomy. In addition to the standard advantages of laparoscopic surgery (smaller incisions, improved vision), most series report lower blood loss and faster patient recovery. Both forms of MIRP are advanced laparoscopic procedures with long learning curves. The robotic platform offers three-dimensional high-definition vision, wristed instruments, and precise instrument maneuvering, which have aided in shortening the learning curve of MIRP. The robotic instrumentation is most beneficial in completing the urethrovesical anastomosis, which is regarded as the most technically challenging portion of laparoscopic radical prostatectomy.

OPERATIVE INDICATIONS

In general, MIRP has the same operative indications as open radical retropubic prostatectomy (RRP). Patients who are believed to have organ-confined prostate cancer, based on Gleason score (grade), clinical stage, prostate-specific antigen (PSA), and staging studies, are appropriate candidates for radical prostatectomy. Patient age, life expectancy, and overall health also are important factors in the clinical decision to treat prostate cancer, but are beyond the scope of this text. Pelvic lymphadenectomy can be performed at the same time as MIRP, if indicated by the above factors. This is a distinct advantage of MIRP over radical perineal prostatectomy, in which lymph node dissection cannot be performed under the same anesthesia or incision.

Patients with obesity, large prostate glands, large median prostate lobes, or prior major pelvic or abdominal surgery tend to be more challenging and should be avoided early in the surgeon's learning curve. In the patient who has had a prior laparoscopic inguinal hernia repair, the initial development of the extraperitoneal space can be extremely difficult and could result in a bladder or pelvic vascular injury. These patients should be counseled about the increased risk for conversion to an open procedure.

All patients should be counseled about other options for treatment of localized prostate cancer, including watchful waiting or active surveillance for appropriate patients, other forms of prostatectomy, external-beam radiation therapy, brachytherapy, and cryotherapy. Focal ablative techniques such as high-intensity focused ultrasound (HIFU) also may be discussed, but currently in the United States these are being performed only under clinical protocols.

PREOPERATIVE EVALUATION, TESTING, AND PREPARATION

Prostate cancer staging studies (such as bone scan, computed tomography [CT] scan, and magnetic resonance imaging [MRI]) should be completed if indicated by the tumor characteristics noted previously. All patients undergoing MIRP should undergo standard medical clearance for major surgery according to their specific health factors. Patients with pulmonary disease may need preoperative pulmonary function testing to ensure they can tolerate insufflation without hypercarbia. All patients should have a blood type and screen before surgery; the rate of transfusion with MIRP, however, has been quite low in most series (about 2.7%). The day before the procedure, the patient completes a bowel preparation of one bottle of magnesium citrate along with a clear liquid diet. Some surgeons also recommend an enema the morning of surgery to evacuate the rectum completely. Recently, some surgeons have advocated omission of any formal bowel preparation.

All patients are counseled preoperatively about possible complications of radical prostatectomy, including erectile dysfunction, stress urinary incontinence, rectal injury, and pelvic nerve or vascular injury. Other general risks include bowel injury, ileus, bleeding, and infection. Patients also should be counseled on whether a nerve-sparing procedure will be performed in light of their pathologic features and risk factors.

PATIENT POSITIONING AND OPERATIVE ROOM SETUP

Sequential pneumatic compression devices or compression stockings are placed preoperatively. A dose of prophylactic antibiotic, such as cefazolin, is administered intravenously. Patients are placed on a large beanbag stabilizer on the operating table. After induction of endotracheal anesthesia, an orogastric tube is placed. The anesthesiologist should ensure that the patient remains completely paralyzed during the entire procedure. To improve intraoperative visualization, intravenous fluids are limited until after the urethrovesical anastomosis is completed to decrease the amount of urine spilling into the field.

The abdomen is clipped of hair, the arms are tucked at the patient's sides, and the elbows are padded with foam. Foam also is placed on top of and underneath the shoulders to prevent excessive pressure on the shoulders after subsequent placement into steep-Trendelenburg position. The beanbag stabilizer then is rolled up around the outside of the arms and shoulders and connected to suction to deflate and hold its position. The beanbag is important in preventing patient movement during steep-Trendelenburg positioning. We do not use any additional taping during positioning.

For standard LRP, the legs remain in the supine position and are secured to the bed with a safety strap. With RARP, the legs are placed in low lithotomy position with Yellowfins stirrups (Allen Medical Systems, Acton, Mass.), taking care not to place excessive strain on the thigh or groin muscles, which can produce postoperative neurapraxia. Alternatively, a spread-leg position (using spreader bars designed for the table) can be used with the patient in supine position. An overview of the patient positioning is shown in Figure 33-1.

For standard LRP, the surgeon stands on the left side of the patient, and the assistant stands on the right. The laparoscopic video monitor is positioned at the foot of the bed at a comfortable height. A robotic camera positioner (Aesop, Intuitive Surgical, Sunnyvale, Calif.) or mechanical holder can be used to provide a stable camera position during the operation. These devices also allow the assistant to use both hands to assist during the procedure. Otherwise, the assistant holds the laparoscope, and a second assistant may be necessary at certain points of the case to perform minor tasks. We find it helpful to place a padded sterile Mayo stand over the patient's head during the procedure. This stand protects the patient's face and provides a surface for the assistant to stabilize his or her left arm while holding the camera.

If a four-arm robot is to be used for RARP, then the assistant generally stands on the patient's right side. The fourth arm can be placed on either side on newer versions of the robotic system; the assistant generally is on the opposite side of the fourth arm. If a three-arm robot is used, then two assistants may be necessary. A laparoscopic video monitor can be positioned on either the right or left side of the patient for the assistant to view, depending on operating room setup and space. Some da Vinci Surgical Systems (Intuitive Surgical) have monitors positioned atop the robotic system for the assistant.

Standard laparoscopic instruments are used in both LRP and RARP. Because the assistant operates the laparoscopic graspers during RARP, bariatric length instruments are helpful for adequate reach and to decrease external collisions with the robotic arms. An ultrasonic scalpel or bipolar dissector is helpful in LRP. The authors generally do not use monopolar cautery during LRP. For RARP, monopolar curved scissors, as well as bipolar graspers, are used on the robotic arms for the dissection.

POSITIONING AND PLACEMENT OF TROCARS

For MIRP, a fan-shaped configuration of trocars in the lower abdomen is used (Fig. 33-2). Five trocars are used during LRP, and six trocars are placed for RARP. A Foley catheter is inserted in a sterile fashion on the field, and the bladder is emptied. Bulb suction is preferred to ensure that the bladder remains empty during the early dissection. After gaining access to the peritoneal cavity, a 12-mm blunt trocar is placed in a supraumbilical midline location for the laparoscope in both types of MIRP. The bed then is placed into Trendelenburg position (13 to 15 degrees, head down).

For standard LRP, a 12-mm trocar is placed 2 fingerbreadths from the left anterior superior iliac spine (ASIS) on a line from the ASIS to the umbilicus (see Fig. 33-2). This trocar is used by the surgeon to pass suture into the abdomen throughout the

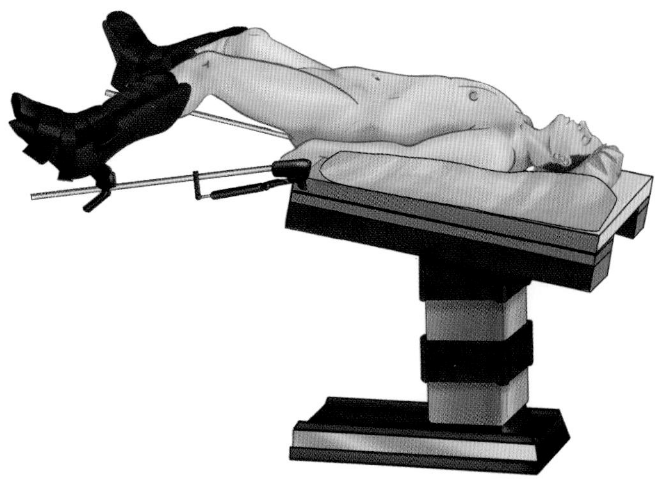

FIGURE 33-1 Patient positioning during robot-assisted radical prostatectomy. Positioning is the same for standard laparoscopic radical prostatectomy except the legs remain in supine position.

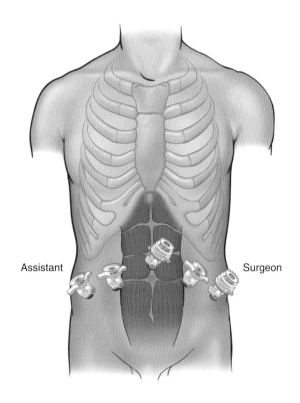

Assistant   Surgeon

FIGURE 33-2 Trocar configuration during laparoscopic radical prostatectomy.

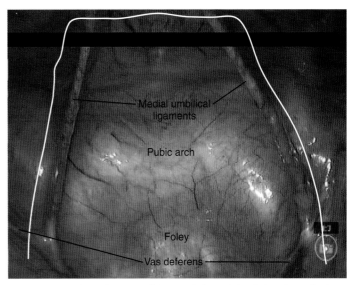

FIGURE 33-4 Outline of peritoneal incision during minimally invasive radical prostatectomy. Incision across medial umbilical ligaments and urachus on anterior abdominal wall continuing lateral to each ligament down past the vas deferens bilaterally.

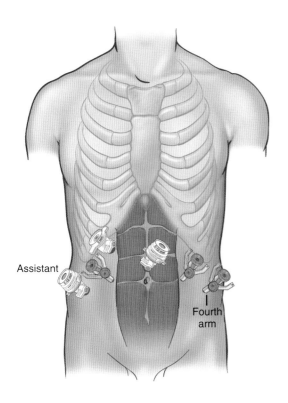

FIGURE 33-3 Trocar configuration during robot-assisted radical prostatectomy (teal blue = robotic 8-mm trocar).

procedure and for the surgeon's grasper during dissection. A 5-mm trocar is placed along this line in the left lower quadrant at the lateral border of the left rectus muscle. The ultrasonic scalpel is used through this trocar during the dissection. Two additional 5-mm trocars are placed in a mirror image in the right lower quadrant for the assistant to use for the suction irrigator and retraction during the procedure. The authors prefer to use low-profile trocars during standard LRP to allow for maximal instrument reach into the pelvis.

For RARP, a similar port configuration is used (Fig. 33-3). Two robot ports are placed in the left lower quadrant as described previously. The third robot port is placed at the lateral border of the rectus in the right lower quadrant on the same line from the umbilicus to the ASIS. A 12-mm port is placed in the right lateral position for the assistant to pass suture into the abdomen and is used for retraction. An additional 5-mm assistant port is placed in the right upper quadrant, between the laparoscope port and right robot port. The suction irrigator is operated through this port by the assistant.

Once all trocars are placed, the robotic arms are docked to robotic trocars, and the instruments are inserted under direct vision. It is imperative that the robot arms have free range of motion without colliding into one another or the patient's extremities; this should be assessed after docking. A Prograsp (Intuitive Surgical) grasper is used for the fourth arm (left lateral robotic trocar). We use a bipolar grasper in the left arm (left medial robotic trocar) and monopolar curved scissors in the right arm (right robotic trocar).

OPERATIVE TECHNIQUE

MIRP can be performed using either a transperitoneal or extraperitoneal approach. The transperitoneal approach is preferred by most surgeons because of a larger working space and greater familiarity with the access technique. Only the transperitoneal approach is discussed in this chapter.

The general steps of MIRP are discussed next. Differences between RARP and LRP will be discussed when applicable. The steps of MIRP can be divided as follows:

1. Creation of the extraperitoneal space
2. Incision of the endopelvic fascia
3. Ligation of the dorsal venous complex
4. Division of the bladder neck
5. Dissection of the seminal vesicles and vas deferens
6. Posterior dissection
7. Nerve-sparing ligation of vascular pedicles
8. Apical dissection
9. Urethrovesical anastomosis
10. Closure

Creation of the Extraperitoneal Space

After gaining safe access to the abdomen and placing all trocars, the surgeon must mobilize the bladder to enter the extraperitoneal space (i.e., the space of Retzius, or retropubic space). The urachus and medial umbilical ligaments are divided high on the anterior abdominal wall using cautery or the ultrasonic scalpel. The peritoneum then is incised lateral to each umbilical ligament down posterior to the vas deferens (Fig. 33-4). The vas deferens is dissected and divided bilaterally. After the bladder has been mobilized from the anterior abdominal wall, the dome of the bladder is retracted cephalad to provide exposure to the pelvis. The assistant's locking grasper retracts the bladder during LRP, whereas the fourth arm of the robot is used for this purpose during RARP.

The retropubic space is further developed in a bloodless plane of loose areolar tissue. Care is taken to identify the iliac vessels and pubic bone early to avoid injury and guide the dissection. Once the pubic bone is identified, the tissue plane along the inferior edge of the bone is defined to completely develop the retropubic space. The endopelvic fascia then is identified, and superficial fat is removed from the dorsum of the prostate and endopelvic fascia bilaterally. The fat overlying the dorsum of the prostate normally contains a superficial dorsal vein, which can be divided with bipolar cautery or the ultrasonic scalpel. Finally, the puboprostatic ligaments are identified and cleaned of all adipose tissue bilaterally. Care should be taken at this point in the procedure to identify and preserve, if possible, any accessory pudendal arteries that may perforate the endopelvic fascia and course into the pelvis. These arteries may play a key role in preservation of postoperative erectile function.

Incision of the Endopelvic Fascia

The prostate is retracted medially, placing the endopelvic fascia on stretch. An incision is made in the posterior aspect of the endopelvic fascia at its most dependent portion, which is where the fascia crosses from prostate to pelvic muscle. If the incision is in the proper location, a potential space is entered that generally is avascular. Cold scissors or the ultrasonic scalpel can be used to extend the fascial incision anteriorly and posteriorly. The levator muscle fibers are swept off the surface of the prostate using sharp and blunt dissection. Care should be taken to avoid cautery in the posterior portion of the fascial incision because neurovascular bundles are in close proximity. In general, a triangular "notch" exists just lateral to each puboprostatic ligament (Fig. 33-5). The ligament is divided at the base of this "notch," which should expose a well-defined muscle at the apex of the prostate as well as the deep dorsal vein. This muscle can be dissected bluntly from the prostate; any tissue enveloping the dorsal vein is dissected sharply until the dorsal vein is completely free. If the puboprostatic ligaments are not adequately incised bilaterally, then ligation of the dorsal vein might fail, which could cause bleeding during the apical dissection.

Ligation of the Dorsal Venous Complex

Multiple techniques have been used for control of the deep dorsal vein during MIRP. Stapler division is advocated by some surgeons, purportedly to decrease apical positive margins. We prefer suture ligation with delayed division until the apical dissection has been completed. A 2-0 polyglycolic acid or other absorbable

suture cut to 22 cm in length on a CT-1 needle is used. For LRP, the suture is introduced through the 12-mm lateral port using a needle driver. Another needle driver is placed through the right medial 5-mm trocar. The assistant must release the bladder grasper retraction to allow for suturing through this but continue to expose the area using the suction irrigator. If the exposure is not adequate, then a locking grasper can be placed through the left medial 5-mm trocar, and the dome of the bladder is retracted cephalad to allow the surgeon to suture. During RARP, the curved scissors and bipolar graspers are exchanged for large needle drivers. The fourth arm maintains its retraction of the bladder. The suture is introduced through the assistant's 12-mm trocar.

The suture is placed beneath the dorsal vein from right to left. If the suture is placed too deeply, then the urethra and possibly the Foley catheter may be included in the stitch. If placed too superficial, then the vein will not be ligated, resulting in bleeding during later division. Normally, a groove between the urethra and dorsal vein can be visualized when the prostate is retracted medially. In addition, the Foley catheter can be manipulated to demonstrate the location of the urethra. The right-hand needle driver is used to load the needle in an upside-down backhand ("frown") orientation (Fig. 33-6). The needle then is passed behind the

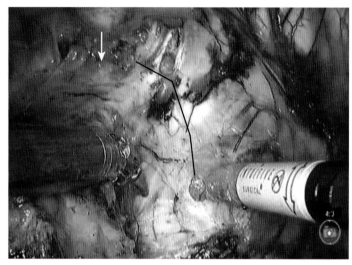

FIGURE 33-5 Incision of endopelvic fascia. Most dependent portion of fascia in the pelvis. Outline of desired incision. *Arrow* indicates dorsal vein.

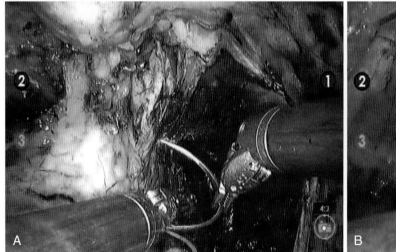
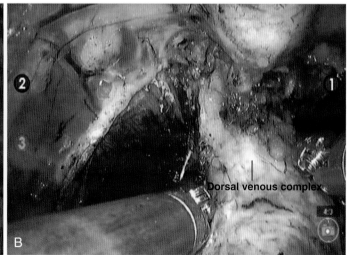

FIGURE 33-6 Suture ligation of dorsal venous complex.

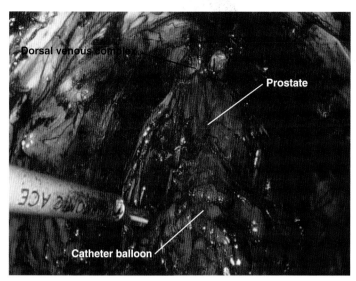

FIGURE 33-7 Identification of bladder neck. Dissection begins in a trough between the prostate and catheter balloon.

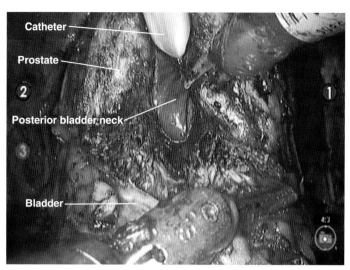

FIGURE 33-8 Division of posterior bladder neck. Catheter is lifted anteriorly by assistant to elevate the prostate and define the posterior bladder neck.

dorsal vein. The assistant retracts the left side of the prostate to expose the needle tip. If the needle tip is difficult to locate, it may be overly rotated posteriorly, or passed too far into the pelvic sidewall musculature. A figure-of-eight suture or two simple sutures can be placed. Some authors recommend anchoring this suture into the pubic bone in an effort to improve urinary continence postoperatively. Regardless, the knot is secured and the needle retrieved.

Division of the Bladder Neck

For standard LRP, the bladder is retracted at the dome by the assistant with a locking grasper, as done previously. The needle drivers are exchanged for a nonlocking grasper and the ultrasonic scalpel. For RARP, the needle drivers are exchanged for a curved monopolar scissors and a bipolar grasper, as before. With the Foley balloon still inflated, the assistant manipulates the catheter to help define the bladder neck. An "hourglass deformity" often can be noted between the Foley balloon and prostate, the narrow portion being the bladder neck (Fig. 33-7). It often is helpful to remove the superficial fat from the dorsum of the prostate and bladder neck junction to better define this area. If the Foley balloon appears to deviate to one side, then a large prostate median lobe may be present. If the Foley is not able to be manipulated easily, then the dorsal vein suture may have inadvertently ligated the urethra, so this suture will need to be removed and replaced. The surgeon also may palpate the bladder neck with the instruments to help define its location.

Beginning anteriorly, the bladder neck fibers are divided using energy (monopolar scissors for RARP or the ultrasonic scalpel for LRP). Care should be taken to avoid extending the incision too far laterally on either side to prevent bleeding, which can be difficult to expose and control in this location. The incision should follow the outline of the prostate, which is generally a frown shape. The Foley catheter can be manipulated intermittently to ensure the proper plane of dissection.

For standard LRP, the Foley balloon is deflated, and the catheter is removed after the bladder neck incision has been defined. A curved Lowsley retractor is placed per urethra into the bladder by the assistant. The tractor is elevated to lift the prostate anteriorly. This helps the surgeon to define the lateral and posterior

aspects of the bladder neck, as well as to enter the bladder precisely at the anterior bladder neck. This anterior traction on the prostate is maintained until the seminal vesicle dissection has begun.

During RARP, the anterior bladder neck is opened, and the Foley balloon is deflated. The catheter is withdrawn and then passed through the opening in the bladder neck. The assistant grasps the eyelet of the catheter with a locking grasper and elevates the catheter anteriorly to the pubic bone. The external portion of the catheter is clamped to the drapes to provide the tension necessary to elevate the catheter. Alternatively, a needlescopic grasper can be placed in the suprapubic area and used to introduce a suture into the field. The suture can be threaded through the eyelet of the Foley catheter and retracted superiorly with the grasper or delivered through the anterior abdominal wall, where it can be secured.

Once the anterior bladder neck is opened, the interior of the bladder is inspected to identify any median lobe tissue as well as the ureteral orifices. If a median lobe of the prostate is present, then it must be delivered through the opening in the bladder neck and elevated anteriorly so that proper division of the posterior bladder neck can be achieved. Extreme care must be taken to avoid injury to the ureteral orifices when dealing with a large median lobe. Intravenous indigo carmine can be given to aid in identification of the ureteral orifices. A suture also may be placed through the median lobe to aid in retraction during division of the posterior bladder neck. The lateral bladder neck then is divided bilaterally. A tissue plane often can be developed posterior to the bladder neck before division of the remaining posterior bladder wall (Fig. 33-8).

The goal of the bladder neck dissection is the preservation of the bladder neck with a circular opening. Care should be taken to ensure equal thickness of the bladder wall around the entire circumference. The bladder neck should be circular, rather than "fish-mouthed" or asymmetrical; otherwise, bladder neck reconstruction may be necessary before the subsequent urethrovesical anastomosis.

Dissection of the Seminal Vesicles and Vas Deferens

After division of the posterior bladder neck, the assistant retracts the bladder neck posteriorly with the suction irrigator. Frequently, a layer of vertically oriented fibers is present; these need to be incised to expose the vasa and seminal vesicles. The vasa are grasped by the surgeon, and the anterior prostatic traction is released. The vasa are dissected posteriorly and then divided using clips, monopolar cautery, or the ultrasonic scalpel. During RARP, it is helpful to have the assistant grasp and elevate the vasa to help expose the seminal vesicles. For standard LRP, the surgeon must elevate the vasa to expose the seminal vesicles. It is most helpful to retract the vasa anteriorly and slightly cephalad to fully expose the seminal vesicles. The seminal vesicles are dissected posteriorly to their tips. Blood vessels are controlled with clips or bipolar cautery. The use of monopolar cautery near the tips of the seminal vesicles should be avoided during nerve-sparing operations because the neurovascular bundles course close to the tips of the vesicles. Once the tips of the seminal vesicles are completely free, both the vasa and seminal vesicles are lifted anteriorly to expose Denonvilliers fascia. Care should be taken to avoid excessive lateral traction to prevent traction injury to the neurovascular bundles.

Posterior Dissection

Denonvilliers fascia is incised with cold scissors just below the prostate and seminal vesicles. Frequently, the reflection of Denonvilliers fascia can be identified, and the incision can be started in the midline just posterior to this reflection. The perirectal fat is identified, and the dissection plane is extended toward the apex of the prostate. Near the apex of the prostate, the rectum courses anteriorly, and care must be taken to avoid both rectal injury and entry into posterior prostate capsule. The incision in Denonvilliers fascia then is widened to the level of the vascular pedicles bilaterally. A gentle, lateral rolling maneuver helps demonstrate the posterior surface of the prostate and may help with the later dissection of the neurovascular bundles.

Nerve-Sparing Ligation of Vascular Pedicles

Any remaining bladder detrusor fibers are divided bilaterally to expose the vascular pedicles. The seminal vesicle is lifted anteriorly to provide adequate exposure. During LRP, the surgeon must provide this exposure, whereas in RARP, the assistant may elevate the seminal vesicle so that the surgeon may work with both hands. Before controlling the vascular pedicles, the lateral prostatic fascia is incised bilaterally along the length of the prostate. This is important to release the neurovascular bundles and prevent injury during the subsequent pedicle division. The lateral prostatic fascia is incised as anterior as possible because the neurovascular bundles lay on the posterolateral aspect of the prostate.

Many techniques exist to control the vascular pedicles, and this aspect of MIRP remains a topic of much debate. Locking plastic or simple titanium clips are used by many surgeons. The ultrasonic scalpel and bipolar cautery also may be used. Other surgeons have advocated vascular bulldog and suture ligation. Whatever method is used, the vascular pedicles should be divided as close to the capsule of the prostate as possible to prevent injury to the neurovascular bundle during nerve-sparing operations. During RARP, we prefer to use locking plastic clips to control the vascular pedicles. The clips are applied by the assistant through the 12-mm trocar while the surgeon provides exposure. After clip placement, the pedicles are sharply divided with cold scissors. During LRP, we prefer to divide the pedicles using the ultrasonic

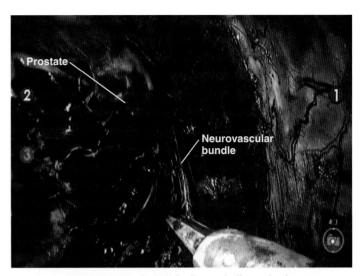

FIGURE 33-9 Neurovascular bundle dissected off capsule of prostate.

scalpel. The pedicles are divided close to the corners of the prostate using brief and judicious applications of the ultrasonic energy source.

After division of the pedicles during a nerve-sparing operation, the capsule of the prostate should be identified. Using sharp dissection with cold scissors, the neurovascular bundles are dissected from the capsule of the prostate proximally to the lateral aspect of the urethra distally (Fig. 33-9). The prostate must be elevated and retracted from side to side to fully accomplish this dissection. Again, it is important to avoid excess lateral traction on the neurovascular bundles during this dissection.

Apical Dissection

The apical dissection includes division of the dorsal vein, urethra, and rectourethralis muscle. Before starting the apical dissection, a Foley catheter is replaced per urethra to aid in identification of the urethra at the apex of the prostate. During LRP, the ultrasonic scalpel is used to divide the previously ligated dorsal venous complex. The initial division is performed with tips of the instrument curved anteriorly to reduce the chance of a positive margin. During RARP, the dorsal vein is divided with monopolar scissors. Some minor bleeding may be encountered during division of the dorsal vein. It is imperative that the assistant maintain a blood-free field to help the surgeon avoid entry into the prostate apex, which could produce a positive margin. Generally, once the venous complex is completely divided, minor bleeding should cease because of the release of tension on the complex. If bleeding persists, then it should be ligated before continuing the apical dissection so that visualization is not impeded.

The anterior wall of the urethra is visualized after dividing the dorsal venous complex. Before dividing the urethra, it is important to release any remaining apical attachments of the neurovascular bundle to the prostate (Fig. 33-10). This helps prevent injury to the bundles when the posterior urethra is divided. The urethra is incised on the anterior surface with cold scissors just beyond the apex of the prostate. The goal is to allow as much urethral length as possible, without entering the apical prostate tissue. Once the anterior wall is incised, the Foley catheter is visualized and withdrawn into the urethral stump to allow division of the lateral and posterior urethral walls. Before division of the lateral walls, the course of the neurovascular bundles should be identified during nerve-sparing procedures to prevent bundle

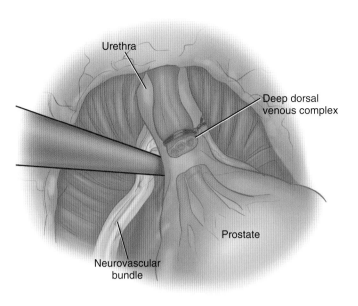

FIGURE 33-10 Before division of the urethra, the neurovascular bundle is mobilized from the apex of the prostate and posterolateral aspect of urethra to prevent injury.

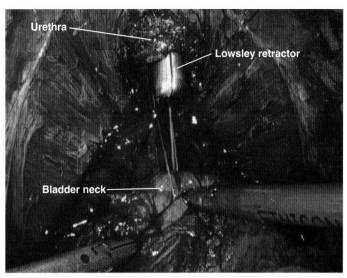

FIGURE 33-11 Interrupted anastomosis. While securing the first posterior anastomotic suture, the bladder traction suture is grasped with the Lowsley tractor to approximate the bladder neck and urethra without tension.

injury. After the posterior wall of the urethra is divided, the rectourethralis muscle is sharply divided, and the specimen should be free in the pelvis. The specimen is inspected for any gross capsular disruptions (potential positive margins) and for the amount of tissue on the capsule (to help assess nerve sparing). The specimen then is placed in an entrapment sac and positioned in the abdomen for later extraction.

Urethrovesical Anastomosis

The urethrovesical anastomosis is regarded as one of the most challenging aspects of MIRP. Numerous anastomotic techniques exist. The goal of the anastomosis is to provide a watertight, tension-free approximation of the urethra and bladder neck. To accomplish this goal, it is beneficial to have complete anterior and lateral bladder mobilization, a long and sturdy urethral stump, and a thick, circular bladder neck. If the bladder neck is large, patulous, or asymmetrical, then it may be necessary to reconstruct this with interrupted sutures.

For standard LRP, we prefer to perform an interrupted anastomosis with 2-0 dyed polyglycolic acid on a CT-3 needle. This needle is robust enough to resist deformity during suturing and has the appropriate length to work within the confines of the pelvis. Standard laparoscopic needle drivers are used. Initially, an undyed 2-0 polyglycolic acid suture is placed in the midline of the posterior bladder neck to function as a traction suture. A Lowsley tractor is placed per urethra. The first anastomotic suture is placed from out-to-in on the posterior bladder neck, and then in-to-out through the posterior urethra. Before tying this initial suture, the bladder neck traction suture is grasped with the jaws of the Lowsley tractor and is retracted toward the urethral stump. The traction suture relieves tension while the anastomotic suture is tied (Fig. 33-11). The suture knot is positioned on the bladder mucosa during tightening to ensure proper approximation of the bladder neck and urethra. After securing the initial anastomosis suture, the traction suture is released from the Lowsley tractor, and the excess suture material is removed from the bladder neck.

Two additional sutures are placed in the posterior bladder neck and urethra at the 5- and 7-o'clock positions, with the knots tied on the lumen side of the bladder. The remaining sutures are then placed circumferentially from posterior to anterior in an interrupted fashion with all knots on the outside of the lumen. Before tying the final two anterior sutures, a new 20-French Foley catheter is placed under direct vision across the anastomosis and into the bladder.

During RARP, we prefer a running (continuous) urethrovesical anastomosis. A running anastomosis can be performed in the same fashion during LRP if desired. A double-armed suture is created by tying together two absorbable sutures with RB-1 needles. Each suture is 15 cm in length, making the entire double-armed suture about 30 cm in length. One suture is dyed and the other undyed to aid in identification during the anastomosis. A Foley catheter is place per urethra through the urethral stump. Both sutures are passed first from *out* to *in* through the posterior bladder neck at the 5- and 7-o'clock positions. Each suture then is placed from *in* to *out* through the posterior urethra. Passes with each suture are continued in this fashion a few more times before cinching down and approximating the bladder neck to the urethra. The sutures act as a pulley system, and each throw is tightened sequentially to provide a tension-free approximation. Each suture is tightened after each pass until the anterior wall is reached. A new Foley catheter is placed under direct vision into the bladder. Both sutures then are tightened and tied to one another to complete the anastomosis.

Closure

The Foley balloon is inflated with 10 mL of water and tested with saline irrigation to verify that the anastomosis is watertight. If any obvious leaks are noted, then additional interrupted sutures can be placed. A closed-suction drain is positioned in the pelvis and brought through one of the 8-mm robotic or 5-mm port sites. All 12-mm port sites are closed at the fascial level with absorbable suture. The supraumbilical midline incision is widened at the skin and fascial level to accommodate specimen extraction, and then this incision is closed. All skin incisions are closed with a subcuticular suture.

POSTOPERATIVE CARE

Patients are admitted to a standard surgical floor. Ambulation the day of surgery is expected and may help to prevent ileus. Clear liquids are initiated on postoperative day 1. Venous thromboembolism prophylaxis with lower extremity compression stockings is maintained. Prophylaxis with low-molecular-weight heparin or low-dose unfractionated heparin is begun on postoperative day 1 as well. Intravenous antibiotics are stopped after 24 hours. Pain control may be managed with ketorolac (assuming normal renal function), oral narcotics, and intravenous morphine for breakthrough pain. If the drain output increases, then a fluid creatinine level is obtained to determine whether there is urine extravasation. If the drain outputs remain low with no evidence of urine extravasation, then the drain is removed before discharge. The Foley catheter is maintained for 7 days; if no urine extravasation is noted, then the Foley is removed at the postoperative visit. The patient is discharged when tolerating liquids, passing flatus, and ambulating with adequate pain control while on oral analgesics (generally 1 to 3 days after the procedure).

MANAGEMENT OF PROCEDURE-SPECIFIC COMPLICATIONS

Rectal injury is a rare but feared complication of prostatectomy. Careful inspection of the rectum before starting the urethrovesical anastomosis is of paramount importance. If significant concern exists, then a finger can be placed per rectum for better intraoperative inspection. Alternatively, a small Foley catheter can be inserted per rectum and the pelvis filled with irrigation. Air then is injected through the intrarectal Foley, and the field is inspected for bubbles in the irrigation. In a previously nonirradiated field with minimal fecal spillage, a small rectal laceration can be closed in two layers. After such a repair, omental or peritoneal interposition may be helpful in preventing rectourinary fistula. Anal dilation is performed at the conclusion of the procedure, and a low-residue diet and laxatives are given postoperatively. In the case of a large laceration, prior irradiated field, or significant fecal contamination, a diverting colostomy may be necessary to facilitate healing. Colostomy takedown generally can be performed in 2 to 3 months.

Anastomotic leakage can lead to ileus, infection, and bladder neck contracture. If the drain fluid creatinine is higher than serum creatinine, then urinary extravasation is present. Adequate bladder drainage is paramount in resolving leaks. The urethral catheter should be irrigated to ensure proper function. A plain film of the abdomen is obtained to identify the position of the drain. If the drain is deep in the pelvis near the anastomosis, then the drain can be withdrawn so that it is not directly overlying the anastomosis. If this fails, then the drain can be taken off suction and placed to dependent drainage. Generally, no further intervention is necessary, and time is required to allow the leak to heal. A cystogram is performed before urethral catheter and drain removal to ensure that there is no persistent extravasation. The surgeon should resist the temptation to reoperate and revise the anastomosis, unless it is determined that the urethral catheter is not in an appropriate position and cannot be replaced endoscopically. A watertight anastomosis with direct visualization of urethral catheter placement is important in preventing anastomotic leakage.

Rarely, urethral catheters may become clogged or nonfunctional. In general, a skilled urologist can attempt gentle replacement with a small Coudé catheter. If any difficulty is encountered, then endoscopic placement is performed over a guidewire. In cases of hematuria, manual and even continuous bladder irrigation may be required to ensure proper bladder drainage and to prevent anastomotic leakage.

Ileus is relatively common after transperitoneal MIRP. Bowel rest and possibly nasogastric decompression usually are all that is necessary. If more serious pathology is suspected or improvement is not seen over time, then a CT scan with oral contrast is performed to evaluate for mechanical obstruction or bowel injury. Missed laparoscopic bowel injury generally presents with low-grade fever, port-site tenderness, neutropenia, and possibly diarrhea. Careful inspection of the bowel on entering and exiting the abdomen is paramount in the identification of bowel injury.

RESULTS AND OUTCOME

The main perioperative outcome measures of radical prostatectomy are estimated blood loss, surgical margins, erectile dysfunction, and urinary incontinence. All of these outcomes are dependent on surgeon experience. Most of the available data come from high-volume centers with surgeons expert in the field of MIRP. Estimated blood loss has been shown to be less with MIRP than RRP. In a recent large retrospective study, the transfusion rate associated with MIRP was 2.7%, compared with 20.8% for radical retropubic prostatectomy.

The incidence of positive surgical margins depends heavily on the final pathologic stage of the tumor. With higher stage disease, the incidence of positive surgical margins increases. The overall incidence of positive surgical margins after MIRP ranges from 6-13%, and is not thought to be different from the rates obtained with RRP.

Erectile dysfunction is a common complication of prostatectomy, regardless of the surgical approach. With a better understanding of the cavernosal nerve anatomy and nerve-sparing techniques, the incidence of erectile dysfunction has decreased compared with historical data. Postoperative erectile function often is difficult to interpret because of a lack of standardized data collection both before and after surgery. More recently, validated questionnaires intended to collect objective data concerning potency have been used with increasing frequency (IIEF-5, SHIM score). Based on several large studies using these validated questionnaires, 66% to 85% of men are able to have intercourse 12 months after prostatectomy.

Similar to erectile dysfunction, stress urinary incontinence also is a common complication of radical prostatectomy. Most men experience at least some degree of postoperative urinary incontinence. Generally, the incontinence improves with time. Kegel exercises and physical therapy may help increase the rate of continence recovery. The use of validated questionnaires to collect data also is important in assessing the incidence of urinary incontinence. In large studies, about 95% of men are continent (no pad use) 6 months after prostatectomy. Surgical techniques that resuspend the urethra anteriorly or reconstruct the posterior support of the urinary rhabdosphincter may improve postoperative continence or hasten early return of continence, but further studies are necessary.

Suggested Readings

Guillonneau B, Cathelineau X, Doublet JD, et al: Laparoscopic radical prostatectomy: Assessment after 550 procedures, *Crit Rev Oncol Hematol* 43:123–133, 2002.

Guillonneau B, el-Fettouh H, Baumert H, et al: Laparoscopic radical prostatectomy: Oncological evaluation after 1000 cases at Montsouris Institute, *J Urol* 169:1261–1266, 2003.

Guillonneau B, Vallancien G: Laparoscopic radical prostatectomy: The Montsouris experience, *J Urol* 163:418–422, 2000.

Joseph JV, Rosenbaum R, Madeb R, et al: Robotic extraperitoneal radical prostatectomy: An alternative approach, *J Urol* 175:945–950, 2006.

Lowrance WT, Elkin EB, Eastham JA: Minimally invasive vs. open radical prostatectomy, *JAMA* 303:619–620; author reply 620, 2010.

Menon M: Robotic radical retropubic prostatectomy, *BJU Int* 91:175–176, 2003.

Menon M, Shrivastava A, Kaul S, et al: Vattikuti Institute prostatectomy: Contemporary technique and analysis of results, *Eur Urol* 51:648–657, 2007.

Menon M, Tewari A, Baize B, et al: Prospective comparison of radical retropubic prostatectomy and robot-assisted anatomic prostatectomy: The Vattikuti Urology Institute experience, *Urology* 60:864–868, 2002.

Patel VR, Thaly R, Shah K: Robotic radical prostatectomy: Outcomes of 500 cases, *BJU Int* 99:1109–1112, 2007.

Secin FP, Savage C, Abbou C, et al: The learning curve for laparoscopic radical prostatectomy: An international multicenter study, *J Urol* 184:2291–2296, 2010.

Jovenel Cherenfant, Tricia Moo-Young, and Richard A. Prinz

CHAPTER 34

Minimally Invasive Retroperitoneal Adrenalectomy

The videos associated with this chapter are listed in the Video Contents and can be found on the accompanying DVDs and on Expertconsult.com.

The frequency of adrenalectomy has increased since 1980. This increase has been due in part to the increased quality and use of abdominal imaging. Incidentalomas account for a substantial number of adrenal lesions identified with abdominal imaging. Although most incidentalomas are nonfunctional and asymptomatic, some patients diagnosed with an incidentaloma ultimately will undergo an adrenalectomy because of changes in lesion characteristics or an increase in its size. Such changes in an incidentaloma raise the possibility of an adrenal neoplasm. The prevalence and incidence of adrenal masses requiring operative removal, however, is not well documented.

The increased frequency of adrenalectomy has been paralleled by an increase in the rate and types of minimally invasive adrenalectomy, including lateral transperitoneal, posterior retroperitoneal, lateral retroperitoneal, robotic, and needlescopic transperitoneal adrenalectomy. In general, the minimally invasive approach has been preferred for the removal of the small to moderate-sized adrenal mass since about 1995. The lateral transperitoneal approach has been the most common minimally invasive technique used in the United States. A less commonly used technique has been the minimally invasive retroperitoneal approach. Posterior retroperitoneoscopic adrenalectomy was popularized in Europe by Walz and coworkers and is the focus of this chapter. The advantages of this approach include direct access to the adrenal gland and the avoidance of intraperitoneal organs and adhesions.

OPERATIVE INDICATIONS

The indications for posterior retroperitoneoscopic adrenalectomy are similar to other minimally invasive approaches, including nonfunctional incidentalomas, functional lesions producing Conn or Cushing syndrome, and pheochromocytoma. Adrenocortical carcinoma usually is considered a contraindication for minimally invasive adrenalectomy because of concerns of local invasion and incomplete resection. The relatively low incidence of adrenal carcinoma limits definitive assessment of these concerns.

Although tumors greater than 6 cm are considered a relative contraindication to minimally invasive adrenalectomy, larger lesions have been removed by the lateral transabdominal approach. An upper size limit for adrenal lesions has not been established for retroperitoneoscopic adrenalectomy. In the era of open surgery, a tumor size greater than 5 cm usually was considered a contraindication for open retroperitoneal adrenalectomy because of the confined operating space. For this reason, it seems reasonable to limit the use of retroperitoneoscopic adrenalectomy to lesions that are smaller than 5 cm.

Morbid obesity (body mass index [BMI] ≥40) complicates proper patient positioning and port placement for retroperitoneoscopic adrenalectomy; in particular, a thick layer of subcutaneous fat hinders port access to the posterior retroperitoneal space. In addition, the morbidly obese patient also is likely to have substantial retroperitoneal fat, which increases the difficulty of dissecting and identifying important structures. For these reasons, a BMI of 40 or greater is a relative contraindication for retroperitoneoscopic adrenalectomy, particularly early on in the surgeon's experience with this technique.

Although the indications for adrenalectomy are the same for essentially all minimally invasive approaches, the retroperitoneoscopic approach offers some advantages compared with other methods to access the adrenal glands. In patients with prior abdominal surgery, retroperitoneoscopic adrenalectomy technique avoids intraperitoneal scar tissue and adhesions, reducing the risk for injury to the intra-abdominal organs. In addition, if the patient requires bilateral adrenalectomy, then repositioning is not necessary, as it would be if the patient were in the decubitus position.

PREOPERATIVE EVALUATION, TESTING, AND PREPARATION

Endocrine evaluation of functional disorders, such as Conn or Cushing syndrome, is performed in the standard fashion and is not reviewed here. The patient with pheochromocytoma should be treated with α-blockade for at least 2 weeks before surgery and should be hydrated during this period to prepare the cardiovascular system for adrenalectomy. Some pheochromocytoma patients also may require β-blockade for tachycardia. This latter treatment should never be started before α-blockade, however, because of the risk for unopposed α-adrenergic stimulation in a patient who already may have severe hypertension. Potassium deficits should be corrected and blood pressure controlled in the patient with an aldosteronoma. Inhibitors of steroidogenesis (e.g., ketoconazole, metyrapone) may be considered for patients with Cushing syndrome.

Although the physiologic changes associated with retroperitoneoscopy are not as well documented as those with pneumoperitoneum, some effects of increased pressure in the retroperitoneal space can be extrapolated from conventional laparoscopy, including decreased venous return from compression of the inferior vena cava, hypercarbia from carbon dioxide insufflation, and decreased renal perfusion. The patient with cardiac dysfunction, chronic obstructive pulmonary disease, or underlying renal disease who undergoes a retroperitoneoscopic procedure should receive the same preoperative optimization, intraoperative management, and postoperative monitoring of their comorbidities as would be done for a laparoscopic procedure.

PATIENT POSITIONING IN THE OPERATING SUITE

Retroperitoneoscopic adrenalectomy is performed with the patient in the prone jackknife position, as shown in Figure 34-1. The upper extremities are flexed at the elbows and pronated. The hips and knees are flexed at a 60- to 90-degree angle. It is important to flex the hips to expose the area between the posterior costal margin and the iliac crest and to permit adequate space for port placement. All pressure points, including the chest, hips, and knees, should be padded. The torso of the patient is kept parallel to the floor.

POSITIONING AND PLACEMENT OF TROCARS

Posterior retroperitoneoscopic adrenalectomy can be performed using either a three-port or a single-port technique. With the three-port approach, the first (10-mm) trocar is placed 1 fingerbreadth below the tip of the 12th rib (Fig. 34-2). If fascia is encountered instead of muscle fibers, then it likely is the thoracodorsal (lumbodorsal) fascia, which invests the erector spinae muscles, meaning that the incision was too medial. If the thoracodorsal fascia is identified and the trocar is passed just lateral to this landmark, then the superior lumbar triangle likely will be traversed (see Fig. 34-2). The musculofascial layers in the region of the triangle are, from superficial to deep, the latissimus dorsi muscle, external oblique muscle, and transversalis fascia (Fig. 34-3). The superior lumbar triangle is the thinnest point of the posterior abdominal wall and is a potential location for incisional hernia. Ideally, therefore, the initial trocar should traverse lateral to this triangle. It often is difficult to ascertain the borders of this

triangle, so this 10-mm port site should be closed securely at the procedure's conclusion.

A properly placed 10-mm port-site incision should sequentially go through skin, subcutaneous fat, external oblique muscle, internal oblique muscle, transversus abdominis muscle, and transversalis fascia before reaching the retroperitoneal space (see Fig. 34-3). If the port is placed slightly cephalad and medial, then the surgeon will sequentially encounter skin, subcutaneous fat, tail of latissimus dorsi overlying the external oblique, external oblique, internal oblique, transversus abdominis, and transversalis fascia. Penetration through the transversalis fascia yields entry

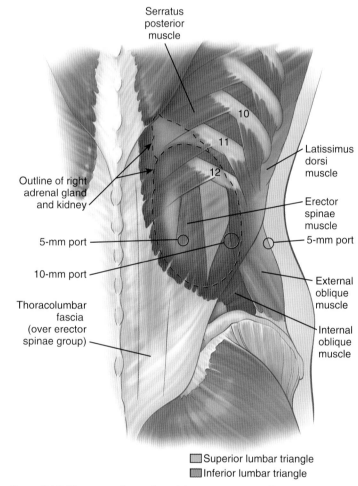

FIGURE 34-2 Placement of ports for a right posterior minimally invasive retroperitoneal adrenalectomy. Ports for a left-sided procedure would be a mirror image.

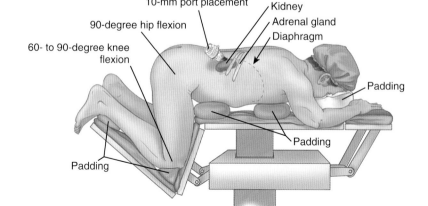

FIGURE 34-1 Prone jackknife positioning for a minimally invasive retroperitoneal adrenalectomy, using a posterior approach.

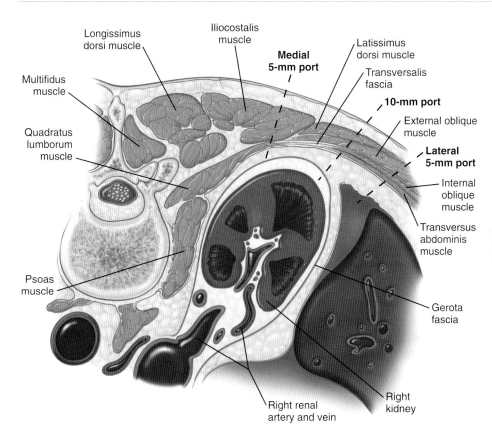

FIGURE 34-3 Transverse section of abdomen showing layers of posterior abdominal wall traversed by the ports in Figure 34-2.

into the retroperitoneum, in particular the posterior pararenal space (see Fig. 34-2). Finger dissection can be performed through the port incision to increase the retroperitoneal working space. The 10-mm port then can be placed, followed by a 30-degree laparoscope; the latter can be used to bluntly dissect additional working space. Alternatively, a balloon dissector can be used to establish this space.

After a working space has been established, carbon dioxide is insufflated to a pressure of 20 to 25 mm Hg. Two additional 5-mm ports then are placed under laparoscopic visualization (see Fig. 34-2). The first is placed medial to the 10-mm port but lateral to the erector spinae muscles. Port traversal through the paraspinous muscles should be avoided because it is difficult to enter the working space and subsequently maneuver the port through this muscle mass. The second 5-mm port is placed lateral to the 10-mm port. The three ports should be aligned horizontally and spaced at least 3 cm apart to prevent interference (Fig. 34-4). The central (10-mm) port typically is used for the laparoscope. If a different dissection angle is desired, however, then a 5-mm laparoscope can be used through the medial or lateral port so that the working ports can be switched.

With the single-port approach, a cutdown technique is performed using the tip of the 12th rib as a landmark, as described previously. The incision is enlarged to accommodate the particular port being used. The port should fit snugly through the incision so that carbon dioxide will not leak and the working space will be maintained. The surgeon should consider the thickness of the patient's posterior abdominal wall when selecting which single port to use. Flank wall thickness may be assessed from cross-sectional computed tomography scans or magnetic resonance images.

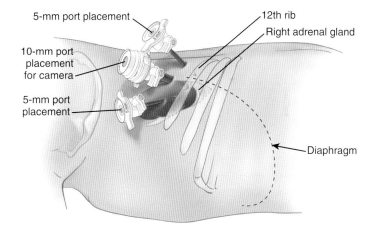

FIGURE 34-4 External view of ports with instruments inserted for a right posterior minimally invasive retroperitoneal adrenalectomy. There needs to be adequate distance between ports to minimize collisions. Note the angle of attack needed to reach the adrenal gland.

OPERATIVE TECHNIQUE

Exposure

The relative positions of the surgical team with respect to the patient are shown in Figure 34-5. The retroperitoneal space is entered inferior to the tip of the 12th rib, which most often corresponds to the hilum or the bottom half of the kidney. To reach the adrenal gland, the instruments and camera must be directed medial and cephalad (see Fig. 34-4). Entry into the posterior pararenal space will position the operator posterior to Gerota

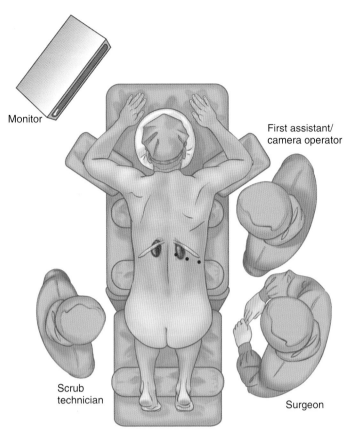

FIGURE 34-5 Positioning of the surgical team with respect to the patient. Note position of the kidneys with respect to the lower costal margin (12th rib).

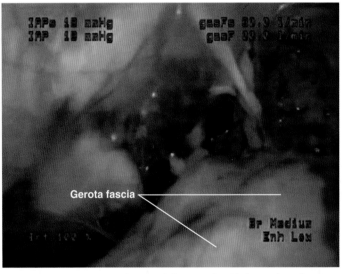

FIGURE 34-6 Intraoperative photograph from a right-sided procedure, showing Gerota fascia, which is seen after the initial entry.

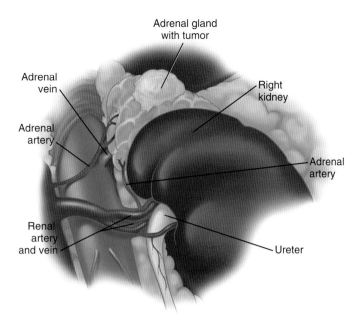

FIGURE 34-7 Relevant surgical anatomy for a right adrenalectomy, as approached posteriorly.

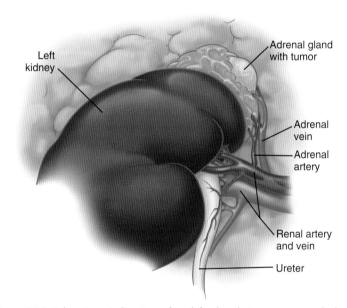

FIGURE 34-8 Relevant surgical anatomy for a left adrenalectomy, as approached posteriorly.

its surrounding fat, along with the kidney and its enveloping fascia, should be free as one unit.

Dissection and Resection

The relevant surgical anatomy for the right and left adrenal glands from a posteroanterior view is shown in Figures 34-7 and 34-8. A key aspect of adrenalectomy is to identify the junction between the adrenal gland and the kidney. To accomplish this, Gerota fascia has to be identified. This dissection can be accomplished with an energy device. Adrenal masses greater than 2 cm may be seen during mobilization of the superior pole of the kidney. In such cases, the demarcation line can be followed with dissection of the fatty tissue surrounding the mass (Fig. 34-9). The adrenal gland or mass should not be grasped because it can tear and bleed, which will obscure the plane of dissection. Avoiding manipulation of the gland is even more crucial when a

fascia (Fig. 34-6). Fibroareolar tissue is swept away bluntly or divided with an energy device. Gerota fascia is identified during this dissection but should not be violated. Lateral fibroareolar attachments are divided using an energy device placed through the lateral port, while counter-traction is placed with an atraumatic grasper through the medial port. The medial and superior renal attachments are transected in the same way to mobilize the superior pole of the kidney. During the lateral dissection, care must be taken to avoid violating the peritoneum. Once the fibroareolar attachments have been dissected, the adrenal gland and

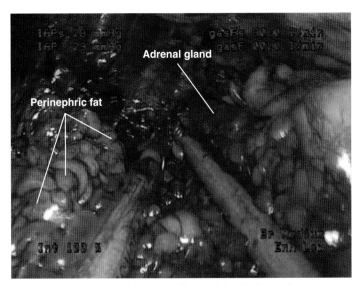

FIGURE 34-9 Intraoperative photograph from a right-sided procedure, demonstrating separation of the adrenal gland from the kidney.

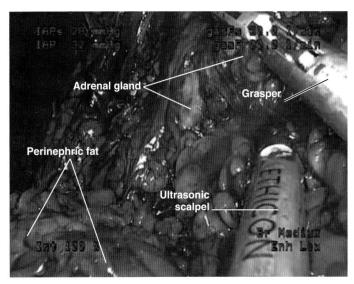

FIGURE 34-11 Intraoperative photograph from a right-sided procedure, demonstrating lateral to medial dissection of the adrenal gland.

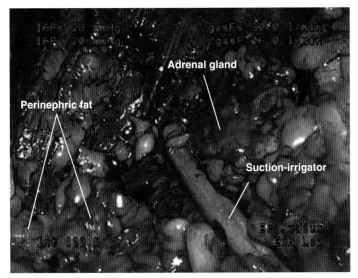

FIGURE 34-10 Intraoperative photograph from a right-sided procedure, demonstrating blunt retraction of the adrenal gland.

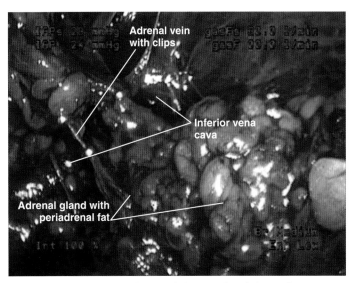

FIGURE 34-12 Intraoperative photograph from a right-sided procedure, demonstrating clips applied to the adrenal vein.

pheochromocytoma is suspected because it is more vascular, and release of catecholamines is a concern. Counter-traction is best provided by grasping periadrenal fat or by gentle blunt retraction without grasping (Fig. 34-10).

Identification of the venous drainage of the adrenal gland is crucial. Dissecting from lateral to medial usually is an easier way to define the course of the main adrenal veins (Fig. 34-11). With a pheochromocytoma, however, dissection should be done medial to the gland to identify and ligate the vein first. Theoretically, this prevents labile hemodynamic changes secondary to hormone release from the tumor. There can be more than one vein draining the gland, and the surgeon must be aware of this possibility.

Inferior vena cava or renal vessel injuries can be avoided by maintaining a three-dimensional orientation of the gland in relation to the surrounding structures. The challenging area of dissection typically is the medial aspect of the gland, where the periadrenal fat and Gerota fascia can obscure the course of the vessels. This region requires meticulous clearing of fat and fibro-areolar tissue. Atraumatic graspers should be applied delicately during this dissection. The periadrenal fat should be gently elevated and dissected one layer at a time, and the tip of the

dissecting instrument should be visualized at all times. Blind entry into the periadrenal fat may lead to injury to the underlying, intertwined vessels.

On the right side, the inferior vena cava should be exposed, with dissection beginning on the medial side of the gland and then proceeding lateral to medial. Any intervening arterial branches are divided with an energy device. Lateral traction may be used on the periadrenal fat to tent the inferior vena cava, which can aid in the exposure of the right adrenal vein. This vessel should be gently elevated to inspect the surrounding attachments because it sometimes bifurcates or trifurcates to other branches. The vein can be ligated with clips (Fig. 34-12), an energy device, or a combination of both. Identification of a single vein should not deter the surgeon from searching for additional venous branches. After the surgeon is certain that all the venous branches have been ligated, the remaining periadrenal fat is divided with the energy device until the gland is free.

Identification of the left adrenal vein is done similarly to the right side, beginning with dissection on the inferomedial aspect of the gland. The left phrenic vein may merge with the adrenal vein before entering the renal vein. The left adrenal vein should be dissected out sufficiently to confirm its entrance into the adrenal gland so that the superior branches of the renal vein will not be injured. After the left adrenal vein has been ligated, the remaining periadrenal fat is divided with the energy device until the gland is free.

Retrieval of the resected adrenal gland is achieved with an endoscopic bag placed through the 10-mm port. The incision may need to be enlarged, depending on the size of the specimen. Some surgeons prefer to morcellate the gland so that they do not have to enlarge the incision to remove the gland. After the gland is removed, the carbon dioxide is partially evacuated, and hemostasis of the working space is evaluated. The ports should be removed under direct vision. The fascia at the 10-mm port site should be reapproximated using sutures placed externally or with a suture-passing device.

POSTOPERATIVE CARE

The surgical management of patients after adrenalectomy depends more on the tumor than the operative approach. Most of our postoperative patients are observed on a non–intensive care unit (ICU) floor; patients with pheochromocytoma are monitored more closely (sometimes in the ICU) until their cardiovascular system and blood glucose levels have stabilized. If urine output has been satisfactory, then the Foley catheter is removed at the end of the procedure. The patient is started on liquids immediately after surgery and is advanced to a regular diet as tolerated. Early ambulation is encouraged. The typical patient requires minimal narcotics and is discharged home within 1 or 2 days. The particular adrenal disorder often will require specific postoperative management, such as perioperative steroids in patients with Cushing syndrome.

MANAGEMENT OF PROCEDURE-SPECIFIC COMPLICATIONS

Bleeding

The retroperitoneoscopic approach to adrenalectomy does not appear to increase the risk for bleeding compared with the other approaches. If bleeding is encountered, however, then an automatic conversion to an open procedure is not mandatory. The bleeding vessel often can be grasped and clamped. The insufflation pressure in the working cavity can be increased to 25 to 30 mm Hg for a tamponade effect, although there is the theoretical concern for gas embolus if a major vessel has been entered. Additional ports may be placed to access the area from other angles that may facilitate exposure and vessel control.

If major bleeding cannot be controlled with the minimally invasive instrumentation, then rapid open conversion can be accomplished in one of two ways. The first is an open retroperitoneal approach with the patient remaining in the prone position. A subcostal incision is made by joining the port-site incisions, and the retroperitoneal space is explored to identify and control the injury. Major bleeding likely is secondary to a vessel injury, although renal or adrenal parenchymal tears also can cause substantial hemorrhage. A large uncontrollable caval injury likely will require an anterior midline peritoneal approach, which is the second type of conversion. The opened retroperitoneum is packed with laparotomy pads, and the patient is flipped into the supine position. Standard technique for exposure and repair of juxtarenal caval injury then is performed.

Renal Vein Ligation

The venous drainage of the adrenal gland and the kidney varies substantially. The superior pole of the kidney may have a high-lying venous branch with a cephalad course that may appear to originate from the adrenal gland. It is important to follow each vein sufficiently along its course to visualize its entrance into either the kidney or the adrenal gland. Ligation of a renal vein can lead to hypertension and renal dysfunction.

Poor Exposure

The retroperitoneal working space is confined, with limited ability for expansion. Exposure can be limited if the ports are not properly placed. If the retroperitoneoscopic exposure is not satisfactory, then additional ports should be placed or repositioned until the area of dissection is exposed. The surgeon should not guess or assume the course of a vessel, the tip of the kidney, or the extent of the mass. Division of any tissue should be done only when it has been positively identified and the mechanism of division has been determined to be safe.

Port-Site Hernia

The risk for port-site incisional hernia appears to be increased in cases in which the incision had to be enlarged for specimen retrieval. The kidney can herniate through such a defect. If the peritoneal layer was inadvertently violated, then bowel also can be incarcerated in a port defect. Although the retroperitoneum is a confined space with fixed organs, this status changes after a retroperitoneal procedure. The kidney is mobile after a retroperitoneoscopic adrenalectomy. For all of these reasons, the fascia at the 10-mm port site should be closed carefully.

RESULTS AND OUTCOMES

Multiple series on retroperitoneoscopic adrenalectomy have reported the feasibility and safety of this technique. The morbidity rate after lateral transperitoneal adrenalectomy has varied from 2.9% to 19%; morbidities have included pneumothorax, bleeding, hypoadrenalism, and wound infection. A mortality rate of 0.4% has been reported for the lateral transperitoneal approach. These rates are comparable to those of retroperitoneoscopic adrenalectomy. Walz and associates (2010) reported zero mortality in a series of 97 cases (Table 34-1). Forty-three operations were completed using the single-port technique, whereas the remaining were done with the three-port approach. These investigators reported no bleeding complications or need to convert to an open procedure. No port-site hernia was observed. They did describe four minor complications of temporary segmental relaxation of the abdominal wall.

Our experience with retroperitoneoscopic adrenalectomy has been similar to that reported in the literature. In our series of 23 patients, we have observed no mortality and 3 complications (13.6%), including one pancreatic fistula, one caval injury (requiring anterior conversion), and one port-site hernia. There was one other conversion (to a lateral transperitoneal approach) secondary to failure to progress. Our average operating time has been 144 minutes.

In comparison with lateral transperitoneal laparoscopic adrenalectomy, posterior retroperitoneoscopic adrenalectomy has advantages of direct access to the adrenal gland, avoidance of

Table 34-1 Results of Minimally Invasive Adrenalectomy

Series	No. of Subjects	Technique	Morbidity (%)	Mortality (%)	LOS (days)	OR Time (min)	Conversion to open, n (%)
Zeh & Udelsman, 2003	100	LT	6	0	2.7	230	13 (13)
Brunt et al, 2001	72	LT	19	0	2.9	176	20 (2.8)
Salomon et al, 2001	39	RT	15.5	0	3.4	116	1 (0.8)
Walz et al, 2010	97	RT	8.5	0	2.7	56	0

LOS, length of stay; LT, lateral transperitoneal; OR, operating room; RT, retroperitoneal.

intraperitoneal organs and adhesions, and ability to perform bilateral adrenalectomy without patient repositioning. In addition, the outcomes of the two approaches appear to be similar, as discussed earlier. Despite these attributes, this technique has not been widely employed in the United States compared with Europe. With respect to retroperitoneoscopic adrenalectomy, some authors have commented on the lack of landmarks in the retroperitoneal space and unfamiliarity with this anatomic approach as reasons for the relative low use of this technique. Indeed, there is a learning curve for this retroperitoneoscopic adrenalectomy. Nevertheless, as more tertiary care centers adopt this approach and more reports are published on the technique and outcome, it is likely that more surgeons will consider this approach for adrenalectomy.

Suggested Readings

Brunt LM: Minimal access adrenal surgery, *Surg Endosc* 20:351–361, 2006.

Brunt L, Moley JF, Doherty GM, et al: Outcomes analysis in patients undergoing laparoscopic adrenalectomy for hormonally active adrenal tumors, *Surgery* 130:629–635, 2001.

Callender GG, Kennamer DL, Grubbs EG, et al: Posterior retroperitoneoscopic adrenalectomy, *Adv Surg* 43:147–157, 2009.

Hirano D, Minei S, Yamaguchi K, et al: Retroperitoneoscopic adrenalectomy for adrenal tumors via a single large port, *J Endourol* 19:788–792, 2005.

Nieman LK: Approach to the patient with an adrenal incidentaloma, *J Clin Endocrinol Metab* 95:4106–4113, 2010.

Salomon L, Rabii R, Soulie M, et al: Experience with retroperitoneal laparoscopic adrenalectomy for pheochromocytoma, *J Urol* 165:1871–1874, 2001.

Walz MK, Groeben H, Alesina PF: Single-access retroperitoneoscopic adrenalectomy (SARA) versus conventional retroperitoneoscopic adrenalectomy (CORA): A case study, *World J Surg* 34:1386–1390, 2010.

Zeh HJ, Udelsman R: One hundred laparoscopic adrenalectomies: A single surgeon's experience, *Ann Surg Oncol* 10:1012–1017, 2003.

Uterus and Adnexa

DENIS QUERLEU AND KRIS JARDON

Laparoscopic Pelvic and Aortic Lymphadenectomy for Gynecologic Malignancy

The development of laparoscopic infrarenal lymph node dissection in the early 1990s represented the last major frontier of nodal dissection in gynecologic oncology. Since then, laparoscopic pelvic exenteration also has been shown to be feasible, although this latter procedure still remains investigational. Pelvic dissection is a component of most procedures in gynecologic oncology and commonly is performed through the transperitoneal route. Laparoscopic pelvic and aortic nodal dissection can be performed using a transperitoneal or extraperitoneal approach.

Credit should be given to the late Daniel Dargent and Joel Childers for their collaboration and interaction in the development of laparoscopic nodal dissection. This operation currently can be performed by a gynecologic oncologist trained in laparoscopic techniques. Of note, robotic assistance has been proposed as an additional technical innovation. The robotic maneuvers essentially are not different from the laparoscopic maneuvers that are described in this chapter; in addition, the robotic approach has not been shown to improve patient outcome.

In experienced hands, the proportion of patients in whom the operation can be completed laparoscopically is more than 90%. Generally, the surgeon must be trained in nodal dissection for gynecologic oncology, management of large vessel injury, and laparoscopic surgery. In addition, the surgeon must be aware of the numerous anatomic variants of the arteries and veins in the aortic area, such as ectopic renal artery and double vena cava. It has been shown that 15 supervised cases of laparoscopic nodal dissection during a surgeon's fellowship is adequate to achieve proficiency in this technique.

OPERATIVE INDICATIONS

Indication for Pelvic Nodal Dissection

Transperitoneal pelvic lymph node dissection typically is performed in gynecologic oncology centers as a staging procedure or as a part of surgical management of cervical and endometrial cancers. In early cervical cancer, pelvic nodal dissection is performed at the time of radical hysterectomy. It is our policy to start with the nodal dissection, in order to select patients for a radical procedure; the patient with positive nodes on frozen section does not benefit from completion of a radical hysterectomy.

The technique of sentinel node dissection is gaining popularity in gynecologic oncology. Removal of a single targeted node from a node-bearing area can be accomplished with minimally invasive technique. Moreover, the identification of minute lymphatic channels located deep in the pelvis is facilitated with magnification, as provided by the laparoscope (Fig. 35-1). Initial attempts at sentinel node detection involved blue dye injection only, with marginal success; subsequently, combined isotope and blue dye mapping improved the detection rate up to 90%. A sentinel node may be found in an unusual area, such as in the region of the common iliac or aorta. Of note, the sentinel node technique does not apply to obviously diseased nodes in which lymphatic flow is blocked, which would make uptake of markers impossible.

Many centers (including ours) consider a positive sentinel node in early cervical cancer as a contraindication for an upfront radical extirpation; rather, it as an indication for aortic nodal dissection and possible definitive chemoradiation therapy. Further pelvic dissection in such a circumstance is not advised because it could increase the risk for a radiation-induced complication. On the other hand, the finding of a negative sentinel node does not necessarily eliminate the need for a pelvic dissection.

In endometrial carcinoma, the performance of a lymph node dissection is not indicated in low-risk patients, is controversial in intermediate-risk patients, and is mandatory in high-risk patients. In the future, pelvic sentinel node sampling could be used as a compromise between performing no dissection versus a full dissection in the intermediate-risk patient. If a patient with endometrial cancer has a positive pelvic sentinel node, then an aortic node dissection or sampling should be performed.

Indications for Aortic Dissection

Aortic node dissection is a component of most gynecologic oncology procedures, for both primary and recurrent gynecologic malignancy, including adnexal cancers. It is controversial in early endometrial cancer but routinely performed by most gynecologic oncologists in the case of positive pelvic nodes or in the high-risk patient (e.g., stage IB G3 endometrioid, or pathologic type 2). In early cervical cancer, some investigators advise routine aortic dissection, whereas others perform aortic dissections only if the patient has positive pelvic nodes. In advanced cervical cancer, the concept of surgical staging is not widely accepted, although an aortic dissection may prevent the node-negative patient from undergoing para-aortic irradiation and may prevent

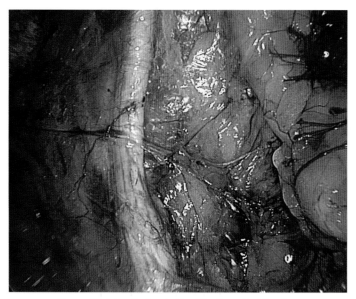

FIGURE 35-1 Sentinel node identification using blue dye.

the node-positive patient from an unnecessary primary procedure or exenteration for pelvic recurrence. An aortic nodal dissection generally is reserved for the patient who has no uptake in the aortic nodes on positron emission tomography (PET).

Indications for Laparoscopic Aortic Dissection

The laparoscopic approach to aortic dissection is the preferred approach if (1) the staging procedure is the only goal of the operation, as in the case of advanced cervical cancer; (2) an early adnexal malignancy has inadequate staging; or (3) the dissection is part of the evaluation before a pelvic exenteration. If simple or radical hysterectomy is feasible, then most stage I uterine cancers can be managed using a minimally invasive approach. As a consequence, aortic dissection may be part of the comprehensive surgical management of early gynecologic malignancy. In some cases, open surgical management of the primary disease is required to remove bulky disease. The laparoscopic management of early ovarian cancer is controversial because it is crucial to avoid tumor rupture and contamination of the abdominal wall. If ovarian tumor size is greater than 5 cm, then extraction through a port incision is not recommended.

Choice of Approach: Transperitoneal versus Extraperitoneal

The main benefits of the extraperitoneal approach are (1) better surgical ergonomics, with easy access to the left infrarenal area and an absence of bowel loops in the way; and (2) a reduction of postoperative adhesions, which has been demonstrated in an experimental study in our laboratory. As a consequence, the patient who is a possible candidate for extended-field radiation may benefit from the extraperitoneal approach. In addition, patients presenting with advanced cervical cancer or with high-risk endometrial cancer may benefit from an extraperitoneal approach.

If the technical conditions are not optimal (e.g., as in obese patients), then it is advisable to try an extraperitoneal approach. If the extraperitoneal approach fails in this situation, then the transperitoneal route can be used. The opposite strategy is not possible because the development of the extraperitoneal space

requires an intact peritoneum. In addition, the extraperitoneal route is preferred if the patient's history suggests the presence of extensive intraperitoneal adhesions.

Considering the improved surgical ergonomics with the extraperitoneal approach, we have favored the extraperitoneal route, even when a transperitoneal procedure is possible. If a reassessment of adnexal malignancy or a hysterectomy is required, then a "combined" approach is used. The first step is a diagnostic transperitoneal laparoscopy. An extraperitoneal aortic dissection (with common iliac and, when indicated, pelvic dissections) is then performed. Finally, the transperitoneal view is reestablished, the trocars used for the extraperitoneal approach are pushed into the peritoneal cavity, and the transperitoneal steps of the operation are performed.

Contraindications

If the patient will not benefit from the pathologic staging of a pelvic malignancy, then laparoscopic staging is not indicated. For example, an elderly patient who is not a candidate for extended-field radiation therapy with concomitant chemotherapy will not benefit from surgical aortic staging. Additionally, a patient with distant metastases identified at the time of PET imaging, or a patient with nodal metastases identified with computed tomography (CT) and then cytologically confirmed, will not benefit from laparoscopic staging.

A relative contraindication is the presence of bulky nodes that are difficult to remove through the laparoscope. Abdominal wall seeding, or spillage of cancer cells in the retroperitoneal space, is a concern in such a case. Although surgical debulking of enlarged nodes is an acceptable procedure, the benefit of such a procedure has never been demonstrated in a randomized trial. In addition, the dissection of fixed nodes may harm large vessels, leading to an emergency laparotomy for vascular repair. Our policy is to laparoscopically remove a diseased node up to 3 cm in diameter, so long as the node may be separated from the associated large vessel without breaking the nodal capsule.

PREOPERATIVE EVALUATION, TESTING, AND PREPARATION

CT and PET are essential for preoperative planning, as discussed earlier. No bowel preparation has been necessary in our experience. Cefazolin (1 to 2 g given intravenously) is used for prophylaxis. For prophylaxis of deep venous thrombosis, we administer a low dose of a low-molecular-weight heparin for 10 days before operation.

PATIENT POSITIONING IN THE OPERATING SUITE

For the transperitoneal approach, the patient is placed in the low lithotomy position without flexion of the hips because thigh elevation may limit instrument movements. Any compression of the legs should be avoided. The surgeon may stand between the legs when exploring the upper quadrants of the abdomen; for this reason, it is advisable to have a monitor at the head of the patient. Shoulder pads are unnecessary and may pose a risk for brachial plexus stretching. For the extraperitoneal approach, the patient is placed supine on the operating table. The senior surgeon stands on the patient's left side, and the assistant stands on the surgeon's left. A monitor is placed on the right side of the patient.

POSITIONING AND PLACEMENT OF TROCARS

The procedure requires scissors, grasping forceps, an irrigation-aspiration device, and bipolar coagulation forceps. We advise the use of bipolar grasping forceps with flat tips for control of smaller vessels that are close to the ureter, bowel, or larger vessels. Endoscopic clips must be available to control larger vessels or to mark fixed nodes for subsequent imaging. We use sponges to clean the operative field and to facilitate suctioning. More sophisticated instruments, such as an argon-beam coagulator, ultrasonic dissectors, or thermal fusion devices, can be used at the surgeon's discretion. In a pilot study, we determined that lymphostasis with the ultrasonic scalpel reduced the rate of postoperative lymph fluid collection after extraperitoneal dissection.

We use a left upper quadrant approach for the Veress needle to create a pneumoperitoneum. In case of previous laparotomy, a syringe test is routinely performed to choose the safest location, usually above the umbilicus. Alternatively, a 10-mm laparoscope is introduced through an umbilical incision (open laparoscopy) in patients without history of laparotomy. As an additional precaution, the direct vision technique using the EndoTIP trocar (Karl Storz, Tuttlingen, Germany) may be used for the introduction of the 10-mm trocar. Subsequent placement of trocars will differ for the extraperitoneal versus transperitoneal dissection, as described later.

OPERATIVE TECHNIQUE

Transperitoneal Pelvic and Aortic Node Dissection

After a laparoscopic survey of the abdomen and pelvis, at least two ancillary 5-mm trocars are placed approximately 10 cm lateral to the umbilicus. An additional 10-mm port is placed, usually in the midline above the symphysis pubis, for the extraction of nodal specimens. In our experience, the protection provided by the trocar sheath is enough to prevent abdominal wall metastases. Only grossly involved nodes that are larger than 10 mm in diameter are removed by an endoscopic bag. The retraction of the bowel may require an additional port (either 5 or 10 mm); we prefer the Endo Retract device (Covidien, Norwalk, Conn.).

Pelvic Node Dissection

The boundaries of dissection are (1) laterally, the external iliac vessels, the psoas muscle, and the pelvic wall; (2) medially, the superior vesical artery; (3) caudally, the circumflex iliac vein as it crosses over the external iliac artery, Cooper ligament, and pubic bone; and (4) cranially, the common iliac bifurcation and the ureter. The arbitrary deep limit is the obturator nerve.

The first step of the pelvic node dissection is the opening of the paravesical space between the round and infundibulopelvic ligaments (Fig. 35-2). The peritoneum is incised in this location. The external iliac vessels are exposed from the circumflex iliac vein caudally, up to the common iliac bifurcation cranially. The superior vesical artery is identified medially, which will be a limit of dissection as described previously. The bladder is mobilized medially. The obturator neurovascular bundle is identified, which will be the inferior limit of dissection.

After these landmarks have been defined, the assistant retracts the superior vesical artery medially to open up the paravesical space. The lymphatic fat pad is grasped at the medial aspect of

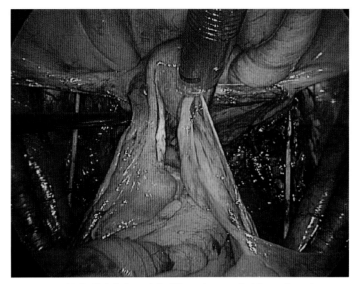

FIGURE 35-2 Global view of the bilateral paravesical fossa dissection.

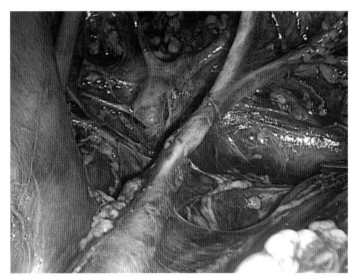

FIGURE 35-3 Clearing of the internal iliac vessels.

the external iliac vessels and is separated from the vasculature. This dissection is performed with atraumatic fenestrated forceps and small-blade monopolar scissors. Large lymphatic or blood vessels are desiccated with bipolar current before division. Clearance of the common iliac bifurcation then is accomplished while the assistant retracts the infundibulopelvic ligament and the ureter cranially.

The extent of nodal tissue resection should encompass the external iliac nodes (lateral to the artery), interiliac nodes (between the external iliac artery and vein, and between the vein and obturator nerve), and superior hypogastric nodes (lateral to the common iliac bifurcation, at the level of the highest root of the sciatic nerve) (Fig. 35-3). The lymphatic fat pad should not be morcellated, in order to avoid a tumor spillage. All specimens are removed through the 10- to 12-mm suprapubic trocar. If the nodes are too large to remove through this port, then a specimen retrieval bag should be used.

Aortic Node Dissection

The operating table is placed in 10 degrees of Trendelenburg position, with leftward tilt as needed. The omentum and intestine are retracted toward the left upper quadrant. The aorta is

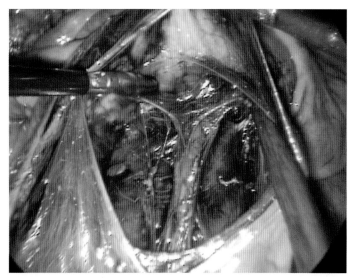

FIGURE 35-4 Transperitoneal aortic dissection; status after incision of the posterior parietal peritoneum.

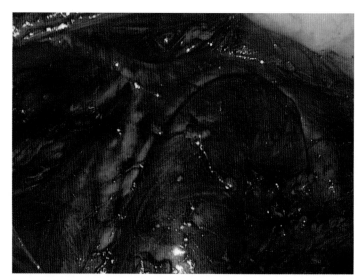

FIGURE 35-5 Transperitoneal aortic dissection; final status demonstrating the left renal vein.

identified under the peritoneum, up to the level of the root of the mesentery. The peritoneum is incised over the lower 5 cm of aorta and the first 2 cm of the right common iliac artery (Fig. 35-4). The left margin of the peritoneal incision is retracted laterally to the left side of the patient, in order to create a "wall" between the operative field and the bowel loops. The anterior aspect of the aorta and of the vena cava is identified with gentle blunt dissection. The retroperitoneal space is developed from the root of the mesentery up to the third or fourth portion of the duodenum. Elevation of the duodenum at this point should allow visualization of the left renal vein.

The retroperitoneal space then is developed laterally under the right and left mesocolon, and both psoas muscles are identified. The ureters and ovarian vessels usually are readily identifiable under the mesocolon and usually are elevated along with the ascending and descending colon. The anterior aspect of the aorta is dissected to above the level of the inferior mesenteric artery. The vena cava is identified on the right side of the aorta. The anterior aspect of the cava is dissected to above the level of the right ovarian vein. To identify the left renal vein, the caval dissection is performed up to the origins of ovarian arteries. Both ovarian arteries may need to be divided to allow elevation of the peritoneum and the viscera, providing space for a panoramic view of the retroperitoneal space and allowing full access to the left renal vein, from the end of the left ovarian vein to the junction with the vena cava (Fig. 35-5).

The para-aortic lymphatic tissue is now ready for removal. The left lateroaortic, precaval, interaorticocaval, and laterocaval nodal areas may be separately dissected from the major vessels and removed. Throughout the operation, blunt dissection with the closed end of atraumatic forceps or with the tip of the aspiration device (used at the same time to clarify the operative field when necessary) can provide a safe dissection method. Electrosurgery with monopolar scissors or desiccation with bipolar electrocautery also may be used. As soon as part of a tissue flap is freed from the great vessels, it may be firmly grasped with a forceps and elevated to show its posterior aspect, overlying the vessels or the prevertebral plane.

All the small vessels going to or coming from the major vessels must be electrodesiccated with bipolar forceps or occluded using clips. The lumbar veins should be identified just anterior to the

prevertebral fascia, particularly beneath the aorta. If moderate bleeding occurs, then compression may be applied with the tip of a closed atraumatic forceps or the irrigation-aspiration device. Such bleeding may stop spontaneously or may require clips (vena cava branches) or electrodessication (aortic branches). At the end of the dissection, the supramesenteric interaorticocaval and the upper left aortic lymph nodes are detached from the left renal vein, using clips to secure hemostasis and lymphostasis. The surgeon should be alert to the presence of large veins from the left renal vein to the lumbar and azygos systems.

Extraperitoneal Para-aortic Node Dissection

The operation starts as a standard laparoscopy. After pneumoperitoneum is established, a 10-mm endoscope is placed at the inferior margin of the umbilicus. An additional 5-mm trocar is placed in the right lower quadrant to accommodate a needle for sampling of the peritoneal fluid or a biopsy forceps in case of suspected peritoneal involvement. A 15-mm incision is made 3 to 4 cm medial to the left iliac spine. The skin, fascia, transverse muscles, and deep fascia are incised, taking care not to open the peritoneum, which can be avoided with simultaneous laparoscopic view of the left lower quadrant.

The surgeon introduces a finger into the incision and dissects the peritoneal sac from the deep surface of the muscles of the abdominal wall, under laparoscopic monitoring. The dissection should reach the psoas muscle and then, medially, the left common iliac artery. These landmarks are identified with touch as a result of shape (psoas muscle) or beating (common iliac artery) and are dissected from the peritoneum as much as possible. The cephalad dissection of the peritoneum is more difficult because it tends to be thinner and more adherent.

It should be possible to develop an extraperitoneal space large enough to allow introduction of two trocars: a 10-mm trocar higher than and posterior to the first incision (in the midaxillary line) and a 5-mm trocar in the anterior axillary line, about 5 cm inferior to the costal margin. Finally, a balloon-tipped port (used for open laparoscopy) is placed through the 15-mm incision, inflated, and secured to the abdominal wall. This port will be used for the endoscope. The peritoneum then is deflated while the extraperitoneal space is inflated with 10 mm Hg pressure of CO_2.

The endoscope is introduced, and the left psoas muscle, left ureter, and left common iliac artery are identified; these will be the three major landmarks of the blunt dissection (Fig. 35-6). The psoas muscle is dissected up to the fascia of the kidney, which can be entered using scissors if the space is too narrow. The lower lumbar and iliac portion of the ureter is separated from the common iliac artery and lifted with the peritoneum. As a result, the ureter forms a "bow" above the operative field throughout the procedure.

The lateral aspect of the common iliac artery is used as a guide to dissect caudally to its bifurcation, and cephalad up to the aortic bifurcation and then to the renal vessels (Fig. 35-7). The anterior aspect of the common iliac artery vessels then is dissected, with the knowledge that small vessels run from the iliac to the ureter and peritoneum. The anterior aspect of the inframesenteric aorta is dissected, preserving the inferior mesenteric artery. After these steps have been completed, the lateroaortic nodes and the lateral

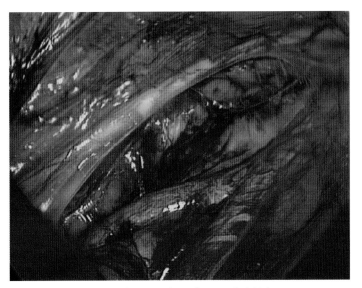

FIGURE 35-6 Left extraperitoneal approach; initial status.

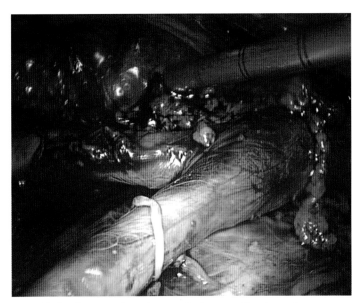

FIGURE 35-7 Left extraperitoneal approach, demonstrating the aortic bifurcation.

common iliac nodes can be detached from these and the lumbar vessels, the prevertebral fascia, and the sympathetic nerves.

The right side of the extraperitoneal space is dissected next. The peritoneum is elevated off the left common iliac vein and then off the sacral promontory. The bifurcation of the inferior vena cava is identified. Care must be taken not to injure the middle sacral vessels. The right common iliac vein and the right common iliac artery are mobilized with blunt dissection. Enlargement of the operative space in this area requires caudal retraction of the sigmoid colon.

The right ureter then is elevated and separated from the iliac vessels and the psoas muscle. The right ovarian vein is identified on the undersurface of the mesocolon. The precaval nodes then are identified and detached from the inferior vena cava. These nodes typically are tethered to the vena cava by small vessels. Gentle elevation of the nodal tissue is used to control these small vessels with monopolar cautery. The inframesenteric preaortic nodes are taken next, followed by the laterocaval nodes. The latter can be dissected within the same plane, with dorsal pushing of the aorta and vena cava.

The infrarenal dissection starts at the lateral aspect of the aorta. The lateroaortic nodes below the left renal vessels are dissected first. The lateroaortic segment of the left renal vein is identified with blunt dissection. The associated venous network, including the lombo-azygos vein and the end of the left ovarian vein, then is dissected. The dissection generally ends with the removal of the high preaortic and left lateroaortic nodes. The dissection of the anterior aspect of the aorta and of the preaortic segment of the left renal vein may require the division of the left ovarian artery, although this is not routinely performed. Separation of the aorta from the prevertebral fascia and the removal of the retrovascular (retrocaval and retroaortic) nodes is feasible but not included in the standard nodal dissection for cervical carcinoma.

At the completion of the operation, a careful check for hemostasis is performed, and the operative field is irrigated and suctioned. An opening in the peritoneum along the left paracolic gutter then is made (either from within the extraperitoneal space or from within the peritoneal cavity) for lymph drainage. Incisions 10 mm and greater are closed with 0-absorbable suture, followed by the skin with sutures or staples. No external drains are placed.

Pelvic Lymph Node Dissection Using a Lateral Extraperitoneal Approach

The development of the extraperitoneal approach for aortic nodal dissection led us to investigate the possibility of using the same approach for pelvic node dissection in the setting of advanced cervical cancer. Starting from a completed extraperitoneal aortic dissection, the left external iliac artery is dissected from the bifurcation of the left common iliac artery to the femoral ring, taking care not to injure the genitofemoral nerve. The lymph nodes of the lateral external iliac chain are removed (Fig. 35-8). The pelvic portion of the ureter is mobilized medially with the peritoneum. The internal iliac artery and the obliterated umbilical artery are identified, and the bladder then is mobilized medially.

At this point, the lymph nodes located at the bifurcation of the common iliac can be removed. The medial aspect of the external iliac vein then is dissected. Direct access to the obturator fossa is difficult because the view of the endoscope from the left

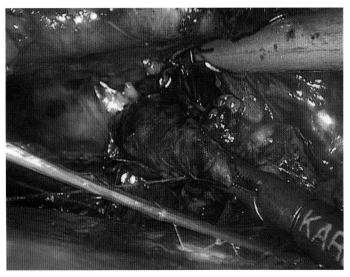

FIGURE 35-8 Extraperitoneal left pelvic dissection, showing removal of an enlarged node.

flank is obstructed by the external iliac vessels where they attach to the psoas muscle. The external iliac vessels can be dissected from the pelvic wall, however, which should produce a view so that the obturator nodes and the underlying obturator nerve can be identified. Dissection and preservation of the obturator nerve often require lateral retraction of the psoas and internal obturator muscles. The obturator nodes then may be dissected from the external iliac vein and obturator nerve.

A right pelvic lymph node dissection may be attempted from the left side. The main obstacle is the mesorectum, which may be pushed caudally, if it has adequate mobility. Alternatively, the plane posterior to the mesorectum may be developed. The extraperitoneal dissection then is extended caudally along the right external and internal iliac vessels. This approach, however, is technically difficult (if not impossible) in most patients.

POSTOPERATIVE CARE

Postprocedure nasogastric intubation and antibiotics are not necessary. Intravenous fluids are stopped on the morning of postoperative day 1. Analgesia is accomplished with oral nonnarcotic medication if possible, with oral narcotic medication being used for breakthrough pain only. The patient is fed as soon as possible and generally is discharged on the first postoperative day.

MANAGEMENT OF PROCEDURE-SPECIFIC COMPLICATIONS

A major risk from lymphadenectomy is venous laceration, which may involve the vena cava, left renal vein, ovarian vein, or a lumbar vein. Minor venous injuries may be managed with 3 minutes of sponge compression; more serious injuries may be controlled with clips. Avulsion of the origin of the ovarian vein may lead to a lateral aortic injury of the aorta, so care should be taken in control of such an injury. Injury to the inferior mesenteric artery may be managed with clip ligation of this vessel. Ureteral injury during para-aortic dissection may be repaired with laparoscopic suturing techniques and cystoscopic placement of a pigtail catheter. The risk for lymphocele formation from an extraperitoneal procedure may be reduced by

opening of the peritoneum after completion of the aortic dissection and by obtaining careful lymphostasis with the ultrasonic scalpel.

RESULTS AND OUTCOME

Our 16-year experience in laparoscopic lymphadenectomy (published in 2006) included 1000 gynecologic cancer patients who underwent laparoscopic pelvic or aortic nodal dissection, or both. A total of 1192 pelvic and aortic lymphadenectomies have been performed, including 415 aortic lymphadenectomies (155 transperitoneal and 260 extraperitoneal). The main indications for laparoscopic lymph node dissection included early cervical carcinoma ($n = 456$), advanced cervical carcinoma ($n = 219$), vaginal carcinoma ($n = 4$), endometrial carcinoma ($n = 182$), and ovarian carcinoma ($n = 139$). There was no perioperative mortality. The open conversion rate was 1.3%.

With experience, the number of nodes retrieved from a laparoscopic dissection has been similar to the number of nodes retrieved from an open dissection. In the German experience, the number of aortic nodes increased from 5.5 to 18.5 from early to later cases. In our experience, the average node yield of an aortic dissection has been 17 for a transperitoneal approach (including our early cases) and 21 for an extraperitoneal approach. Again, this is similar to the average yield of an open aortic dissection.

The rates of intraoperative and postoperative complications in our series were 2.0% and 2.9%, respectively. The overall rate of lymphocele formation was 7.1% and was increased with the extraperitoneal approach. A laparotomy was required to treat a complication in seven patients. There were 11 intraoperative vascular injuries, but none required a laparotomy. Other complications included bowel injury ($n = 7$), urinary tract injury ($n = 5$), and nerve injury ($n = 5$). Of note, since the publication of our series, we incurred a duodenal injury with a retractor during a transperitoneal aortic lymphadenectomy in a nongynecologic cancer patient.

If the complications related to aortic dissection are sorted from the above database, then 9 of 11 vascular injuries and 6 of 17 other complications occurred during an aortic dissection. We concluded that the risk for vascular injury is higher during aortic dissection than pelvic dissection. The overall complication rate in our series decreased with time, with 75% of the complications occurring during the first 5 years of our 16-year experience.

Laparoscopic aortic and pelvic node dissection is feasible and safe in skilled hands. It is useful as a staging procedure. With proper training, an experienced gynecologic oncologist may introduce this operation, including both the transperitoneal and the extraperitoneal approach, into her or his practice.

Suggested Readings

Dargent D, Ansquer Y, Mathevet P: Technical development and results of left extraperitoneal laparoscopic paraaortic lymphadenectomy for cervical cancer, *Gynecol Oncol* 77:87–92, 2000.

Köhler C, Klemm P, Schau A, et al: Introduction of transperitoneal lymphadenectomy in a gynecologic oncology center: Analysis of 650 laparoscopic pelvic and/or paraaortic transperitoneal lymphadenectomies, *Gynecol Oncol* 95:52–61, 2004.

Querleu D, Childers J, Dargent D, editors: *Laparoscopic Surgery in Gynecologic Oncology.* Oxford, 1999, Blackwell.

Querleu D, Ferron G, Rafii A, et al: Pelvic lymph node dissection via a lateral extraperitoneal approach: Description of a technique, *Gynecol Oncol* 109:81–85, 2008.

Querleu D, Leblanc E, Cartron G, et al: Audit of preoperative and early complications of laparoscopic lymph node dissection in 1000 gynecologic cancer patients, *Am J Obstet Gynecol* 195:1287–1292, 2006.

Querleu D, Leblanc E, Ferron G: Laparoscopic surgery in gynaecological oncology, *Eur J Surg Oncol* 32:853–858, 2005.

Rafii A, Camicas A, Ferron G, et al: A comparative study of laparoscopic extraperitoneal laparoscopy with the use of ultrasonically activated shears, *Am J Obstet Gynecol* 201:370e1–e5, 2009.

Scribner DR Jr, Walker JL, Johnson GA, et al: Laparoscopic pelvic and paraaortic lymph node dissection in the obese, *Gynecol Oncol* 84:426–430, 2002.

Sonoda Y, Leblanc E, Querleu D, et al: Prospective evaluation of surgical staging of advanced cervical cancer via a laparoscopic extraperitoneal approach, *Gynecol Oncol* 91:326–331, 2003.

Laparoscopic Hysterectomy for Benign Conditions

Oz Harmanli

It may be intuitive that hysterectomy would best be accomplished through the vagina, the natural orifice to the female genital system. In fact, vaginal hysterectomy (VH) can be traced back to ancient Greek history. Conrad Langenbeck, a German surgeon, presented the first successful VH in 1813. The first documented abdominal hysterectomy was by Charles Clay of England in 1843, albeit this was done without removal of the cervix. Unfortunately, the patient did not survive. The first total abdominal hysterectomy (TAH) was performed by Richardson in 1929 in the United States; TAH subsequently was used for cervical cancer in the ensuing decades. The morbidity and mortality of hysterectomy were reduced with the advent of antibiotics and availability of blood transfusion after World War II. Hysterectomy became one of the most common major surgical procedures performed by gynecologists, second only to cesarean deliveries.

In 1988, Harry Reich performed the first laparoscopic hysterectomy (LH). At this time, TAH accounted for about 75% of hysterectomies, with VH taking up the balance. The rate of LH subsequently increased from 0.3% in 1990 to 14% in 2005, predominantly at the expense of the rate of TAH, which dropped to 64% during the same period. There also was a small drop in the rate of VH, from 24% to 22%. As the laparoscopic approach became more popular, interest in supracervical hysterectomy resurfaced, and its acceptability has increased.

Of approximately 600,000 hysterectomies performed in the United States each year, about 10% are done for malignancy. Although traditionally performed through a midline incision, some gynecologic oncologists have demonstrated that hysterectomy for malignancy can be accomplished with minimally invasive technique, including robotic assistance. The scope of this chapter, however, is limited to LH performed for nonmalignant conditions.

OPERATIVE INDICATIONS

Uterine leiomyoma is the most common indication for hysterectomy, accounting for 30% to 40% of all procedures, followed by abnormal uterine bleeding, pelvic organ prolapse, pelvic pain, endometriosis, and malignant and premalignant conditions. Medical treatment alternatives for uterine leiomyoma include nonsteroidal anti-inflammatory agents and hormonal agents (e.g., progestins and gonadotropin-releasing hormone analogs). Uterus-sparing procedures for uterine leiomyomas include uterine artery embolization or myomectomy. Abnormal uterine bleeding may be controlled with a progestin-releasing intrauterine device or endometrial ablation. Endometriosis may respond well to hormonal agents such as a progestin or a gonadotropin-releasing hormone analog. If the patient has pelvic pain, then a multidisciplinary evaluation that includes gastroenterology, urology, and pain specialists is imperative before consideration of hysterectomy as treatment. Nonoperative management of pelvic organ prolapse may be accomplished with pessaries. In addition, it may be possible to repair a prolapse without a hysterectomy. Successful treatment of precancerous conditions is possible with local excision of cervical intraepithelial neoplasia and with progestin treatment for endometrial hyperplasia; treatment of malignancy is beyond the scope of this chapter.

PROCEDURES

Types of Hysterectomy

For benign uterine disease, the patient's general condition, quality of life, childbearing plans, ovarian reserve, and response to medical therapy will determine the decision between hysterectomy and the alternatives. If the patient opts for hysterectomy, then the surgeon needs to discuss the operative approach with the patient. A systematic review of randomized trials indicated that VH was the first choice of hysterectomy, because of its superior perioperative outcomes. In fact, the American College of Obstetrics and Gynecology has published a committee opinion emphasizing the benefits of the VH. When the vaginal route was not feasible, then the systematic review favored LH over TAH, despite an approximately 25-minute longer operative time with LH. In most cases, however, the gynecologist's comfort level and personal bias have been key factors in the selection of the type of hysterectomy.

Types of Laparoscopic Hysterectomy

A hysterectomy for benign disease may be performed laparoscopically from beginning to end. In total laparoscopic hysterectomy (TLH), all of the steps, including the division of the uterine ligaments, vaginal cuff incision (colpotomy), and vaginal cuff closure, are accomplished through the laparoscope, and the specimen usually is removed from the vagina. If the uterus is too

Table 36-1 Classification System for Laparoscopic Hysterectomy

Type	Laparoscopic Component of Hysterectomy
0	Laparoscopy-directed preparation for vaginal hysterectomy, including adhesiolysis and/or excision of endometriosis
I	Occlusion and division of at least one ovarian pedicle, uteroovarian ligament, or infundibulopelvic ligament, but not the uterine artery
II	Type I plus occlusion and division of one or both uterine arteries
III	Type II plus a portion, but not all, of the cardinal-uterosacral ligament complex, unilateral or bilateral
IV	Complete detachment of the cardinal-uterosacral complex, unilateral or bilateral, with or without entry into the vagina. This category includes total laparoscopic hysterectomy.

Adapted from Olive DL, Parker WH, Cooper JM, et al: The AAGL classification system for laparoscopic hysterectomy. Classification Committee of the American Association of Gynecologic Laparoscopists, J Am Assoc Gynecol Laparosc 7:9–15, 2000.

Table 36-2 Subgroup Classification System for Laparoscopic Hysterectomy

Subgroup	Step Completed Laparoscopically
A	Cases limited to the division of the pedicle(s) containing ovarian or uterine vessels
B	Cases that include dissection of the bladder
C	Cases that include performance of a posterior colpotomy
D	Cases that include both bladder dissection and a posterior colpotomy
E	Applies only to type IV laparoscopic hysterectomies and is reserved for total laparoscopic hysterectomies

Adapted from Olive DL, Parker WH, Cooper JM, et al: The AAGL classification system for laparoscopic hysterectomy. Classification Committee of the American Association of Gynecologic Laparoscopists, J Am Assoc Gynecol Laparosc 7:9–15, 2000.

large, then morcellation may be performed with a specialized morcellator, or by simply cutting the specimen into smaller components with conventional instruments. If laparoscopy is used as an adjunct to VH, then this procedure is considered a laparoscopy-assisted vaginal hysterectomy (LAVH). The American Association of Gynecologic Laparoscopists has standardized the terminology for minimally invasive hysterectomy (Tables 36-1 and 36-2). Based on this classification, TLH is considered a type IVE procedure. Some surgeons have promoted preservation of the cervix and perform a laparoscopic supracervical hysterectomy (LSH).

PREOPERATIVE EVALUATION, TESTING, AND PREPARATION

Preoperative evaluation before hysterectomy depends on the surgical indication. In cases that involve anemia, it has been a common practice to transfuse the patient so that the hemoglobin is 10 g/dL or higher. If a preoperative transfusion is not feasible, then it is prudent to type and crossmatch the patient for the perioperative period. Storing autologous blood for most hysterectomy procedures was not shown to be cost-effective in a large study.

Preoperative Papanicolaou testing and endometrial sampling are indicated in the patient who has abnormal uterine bleeding, cervical intraepithelial neoplasia, or endometrial hyperplasia. If

there is a suspicious pelvic mass or abnormal uterine bleeding, then transvaginal ultrasound also is indicated. More invasive procedures, such as dilation and curettage or hysteroscopy, are needed only if an adequate office biopsy cannot be obtained or, in the postmenopausal stage, if the transvaginal ultrasound demonstrates an endometrial thickness of greater than 4 mm.

Mechanical bowel preparation is prudent for the patient who has a history of previous pelvic surgery, pelvic pain, or endometriosis. Preoperative intravenous antibiotics are administered within 1 hour of skin incision. Spinal or epidural anesthesia is suitable for VH, whereas general anesthesia is necessary for LH.

PATIENT POSITIONING IN THE OPERATING SUITE

The procedure is performed in lithotomy position with padded stirrups. Sequential compression devices are used. The arms are padded and tucked alongside the body. If the patient's bare back is placed against a silicone pad, then steep-Trendelenburg position is possible, which helps keep the intestines away out of the pelvis. The patient's buttocks should overhang the end of the table by 1 to 2 inches to allow easy uterine manipulation, even if the patient slips slightly in Trendelenburg position. An indwelling catheter is placed in the bladder. A uterine manipulator, such as the VCare device (ConMed Endosurgery, Utica, NY) or the RUMI System (Cooper-Surgical, Trumbull, Conn.), is secured inside the uterine cavity so that the uterus can be moved in all directions and the vaginal fornices may be demarcated. Gastric intubation and decompression usually are not necessary, unless there is work planned for the upper abdomen.

POSITIONING AND PLACEMENT OF TROCARS

Veress needle insertion, direct trocar insertion (optical and non-optical), and minilaparotomy for open access are all acceptable techniques for peritoneal access. No definitive study has demonstrated superiority of one access technique over another. Some surgeons prefer an optical trocar that accommodates the laparoscope, allowing visualization of the tissue layers during abdominal wall penetration. A commonly used location for Veress needle or direct trocar insertion is the deepest point within the umbilicus because it provides the shortest distance to the abdominal cavity. For Veress needle or direct trocar insertion, the aim of the instrument may be 45 degrees from horizontal in a patient with a normal body habitus. Elevation of the abdominal wall can help keep the abdominal wall away from the intestines and large vessels. The direction should be increased to up to 90 degrees from horizontal in an obese patient. An intra-abdominal pressure reading below 10 mm Hg is a good indicator for safe peritoneal entry. No return of blood or other fluid and easy flow of the fluid into the abdominal cavity (e.g., the saline drop test) are reassuring signs of peritoneal entry.

After pneumoperitoneum is obtained, the operating ports should be placed under laparoscopic visualization, at least 8 cm lateral to the midline and about 4 to 5 cm cephalad to the pubic symphysis to avoid injury to the bladder and the inferior epigastric vessels (Fig. 36-1). Selection of a point 2 cm above and 2 cm medial to the anterosuperior iliac spine is another method to place the lateral ports (see Fig. 36-1). If the uterus is large or work outside the pelvis is expected, then the lateral ports may be placed more cephalad.

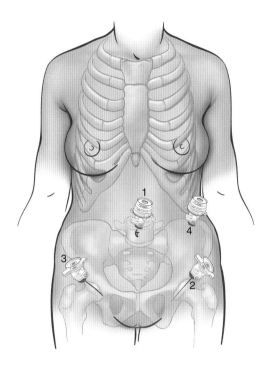

FIGURE 36-1 Trocar placement for laparoscopic hysterectomy. 1, Umbilical port for camera; 2, left operating port (5 mm); 3, right operating port (12 mm); 4, accessory port (5 mm).

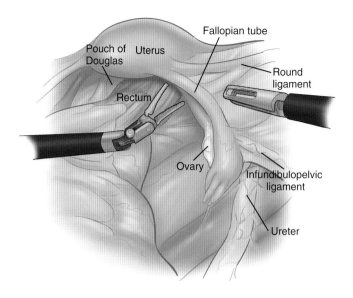

FIGURE 36-2 Laparoscopic view of the right pelvis.

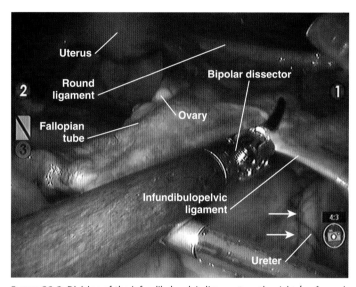

FIGURE 36-3 Division of the infundibulopelvic ligament on the right (performed if salpingo-oophorectomy is planned). The ureter is indicated by the *arrows*.

The operating port can be 5 mm, but the contralateral port should be 12 mm so that the sutures and other devices (e.g., a morcellator) can be introduced. A third 5-mm trocar is placed about 8 cm cephalad to the operating port, on the side that the surgeon has chosen to stand. If specimen removal and cuff closure are planned to be done transvaginally (as in a LAVH), then all ports can be 5 mm. An alternative first insertion site for women who may have adhesions is in the left upper quadrant in the midclavicular line, just below the costal margin. The stomach should be decompressed before inserting a trocar in this location.

OPERATIVE TECHNIQUE

Instrumentation

The key role of the uterine manipulator was emphasized earlier. Most gynecologists prefer bipolar energy, such as the LigaSure sealer and divider (Covidien, Norwalk, Conn.) or PKS OMNI (Gyrus ACMI, Southborough, Mass.) to control the vascular pedicles, instead of using surgical staplers. An ultrasonic scalpel or endoscopic scissors may be used for cutting and dissection. In addition, a suction and irrigation device and endoscopic needle holders are essential tools. In LSH, a morcellator will be necessary to avoid a large extraction incision.

Exposure

The first step in LH is to identify the ureters (Fig. 36-2). The right ureter may be found at the pelvic brim, where it crosses the common iliac vessels. It should be traced along the pelvic side wall until it dives under the cardinal ligament. The sigmoid colon makes it difficult to find the left ureter, but it may be found on the pelvic side wall below the infundibulopelvic ligament. These

steps can be facilitated with traction and counter-traction by a uterine manipulator.

Ligament Division

If salpingo-oophorectomy is planned, then the procedure is begun with occlusion and division of the infundibulopelvic ligament (Fig. 36-3). If the ovary is to be preserved, then the utero-ovarian ligament and the fallopian tube should be dissected and transected. Cauterization and division of the round ligament permits separation of the leaves of the broad ligament (Fig. 36-4). To mobilize the bladder away from the uterus, the anterior leaf of the broad ligament is dissected within the plane of underlying loose areolar tissue (Fig. 36-5). The rim of the cervical cup portion of the uterine manipulator demarcates the uterine border. During this dissection, the peritoneum overlying the bladder is elevated. The bladder has a yellowish hue, which can help the surgeon identify the correct dissection plane (Fig. 36-6).

The ascending branches of the uterine vessels are skeletonized and then transected with a bipolar energy source at a

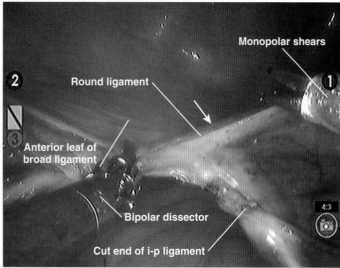

FIGURE 36-4 Division of the round ligament *(arrow)* allows the separation of leaves of the broad ligament. i-p = infundibulopelvic.

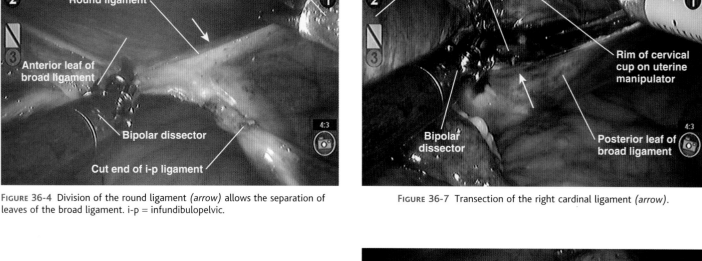

FIGURE 36-7 Transection of the right cardinal ligament *(arrow)*.

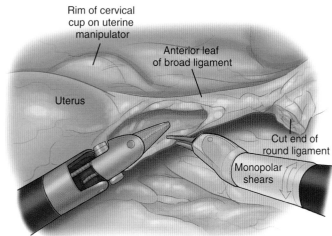

FIGURE 36-5 Dissection of the broad ligament: I, rim of the cervical cup of the uterine manipulator; II, anterior leaf of the broad ligament; III, round ligament.

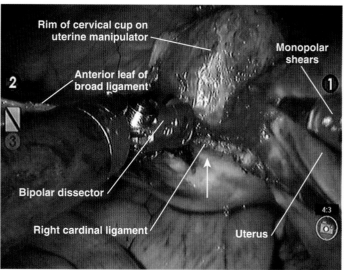

FIGURE 36-8 Transection of the left cardinal ligament *(arrow)*.

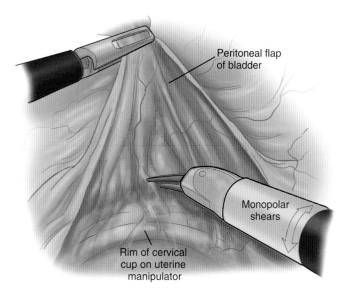

FIGURE 36-6 Elevation of peritoneal flap overlying the bladder. Rim of the cervical cup of the uterine manipulator indicates the vaginal-uterine margin.

perpendicular angle. Starting from this step, the widely open tips of the bipolar grasper should be placed on the uterus. The grasper should be clamped slowly so that it slides off the uterus in order to occlude all the collaterals and protect the ureter from injury (Fig. 36-7). The cardinal ligaments, followed by the uterosacral ligaments, are divided with bipolar energy at their attachment to the uterus. These steps then are duplicated on the other side (Fig. 36-8). When the devascularized uterus acquires a purplish hue, it may be amputated along the rim of the uterine manipulator (Fig. 36-9). If performed in this manner, the hysterectomy specimen will contain the cervix and be considered a TLH. The specimen then is extracted through the vagina unless it is too big, in which case morcellation may be performed.

Vaginal Cuff Closure

Pneumoperitoneum can be maintained after amputation of the uterus by leaving the specimen or placing a gauze-filled glove inside the vagina. The vaginal cuff then should be closed using a 0 absorbable suture with a continuous locking technique, running from one uterosacral-cardinal ligament complex to the other

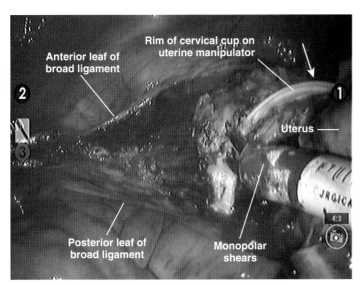

FIGURE 36-9 The devascularized uterus is amputated along the rim of the cervical cup *(arrow)* of the uterine manipulator.

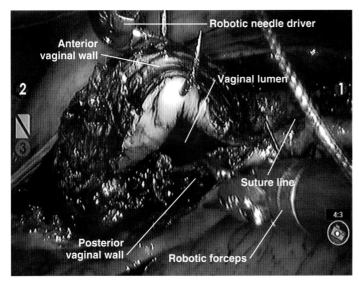

FIGURE 36-10 Closure of the vaginal cuff with full-thickness bites of a 0-0 absorbable suture, running from one uterosacral-cardinal ligament complex to the other.

(Fig. 36-10). Full-thickness suture bites that include fibromuscular tissue not damaged by electrical energy must be obtained to minimize the risk for vaginal cuff dehiscence, which has been reported to be more common with LH than with the TAH and VH. We have used newer suture technology such as barbed sutures and absorbable clips, which minimize the need for tying suture knots. A cuff dehiscence rate of 0.5% was noted in a series of 200 TLHs when barbed suture was used.

After irrigation and a check on hemostasis, all the ports are removed under direct vision. Any port site 10 mm or larger should be closed at the fascial level. We have preferred to use the Carter-Thomason CloseSure System (CooperSurgical) to perform the fascial closure step.

Intraoperative Cystoscopy

Although urinary injury rates are low in hysterectomy, some authors have advocated the use of intraoperative cystoscopy during hysterectomy, especially in patients with complicated anatomy or if uterosacral suspension is planned. A decision analysis indicated that routine use of intraoperative cystoscopy was cost-effective if the urinary injury rate was at least 2%.

Operative Variants of Laparoscopic Hysterectomy

Laparoscopic Supracervical Hysterectomy

The debate about whether to retain the cervix during hysterectomy has been renewed by gynecologic laparoscopists. The main advantage of LSH is that pericervical dissection and suture closure of the cuff are not required. The proponents of cervical preservation argue that maintaining the integrity of the cervix, the vagina, and the uterosacral ligaments simplifies the procedure and reduces the risks for urinary and rectal injury. They also suggest that sexual, urinary, colorectal, and pelvic floor function are more likely to suffer if the cervix is removed during hysterectomy. The opponents of LSH argue that there is a persistent risk for cervical neoplasia and cyclical bleeding, which may necessitate future surgery. The risk for cancer in the cervical stump after LSH has been estimated to be 0.3%.

In the past decade, three randomized trials of open abdominal hysterectomy with up to 2-year follow-up reported improved sexual function and satisfaction after both total and supracervical abdominal hysterectomy but were not able to demonstrate a difference between the total and supracervical technique. An anatomic explanation for this outcome may be that the nerve supply is located in the lateral two thirds of the uterosacral and cardinal ligaments, an area typically disrupted only during a radical hysterectomy. Urinary function was similar in both groups in two of these trials, but increased urge urinary incontinence after supracervical hysterectomy was found in the third. Colorectal function was not affected by the type of hysterectomy in all three trials. Although these trials did not include any LH, it is likely that the results would be similar with the equivalent laparoscopic procedures.

Technically, LSH is similar to TLH until the surgeon reaches the point of transecting the cardinal ligaments. Because the uterus is amputated at the level of internal cervical os, delineation of the cervicovaginal border is not necessary. Therefore, a uterine manipulator without a cervical cup such as the Valtchev Uterine Mobilizer (Conkin Surgical Instruments, Toronto, Canada) may be used. After the uterus becomes ischemic, the uterine corpus is transected above the cervix with either a pair of scissors or a cutting-sealing device. Then 12-mm port is replaced by a morcellator for removal of the specimen. It is crucial to keep the morcellator blade in view at all times. A technique for morcellation through the cervical stump has been described. In these cases, a 12-mm abdominal port is not necessary.

The debate over cervical preservation during laparoscopic hysterectomy is ongoing. In a comparative study, the risk for life-threatening complications or those requiring reoperation was increased twofold for TLH (5.8%) over LSH (2.5%). In addition, TLH was associated with a fourfold higher rate of urinary tract injuries than LSH (2.2% vs. 0.5%, respectively). It appears that laparoscopic supracervical hysterectomy can reduce urinary injury risk, the need for conversion, and the risk for cuff dehiscence. These short-term benefits of LSH should be weighed against long-term risks for continued cyclic bleeding and cervical cancer. Approximately 10% to 25% of women continue to have cyclic bleeding after a supracervical hysterectomy. In one series of LSH, trachelectomy (removal of the cervix) had to be performed in about 20% of all women as a result of continued bleeding. When the patient has had a preoperative diagnosis of pelvic pain or endometriosis, then most laparoscopists have preferred to perform TLH instead of LSH.

Laparoscopy-Assisted Vaginal Hysterectomy

The first LH performed by Reich was an LAVH, which combines laparoscopy with vaginal hysterectomy. He subsequently reported the first TLH in 1993. Compared with TAH, LAVH has a shorter recovery, is associated with less postoperative pain, and has a similar complication rate. LAVH may be more appropriate than VH in women with suspected endometriosis, adhesions, or a pelvic mass. It also is more prudent to perform LAVH in a case of early-stage, grade 1 endometrial carcinoma or complex endometrial hyperplasia if bilateral salpingo-oophorectomy is indicated. LAVH should not, however, be considered a complete substitute for VH. VH should be preferred over LAVH if technically reasonable because adding laparoscopy may increase the perioperative risk profile over VH and definitely will increase the cost.

LAVH can be accomplished with three 5-mm laparoscopic ports because the uterus is removed through the vagina and passing sutures into the abdomen is not necessary. Port placement is otherwise the same as for TLH. Laparoscopy may be used for division of the upper pedicles (including the round, infundibulopelvic, or utero-ovarian ligaments), dissection of the broad ligament leaves, transection of the uterine vessels, and development of the bladder flap, depending on the surgeon's comfort level. Gynecologists who are more comfortable with transvaginal surgery may choose to keep the laparoscopic component shorter, or may prefer to start the procedure vaginally, adding laparoscopy only if they encounter any difficulty.

Robotic Hysterectomy

Laparoscopic surgery with robotic assistance increased in popularity during the first decade of the new millennium. Robotic assistance provides improved depth perception with three-dimensional visualization, improved precision, elimination of tremor, and improved dexterity with articulating instruments. The disadvantages of robotic assistance include higher costs, prolonged operating time associated with equipment setup, relative lack of tactile feedback (an issue under study), and overall bulkiness of the equipment. Once the system is docked, the patient cannot be repositioned.

Although laparoscopic hysterectomy can be performed without robotic assistance, robotic technology has enabled some gynecologists, who lacked advanced endoscopic dissection and suturing skills, to perform LH. Even a skilled laparoscopist may prefer robotic assistance in a case of dense adhesions, severe endometriosis, or malignancy. In short- to medium-term assessment, robotic technology appears to be a useful tool in gynecologic oncology, complex pelvic floor repairs (e.g., sacrocolpopexy), and possibly complex myomectomies. Observational studies showed that robotic-assisted versions of these procedures produced less pain, shorter hospital stays, improved cosmesis, and faster recovery compared with the open versions. Currently, training programs are trying to determine how to incorporate robotic-assisted surgery in the residency and fellowship programs.

Single-Port Hysterectomy

Single-port laparoscopic surgery is a newer technique in which insertion of all instruments, including the laparoscope, occurs through a single 2-cm incision at the umbilicus. In addition to a putative advantage of improved cosmesis with a single incision hidden in the umbilicus, it has been proposed that hernia risk with a single-port procedure may be decreased because it is easier to close a 2-cm minilaparotomy incision than several small incisions. Long-term follow-up data are pending. A major challenge of this new technique is hand collision because of a crowded working space. Instruments with different lengths, articulation, and a flexible or a 30-degree laparoscope may offer a solution to this problem. Although promising, single-port laparoscopy will need more instrument improvements, and well-designed controlled trials will be necessary to substantiate its claimed benefits. At this point, it is not clear whether single-port laparoscopic surgery has any significant advantages over standard laparoscopic surgery.

POSTOPERATIVE CARE

Outpatient laparoscopic hysterectomy is possible if stringent criteria are used and close telephone follow-up is available. If this is practiced, then the surgeon should expect a readmission rate of up to 10% for a variety of temporary postoperative issues, such as ileus. As practiced by most gynecologists, however, most patients can be discharged after an overnight hospital stay. The first follow-up visit usually is 2 to 4 weeks after the procedure. If the patient underwent a cervix-sparing procedure (e.g., LSH), then current cervical pathology screening guidelines should be followed.

MANAGEMENT OF PROCEDURE-SPECIFIC COMPLICATIONS

If malignant and perinatal surgical indications are excluded, then the historical mortality rate for hysterectomy has been in the range of 1 to 3 in 10,000. A serious complication of hysterectomy is vaginal cuff dehiscence. In a series of 7286 hysterectomies, this complication was more frequent after LH (4.93%) than after VH (0.29%) or TAH (0.12%). This may be due to thermal injury to the vaginal cuff during LH. The rate of cuff dehiscence in LH may be decreased by reducing heat energy applied to the cuff and by taking 1-cm full-thickness suture bites with a 1-cm stitch interval. There is an anecdotal association of cuff dehiscence with an early return to intercourse. After TLH, women should be advised to refrain from intercourse for 6 weeks. Conversion to laparotomy in order to complete a procedure safely should not be considered a complication. In most reports of TLH, the laparotomy conversion rate has been 1% to 5%.

RESULTS AND OUTCOME

After hysterectomy for benign disorders, there has been a significant improvement in pelvic pain, urinary symptoms, and psychological and sexual symptoms at 1 year in most women. A large cohort of women who underwent hysterectomy for benign indications in Maryland reported improvements in preoperative symptoms, depression, and quality of life. In the first 2 years after hysterectomy, most women noted no change or improvement in sexual function. Hysterectomy may be associated with early menopause, however, even if the ovaries are not removed. The consequences of early menopause on cardiovascular health, bone metabolism, and general well-being may need consideration. In a nested cohort study from the United Kingdom, however, mortality after hysterectomy was not increased in medium- to long-term follow-up.

In general, VH has been the preferred approach to hysterectomy because it is the least invasive. Laparoscopic hysterectomy is recommended when a vaginal approach is not feasible. Despite the advances in laparoscopy and robotic technology, however, more than 60% of hysterectomies in the United States still are performed through laparotomy.

A Cochrane meta-analysis on various hysterectomy procedures, which included 34 trials with 4495 women, demonstrated that LH prolonged operative time over TAH by 20 minutes. Intraoperative blood loss was about 50 mL less with LH compared with TAH. Postoperatively, LH had less febrile morbidity than TAH (10.6% vs. 13.6%, respectively); not surprisingly, the wound infection rate was higher in TAH compared with LH (6.5 vs. 1.8%, respectively). LH also outperformed TAH with regard to hospital stay and return to normal activities. On the other hand, the meta-analysis indicated that the risk for urinary tract injury was about threefold higher with LH compared with TAH. There were no differences in the rates of bowel injury or venous thromboembolism. In contrast, the Cochrane review confirmed that LH had no specific advantage over VH; in fact, LH extended the operating time by about 40 minutes and had a threefold higher bleeding risk compared with VH.

Hysterectomy remains one of the most common surgical procedures in the United States. The published evidence generally has favored VH as the least invasive approach. LH is recommended when relative contraindications exist for the transvaginal procedure. With adequate training, transition from TAH to LH is possible without increasing the morbidity.

ACKNOWLEDGMENTS

We would like to thank Drs. Elliot Greenberg and James Gebhardt for their support in performing the hysterectomy in the featured video and Dr. Gauri Luthra for her support in preparing and editing the video.

Suggested Readings

Ahmad G, Duffy JMN, Phillips K, Watson A: Laparoscopic entry techniques, *Cochrane Database Syst Rev* 2:CD006583, 2008.

American College of Obstetricians and Gynecologists: ACOG Committee Opinion No. 311: Appropriate use of laparoscopically assisted vaginal hysterectomy, *Obstet Gynecol* 105:929–930, 2005.

American College of Obstetricians and Gynecologists: ACOG Committee Opinion No. 388: Supracervical hysterectomy, *Obstet Gynecol* 110:1215–1217, 2007.

American College of Obstetricians and Gynecologists: ACOG Committee Opinion No. 444: Choosing the route of hysterectomy for benign disease, *Obstet Gynecol* 114:1156–1158, 2009.

Carlson KJ, Miller BA, Fowler FJ Jr: The Main Women's Health Study: I. Outcomes of hysterectomy, *Obstet Gynecol* 83:556–565, 1994.

Einarsson JI, Suzuki Y: Total laparoscopic hysterectomy: 10 steps toward a successful procedure, *Rev Obstet Gynecol* 2:57–64, 2009.

Falcone T, Walters MD: Hysterectomy for benign disease, *Obstet Gynecol* 111:753–767, 2008.

Harmanli OH, Tunitsky E, Esin S, et al: A comparison of short-term outcomes between laparoscopic supracervical and total Hysterectomies, *Am J Obstet Gynecol* 201:536.e1–e7, 2009.

Hartman KE, Ma C, Lamvu GM, et al: Quality of life and sexual function after hysterectomy in women with preoperative pain and depression, *Obstet Gynecol* 104:701–709, 2004.

Hur HC, Guido RS, Mansuria SM, et al: Incidence and patient characteristics of vaginal cuff dehiscence after different modes of hysterectomies, *J Minim Invasive Gynecol* 14:311–317, 2007.

Ibeanu OA, Chesson RR, Echols KT, et al: Urinary tract injury during hysterectomy based on universal cystoscopy, *Obstet Gynecol* 113:6–10, 2009.

Johnson N, Barlow D, Lethaby A, et al: Surgical approach to hysterectomy for benign gynaecological disease, *Cochrane Database Syst Rev* 2:CD003677, 2006.

Lethaby A, Ivanova V, Johnson NP: Total versus subtotal hysterectomy for benign gynaecological conditions, *Cochrane Database Syst Rev* 2:CD004933, 2006.

Olive DL, Parker WH, Cooper JM, et al: The AAGL classification system for laparoscopic hysterectomy. Classification Committee of the American Association of Gynecologic Laparoscopists, *J Am Assoc Gynecol Laparosc* 7:9–15, 2000.

Parker WH: Total laparoscopic hysterectomy and laparoscopic supracervical hysterectomy, *Obstet Gynecol Clin North Am* 31:523–537, viii, 2004.

Sokol AI, Green IC: Laparoscopic hysterectomy, *Clin Obstet Gynecol* 52:304–312, 2009.

Sutton C: Past, present, and future of hysterectomy, *J Minim Invasive Gynecol* 17:421–435, 2010.

Tunitsky E, Citil A, Ayaz R, et al: Does surgical volume influence short-term outcomes of laparoscopic hysterectomy? *Am J Obstet Gynecol* 203:24.e1–6, 2010.

Whiteman MK, Hillis SD, Jamieson DJ, et al: Inpatient hysterectomy surveillance in the United States, 2000-2004, *Am J Obstet Gynecol* 198:34.e1–7, 2008.

ORNELLA SIZZI, ALFONSO ROSSETTI, AND ALESSANDRO LODDO

Laparoscopic Myomectomy

37

A myoma is a benign solid tumor consisting of fibrous tissue; hence, it often is called a *fibroid* tumor. A uterine leiomyoma, or fibroid, refers to a fibrous uterine tumor of smooth muscle origin. A leiomyoma is a well-circumscribed, round solid tumor, pearly white or light tan in color, that may grow as a single nodule or in clusters of varying size. This tumor may be attached to or be within the myometrium and is pseudoencapsulated by fibrous connective tissue. The diameter of a leiomyoma may range from 1 mm to more than 30 cm (Fig. 37-1).

The cumulative risk for the diagnosis of uterine leiomyoma in the age range of 25 to 44 years is about 30 percent. It is not clear whether leiomyoma is a precursor for leiomyosarcoma, the malignant phenotype. The incidence of leiomyosarcoma is extremely low in premenopausal compared with postmenopausal women, in whom leiomyosarcoma accounts for about 1% of uterine malignancies. The cellular morphology of a leiomyosarcoma is similar to normal myometrial smooth muscle cells.

The pathoetiology of leiomyomatous disease has not been determined, but most fibroids develop in women during their reproductive years. A leiomyoma will not develop before the body begins estrogen production; during pregnancy, a leiomyoma may grow quickly because of elevated estrogen levels. Once menopause has been reached, a leiomyoma generally will stop growing, and even can begin to shrink.

Most fibroids are slow growing, cause no symptoms, and do not need to be treated. About 25% of leiomyomas will cause symptoms, however, and may need medical or surgical treatment. Symptoms can include prolonged or heavy menstrual bleeding, anemia, mass effect, low back or pelvic pressure or pain, urinary frequency, constipation, dyspareunia, and in rare cases, reproductive dysfunction. Resection is the most effective treatment for leiomyomatous disease, and this has been the most common indication for hysterectomy.

In addition to hysterectomy and abdominal myomectomy, laparoscopic myomectomy has been developed to treat leiomyomatous disease. Kurt Semm reported the first laparoscopic myomectomy in 1979. This procedure is not without controversy, especially with regard to the volume and number of the myomas that can be removed and the putative risk on a subsequent pregnancy. In this chapter, we discuss the indications, technique, outcome, and controversies of laparoscopic myomectomy for uterine leiomyomatous disease.

OPERATIVE INDICATIONS

Traditionally, symptomatic fibroids have been treated with transabdominal myomectomy or hysterectomy. Hysterectomy is the most common major gynecologic operation in the world, and leiomyomatous disease is the most common cause of hysterectomy. For the patient with symptomatic fibroids who would like to retain her uterus, myomectomy should be considered. The indications for myomectomy include fibroid-associated infertility, tumor enlargement, pelvic pain, and abnormal uterine bleeding. In addition, there needs to be at least one myoma 4 cm or larger that is not accessible by hysteroscopy. Submucosal leiomyomas may be removed by hysteroscopy.

No upper size limit for fibroid resectability exists as long as the myoma can be mobilized. The maximal number of myomas that can be resected is somewhat controversial; some authors suggest no more than three or four myomas with a diameter less than 7 to 8 cm; others suggest eight or more myomas, whereas others suggest that the maximal resection number be based on individual choice, pathologic findings, and surgical expertise. Our experience has indicated that the upper limits of size and number for uterine leiomyoma resection should depend on tumor location, depth of penetration, and ease of mobilization rather than the total number of tumors or the maximal diameter. Nevertheless, it should be recognized that previous studies have indicated that the recurrence and complication rates are higher in cases of myomectomy for multiple fibroids.

If the quantity of myomas favors performance of a hysterectomy, then there are a number of less invasive approaches that can be offered to the patient, such as: (1) laparoscopic or percutaneous cryoablation; (2) laparoscopic or percutaneous myolysis with a variety of energy sources; (3) uterine artery embolization (UAE); or (4) magnetic resonance imaging (MRI)-guided focused ultrasound. All these procedures work to decrease fibroid blood supply, which can produce a tumor volume shrinkage between 40% and 80% but will not eliminate the fibroid.

UAE is a percutaneous, image-guided procedure performed by an interventional radiologist and may be performed in the patient who wishes to avoid surgery, is a poor surgical candidate, or wishes to retain her uterus. During UAE, a transfemoral angiographic catheter is placed sequentially into each uterine artery for injection of embolic agents (e.g., polyvinyl alcohol particles

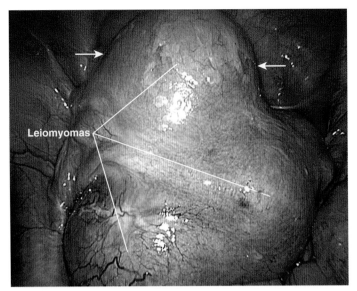

FIGURE 37-1 Laparoscopic view of the pelvis demonstrating a uterus that is laden with leiomyomas. *White arrows* delineate lateral extent of a large anterior myoma.

or trisacryl gelatin microspheres). This embolization is intended to produce uterine ischemia that will cause some fibroid necrosis and involution. The normal myometrium, which receives blood supply from the vaginal and ovarian arteries in addition to the uterine arteries (myomas typically are vascularized only by the latter), is expected to recover from the ischemic insult of a UAE. Large leiomyomas may be treated with UAE before laparoscopic myomectomy to facilitate the operation and reduce the risk for intraoperative hemorrhage. Of note, UAE is a relatively new procedure; there currently is little information on its efficacy, recurrence, incidence of premature menopause, effect on future pregnancy, and so forth.

In MRI-guided focused ultrasound, the clinician uses MRI to guide ultrasonic energy directly into the fibroid. The focused ultrasound beam (different from ultrasound used for clinical imaging) causes the temperature in the target tissue to rise to 55° to 90° C, which induces coagulative necrosis within a few seconds. The clinician can monitor the thermal destruction of the fibroid in real time with MRI, minimizing the risk to nearby tissue or structures. Each fibroid is treated separately, and total treatment times are generally longer than 1 hour for most patients.

Medical management of leiomyomatous disease includes oral contraceptives, menopausal hormone replacement therapy, gonadotropin-releasing hormone (GnRH) agonists, antiprogestins, progesterone-containing intrauterine devices, nonsteroidal anti-inflammatory drugs, and danazol. For example, therapy with a GnRH agonist often is used as neoadjuvant treatment before surgery. GnRH agonist therapy can down-regulate estrogen receptors, which can decrease fibroid growth and may increase the hematocrit that declined secondary to fibroid-associated menorrhagia. Mifepristone is a synthetic steroid that competitively binds to the intracellular progesterone receptor, thereby blocking the effects of progesterone and causing fibroid shrinkage. Raloxifene is a selective estrogen receptor modulator (SERM) that has been reported to decrease fibroid size. These medical treatments may be useful in the short-term for some cases, but none of these treatments is curative.

PREOPERATIVE EVALUATION, TESTING, AND PREPARATION

Routine preoperative evaluation for a myomectomy should include an ultrasound and hysteroscopy. A hysteroscopy will give information about the degree of submucosal involvement and whether a hysteroscopic resection would be appropriate. An ultrasound examination should determine the number and location of the myomas. Particular attention has to be paid regarding the distance of intramural myomas from the serosa and from the endometrium. The ultrasound may be able to rule out an adenomyoma or a sarcoma or may indicate the need for an MRI. Signs of adenomyosis include uterine enlargement in the absence of myomas, asymmetrical enlargement of the posterior or anterior abdominal wall, anechoic lacunae or cysts of various size, lack of contour abnormality or mass effect, hyperechoic islands or nodules, finger-like projections or linear striations, and increased echotexture of the endometrium. The vascular architecture of a myoma typically circumscribes the tumor, whereas the architecture associated with diffuse or focal adenomyosis will appear unremarkable, with the vessels following their normal course perpendicular to the endometrial interface.

A uterine conservation procedure is difficult in the presence of adenomyosis, because of the uncertainty in defining the site and extent of the disease. Unless the adenomyosis is well defined (as in an adenomyoma), it may not be possible to obtain cure with a local excision. Even a focal adenomyoma can have poorly defined margins where the tumor intertwines with the surrounding myometrium. In contrast, a leiomyoma compresses the surrounding myometrium and has well-circumscribed margins. A leiomyoma can be enucleated, whereas an adenomyoma cannot. When a uterine fibroid is removed, a capsule demarcates it from normal myometrium.

If the patient has rapidly growing or degenerating myomas that are not responsive to GnRH agonist therapy, then an MRI and lactate dehydrogenase (LDH) assay (total and isozyme type 3) are recommended to address the possibility of a uterine sarcoma. If the patient has a large myoma or the surgeon anticipates intraoperative difficulty with mobilization, or if the patient has anemia from menometrorrhagia, then 3 weeks of preoperative GnRH agonist therapy may be prescribed. One week before surgery, the patient may be given the option for collection of autologous blood for perioperative transfusion. A standard bowel preparation may be given. Administration of short-term antibiotic prophylaxis (e.g., a second-generation cephalosporin) is routine.

PATIENT POSITIONING IN THE OPERATING SUITE

Under general endotracheal anesthesia, the patient is positioned in lithotomy position with arms tucked at the sides to allow for surgeon mobility and to avoid brachial plexus injury (Fig. 37-2). A Foley catheter is placed. Two video monitors are placed at the foot of the bed. The cervix is grasped with a tenaculum and dilated with Hegar cones, and a uterine manipulator is inserted to assist with exposure and removal of the myomas. The surgeon stands on the patient's left, the first assistant stands to the right, and the second assistant is between the legs. A Veress needle is inserted at the umbilicus, and the abdomen is insufflated with carbon dioxide to a pressure of 18 mm Hg.

POSITIONING AND PLACEMENT OF TROCARS

A 10-mm optical trocar is inserted at the umbilicus, and the laparoscope is placed through this port (Fig. 37-3A). Two 5-mm trocars are inserted in the lower abdomen, lateral to the inferior epigastric arteries. A third 5-mm trocar is inserted in the midline, level with or higher than the first two. If the patient has a large myoma that extends toward the umbilicus, then the surgeon may consider an open supraumbilical abdominal entry to establish pneumoperitoneum (Fig. 37-3B). The midline operative port then should be placed through the umbilicus or even higher. In the presence of large pathology, the optimal insertion points for the lateral 5-mm trocars can be determined after laparoscopic inspection of the pelvis.

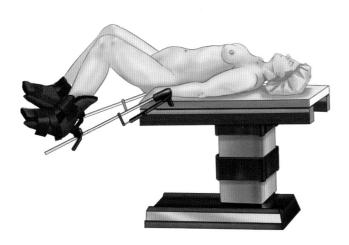

FIGURE 37-2 Dorsal lithotomy position, both arms tucked.

OPERATIVE TECHNIQUE

The basic operative instruments for a laparoscopic myomectomy include a bipolar coagulation forceps, monopolar hook, hook scissors, grasping instruments (e.g., tenaculum, crocodile forceps, screwdriver; Fig. 37-4), suction-irrigator, needle drivers, and a uterine manipulator. In addition, an electromechanical morcellator will be necessary.

Pedunculated Myomas

For a small pedunculated myoma, a tenaculum is used to grasp the body, and the pedicle is coagulated with the bipolar forceps next to the tumor (not the uterus). Coagulation of the myometrium should be avoided. The pedicle then is cut, and the specimen is extracted. The same technique may be employed for a large pedunculated myoma, except that the coagulation may be preceded by injection of a vasoconstrictive agent (see later) into the pedicle (Fig. 37-5). Alternatively, the pedicle may be secured on the uterus side with a suture loop before the coagulation step. If a knot pusher is used, then the first throw of the suture can be progressively cinched down as the pedicle coagulation proceeds. After the pedicle has been transected, the surrounding uterine serosa should be closed over the top of the pedicle with a running absorbable suture.

Subserosal and Intramural Myomas

The technique for removal of subserosal or intramural myomas consists of five steps.

1. *Infiltration of vasoconstrictive agents.* To constrict the vascular supply and reduce blood loss, we perform an injection with diluted ornithine-vasopressin or arginine-vasopressin (20 IU in 500 mL saline) using a laparoscopic needle (a

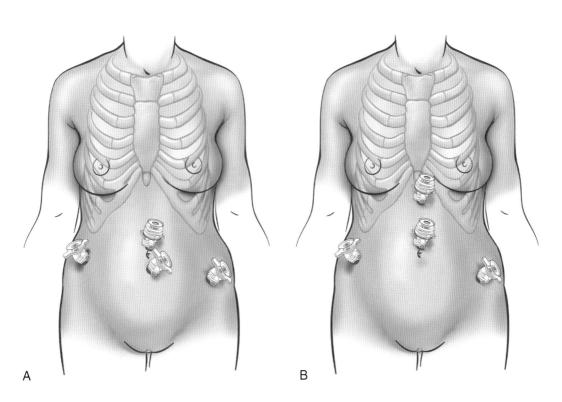

FIGURE 37-3 Port positions for a laparoscopic myomectomy. **A,** Standard positions. **B,** Positions for large pathology that extends to the umbilicus.

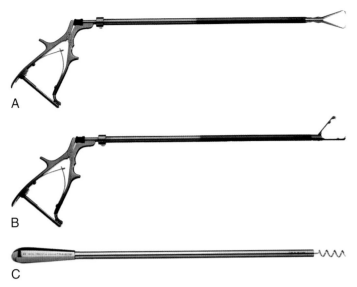

FIGURE 37-4 Grasping instrumentation for a laparoscopic myomectomy. A, Tenaculum. B, Crocodile forceps. C, Screwdriver.

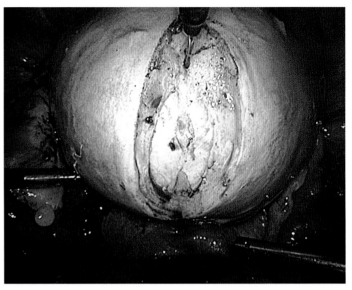

FIGURE 37-6 Vertical hysterotomy for excision of an intramural leiomyoma.

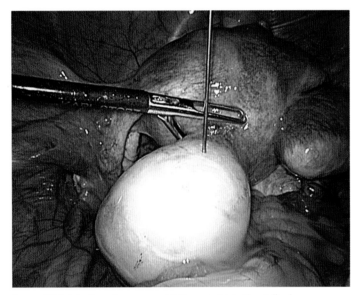

FIGURE 37-5 Injection of a vasoconstrictive agent into the stalk of a pedunculated myoma, in preparation for excision.

transabdominal epidural needle also may be used). The substance is injected between the normal myometrium and the myoma capsule, looking for the cleavage plane, around the accessible surface of the tumor, until blanching occurs. It is not helpful to directly inject the vasopressin inside the myoma. The use of the intraoperative ultrasound can help detect and isolate smaller myomas.

2. *Incision.* For both subserosal and intramural myomas in the anterior or posterior myomas, a vertical incision (hysterotomy) is made on the serosa overlying the myoma and carried through the myoma pseudocapsule, using a monopolar cautery hook or scissors with high cutting current (Fig. 37-6). Alternatively, an ultrasonic scalpel may be used for this step. The incision is continued into the uterus until the cleavage plane is found between the fibroid and the surrounding pseudocapsule and myometrium. The vertical hysterotomy typically is closed by suturing through the midline port. A transverse hysterotomy may be used as an alternative; this incision typically is closed using a lateral port.

3. *Enucleation.* After the myoma has been exposed through the hysterotomy, traction is applied on the tumor with a grasping forceps (or a tenaculum or screwdriver, as in Fig. 37-4). With the second assistant providing additional traction on the uterine manipulator, a laparoscopic grasper bluntly develops the plane between the tumor and the myometrium. Some bands of tissue and vascularized attachments between the fibroid and the myometrium will need to be divided with electrical or ultrasonic energy. Using this type of dissection, the myoma is enucleated. If unsuspected adenomyosis is discovered (typically manifested by a lack of a cleavage plane), then the excision will need to be performed sharply, with monopolar cautery or an ultrasonic scalpel.

4. *Hysterotomy closure.* For subserosal or intramural myomas, the uterine incision is sutured in one or two layers, depending on the incision depth. A careful closure is important to prevent the formation of a hematoma. Large, curved needles (CT-1, 30 to 40 mm) swaged to polyglactin suture (1-0 or 0-0) are used. For one-layer sutures, we use interrupted, simple, or (more frequently) cross-stitches, commonly known as figure-of-eight stitches, tied intracorporeally. In most cases, however, a two-layer closure will be necessary. One method to accomplish this is to catch different layers of tissue with each loop of a cross-stitch, as shown in Figure 37-7. The first loop is full thickness; the second loop is a superficial bite that inverts the serosa (a "vertical mattress" configuration) as the stitch is tied. Each stitch should be tied so that the tissue is approximated but not strangulated. After the incision has been closed, additional serosal stitches may be placed as needed to invert the serosa. Alternatively, a running suture may be employed, using the same pattern of tissue bites shown in Figure 37-7 (i.e., full-thickness alternating with serosal bites). In any case, it is imperative to obliterate dead space during the hysterotomy closure, which should minimize the risk for intramural hematoma.

The suturing technique to close the hysterotomy will differ according to myoma location. If a posterior vertical hysterotomy was made, then the needle is positioned in the needle holder with the convexity toward the uterus; that is, the needle is upside-down (Fig. 37-8). The midline port typically is used

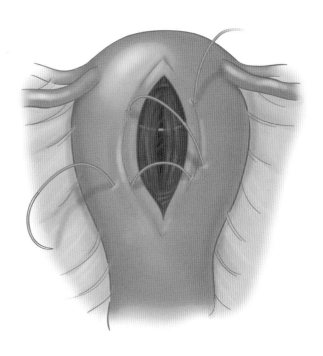

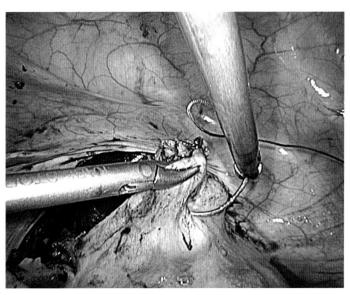

FIGURE 37-9 Suture closure of an anterior vertical hysterotomy.

FIGURE 37-7 Cross-stitch for hysterotomy closure. The first loop is full-thickness; the second loop is a vertical mattress of serosa.

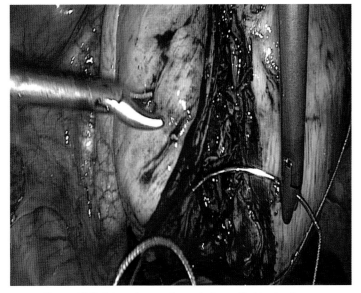

FIGURE 37-8 Suture closure of a posterior vertical hysterotomy.

without the need for a large abdominal incision. There are multiple available configurations for a morcellator; a typical version consists of a 10-mm diameter cylindrical tube with a coring knife at the end that is rotated by an electrical micro-engine attached to the trocar. With the specimen stabilized between grasping forces, cylindrical tissue blocks are cut sequentially out of the main specimen and are removed from the peritoneal cavity through the morcellator with a grasping forceps. Alternatively, the specimen may be cut up with a morcellating blade and then extracted through a posterior culdotomy or an enlarged port incision. Newer morcellator technology has included bladeless devices that use bipolar energy. After morcellation, the specimen pieces are sent for histologic examination. Myoma morcellation is the most time-consuming part of laparoscopic myomectomy. Morcellation time is directly influenced by the myoma diameter and number; the surgeon should remember that tumor volume increases geometrically with the radius [i.e., sphere volume = $\frac{4}{3}\pi(r)^3$].

Infraligamentous Myomas

An infraligamentous myoma usually is a pedunculated or subserosal fibroid arising in the broad ligament. It can involve the anterior, posterior, or both leaves of the ligament. Excision of an infraligamentous myoma can be difficult secondary to their proximity to vital structures. The peritoneum surrounding the myoma is incised with cold scissors or bipolar forceps, or both. The myoma is gently enucleated from the surrounding areolar tissue with the scissors, bipolar forceps, and graspers. Hemostasis of vessels feeding the fibroid can be achieved with ultrasonic energy or bipolar coagulation, taking care to avoid thermal injury to nearby structures such as the ureter or uterine vessels. When the base of the myoma has been reached, coagulation of the vasculature is performed with bipolar forceps. If an infraligamentous myoma extends up into the uterine body (i.e., has a subserosal-intramural component; Fig. 37-10), then the uterine body should be closed with suture after fibroid excision, as described earlier. Otherwise, there is no need to close the peritoneum if hemostasis has been achieved.

to sew. If an anterior vertical hysterotomy was made, then the needle also is positioned with the convexity turned toward the uterus, but this time a right-side-up needle configuration will result (Fig. 37-9). To facilitate the suturing, the second assistant should maintain the uterus in an upright position with the manipulator. Some products have been introduced to facilitate closure of the hysterotomy during laparoscopic myomectomy, including unidirectional or bidirectional knotless barbed suture, the strands of which penetrate the tissue and lock the suture in place. Although further studies are needed, knotless barbed suture may reduce the time required to close the hysterotomy, thus possibly decreasing intraoperative blood loss.

5. *Morcellation.* Cutting the myomectomy specimen into small pieces (morcellation) allows extraction of the specimen

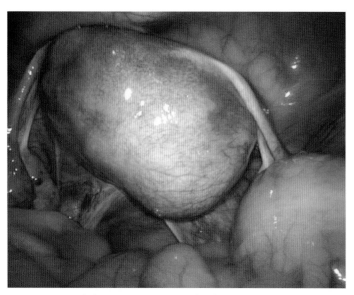

FIGURE 37-10 Infraligamentous myoma with subserosal/intramural extension.

Table 37-1 Complications of Laparoscopic Myomectomy in 2050 Procedures

Complications	No. of Patients (%)
Major	
Hematoma*	10 (0.48)
Intraoperative hemorrhage	14 (0.68)
Sarcomas	2 (0.09)
Postoperative hemorrhage	2 (0.09)
Postoperative renal failure	1 (0.04)
Bowel injury	1 (0.04)
Uterine rupture in subsequent pregnancy†	1 (0.26)
Procedure failure	7 (0.34)
TOTAL	**38 (2.02)**
Minor	
Urinary tract infection	70 (3.41)
Fever >38° C, unknown origin	105 (5.11)
Minor manipulator lesion	12 (0.58)
TOTAL	**187 (9.11)**
TOTAL MAJOR AND MINOR COMPLICATIONS	**225 (11.1)**

*Concurrent diagnosis of adenomyosis.
†Data on uterine rupture are reported using the number of subsequent pregnancies (386 cases) as the denominator.

POSTOPERATIVE CARE

The postoperative course is typical for a minimally invasive procedure that does not involve a gastrointestinal anastomosis. The Foley catheter is removed on postoperative day 1. Bowel function typically resumes after day 1. Perioperative antibiotic prophylaxis is routine. The patient usually is discharged on postoperative day 1 or 2 and may return to work in 2 weeks.

MANAGEMENT OF PROCEDURE-SPECIFIC COMPLICATIONS

The risk for uterine rupture may be minimized with a meticulous closure of the hysterotomy, as described earlier. The use of injected vasoconstrictors can help minimize the use of electrosurgery for hemostasis, thereby resulting in less tissue damage. The occurrence of febrile morbidity (temperature >38° C) after myomectomy is quite common and almost always resolves spontaneously. This latter complication appears to be less frequent after laparoscopic myomectomy compared with the open procedure.

RESULTS AND OUTCOME

In 2007, we published a multicenter study on complications of 2050 laparoscopic myomectomies. The overall complication rate was 11.1%. Minor complications occurred in 187 cases (9.1%) and major complications in 38 cases (2.0%), as listed in Table 37-1. A regression analysis of these data demonstrated that the complication risk for laparoscopic myomectomy correlated positively with both the number and diameter of myomas (odds ration [OR], 2, 11; $P < .01$), and also with infraligamentous location (OR, 2,19; $P < .05$).

Regarding the cases listed in Table 37-1, only one of the patients with intraoperative hemorrhage required a transfusion. One patient with postoperative hemorrhage was treated with a laparoscopic hysterectomy, and the other underwent drainage of a broad ligament hematoma with ultrasound guidance. All the cases of unexplained pyrexia resolved quickly. Hematoma at the uterine incision was detected by postoperative transvaginal ultrasound.

Failure to complete the planned operation occurred in seven cases (0.34%). In one case, conversion to a laparoscopic hysterectomy was necessary because of a large infraligamentous myoma. Conversion to laparotomy was necessary secondary to anesthetic issues ($n = 3$), insufficient operative space ($n = 2$), and a suspected sarcoma ($n = 1$). A bowel injury occurred in one patient (0.04%) who had a previous laparoscopic myomectomy and presented with multiple myomas in the right round ligament, the right uterosacral ligament, and the pouch of Douglas. A bowel perforation was diagnosed on postoperative day 13; the patient underwent a laparoscopic repair, including suture of the perforation, irrigation, and drainage, but no colostomy.

Our incidence of unexpected sarcoma (0.09%) in this series was low relative to the historical rate of leiomyosarcoma within uterine myomas, which has been estimated to be 0.13% to 0.29%. The same rate in hysterectomy for presumed benign disease is about 0.49%. Our low incidence of leiomyosarcoma may be due in part to the preoperative evaluation (ultrasound, with MRI and LDH testing as indicated) or to the younger age of our patient population (the incidence of sarcoma increases during the fourth to seventh decade), or both. Morcellation of unsuspected or misdiagnosed sarcoma may predispose the patient to a local recurrence.

In this series of 2050 myomectomy patients, 386 patients (22.9%) conceived during the follow-up period. The pregnancy rate in the subgroup of patients ($n = 553$) who were trying to conceive was 69.8%. The miscarriage rate in this subgroup was 20%; of the patients going on to delivery, 81% had a cesarean delivery, with the balance having a vaginal delivery. These data are in accordance with other studies of pregnancy outcome after laparoscopic or open myomectomy, which have demonstrated an improvement in fertility rate after removal of fibroid tumors.

One patient in our subgroup of patients who became pregnant had spontaneous uterine rupture (0.26%) at 33 weeks' gestation; she previously had removal of an 8-cm adenomyoma. It is likely that removal of this adenomyoma weakened the uterine wall because the normal myometrium typically is intermingled with the adenomyosis. Nineteen reports of uterine rupture after laparoscopic myomectomy had been reported in the literature up to 2010; the precise frequency of postmyomectomy rupture is difficult to determine because these were case reports without mention of a denominator. There was one study of more than 100 pregnancies after laparoscopic myomectomy ,which documented a uterine rupture rate of 1%. Possible risk factors for uterine rupture after myomectomy include excessive use of electrical energy, small suture size for hysterotomy closure, uterine wall hematoma, and uterine fistula.

Analysis of our data has shown that laparoscopic myomectomy, in comparison with the open procedure, resulted in a smaller decrease in hemoglobin (1.3% vs. 2.2%), less postoperative pain, less febrile morbidity (12.1% vs. 26.2%), and faster recovery. No difference was found between laparoscopic and open myomectomy regarding the pregnancy rate or abortion rate. Other authors have found that laparoscopic myomectomy results in fewer adhesions than the open procedure.

Laparoscopy-assisted myomectomy, in which the hysterotomy is closed through a small open incision, has been advocated as more effective in the prevention of uterine rupture, but the data on this procedure are incomplete. In open myomectomy, the rate of postmyomectomy uterine rupture during pregnancy was 0.24% in one 14-year retrospective study; the companion rate of uterine rupture during pregnancy in patients with previous cesarean delivery was 4.1%. Incidentally, it should be noted that pregnancy-associated uterine rupture can occur even in the unscarred uterus or after a hysteroscopic resection.

We have evaluated the morphology and vascularization of the uterus after laparoscopic compared with open myomectomy (15 patients in each group) with transvaginal color Doppler ultrasonography. Using this technique, a careful assessment of the scar morphology and surrounding blood supply is possible. Sonographic evaluation performed 7 to 15 days after the myomectomy demonstrated a marked increase in vascularity around the myomectomy scar; this increase was gone by day 45. A progressive reduction in scar volume also was noted, and no hematoma was noted. There were no significant differences in the vascularity or morphology between the laparoscopic compared with open myomectomy patients. The results of this study provided us with evidence that our laparoscopic and open techniques were equivalent with respect to the sutured hysterotomy closure.

Our overall recurrence rate after laparoscopic myomectomy during a 14-year period has been 21.3% (Fig. 37-11). Most recurrences were diagnosed with ultrasound at a mean of 29 months (range, 2 to 105 months) after surgery. The risk for recurrence was independently associated with the number of myomas removed, the depth of myoma penetration into the myometrium, or the use of preoperative GnRH analogs. Notably, the risk for residual fibroids increased with the number of fibroids actually excised; almost all patients with 10 or more fibroids removed had residual tumors.

We had three cases of leiomyomatosis peritonealis disseminata (LPD) in patients who had previous laparoscopic myomectomy in the early 1990s, when manual morcellation was in use. As its name suggests, LPD involves widespread implants of leiomyomas on the peritoneal surfaces. It is conceivable that the surgical technique early in the experience of laparoscopic myomectomy fostered the disseminated disease in these cases.

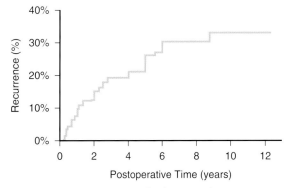

FIGURE 37-11 Recurrence rate after laparoscopic myomectomy.

Laparoscopic myomectomy appears to be a safe technique with a low intraoperative failure rate and satisfactory long-term results with respect to recurrence rate and future pregnancy. The complication rate of laparoscopic myomectomy appears to be comparable to or even less than that of open myomectomy. Regardless of the approach, the recurrence rate of myomectomy is relatively high. Therefore, if the expertise is available, then it would be reasonable to offer the patient a minimally invasive myomectomy, particularly for a primary procedure.

Suggested Readings

Blake RE: Leiomyomata uteri: Hormonal and molecular determinants of growth, *J Natl Med Assoc* 99:1170–1184, 2007.

Dubuisson JB, Chapron C: Laparoscopic myomectomy today: A good technique when correctly indicated, *Hum Reprod* 11:934–935, 1996.

Dubuisson JB, Chapron C, Fauconnier A: Laparoscopic myomectomy: Operative technique and results, *Ann N Y Acad Sci* 828:326–331, 1997.

Dubuisson JB, Chapron C, Fauconnier A, et al: Laparoscopic myomectomy fertility results, *Ann N Y Acad Sci* 943:269–275, 2001.

Dubuisson JB, Chapron C, Verspyck E, et al: Laparoscopic myomectomy: 102 cases, *Contracept Fertil Sex* 21:920–922, 1993.

Goto A, Takeuchi S, Sugimura K, et al: Usefulness of Gd-DTPA contrast-enhanced dynamic MRI and serum determination of LDH and its isozymes in the differential diagnosis of leiomyosarcoma from degenerated leiomyoma of the uterus, *Int J Gynecol Cancer* 12:354–361, 2002.

Lumsden MA: Embolization versus myomectomy versus hysterectomy: Which is best, when? *Hum Reprod* 17:253–259, 2002.

Mais V, Ajossa S, Guerriero S, et al: Laparoscopic versus abdominal myomectomy: A prospective, randomized trial to evaluate benefits in early outcome, *Am J Obstet Gynecol* 174:654–658, 1996.

Miller CE, Johnston M, Rundell M: Laparoscopic myomectomy in the infertile woman, *J Am Assoc Gynecol Laparosc* 3:525–532, 1996.

Morice P, Rodriguez A, Rey A, et al: Prognostic value of initial surgical procedure for patients with uterine sarcoma: Analysis of 123 patients, *Eur J Gynaecol Oncol* 24:237–240, 2003.

Ostrzenski A: Uterine leiomyoma particle growing in an abdominal-wall incision after laparoscopic retrieval, *Obstet Gynecol* 89:853–854, 1997.

Rossetti A, Paccosi M, Sizzi O, et al: Dilute ornitin vasopressin and a myoma drill for laparoscopic myomectomy, *J Am Assoc Gynecol Laparosc* 6:189–193, 1999.

Seracchioli R, Rossi S, Govoni F, et al: Fertility and obstetric outcome after laparoscopic myomectomy of large myomata: A randomized comparison with abdominal myomectomy, *Hum Reprod* 15:2663–2668, 2000.

Takeuchi H, Kuwatsuru R: The indications, surgical techniques, and limitations of laparoscopic myomectomy, *JSLS* 7:89–95, 2003.

Tropeano G, Amoroso S, Scambia G: Non-surgical management of uterine fibroids, *Hum Reprod Update* 14:259–274, 2008.

Viswanathan M, Hartmann K, McKoy N, et al: Management of uterine fibroids: An update of the evidence, *Evid Rep Technol Assess* 154:1–122, 2007.

Sejal Dharia Patel, Nora Alghothani, and Olga A. Tusheva

Robot-Assisted Tubal Anastomosis

Worldwide, more than 153 million women have chosen sterilization as their contraceptive method. As many as 20% will subsequently regret their decision because of a change in family circumstances such as the death of a child, improved economic situation, or change in marital status. Of these patients, 1% to 5% will express interest in sterilization reversal. Tubal anastomosis is a surgical approach to sterilization reversal and can be performed with robotic assistance. Robotic technology combines the benefits of open microsurgery with a laparoscopic approach. This chapter describes the evolution of robotic technology, instrumentation, essential components of the system, and technique of robotic tubal anastomosis.

OPERATIVE INDICATIONS

The ideal candidate for tubal reversal has normal ovulatory function, intrauterine anatomy, and seminal parameters (in the partner). *In vitro* fertilization (IVF) is a nonsurgical option for couples desiring fertility after tubal ligation. Surgical reversal of tubal ligation with tubal anastomosis can be performed by laparotomy, by laparoscopy, or with robotics.

In Vitro Fertilization

IVF is an alternative procedure to surgical tubal anastomosis. It requires medication to recruit the development of multiple follicles. Once the follicles are of a certain diameter (as determined by serial ultrasound and serum estradiol), medication is given to induce ovulation. Before ovulation, the oocytes are harvested from the follicles through a transvaginal ultrasound-guided oocyte aspiration. The aspirated oocytes are incubated with sperm, and fertilization is assessed 17 to 25 hours later. These fertilized oocytes are monitored for growth and development. Of the resulting embryos, the most functional ones are transferred. Pregnancy rates have varied based on maternal age. For a good-prognosis patient younger than 35 years, the IVF pregnancy rate in our clinic (reported to the Centers for Disease Control and Prevention in 2009) is 58.6%, if the patient underwent a blastocyst transfer. One advantage of IVF includes correction of concomitant infertility factors. In addition, use of IVF avoids a major surgical procedure and does not require the patient to address contraception after delivery. IVF reduces the risk for ectopic pregnancy to that of the general population. IVF does involve, however, a defined cost per cycle, as well as the risk for twin gestation if more than one embryo is transferred.

Laparotomy

The first report to document microsurgical technique for tubal anastomosis was published in 1977. Pregnancy outcomes were improved compared with macrosurgical techniques. The reported pregnancy rates were 30% to 63% at 6 months and 53% to 80% at 12 months. Subsequent microsurgical tubal anastomosis by minilaparotomy yielded pregnancy rates of 72% to 78%.

Laparoscopy

Early laparoscopic unilateral sterilization reversal used biologic glue with intraluminal guidance and resulted in low pregnancy rates. In 1992, Charles Koh applied the principles of microsurgery to laparoscopic tubal anastomosis, resulting in improved pregnancy rates over time (up to 83.3%) at 18 months. These results were comparable to those achieved by open microsurgery.

Several laparoscopic surgical techniques have been described for laparoscopic tubal anastomosis. Many authors reapproximate the muscularis layer with four interrupted sutures at the 3-, 6-, 9-, and 12-o'clock positions and close the serosa with two or three interrupted sutures. Others prefer a one-stitch, two-stitch, or three-stitch technique, closing both muscularis and serosal layers. Regardless of the anastomotic technique, laparoscopic tubal anastomosis does offer the benefits of minimally invasive surgery. This approach is limited, however, by the absence of stereoscopic vision and the difficulty of handling fine suture with laparoscopic instruments.

Robotic Approach

The feasibility of robotically assisted tubal anastomosis was demonstrated in 1998 in animal models using the Zeus system and then followed by a pilot study in women. The procedure was successfully completed in all patients without complications. Subsequent studies have confirmed the feasibility of this technique.

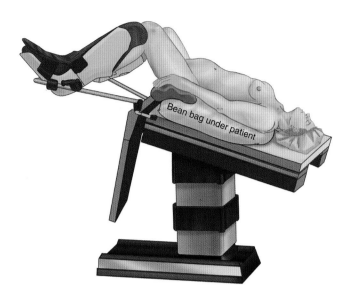

FIGURE 38-1 Patient positioning for a robotic tubal anastomosis.

PREOPERATIVE EVALUATION, TESTING, AND PREPARATION

Patients who desire robotic tubal reversal must show documentation of a competent oocyte, partner sperm, and a patent uterine cavity. Each patient has serum progesterone measured in the luteal phase to document evidence of ovulation. The partner must undergo a semen analysis showing adequate sperm (moderate oligoasthenoteratozoospermia is permitted). Finally, the patient undergoes a hysterosalpingogram to confirm a normal uterine cavity and to rule out isthmic or ampullary obstruction. If there is evidence of distal ampullary or fimbrial obstruction, the patient is not offered a robotic tubal reversal.

PATIENT POSITIONING IN THE OPERATING SUITE

The patient initially is placed in the supine position with the buttocks at the table break and the arms tucked to the sides. The caudal end of the table then is removed, and the legs are then placed into Allen stirrups (Allen Medical Systems, Acton, Mass.), with the knees flexed and lowered (Fig. 38-1). Gel pads are placed under the patient to minimize trauma at pressure points. The patient is held into position with a desufflated "bean bag" (Olympic Vac Pac, Olympic Medical, Seattle, Wash.). The elbows, shoulders, and chest are cushioned before the patient is taped to the table to prevent movement in steep-Trendelenburg position. A uterine manipulator is inserted to facilitate performance of chromopertubation during the anastomotic construction.

POSITIONING AND PLACEMENT OF TROCARS

A Veress needle is used to establish pneumoperitoneum before inserting a 12-mm primary trocar at the level of the umbilicus (Fig. 38-2). Two lateral 8-mm da Vinci ports are placed in the midaxillary line, 2 cm below the level of the umbilicus and separated by a minimum of 8 cm between the port sites. The patient is placed into steep-Trendelenburg position (see Fig. 38-1). After

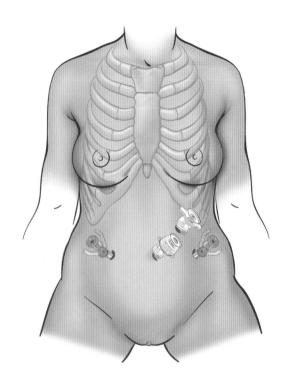

FIGURE 38-2 Port placement for a robotic tubal anastomosis.

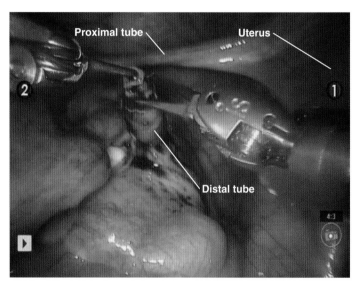

FIGURE 38-3 Serosal stripping of the distal segment (left tubal anastomosis).

confirming the feasibility of tubal anastomosis, an accessory 8-mm port is placed on the left side about 2 cm superior and 5 cm lateral to the primary port; the accessory port is used for irrigation and for introduction and retrieval of suture material. The robot then is positioned at the left knee (also known as *side-docking*) to permit vaginal access for chromopertubation. The robotic arms then are connected to the respective ports.

OPERATIVE TECHNIQUE

Instruments for robot-assisted tubal anastomosis include a Black Diamond microforceps and Potts scissors, which initially are used to strip the serosa off the distal segment (the ovarian side) of the fallopian tube (Fig. 38-3). The distal segment may vary in length; the amount of serosa that should be removed, however, is approximately 1 to 2 mm. The goal of these maneuvers is to acquire the ability to perform a two-layer closure: (1) the mucosa/muscularis and (2) the serosa. Once the serosa has been stripped, the distal tubal is milked until the obstructed lumen bulges from pressure. The tip then is transected with the scissors, exposing the lumen of the distal tube. The distal lumen is identified by its mucosal rugations. If there is difficulty in the identification of the distal lumen, then the lumen is distended by fluid injected with a 5-mm irrigator inserted into the fimbria. Alternatively, a pediatric Foley catheter can be threaded through the fimbria to distend the proximal obstructed lumen of the distal segment.

After preparation of the distal segment of the fallopian tube, the mesosalpinx of the proximal segment (the uterine side) is cauterized and transected for a few millimeters with a microbipolar instrument (Fig. 38-4) to mobilize the proximal segment and decrease tension on the future anastomotic site. The tip of the proximal segment then is mobilized and transected (Fig. 38-5), as was done with the distal segment, to demonstrate the lumen of the proximal tube. Chromopertubation (transcervical injection of dye) is used to confirm patency of the proximal tubal segment. If the chromopertubation balloon is displaced or otherwise malfunctions, then the robotic system is docked, and the chromopertubation device is replaced. After proximal tubal patency has been confirmed, the mesosalpinx is reapproximated to minimize tension at the level of the anastomosis (Fig. 38-6), using one or two interrupted 6-0 polyglactin sutures on an S-14 needle.

The fallopian tube anastomosis is constructed in two layers. Placement of the mesosalpingeal sutures should have brought the proximal and distal tubal lumens in apposition. With the first layer, the initial suture is placed at the 6-o'clock position, incorporating muscularis and mucosa, going from outside-in to inside-out, such that the knot is on the serosal side (Figs. 38-7 and 38-8). This first layer is sutured with interrupted 7-0 polyglactin suture on a TG-140 needle. The second suture of the first layer is placed at the 12-o'clock position (Fig. 38-9). If the tubal lumen can tolerate additional suturing, then a stitch is placed at the 3- and 9-o'clock positions. For this first layer, the mucosal layer and half the diameter of the muscularis layer are incorporated into each suture. For the second layer of the anastomosis, the serosa is closed with a running 7-0 polyglactin suture (Fig. 38-10). The intent of the second layer is to decrease tension at the mucosal layer and to minimize formation of adhesions to the anastomosis.

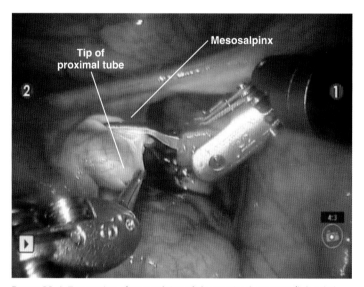

FIGURE 38-4 Transection of mesosalpinx of the proximal segment (left tubal anastomosis).

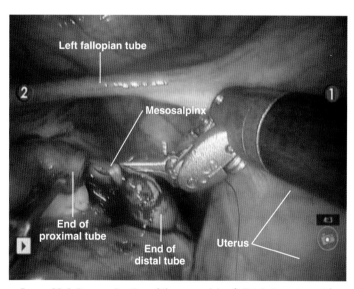

FIGURE 38-6 Reapproximation of the mesosalpinx (left tubal anastomosis).

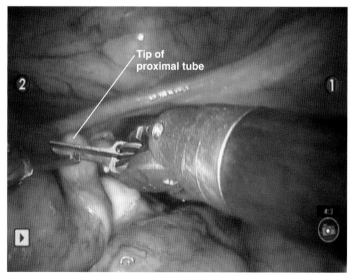

FIGURE 38-5 Serosal stripping of the proximal segment (left tubal anastomosis).

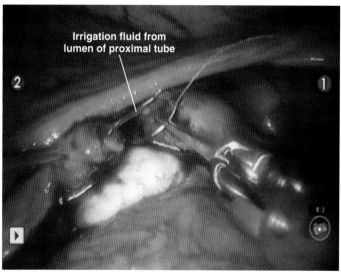

FIGURE 38-7 Initial stitch of first layer of left tubal anastomosis, showing jet of irrigation fluid from lumen of proximal tube.

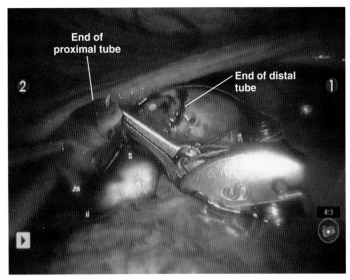

FIGURE 38-8 Initial stitch of first layer of left tubal anastomosis, taking a bite of muscularis and mucosa.

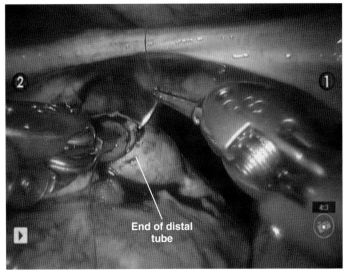

FIGURE 38-9 Second stitch of first layer of left tubal anastomosis.

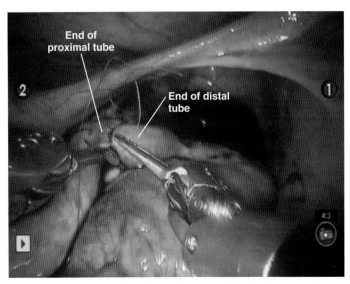

FIGURE 38-10 Second layer (serosal closure) of left tubal anastomosis.

The patency of the surgical repair is determined by another chromopertubation test.

If the chromopertubation reveals obstruction, then the level of obstruction should be determined. If there is patency both proximal and distal to the anastomosis, then the anastomosis should be taken down and redone. If the proximal lumen is obstructed at the level of the tubal ostia, then hysteroscopic tubal cannulation with a Novy cannula can be performed. If there is distal obstruction, then either a Novy cannula can be used to cannulate the tube proximally or a 5-French pediatric Foley catheter can be used to cannulate the tube distally.

POSTOPERATIVE CARE

Once the procedure is completed, the patient is taken to the recovery unit, where she will remain until she is able to ambulate, tolerate oral intake, and urinate without difficulty. Each patient is discharged home the same day. Small adhesive dressings overlying the incisions may be removed the following day, and patients are able to resume normal activities of daily living. Patients may use a nonsteroidal anti-inflammatory medication for pain control. A narcotic prescription is made available, but most patients use only about one third of the pills prescribed. Patients are cautioned to refrain from sexual intercourse until the first postoperative visit. Attempts at conception are permitted with the start of the next menstrual cycle, or at least 3 weeks from the date of the surgery.

MANAGEMENT OF PROCEDURE-SPECIFIC COMPLICATIONS

Procedure-specific complications from a robotic tubal reversal include ectopic pregnancy and tubal obstruction. These complications may be avoided by limiting the number of luminal sutures during the anastomosis to prevent constriction of the lumen. Another important precaution is the abstention from sexual intercourse for one menstrual cycle after the surgical procedure to prevent conception during the immediate postoperative period.

RESULTS AND OUTCOME

Tubal patency rates after robotic tubal anastomosis have varied from 89% to 95%. Pregnancy rates after robotic tubal reversal have ranged from 50% to 71%, with ongoing pregnancy rates of 30% to 62%. Ectopic pregnancy rates have ranged from 11% to 22%, and spontaneous pregnancy loss rates have ranged from 11% to 26%. Most pregnancies have occurred in the first 6 months after surgery.

Some authors have advocated the use of IVF as first-line therapy for any patient with tubal damage. Pregnancy rates with sterilization reversal are comparable to those achieved with IVF technology. Conception with IVF treatment, however, can occur more quickly than with surgical reversal. IVF allows for correction of multiple infertility factors but carries the risk for multiple gestation and medication side effects. On the other hand, surgical tubal reversal can result in several pregnancies over time but is associated with a risk for ectopic gestation and tubal reocclusion. IVF and tubal reversal may be considered as complementary procedures, and selection of the appropriate therapy should be based on the individual patient.

Suggested Readings

Botros DK, Rizk RMB, Falcone GT: *Human Assisted Reproductive Technology: Future Trends in Laboratory and Clinical Practice*, Cambridge, UK, 2011, Cambridge University Press.

Caillet M, Vandromme J, Rozenberg S, et al: Robotically assisted laparoscopic microsurgical tubal reanastomosis: A retrospective study, *Fertil Steril* 94:1844-1847, 2010.

Dharia Patel SP, Steinkampf MP, Whitten SJ, Malizia BA: Robotic tubal anastomosis: Surgical technique and cost effectiveness, *Fertil Steril* 90:1175-1179, 2008.

Rodgers AK, Goldberg JM, Hammel JP, et al: Tubal anastomosis by robotic compared with outpatient minilaparotomy, *Obstet Gynecol* 109:1375-1380, 2007.

Rodgers AK, Goldberg JM, Hammel JP, Falcone T: Tubal anastomosis by robotic compared with outpatient minilaparotomy, *Obstet Gynecol* 109:1375-1380, 2007.

Rotman C, Rana N, Song J, Sueldo C: Laparoscopic tubal anastomosis. In *Textbook of Infertility and Reproduction*, Cambridge, UK, 2007, Cambridge University Press.

Tulandi T, Advincula A: Robotic surgery in gynecology. In *Emerging Technologies in Women's Health* (Bentham Science eBook series). Available at http://www.benthamscience.com/ebooks/9781608052721/index.htm.

Pediatrics

Shahab F. Abdessalam, Kenneth S. Azarow, Robert A. Cusick, Stephen C. Raynor, and Adam S. Gorra

Associate Editor for Chapter 39: Shahab F. Abdessalam

Minimally Invasive Pediatric Procedures

LIST OF MINIMALLY INVASIVE PEDIATRIC PROCEDURES

The videos associated with this chapter are listed in the Video Contents and can be found on the accompanying DVDs and *on Expertconsult.com.*

Since the initial application of laparoscopy in children in the early 1990s, an increasing number of procedures have been performed with a minimally invasive approach in patients as small as 1 to 1.5 kg and as young as 1 day. We have arrived at a point at which procedures are being performed in newborns almost without size limitation, depending on the skill of the surgeon and the precision of the instrumentation. This chapter highlights some of the more common procedures that can be performed in the pediatric population.

Each procedure will be discussed in detail, but there are some general principles specific to pediatrics that should be mentioned first. Because of variability in patient size, port placement and patient positioning must be individualized in each case. Each section will discuss recommendations for patient positioning and port placement. For thoracoscopic procedures, we do not recommend double-lumen endotracheal tube placement because patient size limits their use. A low insufflation pressure (in the range of 3 to 6 mm Hg) deflates the lung adequately for enough visualization to perform the procedure. In general, children have enough pulmonary "reserve" to tolerate low pressure, intrapleural insufflation.

Patients with congenital heart disease deserve special mention for both thoracoscopic and laparoscopic procedures. These patients may require several stages to repair a heart defect, and they may have a shunt that that is dependent on venous return to the heart, which will be adversely affected by the pressures introduced during insufflation. For these patients, we start with lower than normal pressures (8 to 10 mm Hg); adjustments are made thereafter, depending on patient stability and the surgeon's visualization. In children younger than 1 year, we recommend using "neonatal" settings for the insufflation machine. The maximal pressure is set in the 8 to 10 mm Hg range. The CO_2 is delivered at much lower flow rates (0.1 to 0.5 L/minute); the machine will make adjustments at slower intervals because changes in pressures will vary dramatically during ventilation.

In both the congenital heart patients and the neonatal population, ventilator adjustments such as lower tidal volumes and faster ventilatory rates will be necessary by the anesthesiologist, in order to prevent acidosis secondary to carbon dioxide retention. Port sizes for children are variable, and will be addressed with each procedure. The option of direct instrument placement without a port exists for a variety of procedures.

As listed in the Index, this chapter describes minimally invasive thoracic procedures for pectus excavatum, congenital cystic adenomatoid malformation and pulmonary sequestration, mediastinal cysts, and Bochdalek congenital diaphragmatic hernia. In addition, we discuss minimally invasive abdominal procedures for urachal anomalies, pyloric stenosis, Meckel diverticulum, feeding difficulties, Hirschsprung disease, undescended testicle, ovarian cysts and torsion, and diaphragmatic defects.

Although commonly performed in pediatrics, cholecystectomy, appendectomy, splenectomy, colectomy, and adrenalectomy have been well described elsewhere in this and other atlases. These procedures are not appreciably different in children, so their description will not be repeated here. Laparoscopy for malrotation and intussusception also will not be described; we believe that there is no added benefit for laparoscopy in these procedures because they can be completed with a relatively small incision.

I. Pectus excavatum

Preoperative Considerations

Pectus excavatum is the most common defect of the chest wall in infants. The incidence is estimated to be up to 38 per 10,000 births in white infants. The incidence appears to be less in other races, estimated at 7 per 10,000 black infants. The precise etiology of the defect is unknown, and there appears to be genetic transmission of the condition. This defect also is associated with Marfan disease and other connective tissue disorders. The appearance and severity of pectus vary among individuals. There may be a localized defect in the lowermost portion of the sternum, or a longer trench. These defects may be symmetrical, localized to one side of the chest wall, or mixed excavatum and carinatum defects.

Children with this defect often are self-conscious about their body image. This is not an inconsequential problem, and studies have demonstrated improvement in self-image after repair. These children also can complain of exercise intolerance. Although there has been controversy about the physiologic effects of repair of the defect, some studies support an improvement in postoperative pulmonary performance when preoperative cardiac compression exists. Many patients report an improved perception of their tolerance for exercise.

Because of the lack of consistent, reproducible, postoperative improvements in pulmonary function, and the perception by some that this defect is only a cosmetic one, there have been efforts to define which patients will benefit from operative correction. Preoperative evaluation should include a chest radiograph, computed tomography (CT) of the chest, pulmonary function studies, and echocardiography. The CT scan can demonstrate the defect, including morphology of the cartilaginous component, and cardiac or pulmonary compression. It also allows for accurate measurement of the Haller index, a ratio between the anteroposterior and transverse dimensions of the chest (Fig. 39-1A). An index of greater than 3.25 is considered severe. Echocardiography can demonstrate mitral valve prolapse or other pathology that results from cardiac compression.

Not all children who have a pectus excavatum defect need repair. The decision to offer surgical repair should be based on objective criteria from the preoperative evaluation as well as the patient's desire to undergo the operation. As for every operation, a detailed discussion of the risks, benefits, and potential complications of the procedure should take place in the preoperative period.

Operative Technique

Minimally invasive pectus repair has gained popularity since its introduction and probably is the most frequently done corrective procedure for pectus excavatum at this time. This approach is best suited for the more symmetrical defects, although it has been applied to different chest morphologies. There have been many reported modifications to the original procedure, including asymmetrical bar bending, a subxiphoid incision, sternocostal relaxing incisions, and use of multiple bars. The open or Ravitch repair still is used but has become less common than the minimally invasive approach and is not discussed here.

The patient is positioned supine on the operating room table, with the shoulders abducted, elbows flexed, and arm slightly rotated externally (Fig. 39-1B). Great care should be taken to properly pad the arms and avoid a stretch injury to the brachial plexus. Antibiotics are administered and continued for 24 hours after the procedure. After a sterile preparation and draping, appropriate sites are chosen for skin incisions, as well as for the entry and exit sites of the thoracic cavity. The thoracoscope is introduced through a port placed two interspaces below the lowermost skin incision on the right side in the midaxillary line. We use an insufflation pressure of 4 to 6 mm Hg. This provides good visualization when the pectus tunneler is passed across

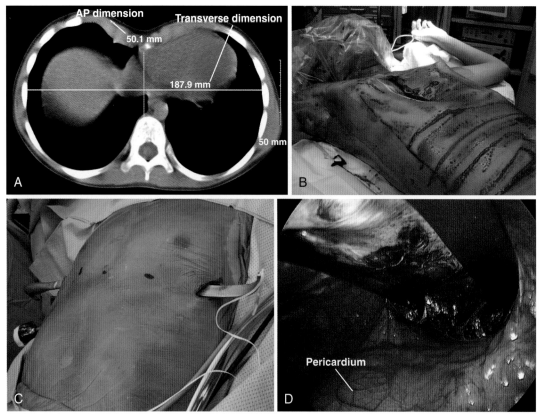

FIGURE 39-1 Pectus excavatum. **A,** Computed tomography scan demonstrating calculation of the Haller index. **B,** Positioning of the patient in the operating room. **C,** External image of tunneler placement. **D,** Thoracoscopic view of bar placement.

the mediastinum, anterior to the pericardium, exiting on the opposite side in a predetermined location (Fig. 39-1C).

We make a subxiphoid incision to remove the xiphoid, and then use blunt finger dissection to help create the plane between the sternum and pericardium, as well as to guide the tunneler across the mediastinum. At completion of placement of the bar or bars (Fig. 39-1D), a stabilizer is placed on the left side, while on the right side, the thoracoscope is used to guide placement of a 0-0 PDS suture around the bar to secure it to two separate ribs. The pneumothorax then is evacuated out the insufflation tubing, which is held under water as the anesthesiologist gives positive-pressure breaths. A small postoperative pneumothorax is to be expected but rarely requires placement of a chest tube.

Postoperative Considerations

Although done as a minimally invasive procedure, there is still a significant amount of postoperative pain associated with this procedure, so effective pain relief is essential. This is achieved with various modalities, including thoracic epidurals, patient-controlled analgesia (PCA) of narcotics, nonsteroidal anti-inflammatory drugs (NSAIDs), oral muscle relaxants, and oral narcotics. Patients are kept supine for the first 24 hours. On postoperative day 1, they are encouraged to be up in a chair most of the day, with precautions to avoid any twisting or rotation of the trunk. The Foley catheter is removed on postoperative day 1.

On postoperative day 3, all patients are ambulating with assistance in the hallways. Incentive spirometry is taught preoperatively and started in the immediate postoperative period. The major complication of this operation is injury to the pericardium or the heart during passage of the tunneler. This can be avoided with the combination of the thoracoscopic guidance of the tunneler and subxiphoid dissection and guidance. The bar or bars are removed 2 or 3 years after the procedure.

II. MEDIASTINAL CYSTS

Preoperative Considerations

Cystic lesions of the mediastinum in children often are asymptomatic and usually benign. They commonly are found incidentally on chest radiograph. Because they compress adjacent structures, they can be associated with cough, chest pain, dyspnea, and dysphagia. Rarely, the cystic cavity can become infected, resulting in fever and general malaise. Regardless of the location of the lesion, excision is indicated to (1) eliminate symptoms, if present; (2) prevent progression to symptoms, if not yet present; (3) prevent infection; and (4) rule out malignancy. The operation can be scheduled on an elective basis. In the event of infection, resection should be deferred for 6 to 8 weeks to allow for resolution of the inflammatory process.

The mediastinum is divided into three parts: the anterior mediastinum between the sternum and the anterior pericardium, the middle mediastinum between the anterior pericardium and the prevertebral fascia, and the posterior mediastinum behind the prevertebral fascia. The location of the lesion in relation to these compartments can provide clues to the pathology. Thymic cysts occur exclusively in the anterior mediastinum. Esophageal duplication cysts, pericardial cysts, and bronchogenic cysts are located in the middle mediastinum. Neuroenteric cysts arise from incomplete separation of the foregut and primitive notochord. Cystic teratomas and lymphangiomas can arise in any mediastinal compartment. Magnetic resonance imaging (MRI) or CT of the chest helps delineate the anatomy of a mediastinal cyst. When there is suspicion of esophageal or airway involvement, endoscopy may be indicated. In many of these cases, however, operative exploration and resection are necessary to obtain a diagnosis.

Thoracoscopy provides excellent exposure to important normal structures, minimizes postoperative pain, and is the preferred approach to resection of many mediastinal cysts. The objective should be to remove the lesion in its entirety, with as little disruption of adjacent structures as possible.

Operative Technique

A first-generation cephalosporin is given just before the operation. As with most thoracoscopic procedures, patients are positioned in the decubitus position with the uninvolved side against the operating room table. Depending on the location of the lesion, adjustments should be made to optimize exposure. For posterior mediastinal lesions, the patient can be placed in the anterior oblique position to allow mediastinal structures to fall forward with gravity. For anterior mediastinal lesions, the posterior oblique position allows mediastinal structures to fall away from the sternum.

Many lesions can be excised with two working ports and one camera port. Sometimes, a third working port is necessary to help with retraction by an assistant. Port positioning is individualized for each operation, depending on the specific location and dimensions of the lesion. When possible, the ports should be triangulated, and the camera should be placed between the two working ports. Once the mass is identified within the mediastinum (Fig. 39-2A), the next step is to incise the mediastinal pleura that overlies it. The cyst then is mobilized off adjacent structures, using blunt dissection and cautery when necessary (Fig. 39-2B). Most benign mediastinal cysts have little collateral circulation and can be removed with little risk for blood loss.

Care should be taken to preserve the phrenic nerve that runs longitudinally, deep to the pleura of the middle mediastinum. For lesions in the area of the esophagus, an appropriately sized bougie can help clarify the anatomy to avoid inadvertent esophageal perforation. The bougie also can help define an esophageal defect in the event that a foregut duplication cyst shares a common wall with the normal esophagus. In the region of the aortic arch, the recurrent laryngeal nerve should be identified and spared. Special attention should be given to maintaining the integrity of the cyst wall because, if a cyst is ruptured, the tissues planes can become obscure. Whether ruptured or not, the entire cyst wall should be removed, or the lining stripped, to minimize the chances of recurrence.

The specimen should be placed in an endoscopic retrieval bag and removed through a port site that has been enlarged by blunt spreading of the intercostal muscles. Large cysts may require decompression within the retrieval bag before they are pulled through the chest wall. A lesion with solid components (such as a teratoma) may require a larger intercostal incision to allow enough space for retrieval between the ribs. A thoracostomy tube should be inserted through the most convenient port wound, positioned adjacent to the bed of the resection, secured at the skin with sutures, and attached to the suction drainage system.

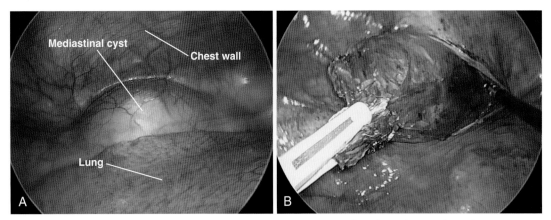

FIGURE 39-2 Mediastinal cysts. **A**, Thoracoscopic appearance. **B**, Incision of overlying pleura and cyst dissection.

Postoperative Considerations

After surgery, the patient is started on a regular diet with oral pain medications. Scheduled NSAIDs can be added as an adjunct. The chest tube can be removed when there is resolution of the pneumothorax on chest radiograph, no air leak, and minimal serous fluid output. In many cases, patients can be discharged as soon as 48 hours after the operation, with minimal activity restriction.

III. CONGENITAL LUNG LESIONS

Preoperative Considerations

Congenital lung lesions that can be managed thoracoscopically include congenital cystic adenomatoid malformations (CCAMs) and pulmonary sequestrations. A CCAM arises from an abnormal overgrowth of the terminal respiratory structures, forming an intercommunicating cyst of varying size. CCAMs are categorized by cyst size: type 1 (>2 cm), type 2 (1 to 2 cm), and type 3 (microscopic). These lesions are being diagnosed more frequently by prenatal ultrasound and should be followed prenatally and postnatally because occasionally such a lesion may resolve spontaneously. The primary symptom is respiratory distress, but a significant number are asymptomatic.

If respiratory distress exists, then the infant should be prepared for operative removal. If the child lacks any symptoms, then we prefer to obtain an MRI or CT scan of the chest at 3 to 6 months of age. If the lesion still is present, then the child should be prepared for operative removal because the goal is resection before the onset of infection. If the child does not have symptoms at birth and the diagnosis was not made prenatally, the typical presentation is recurrent pulmonary infection. Operative resection should be performed 6 to 8 weeks after treatment of the infection to optimize the chance for thoracoscopic removal.

A pulmonary sequestration is composed of nonfunctioning lung that lacks normal communication with the tracheobronchial tree and has an anomalous systemic arterial supply. A sequestration can be either intralobar (75%) or extralobar (25%). Similar to CCAMs, a sequestration is diagnosed more frequently prenatally by ultrasound and also can possibly involute. The primary symptom is respiratory distress, and, if present, the infant should be prepared for the operating room. If the patient is asymptomatic, then an MRI or CT scan of the chest should be performed at 3 to 6 months of age; if the sequestration still is present, then resection is indicated. If the patient escapes perinatal diagnosis,

the primary symptom usually is recurrent infection. CT or MRI often will show the underlying lesion, and resection should be planned 6 to 8 weeks after treatment of the infection.

The presence of either a CCAM or a sequestration mandates an operation because no other treatment has been shown to be effective. Even if the patient is asymptomatic, both types of lesions have been associated with recurrent infections and even malignant transformation later in life, so these lesions should be removed. If a patient experienced recurrent infections before the discovery of the lesion, then the operation can be very challenging because the anatomy likely will be obscured. In such cases, it may be safer to convert to an open thoracotomy or simply to proceed with an open thoracotomy from the start.

Operative Technique

The infant or child is placed in the lateral decubitus position with the side of the lesion facing upward. A single dose of prophylactic antibiotics is administered. The initial port placement (5 mm) is in the midaxillary line in the fifth intercostal space. The chest is insufflated to 4 mm Hg. Depending on which lobe is involved, two or three additional 5-mm ports are placed to optimize removal and visualization. The ports should be spaced as far apart as possible to prevent "sword fighting" between the cannulas.

For a sequestration, the inferior pulmonary ligament should be divided first with a clip applier to control any aberrant vessels (Fig. 39-3A). This will be the extent of dissection for an extralobar sequestration; the lesion then can be removed after placement into a 10-cm retrieval bag. If the lesion is large, then the port site may need to be extended 1 to 2 cm. For CCAMs (Fig. 39-3B) and intralobar sequestrations, a lobectomy is the preferred treatment to ensure complete removal.

The pleural is incised completely around the involved lobe with cautery. Care should be taken to identify the phrenic nerve. A tissue sealing device then is used to separate the parenchyma down to the hilum. Each of the pulmonary vessels is individually dissected out and divided with the clip applier. For smaller vessels (1 to 3 mm), the tissue sealing device usually is sufficient, but we do not hesitate to put a clip on as well. With just the bronchus remaining, one of the 5-mm ports is converted to a 12-mm port for an endostapler. The port farthest from the bronchus should be used to ensure adequate room for stapler deployment, particularly in the neonate.

To ensure that the bronchus is supplying only the involved lobe, the stapler is clamped down, and large sustained breaths are

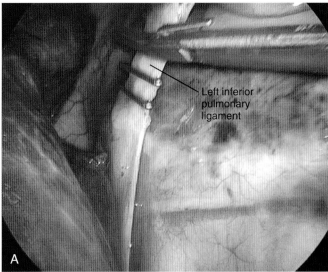

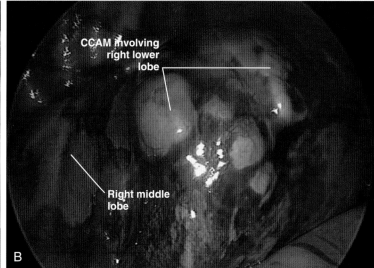

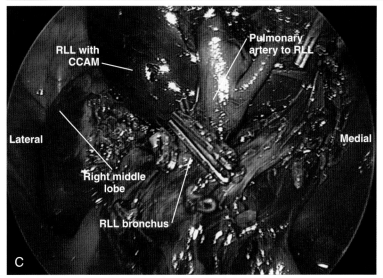

FIGURE 39-3 Congenital lung lesions. **A,** Clipping of inferior pulmonary ligament. **B,** Right lower lobe congenital cystic adenomatoid malformation. **C,** Clipping of right lower lobe bronchus.

given to ensure that the remaining lobes are not supplied by the bronchus that is about to be divided. The stapler is fired (Fig. 39-3C), and the lobe is placed into a 10-cm retrieval bag, which then is brought out through the 12-mm port site (extended as needed). The chest is filled with saline to cover the bronchial stump, and another sustained breath (to about 30 cm H_2O pressure) is given to ensure that there is no leak. A chest tube is inserted through one of the port sites, and the remaining port sites are closed.

Postoperative Considerations

As soon as the child is awake, formula or a regular diet is resumed. The chest tube is put on 20 cm H_2O suction until any air leak is resolved and the chest radiograph shows no pneumothorax, which should take 2 to 5 days. Chest tube output should be minimal. The risk for prolonged air leak can be minimized with removal of the entire lobe. If a segmental resection is performed for a more peripheral lesion, then a persistent air leak can result. The surgeon then must decide whether to proceed with a formal lobectomy or to release the patient with a Heimlich valve. A follow-up visit with a chest radiograph should be done 2 to 4 weeks after resection. Results of CCAM or sequestration resection generally are excellent, with essentially no chance of recurrence.

IV. CONGENITAL DIAPHRAGMATIC HERNIA AND DIAPHRAGMATIC EVENTRATION

Preoperative Considerations

Congenital diaphragmatic hernia results from the lack of fusion of the diaphragmatic musculature. This defect typically occurs in two distinct areas: (1) a posterolateral location, either left (85%) or right (15%); or (2) a central-anterior location. A posterior-lateral hernia commonly is referred to as a *Bochdalek hernia*, and the central-anterior defect is referred to as a *foramen of Morgagni hernia* (Fig. 39-4A).

Bochdalek hernia often is diagnosed prenatally and can cause a variable degree of respiratory distress shortly after birth. The primary problem is pulmonary hypoplasia and resultant pulmonary hypertension. The severity of pulmonary hypoplasia ranges from mild (asymptomatic) to incompatible with life. Patients with mild pulmonary hypoplasia, however, can present after the neonatal period with extremes of symptoms, ranging from persistent cough to near death from strangulated intestine. The hernia also may be discovered incidentally with a chest radiograph.

Regardless of the intensity of symptoms, an operation is indicated. The timing of the operation for patients who are symptomatic at birth is dependent on the degree of pulmonary

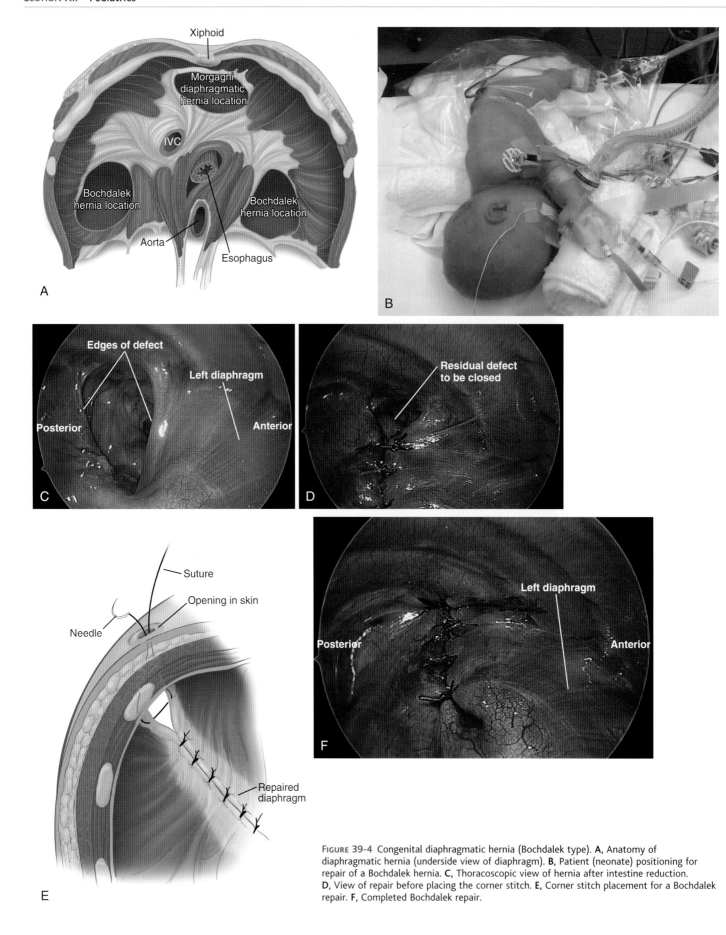

FIGURE 39-4 Congenital diaphragmatic hernia (Bochdalek type). **A,** Anatomy of diaphragmatic hernia (underside view of diaphragm). **B,** Patient (neonate) positioning for repair of a Bochdalek hernia. **C,** Thoracoscopic view of hernia after intestine reduction. **D,** View of repair before placing the corner stitch. **E,** Corner stitch placement for a Bochdalek repair. **F,** Completed Bochdalek repair.

hypoplasia and pulmonary hypertension. Current recommendations are to repair the diaphragm after the patient has demonstrated cardiorespiratory stability.

A foramen of Morgagni hernia rarely produces respiratory symptoms because the lungs have developed normally. This hernia type usually is noted incidentally while obtaining a chest radiograph for vague complaints of substernal pressure, chest pain, or cough. If the stomach is herniating through the defect, then the patient may experience unexplained emesis or even intermittent hematemesis. Strangulation of the contents within a Morgagni hernia is rare. The existence of a foramen of Morgagni hernia also mandates repair, but this generally can be done electively.

Eventration of the diaphragm is believed to result from either a congenital or a traumatic injury to the phrenic nerve. Without the phrenic nerve, the diaphragm undergoes weakening and atrophy. Paradoxical motion occurs when the abdominal contents push up on the diaphragm and negative inspiratory pressure within the chest pulls the diaphragm upward. This situation can impair pulmonary function. It can be difficult to distinguish between an eventration and a hernia on a plain chest radiograph. Fluoroscopy or ultrasound can show the paradoxical motion of the diaphragm, but a diaphragmatic hernia with an intact sac can have a similar appearance.

Symptoms from an eventration generally are mild unless pneumonia develops from the underexpanded lung, or the contents push on the mediastinum, causing a tracheal shift that produces stridor or wheezing. If any symptoms can be attributed to the eventration, or there is considerable lung compression from a large eventration, then elective operative repair is indicated.

Operative Technique

The minimally invasive repair of a Bochdalek hernia is best approached with a thoracoscope. The neonatal patient is placed transversely across the operating table, with bumps placed beneath the patient to elevate the body another 4 to 6 inches off the table. The patient then is placed in the lateral decubitus position with the hernia side facing up (Fig. 39-4B). For an older patient who will not fit transversely across the table, the head is positioned at the top of the bed, and the bed is turned 90 degrees. The goal is to position the surgeon at the patient's head, facing the feet.

The first of three 5-mm ports is placed in the midaxillary line at the third intercostal space, and the chest is insufflated to 4 mm Hg. The remaining two ports are placed as far anterior and posterior in the third intercostal space as possible to maximize room for movement. The only visible structure for left-sided defects usually is the intestine, with the hernia being obscured. Using soft-tipped grasping instruments, the intestine is pushed gently toward the posterior lateral aspect of the diaphragm. This is continued until the intestine begins to reduce and the hernia is visualized.

The remainder of the hernia contents are pushed through the defect under direct vision, including the liver and spleen, if present. After the contents have been reduced, they should stay in the abdomen secondary to the insufflation pressure (Fig. 39-4C). If the contents are not retained in the abdomen, then a fourth port can be inserted just above the diaphragm for additional retraction. Cautery then is used to mobilize the posterior leaflet of the diaphragm from the retroperitoneum as much as possible.

Braided nonabsorbable sutures (0-0 or 2-0) are used to close the defect from a medial to lateral direction. For the most lateral suture, we have found that diaphragmatic tissue typically is lacking (Fig. 39-4D). Because this is the most likely site for recurrence, we now employ an external suture to secure this corner (Fig. 39-4E). A stab incision is made in the skin just under the rib at the corner of the diaphragm. The suture is brought through the skin and under the rib, and then grasped inside the chest using the thoracoscopic needle drivers. Next, the suture is placed

through the upper rim of the diaphragm and the lower rim of the diaphragm, and then back out through the chest wall above the rib where it originally came under, in a triangular configuration. The suture is tied down with the knot just under the skin (Fig. 39-4F). For right-sided defects, care must be taken to avoid injury to the hepatic veins along the medial aspect of the defect.

The pneumothorax is evacuated through the ports, and they are removed. The port sites are closed with absorbable suture. If the defect is too large for primary closure, placement of a patch should be done with a thoracotomy.

A foramen of Morgagni hernia is repaired through a laparoscopic approach. The patient is placed supine on the operating table as close to the foot of the bed as possible. For infants and small children, the legs can be placed in a squatting position. For older children, lithotomy is the preferred position, with the surgeon standing between the legs. The first of three 5-mm ports is placed through the umbilicus, and the remaining two are placed in the right and left lower quadrants. The abdomen is insufflated to 15 mm Hg.

The contents of the hernia are reduced into the abdomen (Fig. 39-5A). The falciform ligament is mobilized with cautery all the way to the lower edge of the hernia defect so that the entire defect can be visualized. The hernia sac is grasped at the apex and inverted into the abdomen. The sac then is removed circumferentially from the edges of the diaphragm with a tissue sealing device or cautery.

The abdominal wall is palpated just below the xiphoid, visualizing with the laparoscope until the probing finger is centered over the defect. A 1-cm incision is made transversely in the skin. Braided, nonabsorbable 0-0 or 2-0 sutures then are placed full thickness through the abdominal wall and grasped with the laparoscopic needle drivers. We generally start on the right side of the defect and proceed sequentially to the left, placing five or six sutures to close the entire defect (Fig. 39-5B and C). Each suture is placed in a U-type fashion through the posterior aspect of the diaphragmatic defect. The needle then is directed back out through the anterior abdominal wall. All sutures are placed before tying the knots.

After the sutures have been placed, the air is released from the abdomen, and all the knots are tied while the assistant holds the untied sutures under tension. After all the knots have been tied, the abdomen is reinsufflated (but only to 10 mm Hg), and the repair is inspected (Fig. 39-5D). The ports are removed, and the sites are closed with absorbable sutures.

Diaphragmatic eventration also is approached through laparoscopy. We perform a plication instead of an imbrication; the latter commonly is used when a chest approach is used. The patient is positioned supine on the operating table. A 5-mm camera port is placed in the umbilicus, and the abdomen is insufflated to 15 mm Hg. For a right-sided eventration, a 12-mm port is placed in the left upper quadrant in the anterior axillary line just below the rib, and a 5-mm port is placed in the right lower quadrant. For left-sided eventration, the 12-mm and 5-mm port sites are reversed. The falciform ligament is mobilized with cautery up to the hepatic veins.

The apex of the eventration is visualized easily because it is nearly transparent. A 2-0 suture is advanced through the 5-mm lower quadrant port and grasped inside the abdomen. The suture is placed through the apex of the eventration and then extracted through the same 5-mm port. This is repeated with an additional 2-0 suture to help disperse the tension on the thin tissue. Tension is applied to the sutures to invert the diaphragm into the abdomen

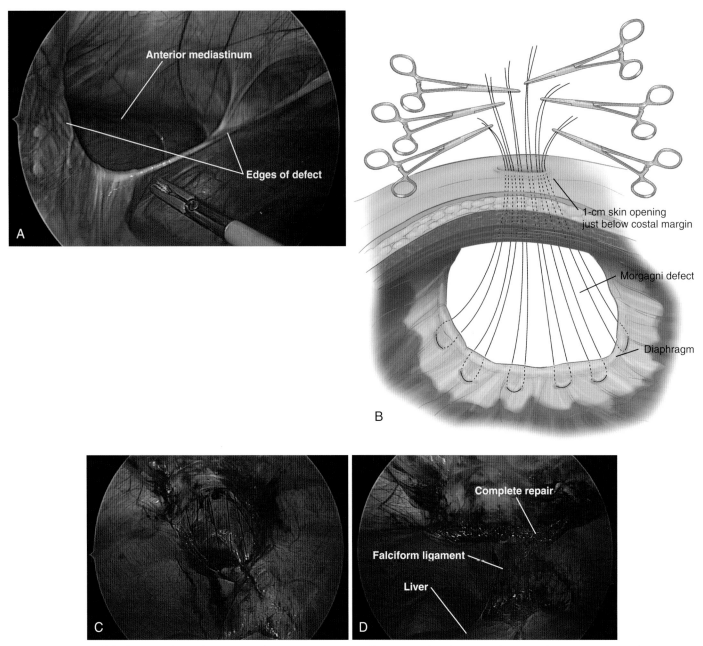

FIGURE 39-5 Congenital diaphragmatic hernia (Morgagni type). **A,** Laparoscopic view of hernia. **B** and **C,** Placement of Morgagni hernia repair sutures (drawing and photo). **D,** Completed Morgagni repair.

(Fig. 39-6A). An endostapler then is inserted through the 12-mm port in the upper lateral abdomen, and the redundant diaphragm is divided from medial to lateral (Fig. 39-6B). The plication typically requires three or four stapler loads to transect the atrophied muscle (Fig. 39-6C). The ports are removed, and the sites are closed with absorbable sutures.

Postoperative Considerations

For the neonate who has undergone repair of a Bochdalek hernia, the postoperative recovery is dependent on the degree of pulmonary hypoplasia and any associated defects. For repairs that are performed outside of the neonatal period, the patient generally is fed that same day and discharged the following morning. Oral pain medication usually is all that is needed. All repairs are followed closely with a chest radiograph every 3 months for the first year and then yearly for the next 4 years to rule out recurrence. Recurrence is the major postoperative complication and should

be less than 10%. It should be noted, however, that minimally invasive repair of this hernia does not have a long history, so the true recurrence rate is not yet known. Steps to avoid recurrence include meticulous suturing technique, gentle handling of the diaphragm, and successful placement of the corner, triangular, extracorporeal suture.

A patient who has had a repair of a foramen of Morgagni hernia is started on a regular diet, and pain is controlled with oral pain medications only. The patient is discharged the following morning. Follow-up occurs at 2 weeks with a chest radiograph. Additional follow-up with a chest radiograph is performed at 1 year to ensure that no recurrence has developed. The upper abdomen initially may appear slightly indented, but this should resolve within several months.

After repair of an eventration, the patient is started on a regular diet and then discharged the following morning. Oral pain medication is all that is needed for postoperative pain control. Initial follow-up is obtained at 2 weeks with a chest

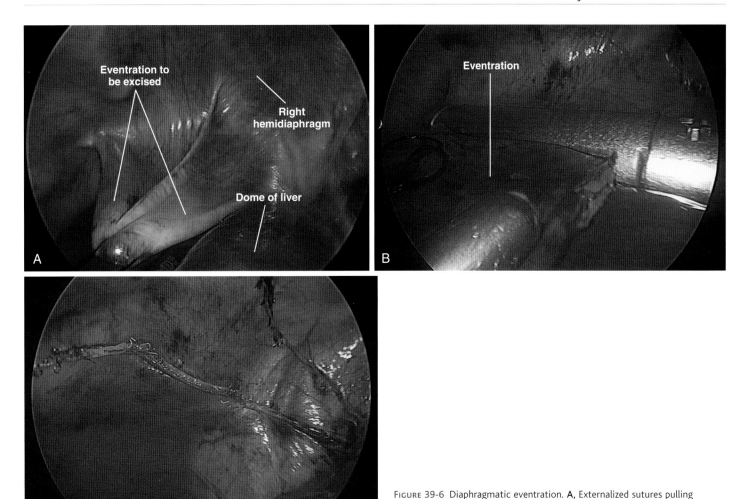

FIGURE 39-6 Diaphragmatic eventration. **A,** Externalized sutures pulling eventration into the abdomen. **B,** Placement of endostapler to resect the eventration. **C,** Completed resection of eventration.

radiograph and then yearly for the next 4 years. Depending on the degree of phrenic nerve dysfunction, the remaining diaphragm may continue to atrophy during follow-up.

V. FEEDING DIFFICULTIES

Preoperative Considerations

Gastrostomy and jejunostomy are invaluable interventions that can assist in both venting the gastrointestinal tract and as a conduit for enteral nutrition. With the advent of the percutaneous endoscopic gastrostomy (PEG), minimally invasive approaches to these surgical adjuncts have become a mainstay of treatment for a variety of conditions. Percutaneous approaches with or without endoscopic assistance, as well as laparoscopic approaches, have emerged as quick and safe. The intraoperative use of fluoroscopy has enabled jejunal advancement of a tube inserted into the stomach without the use of endoscopic guidance. This is particularly helpful in small infants, in whom endoscopy can be technically difficult and instrumentation may be limited by size.

Operative indications include failure to thrive for multiple reasons. Nutritional supplementation for children who do not or cannot eat enough is managed best with enteral feeding. If severe reflux is a concern, or there is concern that creating a gastrostomy will worsen mild to moderate reflux, then a gastrojejunostomy with direct jejunal feeds has become an option to an antireflux procedure in association with a gastrostomy. For most

infants and children who are severely refluxing, however, a fundoplication still is the treatment of choice.

Before any operative manipulation of the upper gastrointestinal (GI) tract, an upper GI contrast study should be obtained to rule out any anatomic reason for reflux, gastric outlet obstruction, or duodenal obstruction. Although malrotation is the most common anomaly that is diagnosed on such an evaluation, the presence of gastroparesis, duodenal webs, or abnormal caliber of the proximal small bowel may lead to a surgical or medical option other than a gastrostomy or gastrojejunostomy. In addition, when reflux is a concern, we obtain an impedance study to quantitate the severity of reflux.

For children who can protect their airway, a trial of nasogastric bolus feeds can be used to predict problems associated with a gastrostomy alone. As indicated earlier, a gastrostomy can worsen existing reflux and may cause reflux in a child who previously did not have any. In patients with reflux complications (i.e., pneumonia, Barrett esophagus, esophagitis, laryngeal edema), a fundoplication always should be done with the gastrostomy, or a gastrojejunostomy should be performed as an alternative.

Operative Technique

The patient is positioned supine. A prophylactic antibiotic is administered. Positioning of ancillary equipment is critical for gastrojejunostomy tube placement because the surgeon needs to have visualization of the laparoscopic tower and the fluoroscopy screen. The site for either the planned gastrostomy or

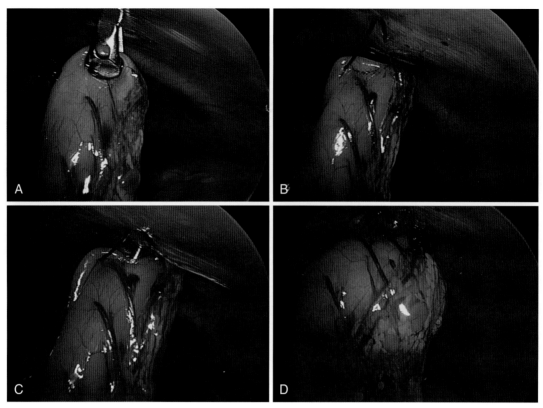

FIGURE 39-7 Gastrostomy and gastrojejunostomy. **A,** Babcock instrument elevating the stomach at the planned gastrostomy site. **B,** Stay suture placement. **C,** Needle entering stomach for passage of guidewire. **D,** Insufflated balloon of gastrostomy button.

gastrojejunostomy is about 1 fingerbreadth below the left costal margin in the midaxillary line. This spot is marked before insufflation of the abdomen. A 5-mm camera port is placed at the umbilicus, and the abdomen is insufflated to 10 to 12 mm Hg.

A nasogastric tube is used to insufflate the stomach, and the previously placed left upper quadrant mark is inspected to confirm optimal gastrostomy site placement. The stomach is suctioned, and a second 5-mm port then is placed at the left upper quadrant mark. Alternatively, a full-thickness 5-mm incision is made under direct vision through the abdominal wall, and a Babcock instrument is placed directly into the abdomen. The greater curvature of the stomach is grasped with the Babcock, directly across from the lesser incisura vessels and well away from the pylorus, and brought up to the anterior abdominal wall (Fig. 39-7A). If a trocar was placed, then it is removed as the stomach is elevated.

The stomach will seal the site and prevent leakage of carbon dioxide. We commonly increase the insufflation flow to 1 to 5 L/minute to compensate for leakage. Next, three or four small stab incisions are made through the skin around the left upper quadrant site. A 0-0 or 2-0 PDS suture on a CTX or CT-1 needle (depending on patient size) is placed full thickness through the abdominal wall through one of the upper stab incisions. The anterior wall of the stomach, immediately adjacent to the Babcock grasper, is incorporated in the suture before extracting the suture through the inferior stab incision. The needle is protected and left on the suture for future use.

The same maneuver is performed through the remaining stab incisions so that the two sutures are on opposite sides of the Babcock grasper. The Babcock is released and removed. The stomach now can be held securely to the anterior abdominal wall with these stay sutures (Fig. 39-7B). The stomach is insufflated by the anesthesiologist, and an 18-gauge needle is placed through

the trocar site into the stomach between the two PDS sutures (Fig. 39-7C). This is followed with a guidewire using the Seldinger technique. The needle then is removed, and the tract is dilated over the wire until an appropriately sized gastrostomy button can be placed.

Under direct visualization, the balloon is insufflated (Fig. 39-7D), and the gastrostomy is checked for intraluminal placement by gravity drainage of saline into the stomach and also by aspiration of gastric contents. The suture needles, which still are attached to the stay sutures, are passed back through their respective stab incisions, but this time remaining in the subcutaneous location. When the needle and free ends emerge from the same stab incision, the sutures are tied with the knots buried in the subcutaneous space. This portion of the procedure is somewhat "scarless" because each stab incision is about 1 mm. The umbilical trocar then is removed, and the site is closed with absorbable sutures.

A gastrojejunostomy is placed in the same manner with the exception that fluoroscopy is used to guide a wire with a soft, flexible tip around the duodenum to the ligament of Treitz. If finding the pylorus is a challenge, then a Bart catheter can be used. This device has a slight angle and has the propensity to slide along the distal antrum and into the pylorus. When in the pyloric channel, the wire is advanced under fluoroscopic guidance so that its tip is well within the distal duodenum or proximal jejunum. With the wire in place, the tract is sequentially dilated to the appropriate size, and the previously chosen gastrojejunostomy button is placed. The wire is removed after the balloon is inflated under laparoscopic visualization and shown to be within the stomach. If there is any question about the jejunal positioning, then contrast can be injected through the J port, but usually this is not necessary.

Postoperative Considerations

For both buttons, postoperative management consists of placing the gastrostomy or gastric portion of the G-J button to gravity for about 6 to 12 hours, and then commencing the feeds through the appropriate channel. We have found that jejunal feedings can begin as soon as the patient has left the recovery room. Pain management with oral narcotics or NSAIDs for the 24 hours is adequate. Most patients can be discharged the following day after appropriate parental teaching has been completed.

Procedure-specific complications are categorized into intraoperative and postoperative. Intraoperative complications include failure to enter the stomach (including tangential needle placement), failure to gain an adequate seal with stay sutures, and bleeding. The best way to avoid placing the wire through a tangentially inserted needle is to remember that needle direction typically is more superior than apparent, and to listen for air return from the distended stomach. Failure to gain a complete seal with two stay sutures is not uncommon and may not be avoidable, especially in a patient with a thick abdominal wall, because the needle may not be large enough to take an adequate bite of the stomach. The critical element is to recognize this possibility and place additional stay sutures. Three- or four-point fixation can be performed through the same stab incisions. Bleeding can be avoided by visualization of the stay suture needle as it traverses the abdominal wall and stomach.

Postoperative complications include a leak in the first several days, tube displacement resulting in loss of the tract, and site issues usually secondary to granulation tissue. Leaks are sometimes unavoidable; however, there are some preventable causes. First, an incompetent balloon will result in a leak because the balloon is the primary device that prevents a leak. The balloon always should be tested and inflated to the manufacturer's suggested level before placement. Next, the surgeon should ensure that a proper seal exists between the stomach and the anterior abdominal wall. If any portion of the button can be seen through the laparoscope, then additional stay sutures should be placed. Finally, the wrong choice of procedure may lead to a leak. For example, a child who is a severe retcher should not have a simple gastrostomy button. In such a patient, further evaluation should be done to determine whether a fundoplication with a gastrostomy button or gastrojejunostomy button would be a better option.

We have not found a way to prevent granulation tissue. It can result in redness around the site but rarely produces an infection. Granulation tissue can lead to leakage of gastric contents and resultant skin erythema. The same applies for bleeding from the site. Bleeding rarely is from the stomach proper, but usually derives from granulation tissue. Silver nitrate applied locally will resolve most issues resulting from granulation tissue. In extreme cases, surgical resection of the granulation tissue may be necessary.

The results from G and G-J button placement are excellent for the most part, and complications more often are related to the underlying disease and indication for placement than to the actual procedure. Although most manufacturers recommend button replacement every 3 months, we have had several patients go 1 to 2 years between button replacements. For dislodgment, most parents can easily replace a gastrostomy button themselves at home if they have received instructions. We generally wait 8 to 12 weeks to teach the parents button change and replacement methods to allow sufficient time for the tract to mature.

For G-J dislodgment, fluoroscopic or endoscopic replacement will be necessary, but such an occurrence should not be an emergency if the parents can maintain the site with a gastrostomy button. When the button is no longer needed, we have the parents remove it at home; the site tends to close within hours. If there is still leakage after a week (15% to 20%), then the patient will be set up for elective, outpatient closure of the gastrocutaneous fistula.

VI. GASTROESOPHAGEAL REFLUX DISEASE

Preoperative Considerations

Gastroesophageal reflux disease (GERD) is common in children. The true incidence is difficult to determine because, in most infants, gastroesophageal reflux is physiologic and will be outgrown by 2 years of age. Medical management will control symptoms in most infants, even those with severe disease. Treatment begins with upright positioning and thickened feeds and progresses to the use of acid-suppressive and motility medications. Operative intervention usually is reserved for the most severe cases and usually is in the setting of other medical issues, such as prematurity, chronic lung disease, cerebral palsy, and congenital heart disease. Unfortunately, these patients also have a higher operative risk and can have a worse outcome.

Presentation of GERD in children can occur with emesis, which can lead to failure to thrive that is manifested by a fall off the growth curve. Other patients present with respiratory symptoms such as coughing with feeds. This can lead to recurrent aspiration pneumonia. In the infant, laryngospasm from GERD and aspiration can lead to an acute life-threatening event. Silent GERD may be associated with asthma, sinusitis, recurrent otitis media, and hoarseness.

Preoperative evaluation varies among practitioners; most agree that an upper gastrointestinal contrast study is indicated. This study delineates the anatomy, evaluates gastric emptying, and can demonstrate GERD. Anatomic variants that can be detected with this study include malrotation and duodenal stenosis. Esophagogastroduodenoscopy may demonstrate stricture or inflammation, but is not mandatory for evaluation. Additional studies include pH probes, impedance probes, deglutition studies, and gastric emptying studies, but these should be individualized according to the clinical situation. In children younger than 1 year, physiologic studies can be difficult to interpret because normal values range widely. Indications for an operation include an acute life-threatening event from aspiration associated with GERD, recurrent aspiration, recurrent esophageal stricture, failure to thrive despite GERD medical management, and need for a gastrostomy tube in an infant with GERD.

Operative Technique

Laparoscopic fundoplication can be performed safely at almost any size or age. A prophylactic antibiotic is administered, and the child is moved to the end of the short operating table. The surgeon stands at the patient's feet; stirrups can be used in teenagers. An assistant stands on either side. Access to the abdomen is gained at the umbilicus with a 5-mm trocar. Insufflation is begun at 10 to 12 mm Hg, with a flow rate of 1 to 2 L/minute. Two additional 5-mm trocars are placed on each side of the abdomen. A liver retractor is placed through a stab wound or a 5-mm trocar just under the right costal margin in the midclavicular line. A locking

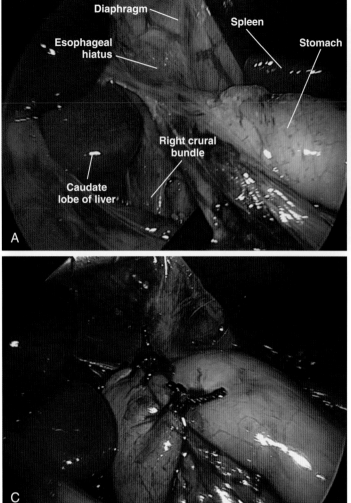

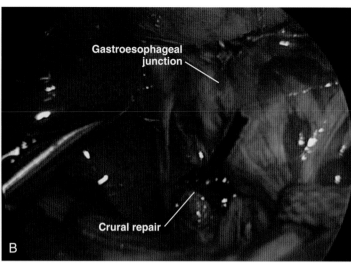

FIGURE 39-8 Gastroesophageal reflux disease. **A,** Minimal dissection of the esophagus during a Nissen fundoplication. **B,** Crural sutures. **C,** Completed fundoplication.

grasper then is inserted and advanced under the left lobe of the liver to the diaphragm. In larger babies and children, a triangle retractor is used to retract the left lobe of the liver.

The two trocars at the level of the umbilicus are used by the surgeon for dissection and sewing the wrap. The final trocar is placed in the left midclavicular line, 1 fingerbreadth below the left costal margin. As discussed in the preceding section, this is marked *before* insufflation because it will serve as the site for the gastrostomy button (which is needed in most patients). If a gastrostomy button is not required, this trocar can be placed more laterally to avoid the other trocars. In small infants, these trocars tend to slide in and out. Various methods are described for sewing these in place to prevent the sliding.

After the trocars have been placed, the dissection begins with division of the short gastric vessels. This allows for mobilization of the fundus and aids in the identification of the left crus. The dissection begins at the inferior pole of the spleen and can be completed with a tissue sealing device or cautery in small infants. The left-handed instrument retracts the stomach while the right-handed instrument divides the vessels. The assistant gently retracts the spleen. A posterior row of short gastric vessels can be identified in some cases and should be divided.

After the left crus has been identified, the dissection proceeds to the right side of the stomach, and the gastrohepatic ligament is divided. Care is taken to look for a replaced left hepatic vessel. If identified, the dissection usually can be continued without division of this vessel. If this is not possible, then it should be safe

to divide this vessel. The dissection then is carried up to the right crus. Secondary to the complication of posterior migration of the wrap and stomach, we perform a "minimal dissection" of the esophagus (Fig. 39-8A) and do not mobilize the esophagus off the diaphragm or crura (this method has been supported by prospective randomized studies). The assistant pulls the stomach to the left, and the retroesophageal plane is developed. This should be done posterior to the vagus nerve (to prevent esophageal injury) and cephalad to the left gastric pedicle. An appropriate-sized bougie (there are published charts based on weight) is placed to facilitate identification of the esophagus. Again, minimal dissection to allow passage of the wrap is recommended to prevent posterior wrap migration.

The hiatus is repaired if a significant defect is present. This is performed with 2-0 or 3-0 nonabsorbable, braided suture on an RB-1 needle, which will pass through a 5-mm trocar. The suture is cut to 12 cm to facilitate suturing. One or two stitches usually are required (Fig. 39-8B). At this point, the left-handed instrument is passed posterior to the esophagus, and the assistant passes the fundus into the instrument. If appropriate division of the short gastric vessels has been performed and the appropriate location on the fundus has been identified, then the fundus should pass easily to the right side of the esophagus, even in small infants.

Suturing of the fundoplication begins with the bougie in place. The first suture is placed though the left fundus, then through the esophageal hiatus anteriorly, incorporating the anterior wall of the esophagus, and then through the fundus on the right. Two additional sutures are placed through the fundus on the left, then the esophagus, and finally the fundus on the right. This completes a 360-degree wrap measuring 1 to 3 cm in length (Fig. 39-8C). In most cases, a gastrostomy tube is placed next, using techniques described in the previous section. The bougie then is removed, along with the nasogastric tube. The port sites are closed with absorbable sutures.

Postoperative Considerations

Pain is managed with a combination of intravenous narcotics (until feeds are started) and NSAIDs. The gastrostomy is left to dependent drainage for the first night. Feeding generally is begun on postoperative day 1 and advanced to goal over the next 24 hours. Most patients can be discharged on postoperative day 2 if their underlying comorbidities allow. Parents are encouraged to vent the gastrostomy tube as needed for abdominal distention, retching, and fussiness.

Complications from laparoscopic fundoplication are rare in the perioperative period but are more common in the long-term. Early complications tend to be related to underlying disease processes (cardiac, seizures, respiratory) rather than the procedure itself. Transfusions and conversions to open procedures are rare. Long-term issues include retching, wrap failure, wrap migration, and delayed gastric emptying; 5% to 10% of patients will require reoperation, and others will require ongoing acid suppression.

VII. HYPERTROPHIC PYLORIC STENOSIS

Preoperative Considerations

Hypertrophy of the pyloric muscle is one of the most common diseases treated with a laparoscopic procedure in infants. The procedure can be performed quickly with minimal complications and excellent results. Performing the myotomy with an open technique is a classic pediatric surgical procedure and can be taught at the intern level. The simplicity makes it a natural procedure to transition to the laparoscopy; however, the haptics required makes this procedure more difficult to teach.

The etiology of pyloric stenosis is not known. There is a predominance in males, and it can cluster in families. It presents at 2 to 6 weeks of age with nonbilious emesis, which tends to be progressive and projectile in nature. Occasionally, there will be blood in the emesis, particularly if gastritis is present. These babies tend to look well early in the course and are vigorous eaters even after episodes of emesis. Over time, they can become progressively lethargic from dehydration and electrolyte imbalances. The principal differential diagnosis includes formula intolerance and GERD, and therefore formula changes and acid suppression usually occur before surgical involvement.

The diagnosis can be made with a simple physical examination, palpating for a mobile, smooth-walled, 2-cm mass midway between the umbilicus and the xiphoid. If the pyloric mass is not palpable, then an ultrasound can be used to make the diagnosis. Ultrasound criteria include a minimal pyloric wall thickness of 4 mm and minimal length of 14 mm, as well as pyloric nonemptying. Laboratory studies are limited to a chemistry panel to determine whether the infant has developed a hypochloremic, hypokalemic metabolic alkalosis. Electrolyte imbalance must be corrected before a general anesthetic is used; otherwise, the child can develop postoperative apnea requiring prolonged intubation.

Electrolyte correction may require 1 to 2 days of aggressive rehydration. A nasogastric tube should be placed preoperatively so that the child will have an empty stomach during intubation. An experienced anesthesiologist is critical in presence of dehydration and a full stomach in a small infant.

Operative Technique

The infant is intubated and placed in the supine position transversely on the bed. This allows easy access to both the airway and the abdomen. The surgeon is positioned at the feet. A small bump should be placed at the middle back to bring the pylorus more anterior. The monitor is set above the infant's head. A 5-mm incision is made at the umbilicus. The umbilical ring often is open, allowing access for a hemostat, followed by a 5-mm trocar. Insufflation is set at 8 to 10 mm Hg with a flow rate of 1 L/minute. Some prefer a 3-mm scope and trocar, but the image is smaller. Because the cosmetic result is no different, we prefer to use a 5-mm port and camera.

A 2-mm full-thickness abdominal wall stab incision is made with a no. 11 blade in the right flank at the level of the umbilicus in the anterior axillary line. A pyloric grasper inserted through this incision (Fig. 39-9A) is used to steady the pylorus (Fig. 39-9B). A similar 2-mm full-thickness stab incision then is made in the left upper abdomen at the level of the pylorus in the midclavicular line. A beaver blade with an adhesive strip covering all but the distal 2 mm of blade is inserted through the second site (see Fig. 39-9A). The pyloromyotomy is begun just proximal to the duodenum and extending up onto the stomach (2 to 3 cm in most infants). The starting point may be marked by the pyloric vein of Mayo; care should be taken because the pylorus is thinnest at this point, which also is the most common location for perforation. It is preferable to leave a few pyloric muscle fibers distally rather than risk a perforation. The incision is 2 mm in depth.

The blade is exchanged for a pyloric spreader (Fig. 39-9C). Spreading is started in the middle of the incision with constant uniform downward and outward pressure. When the surgeon can see the shiny white external surface of the mucosa bulging along the entire length of the incision, the myotomy is complete (Fig. 39-9D). The spreader and grasper then are removed, and two blunt tip graspers are used to grab the edges of the myotomy and show they move independently. This also confirms a complete myotomy.

Finally, a grasper is gently used to occlude the duodenum. The anesthesiologist inflates the stomach using an orogastric tube and bulb syringe. The myotomy is observed for any signs of a leak. Bleeding from the edges usually stops; cautery near the mucosa is discouraged. The omentum then is placed in the myotomy. All instruments are removed. The only suture used for closure is a 3-0 absorbable suture on an RB-1 needle, for the fascia at the umbilicus. This stitch is critical to prevent postoperative hernias at the umbilicus. Adhesive strips are applied.

Postoperative Considerations

Postoperatively, the orogastric tube is removed when the child is extubated in the operating room. Narcotics must be avoided because of the concern for postoperative apnea. An apnea and bradycardia monitor is used for the first 24 hours. The entire allowable dose of local anesthesia is given during the operation, which should eliminate the need for pain medicine beyond

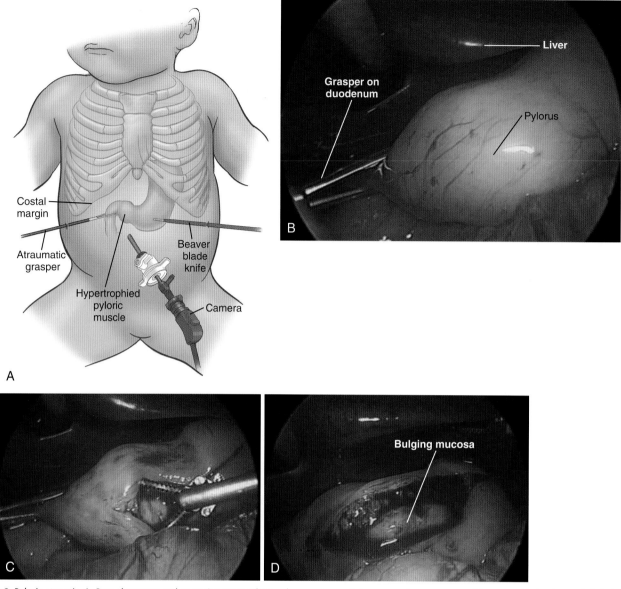

FIGURE 39-9 Pyloric stenosis. **A**, Port placement and operative approach to pyloromyotomy. **B**, Laparoscopic appearance of hypertrophied pylorus. **C**, Pyloric spreader disrupting the pyloric muscle. **D**, Completed pyloromyotomy.

acetaminophen. Frequent small feedings are given when the infant is alert and interested in eating. Upright positioning and frequent burping are encouraged. Parents are reassured that although some emesis will continue, it will resolve. Most patients can be discharged at 24 hours, although some may require longer hospitalizations if there is a component of GERD.

Complications are infrequent and may include incomplete myotomy, open conversion, perforation, infection, and umbilical hernia. Concern for a perforation should be raised if the abdomen is distended with peritoneal signs, tachycardia, and emesis in the postoperative period. This complication typically is identified 2 to 3 days postoperatively, making the repair more difficult and potentially leading to more morbidity. If diagnosed early, a simple repair of the mucosa can be performed, followed by a short duration of nasogastric decompression. If diagnosed late, closure of the myotomy over the mucosal repair is followed by rotation of the pylorus 90 degrees, and a new myotomy is performed. Overall, outcomes are excellent. In general, no long-term effects should occur after a successful myotomy.

VIII. MECKEL DIVERTICULUM

Preoperative Considerations

Meckel diverticulum is defined as an embryologic remnant of the vitelline duct, which connects the fetal intestine to the yolk sac through the umbilical cord. When a remnant persists, it may be in the form of an antimesenteric diverticulum, an ileal-umbilical fistula, an umbilical sinus with or without a cyst, or a fibrotic band between the ileum and the umbilicus. It may harbor ectopic tissue (gastric or pancreatic) in a small percentage of patients. If the lining of the Meckel diverticulum secretes acid, bicarbonate, or pancreatic enzymatic fluid, then the ileum surrounding the diverticulum can have an inflammatory response because this region does not contain goblet cells that provide a mucosal protective function. The outcome can be bleeding from an adjacent ulcer, perforation, or Meckel diverticulitis.

The Meckel diverticulum also can become inflamed as a result of intestinal contents becoming trapped, similar to appendicitis

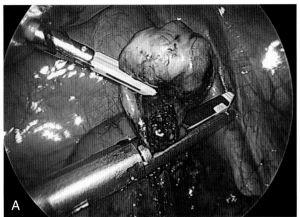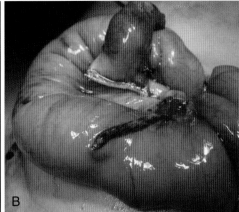

FIGURE 39-10 Meckel diverticulum. **A,** Endostapler resection of the diverticulum. **B,** Intestine appearance after resection.

or colonic diverticulitis. These diverticula usually have a narrow opening into the ileum. If a connection between the ileum and the umbilicus persists, then this may serve as a nidus for a volvulus of a portion of small intestine. Finally, the diverticulum can serve as a lead point for intussusception with resultant bowel obstruction. Despite these multiple pathologic states, most Meckel diverticula will be asymptomatic. A common scenario is the finding of a Meckel diverticulum incidentally when operating for another indication.

Operative indications include bleeding, bowel obstruction, peritonitis, and perforation. For most indications, a laparoscopic exploration is preferred. Preoperative evaluation, testing, and preparation depend on the indications for surgery. In the case of complete bowel obstruction, perforation, or peritonitis, a physical examination and abdominal radiographs are all that is needed. In these scenarios, however, CT or ultrasound of the abdomen often is obtained before a surgical consultation. An obstructive pattern of the small bowel with free fluid in the pelvis and a normal appendix should prompt the diagnosis of a Meckel diverticulum. Additionally, any complete bowel obstruction in someone who has never had an abdominal operation should prompt the diagnosis of a Meckel diverticulum as the etiology. In the case of intermittent blood per rectum, a Meckel scan (technetium-99 nuclear scan), which can indicate ectopic gastric mucosa, is the most common method of making the diagnosis. Preoperative transfusions may be necessary because a Meckel diverticulum is the number one cause of a gastrointestinal bleed that requires a transfusion in the small child.

Operative Technique

The patient is placed in the supine position, and a prophylactic antibiotic is administered. A 5-mm umbilical trocar is used for initial camera placement. We prefer to place the remaining two trocars (one 5 mm and one 12 mm) in the suprapubic location and in the left lower quadrant. An additional fourth port may be necessary in the right flank for the assistant to help with retraction. In the case of a complete small bowel obstruction, the nidus for the obstruction can be an umbilical band or an intussusception, so care should be taken when placing the initial umbilical port.

Atraumatic graspers are used to run the small bowel from the ileocecal valve proximally. The choice of operation depends on the pathology caused by the Meckel diverticulum. For bleeding, diverticulitis, and an intussusception that has reduced, a transverse diverticulectomy is sufficient. Ulcers in the adjacent jejunum

will heal after the focus of acid production (the diverticulum) has been removed. To accomplish this, an endostapler inserted through the 12-mm trocar is positioned transversely across the base of the diverticulum (Fig. 39-10A and B). The remaining one or two trocars are used to hold the bowel in position. The stapler is deployed, and the resected diverticulum is placed in an endoscopic retrieval bag and removed.

For patients with a volvulus, the band connecting the Meckel diverticulum to the umbilicus is first divided with cautery as close to the umbilicus as possible, and the intestine is untwisted. The intestine is inspected for viability. If viable, then the diverticulum is resected (with the attached band), as described previously. If there is intestinal necrosis, then either the suprapubic incision or the umbilical incision is enlarged, the intestine is exteriorized, and an extracorporeal resection with anastomosis is performed.

A similar approach is used for perforations associated with the Meckel diverticulum. If the perforation is contained within the diverticulum, then a simple diverticulectomy can be performed. If the adjacent ileum contains the perforation, we again enlarge either the suprapubic or umbilical port sites, deliver the intestine through the opening, and perform an extracorporeal resection and anastomosis. For most cases of Meckel diverticulum, we also remove the appendix because it may serve as a nidus for problems in the future, and there is little additional risk or operative time added. After resection, the appendix and the diverticulum can be placed in the same retrieval bag and extracted together.

Postoperative Considerations

Postoperative care depends on the operation performed and the degree of preoperative obstruction. For a transverse diverticulectomy without significant preoperative obstruction, the patient leaves the operating room without any tubes and is begun on oral intake on postoperative day 1. Proton pump inhibitors are continued for 2 to 4 weeks while the ulcers in the jejunum continue to heal. If the patient had a significant bowel obstruction or peritonitis, or underwent a small bowel anastomosis, then feeding is held until return of gastrointestinal function. A nasogastric tube may be necessary in the patient with a complete bowel obstruction because postoperative ileus may be an issue. One additional dose of antibiotic is administered postoperatively; in a patient with a perforation, however, a week of intravenous antibiotics may be needed.

Specific complications included negative exploration, injury to the bowel during examination, and stricture of the small bowel due to the resection or anastomosis. If the Meckel diverticulum is not seen after examining the bowel, then a repeat examination in the reverse direction (from the ligament of Treitz to the ileocecal valve) is performed with the camera in the suprapubic position. Atraumatic graspers should be used on the pediatric intestine because standard grasping instruments can cause full-thickness bowel injuries. When performing a diverticulectomy, the stapler should be oriented 90 degrees to the intestinal lumen, which should result in less narrowing of the ileum. Finally, when performing an anastomosis for a perforation, inspect the bowel lumen at the margins. Sewing an ulcer into an anastomosis can cause a leak or result in a stricture of the lumen. Overall, the results of Meckel procedures are excellent. As with any abdominal operation, the only long-term sequelae of which to inform parents is a 5% lifetime risk for postoperative adhesive bowel obstruction.

IX. URACHUS

Preoperative Considerations

The urachus is an embryonic connection between the cloaca and the allantois. As the allantois involutes and the cloaca separates into hindgut and genitourinary systems, a connection persists between the urinary bladder and the umbilical cord (Fig. 39-11A). The natural history of this structure is to undergo fibrosis and regression. Failure to do so may lead to a persistent vesicoumbilical fistula, diverticulum of the bladder, sinus of the umbilicus, or cyst anywhere along the path. Epithelial overgrowth at the umbilicus may result in a granuloma of the cord, which is to be distinguished from a true urachal anomaly.

Operative indications for urachal disease include abscess of a urachal cyst, chronic bladder infections, and persistent umbilical drainage. Persistent umbilical drainage is not an operative emergency, and the timing of surgery has been the subject of debate in the literature. An operation as early as 2 months, to waiting for 1 to 2 years, and in some cases observational management all have had support in the literature. If the patient has symptoms, then we usually recommend an operation. For patients who present with erythema of the umbilicus (or anywhere along the urachal tract), tenderness, and fever, a 10- to 14-day course of antibiotics usually is sufficient to treat the infection before surgery. Occasionally, an incision and drainage are necessary for a true umbilical or urachal cyst abscess. We wait 4 to 6 weeks to allow the inflammatory process to resolve, and then proceed with a resection.

Preoperative preparation should include urinalysis. An undiagnosed urinary tract infection should be treated before an operation. Ultrasound commonly has been used to make the diagnosis in an infant with umbilical drainage, but this diagnosis can be made on physical examination; we have only used ultrasound for cases in which the diagnosis was in doubt. In the case of recurrent bladder infections, an ultrasound or voiding cystourethrogram can be used to determine whether a bladder diverticulum is present.

Operative Technique

Patient positioning in the operating suite is supine. Most of these cases can be performed with umbilical exploration alone. The approach is identical to an umbilical hernia repair. When the umbilical stalk is cut, the inferior preperitoneal space is inspected and the urachal remnant grasped, usually along with the urachal artery remnants. With blunt dissection in the preperitoneal plane, the bladder usually can be brought to the umbilicus, and the tract can be excised at the level of the dome of the bladder.

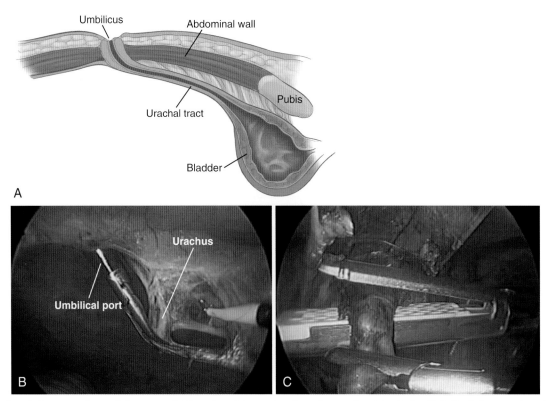

FIGURE 39-11 Urachus. **A,** Anatomy of a urachal remnant. **B,** Dissection of the urachus from the anterior abdominal wall. **C,** Urachal transection with endostapler over the dome of the bladder.

In cases in which there is a diverticulum or a history of cyst abscess, mobilization of the bladder may be difficult, and this is where laparoscopy has a role. Another role for laparoscopy in urachal disease is for the teenager, in whom the distance between the umbilicus and bladder is greater.

If laparoscopy is to be used, then a supraumbilical approach to the umbilical stalk is used. A Veress needle or trocar can be placed here, avoiding the urachal remnant on the inferior border of the umbilicus. Another option is to place the initial trocar in the right upper quadrant, just below the costal margin. After the abdomen has been insufflated (10 to 12 mm Hg), two or three other ports will be necessary and generally are placed along the flanks and lower quadrants to triangulate the camera and working ports. One of these ports should be 12 mm in the right lower quadrant, for stapler deployment.

The dissection is begun at the umbilicus. Cautery is used to divide the tract at the umbilicus, off the abdominal wall. If the urachus is extending to the skin of the umbilicus, then this must be removed with the specimen. The tissue is used as a handle, and the remainder of the urachus is dissected off the abdominal wall (Fig. 39-11B) until the dome of the bladder is reached. The endostapler then is fired across the dome of the bladder (Fig. 39-11C), and the specimen is removed through the 12-mm port site.

Postoperative Considerations

Postoperative care is identical to any other laparoscopic procedure in a child, with the exception that a Foley is left in overnight. Oral narcotics and NSAIDs usually are sufficient for pain control. A regular diet is resumed immediately. The Foley catheter is removed the following morning; the patient may be discharged after voiding.

Most complications involve the umbilical wound. Complete excision or fulguration of the tract going through the umbilical skin is required; otherwise, persistent drainage and infection can be expected. The surgeon should resist the urge to leave the umbilical skin alone. In the long run, the cosmetic deficit will be better if the tract is completely eliminated at the initial definitive procedure.

X. Hirschsprung disease

Preoperative Considerations

Since Orvar Swenson characterized the absence of ganglion cells as the reason for a dysfunctional distal segment of bowel, there have been several operations developed to treat Hirschsprung disease. Each of these operations has been modified several times, and now minimally invasive approaches are available. The three original operations that are considered potentially curative are the Soave, Swenson, and Duhamel procedures. For the purposes of this chapter, the laparoscopic Duhamel and the laparoscopy-assisted perineal pull-through procedures are described. It should be emphasized that there may be no other operation in all of pediatric surgery that is dependent on an experienced pediatric pathologist to (1) make the original diagnosis and (2) guide therapy (by locating the transition point where ganglion cells appear).

There are three major presentations for patients with Hirschsprung disease. Most common is the newborn who fails to pass meconium in the first 24 hours of life and does not tolerate initial feedings. Second is the infant who actually does tolerate

feedings initially, but then presents with enterocolitis (the most severe form of which is toxic megacolon). Third, there is the chronically constipated infant, toddler, or child. Typically, a patient in this last group will present either at weaning off breast milk or conversion to solid food. The diagnosis of Hirschsprung disease can be suspected if a transition zone is seen on a barium enema but requires a rectal biopsy for confirmation. Suction rectal biopsy, partial-thickness punch biopsy, and full-thickness biopsy have all been described and are all acceptable means of making a diagnosis.

After the diagnosis has been made, the next decision is whether to perform a staged or primary repair. Historically, all of these patients received colostomies, and the definitive procedure was delayed until appropriate weight gain and nutritional status could be confirmed. This colostomy was combined with a staging procedure in which multiple seromuscular biopsies were taken to identify the transition zone where ganglion cells could be definitively identified. It was at this location that the colostomy was created (also known as the *leveling colostomy*). This not only ensured intestinal function but also located the point of the future pull-through procedure. In the past 20 years, however, a primary pull-through option without a stoma commonly has been offered in the neonatal period.

Depending on the age and type of presentation, the preoperative evaluation and planning will differ. For the newborn who is vomiting and fails to pass meconium, but who otherwise is not ill and has a normal abdominal examination, a barium enema followed by a rectal biopsy is all that is necessary. A primary pull-through in the first week of life or a short course of rectal irrigations followed by a primary pull-through is our preferred approach. For the older infant who presents with enterocolitis, intravenous antibiotics, in combination with rectal irrigations, are required before considering an operation. A rectal biopsy is performed to make the diagnosis. It is our preference to stage these patients with a colostomy or ileostomy. For the constipated toddler, anorectal manometry becomes useful along with a barium enema to decide which patients require a rectal biopsy. These patients also will need a staged repair with a leveling colostomy to decompress the dilated colon, which can become massively enlarged secondary to the chronic distal obstruction.

Operative Technique

For laparoscopic *staging* procedures, a 5-mm umbilical trocar and two additional 5-mm trocars in the bilateral upper quadrants are inserted. The procedure is started with an appendectomy. Serial seromuscular biopsy specimens then are obtained every 10 cm, starting at the most distal dilated colon, until ganglion cells are found on frozen section. Intracorporeal suturing may be accomplished as a figure-of-eight or a pursestring suture around the biopsy sites, or alternatively a PDS Endoloop (Ethicon Biosurgery, Cincinnati, Ohio) is used to obtain a full-thickness biopsy (Fig. 39-12A). This process can be very time-consuming because each specimen takes about 25 to 30 minutes to process and examine by an experienced pathologist. The leveling colostomy then is made in a standard fashion at the site where ganglion cells are identified.

An alternative approach to identify the usual rectosigmoid location of the transition zone is to perform a small muscle-splitting incision on the left side of the abdomen and to pull up the sigmoid colon through this small opening. Biopsies then are performed until ganglion cells are confirmed. This small incision

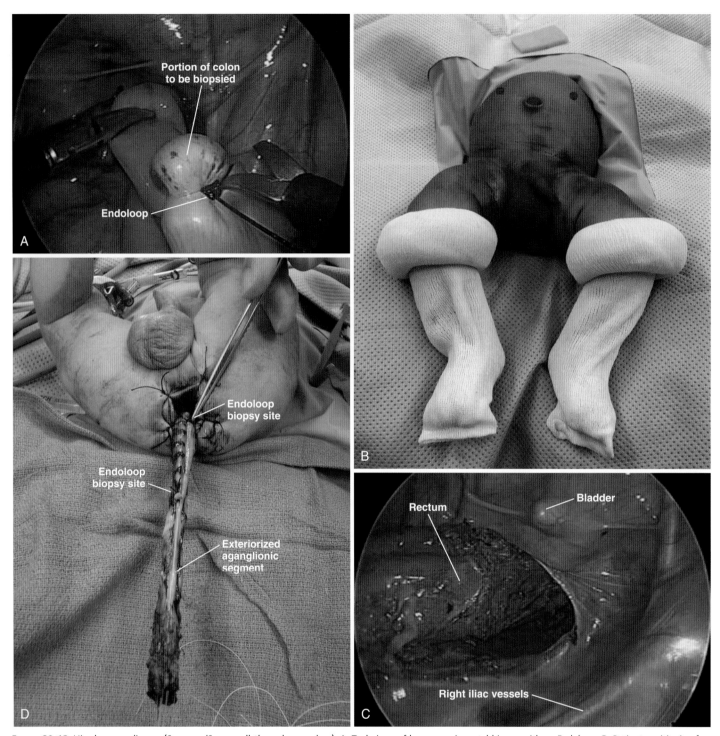

FIGURE 39-12 Hirschsprung disease (Swenson/Soave pull-through procedure). **A,** Technique of laparoscopic rectal biopsy with an Endoloop. **B,** Patient positioning for a pull-through procedure. **C,** Completed rectal dissection before pull-through. **D,** Perineal exteriorization of aganglionic colorectal segment.

subsequently is used as the colostomy site. If a transition zone is not found through this small incision, then a 12-mm trocar can be placed through this site, and a laparoscopic exploration is done as described previously.

If a separate staging procedure is not required, then a one-stage pull-through reconstruction is performed. Our preferred approach is to perform either (1) a laparoscopic mobilization with serial biopsies, combined with a perineal dissection (either a Soave, in which only the mucosa is dissected above the dentate line, or a Swenson, in which the full thickness of the rectum is dissected above the dentate line); or (2) a laparoscopic Duhamel procedure. These two approaches are described next.

Regardless of the procedure, the patient is placed into a modified lithotomy position at the end of the table (Fig. 39-12B). The surgeons will need access to the anus and abdomen and should have freedom of instrument movement with respect to the legs. No intravenous lines should be placed in the lower extremities. The child is prepared circumferentially from the nipples to the toes, and stockinets wrapped in Coban (3M, St. Paul, Minn.) are used to cover the legs. A prophylactic dose of antibiotics is administered. The lower half of the infant's body may be placed through the opening of an extremity drape, which will protect the prepped area. A Foley catheter is inserted after the drapes have been placed.

For both the Swenson and Soave pull-through procedures, the operation is started in the abdomen. A 5-mm camera port is inserted at the umbilicus, and two additional 5-mm ports are placed in the bilateral upper quadrants. The colon is examined for a dilation transition point, which usually is at the rectosigmoid or distal sigmoid. We then proceed with staging as previously described. While awaiting pathology, the intra-abdominal mobilization and dissection are performed. The ureters are identified bilaterally as they cross over the iliac arteries and down into the pelvis. The mesentery immediately beneath the most proximal PDS suture biopsy site is opened with a tissue sealing device. The mesenteric dissection is continued distally to the peritoneal reflection. The peritoneum around the rectum is opened circumferentially.

The posterior dissection down to the pelvic floor is performed with blunt instrumentation to avoid injury to the pelvic nerves. Anteriorly, the rectum is mobilized from the bladder and vagina, staying directly on the rectal wall. When 1 cm of the dissection has been completed, the rectum should be easily separable, and the dissection can be carried down to the pelvic floor (Fig. 39-12C). The vascular pedicles then are divided along the lateral walls of the rectum.

By this time, the pathologist should have the frozen section results. If ganglion cells are identified, then no further dissection is required. If ganglion cells are not identified, then an additional biopsy is taken 10 cm more proximal on the descending colon. While awaiting the secondary results, more proximal colonic mobilization is performed along the white line of Toldt. The splenocolic ligament is divided. The mesentery is divided up to the biopsy site. The laparoscopic dissection may need to be performed at 10-cm intervals all the way to the ileum, if necessary, until ganglion cells are identified.

After normal colon has been identified, the perineal portion of the procedure ensues. The pneumoperitoneum is released with the ports in place. The legs are elevated up onto the abdomen to expose the anus, and the surgeon stands at the foot of the bed. A self-retaining retractor, or 3-0 silk perianal sutures, are used to evert the dentate line. Cautery is used to circumferentially incise the mucosa about 5 mm above the dentate line. For a Soave pull-through, the mucosal plane is dissected for another 5 to 7 cm proximally. At this point, the rectal wall is divided, thus entering into the pelvic dissection from the abdominal portion of the operation.

For a Swenson pull-through, the rectal wall is divided full thickness just above the dentate line. It is safest to start at the posterior half of the anal opening, and after the pelvic dissection from above has been entered, the anterior half is completed. This is done to avoid injury to the prostatic urethra; care is taken to stay on the rectal wall. With the rectum now completely mobile, the abdomen is reinsufflated. The camera is inserted to help guide the colon down to the perineum, ensuring that it is not twisted during its descent (Fig. 39-12D). The PDS sutures at the biopsy sites are kept anterior, and the mesentery is kept posterior.

After the final PDS has been pulled down past the anal opening, the colon is inspected for tension and twisting. If there is excessive tension on the colon, then further mobilization should be performed. If the colonic length is deemed adequate, then the pneumoperitoneum is released again, and attention returns to the anus. The colon is divided just above the PDS biopsy site that demonstrated ganglion cells, and a hand-sewn coloanal anastomosis is completed with interrupted 4-0 absorbable sutures, using the mucosa 5 mm above the dentate line. The

abdomen is reinsufflated, and the camera is inserted. A 10-mm Hagar dilator is inserted gently through the anastomosis while visualizing with the laparoscope from above. This is the final check to make sure that the colon was not twisted as it was pulled down. The dilator is removed, the anal sutures and self-retaining retractor are released, the camera and ports are removed, and the ports sites are closed with absorbable sutures.

If performed as a staged procedure, the Duhamel procedure involves closure of the prior staging stoma with placement of a 12-mm trocar through that site. If a primary Duhamel pull-through will be performed, then a 5-mm camera port is placed at the umbilicus, and two 5-mm ports are placed in the right mid and upper abdomen. A 12-mm port is placed in the left upper abdomen. The sigmoid colon is mobilized, with creation of a mesenteric window. The mesentery is divided with cautery down to the peritoneal reflection. A 45-mm articulating stapler is used to divide the distal sigmoid colon at the peritoneal reflection.

The proximal rectum is retracted anteriorly and superiorly, exposing the retrorectal plane. A Kittner dissector is used to develop this plane down to the levators, staying on the posterior midline. An articulating stapler (in the closed position, without a cartridge) is placed through the 12-mm port and aimed into the retrorectal plane (Fig. 39-13A). When the stapler has been passed as distal as possible, it is opened to enlarge the dissection space so that the pull-through section of intestine may be accommodated.

At this point, the surgeon moves to the perineal position while the assistant continues to help from above. A Kittner dissector is place into the retrorectal space and elevated anteriorly, so that it

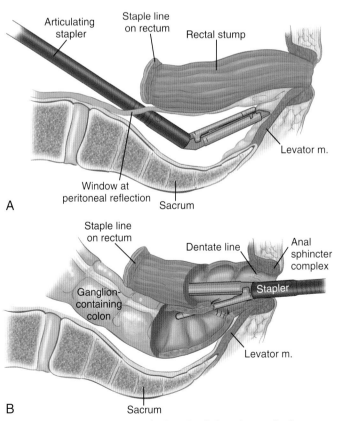

FIGURE 39-13 Hirschsprung disease (Duhamel pull-through procedure). A, Retrorectal dissection with empty stapler. B, Creation of channel between ganglion-containing colon and rectal stump using transanally inserted endostapler.

can be felt with a finger in the anus. The dentate line is exposed as previously described. A posterior rectotomy within 1 cm of the dentate line is performed with cautery, exposing the Kittner dissector. A transanal locking grasper grabs the Kittner, and the Kittner is withdrawn back into the abdomen, bringing the grasper with it (the surgeon's finger may need to occlude the rectotomy to maintain pneumoperitoneum). A Babcock then is used to grasp either the prior stoma or the stapled proximal segment of sigmoid colon and delivers this segment to the transanal grasper. The transanal grasper is withdrawn, exteriorizing the colon through the posterior rectotomy and out the perineum.

After the segment has been pulled through the posterior rectum, serial full-thickness biopsy specimens are taken and sent for frozen section until ganglion cells are identified (if a prior leveling colostomy was performed in which ganglion cells were identified, then no additional biopsy or resection will be needed). Further mobilization may be necessary by individually ligating and dividing mesenteric vessels, which are oriented posteriorly on the pulled-through segment. When ganglion cells are confirmed, the aganglionic segment is resected, and a single-layer, hand-sewn, end-to-side anastomosis is performed with absorbable sutures between the ganglionic colon and the rectal stump.

After the end-to-side anastomosis has been completed, a 45-mm endo-GIA stapler is inserted transanally, with a jaw into each limb of this anastomosis (Fig. 39-13B). The stapler is fired, creating a side-to-side anastomosis with a pouch. Two loads are necessary to make an 8- to 10-cm common wall and pouch. The finished anastomosis is inspected with the laparoscope, and any anterior rectal remnant greater than 1 cm and not incorporated into the anastomosis (i.e., a spur) is excised with an additional stapler load through the 12-mm port. The trocars then are removed, and the sites are closed with absorbable sutures.

Postoperative Considerations

Postoperative care includes 1 to 3 days of NPO, a Foley catheter for 1 to 2 days, and perineal barrier cream to prevent severe diaper rash, especially for the patient who had a colostomy. Pain management with intravenous narcotics is required for 48 hours, or until the patient is tolerating oral intake; in the neonatal population, however, oral acetaminophen may be all that is needed. Perineal wound complications are rare, so a protective stoma is not mandatory.

Before discharge, the parents should be instructed to perform rectal irrigations as needed, but this never should be done within 3 weeks of the operation. If a rectal irrigation is needed for any reason within 2 to 3 weeks of the procedure, then an extensive evaluation for pelvic abscess or leak needs to be undertaken. For the Soave or Swenson procedures, we begin daily rectal dilations with Hagar dilators 2 to 3 weeks after the operation. This is performed for 2 to 3 months to prevent postoperative anastomotic stricture. It is far better to prevent the stricture with simple daily dilation than to treat a stricture that might develop later.

Postoperative enterocolitis occurs in up to 40% of the population with Hirschsprung disease after a pull-through procedure. It may be triggered by a viral gastroenteritis, or it may occur spontaneously. Total colonic Hirschsprung disease is predictive of a higher risk for enterocolitis, but any patient is at risk. Enterocolitis is treated with rectal irrigations and antibiotics. For recurrent enterocolitis, rectal irrigations may be used as prophylaxis. Investigations currently are evaluating the microbiome of the pouch and proximal colon with respect to this complication, and trials of probiotics also are being performed.

Internal anal sphincter achalasia occurs in up to 15% of patients after procedures for Hirschsprung disease. Intermittent Botox injections, sphincterotomies, and myotomies have all been described to treat this problem, which is associated with chronic constipation and enterocolitis. Although the operations described are anatomically "curative," parents of children with Hirschsprung disease need to be counseled that this is a lifelong diagnosis and that patients may experience complications at any age (although such complications decrease in frequency by the teenage years).

XI. UNDESCENDED TESTICLE

Preoperative Considerations

Cryptorchidism results from the lack of normal descent of the testicle following its formation near the kidney to its final resting place in the scrotum. The descent is dependent on endocrine, neural, and mechanical factors. The incidence varies in reported series between 1% and 5% of male births. In 75% to 95% of cases, the undescended testicle is located within the inguinal canal or just outside of the external inguinal ring. This is repaired as a single-stage operation through a groin and scrotal incision. A testicle that is located within the abdomen (or that is nonpalpable) is best approached by laparoscopy, and correction typically is performed as a two-stage operation, that is, a Fowler-Stephen procedure. If the testicle is not palpable within the scrotum by 6 months of age, most experts agree that an orchiopexy is indicated to bring the testicle into the scrotum. Hormonal therapy has not been shown to be effective treatment for the true undescended testicle.

The most critical part of the preoperative evaluation is the physical examination. If the testicle is palpable and can be brought to the bottom of the scrotum, then the child is diagnosed with a retractile testicle, which requires no intervention. If the testicle is either palpable at the external ring or within the inguinal canal, and the child is older than 6 months, then the child should undergo a single-stage orchiopexy through a groin incision. If the testicle is nonpalpable, then the next step in the evaluation should be an ultrasound. If the testicle is identified in the inguinal canal, then a single-stage orchiopexy still can be performed. If the testicle is identified within the internal ring or cannot be found, then the patient should be prepared for a laparoscopic exploration.

Operative Technique

The patient is placed in the supine position. The initial 5-mm camera port is placed at the umbilicus, and two 5-mm working ports are placed in the left and right upper quadrants under direct vision. If a testicle is identified (Fig. 39-14A), then it usually is located immediately next to the internal ring or in the pericolic gutters. If the testicle cannot be found in these locations, then the spermatic cord and testicular vessels should be identified and traced. If only a minuscule testicle is found, then an orchiectomy should be performed by laparoscopy with either cautery or a clip. If a normal-appearing testicle is identified, then the first stage of the operation should be completed.

The testicular vessels are identified and dissected for 1 to 2 cm away from the testicle, and then the vessels are ligated with two 10-mm clips (Fig. 39-14B). The vessels may be divided between the clips or left in continuity. No further dissection or

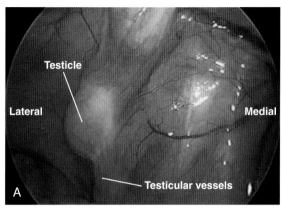

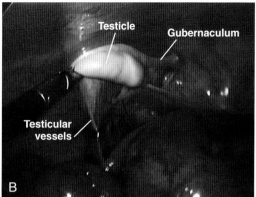

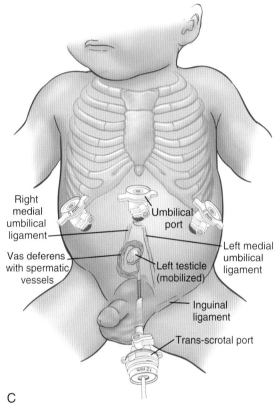

FIGURE 39-14 Undescended testicle. **A,** Laparoscopic appearance. **B,** Clipping of testicular vessels. **C,** Insertion of scrotal trocar to retrieve intra-abdominal testicle during the second stage.

manipulation should be performed. The port sites are closed, and the patient is discharged the same day. In 4 to 6 months, the child should be prepared for the next stage of the operation. The parents should be counseled that in about 5% of patients, the previous ligation of the testicular vessels will result in testicular loss. If the testicle is found to be nonviable, then an orchiectomy will be performed. The parents also should understand that another 5% to 10% of testicles will undergo atrophy after the second-stage operation.

The second-stage operation starts with the port placement at the previous three port sites. The testicle is examined for viability and size. If the testicle is determined to be adequate, then cautery or a tissue sealing device is used to dissect the testicle away from the peritoneal lining, maintaining the pedicle around the spermatic cord. A 1-cm swath of peritoneum is taken around the testicle and the vas deferens to avoid disruption of the testicular revascularization process, which is associated with the vas deferens.

After the testicular mobilization has been completed, a 1-cm transverse incision is made in the base of the scrotum, just lateral to the median raphe on the ipsilateral side. Blunt dissection is carried down to dartos fascia. Sutures (5-0 polypropylene) are placed in the medial and lateral aspects of dartos fascia about 1 cm apart, and the fascia is opened between the two sutures. The abdomen then is reinsufflated to guide the trocar entrance into the abdomen.

A blunt-tipped 12-mm trocar is slowly advanced through the opening in the dartos fascia and is advanced into the abdomen under the guidance of the laparoscope through the floor of the canal, just lateral to the bladder at the medial umbilical remnant (Fig. 39-14C). A blunt grasper is used to grasp the tissue just outside of the testicle, the testicle is brought into the scrotum through the 12-mm trocar, and the trocar is removed. Because there usually is no tension, the testicle should rest easily outside of the dartos fascia. Care must be taken to avoid twisting the spermatic cord in its descent through the trocar.

The testicle is secured with the previously placed polypropylene sutures through the tunica of the testicle. The scrotal skin incision is closed with a chromic suture. The inguinal hernia, which often accompanies an undescended testicle, then can be repaired by a pursestring suture of the peritoneum around the internal ring with a 3-0 Vicryl suture. The ports are removed, and the port sites are closed.

Postoperative Considerations

The patient is dismissed the same day, and the parents are instructed to avoid straddle-type toys for the next 2 weeks, at which time the patient is reexamined for testicular loss. The patient then should be reexamined at 3 months, and yearly thereafter. The major complication of this procedure is testicular loss. The best way to avoid this is to ligate the testicular vessels well away from the testicle during the first stage and then to stay far away from the testicle during the dissection of the second stage. In addition, great care must be taken to avoid any rotation of the spermatic cord during its descent through the trocar into the scrotum.

Greater than 85% testicular survival is expected following the two-stage approach, although it generally is accepted that the growth of the operated testicle most likely will not equal that of its counterpart. Fertility rates are about 80%, and the risk for malignancy is fivefold that of the general population. It is imperative to perform follow-up examinations on a yearly basis, as well as to instruct the patient to perform self-examination when he reaches the early teenage years.

XII. OVARIAN MASSES AND TORSION

Preoperative Considerations

Ovarian disease in children is variable in terms of presentation age, pathology, and management. Most of the pathology is benign, but malignant potential cannot be ignored. During pregnancy, the female fetus undergoes maternal estrogen stimulation, which can lead to ovarian cysts. These cysts generally are small and asymptomatic. Larger cysts can undergo prenatal torsion with ovarian loss. Historically, some experts have recommended intervention based on size, either prenatally or after birth. More current recommendations include a nonoperative approach with intervention only for symptoms, or if there is a diagnostic dilemma. Before 1 year of age, ovarian cancer is almost unheard of, with one case report in the literature, so malignancy is not a factor in determining the need for intervention in this situation. Torsion or a complex mass is not an indication for intervention because this likely occurred in utero, and ovarian salvage is unlikely.

Dermoid cysts, also called teratomas, are the next most common pediatric ovarian pathology. These have a combination of cystic and solid elements and possess at least two germ cell lines. They can be malignant, but most are benign and require simple excision. A dermoid cyst of the ovary often presents with ovarian torsion.

Simple ovarian cysts are common in adolescence. This pathology is part of the differential of abdominal pain in this age group, along with appendicitis. Severe peritoneal signs may be noted with hemorrhagic cysts after rupture. The typical patient presents 2 weeks after her last menstrual cycle (though in an adolescent, the cycles may be irregular). If the diagnosis is confirmed with abdominal imaging, nonoperative management with NSAID administration for pain control is preferred. In the case of a diagnostic dilemma, a laparoscopy is performed. In the setting of a rupture of a simple ovarian cyst, appendectomy at the time of laparoscopy should help prevent future diagnostic confusion.

Adolescence also is the typical age for presentation of ovarian torsion. Such a patient can present with acute onset of symptoms (the patient often can tell you the exact time of symptom onset) localized to either side of the lower abdomen, although two thirds are on the right. Ultrasound is the diagnostic study of choice. Torsion generally occurs in the setting of an abnormal ovary. This may be a simple cyst, a teratoma, or a malignancy. Torsion also can be associated with a long pedicle. The surgeon should maintain an interest in ovarian preservation even in the setting of torsion, if at all possible.

Operative Technique

The child is placed in the supine position. General anesthesia is initiated, and a prophylactic antibiotic is given. The monitor is placed at the foot of the bed. Access is gained through the umbilicus with a 5-mm trocar, and insufflation to 12 mm Hg is initiated. In infants, 3-mm instruments without trocars are used; in adolescents, 5-mm instruments with trocars are used. In general, two additional trocars are placed on either side of the umbilicus.

For an ovarian mass in the infant, a simple cyst may be encountered that requires drainage. This can be done percutaneously with a spinal needle under ultrasound visualization, or laparoscopically. The wall can be biopsied, although malignancy is not a concern. Sometimes a "chocolate cyst" is encountered (Fig. 39-15A), which is an in utero torsion that has become hemorrhagic and filled with brown fluid. This type of cyst often has separated completely from its pedicle and can be free-floating in the abdomen. It may have minimal attachments, which can lead to a bowel obstruction. The cyst can be aspirated and removed through the umbilicus.

Older children who present with an ovarian mass usually have a teratoma (Fig. 39-15B) or other large, predominately cystic mass, but malignancy must be considered. These masses can be the size of a basketball but still can be approached laparoscopically. In this setting, an open umbilical approach for trocar placement is used. Before placement of the trocar, the large mass often is visualized immediately beneath the incision. A pursestring suture then is placed in the exposed wall, and fluid is aspirated in a controlled fashion using a pool sucker.

After most of the fluid has been drained, the pursestring is secured. The 12-mm port is placed at the umbilicus, and two additional 5-mm trocars are placed on opposite sides of the abdomen. The mass and the ovary from which the mass arises are identified. The ovarian pedicle is divided with a vascular stapler. The fallopian tube is either dissected off or divided at the junction of the uterus with a laparoscopic stapler. The teratoma can now be placed in a laparoscopic bag and removed.

Extraction through the umbilical port may not be possible for a larger mass; in such a case, removal may require extension of the umbilical incision or creation of a Pfannenstiel incision. The rest of the abdomen should be examined in case the teratoma is malignant. Pelvic peritoneal studding with glial elements is not uncommon and generally is not considered a sign of malignancy. Ovarian preservation should be considered if normal ovarian tissue can be identified separately from the mass. The ovarian vessels are not divided in this instance. The dissection to excise the teratoma can be performed with a tissue sealing device, staying outside of the wall of the mass (Fig. 39-15C). The ovarian remnant is imbricated after excision of the mass (Fig. 39-15D). Even if only a small portion of the ovary remains, it still has

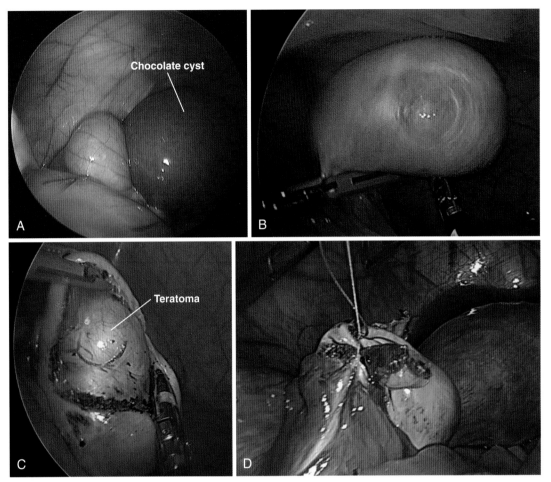

FIGURE 39-15 Ovarian masses and torsion. **A**, Chocolate ovarian cyst. **B**, Ovarian teratoma. **C**, Ovary-preserving resection of an ovarian teratoma. **D**, Imbrication of ovarian remnant after teratoma excision.

potential for function. The opposite ovary should be thoroughly examined, and any lesion should be excised for biopsy. With or without ovarian preservation, the family should be counseled that additional surgery may be necessary after the final pathology is reviewed.

A simple cyst is managed by unroofing and biopsy of the cyst wall. An appendectomy also should be considered to prevent future diagnostic confusion. Hemorrhagic cysts may require cautery for control of bleeding. For torsion without a mass, the ovary should be detorsed and observed for viability. Even if viability is questionable, the affected ovary only should be biopsied and left alone after detorsion. Future ultrasonic studies have demonstrated ovulation in ovaries that had been believed to be nonviable. If the pedicle is long and identified to be the cause of the torsion, then a pexy procedure should be done, attaching the ovary to the pelvic side wall with a polypropylene suture.

Postoperative Considerations

Outcomes in children with benign ovarian pathology are excellent, and complications can be minimized with the previously mentioned precautions taken during the operation. Simple cysts in adolescents are associated with recurrence, and some experts have recommended hormonal therapy in these patients.

Suggested Readings

Ashley RA: Cryptorchidism: Pathogenesis, diagnosis, treatment and prognosis, *Urol Clin North Am* May 37:183–193, 2010.

Bryant AE, Laufer MR: Fetal ovarian cysts, *J Reprod Med* 49:329–337, 2004.

Cass DL, Hawkins E, Brandt ML, et al: Surgery for ovarian masses in infants, children, and adolscents, *J Pediatr Surg* 36:693–699, 2001.

Cilento B, Bauer S, Retik A, et al: Urachal anomalies: Defining the best diagnostic modality, *Urology* 52:120–122, 1998.

Cusick RA, Arkovitz MS: Ovarian cysts in the fetus, infant, and child. In Altcheck A, Deligdisch L, editors: *Pediatric, Adolescent, and Adult Gynecology*, 2009, Wiley Online Library, pp 87–96.

Friedman J, Ahmed S, Connolly B, et al: Complications associated with image-guided gastrostomy and gastrojejunostomy tubes in children, *Pediatrics* 114:458–461, 2004.

Georgeson KE, Fuenfer MM, Hardin WD: Primary laparoscopic pull-through for Hirschsprung's disease in infants and children, *J Pediatric Surg* 30:1017–1022, 1995.

Goldin AB, Sawin R, Seidel KD, et al: Do antireflux operations decrease the rate of reflux-related hospitalization in children? *Pediatrics* 118:2326–2333, 2006.

Johnson JN, Hartman TK, Pianosi PT, Driscoll DJ: Cardiorespiratory function after operation for pectus excavatum, *J Pediatr* 153:359–364, 2008.

Kandalakis JE, Gray SW, Ricketts R, Richardson DD: The small intestines. In *Embryology for Surgeons: The Embryologic Basis for the Treatment of Congenital Anomalies* (2nd ed.), Baltimore, 1994, Williams & Wilkins, pp 214–222.

Kelly RE Jr: Pectus excavatum: Historical background, clinical picture, preoperative evaluation and criteria for operation, *Semin Pediatr Surg* 17:181–193, 2008.

Kelly RE Jr, Cash TF, Shamberger RC, et al: Surgical repair of pectus excavatum markedly improves body image and perceived ability for physical activity: Multicenter study, *Pediatrics* 122:1218–1222, 2008.

Kokoska ER, Keller MS, Weber TR: Acute ovarian torsion in children, *Am J Surg* 180:462–465, 2000.

Langer JC, Minkes RK, Mazziotti MV, et al: Transanal one-stage Soave procedure for infants with Hirschsprung's disease, *J Pediatr Surg* 34:142–158, 1999.

Michel JL, Revillon P, Montupet P, et al: Thoracoscopic treatment of mediastinal cysts in children, *J Pediatr Surg* 33:1745–1748, 1998.

Nuss D: Minimally invasive surgical repair of pectus excavatum, *Semin Pediatr Surg* 17:209–227, 2008.

Panteli C: New insights in the pathogenesis of infantile pyloric stenosis, *Pediatr Surg Int* 25:1043–1052, 2009.

Ponsky T, Lukish J: Single site laparoscopic gastrostomy with a 4-mm bronchoscopic optical grasper, *J Pediatr Surg* 43:412–414, 2008.

Rothenberg S, Chang J, Bealer J: Experience with minimally invasive surgery in infants, *Am J Surg* 176:654–658, 1998.

Smeith BM, Steiner RB, Lobe TE: Laparoscopic Duhamel pullthrough procedure for Hirschsprung's disease in children, *J Laparoendo Surg* 4:273–276, 1994.

Snyder ME, Luck SR, Hernandez R, et al: Diagnostic dilemmas of mediastinal cysts, *J Pediatr Surg* 20:810–815, 1985.

St. Peter SD, Barnhart DC, Ostlie DJ, et al: Minimal vs extensive esophageal mobilization during laparoscopic fundoplication: A prospective randomized trial, *J Pediatr Surg* 46:163–168, 2011.

St. Peter SD, Holcomb GW, Calkins CM, et al: Open versus laparoscopic pyloromyotomy for pyloric stenosis: A prospective randomized trial, *Ann Surg* 244:363–370, 2006.

St-Vil D, Brandt ML, Panic S, et al: Meckel's diverticulum in children: A 20-year review, *J Pediatr Surg* 26:1289–1292, 1991.

Tovar JA, Luis AL, Encinas JL, et al: Pediatric surgeons and gastroesophageal reflux, *J Pediatr Surg* 42:277–283, 2007.

Valusek PA, St Peter SD, Keckler SJ, et al: Does an upper gastrointestinal study change operative management for gastroesophageal reflux? *J Pediatr Surg* 45:1169–1172, 2010.

Vane DW, Kest KW, Grosfeld JL: Vitelline duct anomalies: Experience with 217 childhood cases, *Arch Surg* 122:542–547, 1987.

Wright CD: Mediastinal tumors and cysts in the pediatric population, *Thorac Surg Clin* 19:47–61, 2009.

Zani A, Eaton S, Rees C, Pierro A: Incidentally detected Meckel diverticulum: To resect or not to resect? *Ann Surg* 247:276–281, 2008.

Zenn MR, Redo SF: Infantile hypertrophic pyloric stenosis, *J Pediatr Surg* 28:1577, 1993.

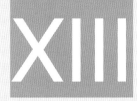

General Topics

MARK A. CARLSON

Complications of First Entry into the Peritoneal Cavity

40

For laparoscopic procedures on the abdomen, initial entry usually entails gaining access to the peritoneal cavity so that carbon dioxide can be insufflated. This initial entry into the operative space is a necessary but potentially risky maneuver in minimally invasive surgery. In the normal state, the peritoneal cavity is a potential space, so successful insertion of an insufflation device necessitates insinuation of the device between contiguous organs and structures without causing injury. Depending on the type of procedure, first entry complications can account for up to 40% to 50% of all complications associated with minimally invasive surgery and up to half of the fatalities[1,2] and can produce a serious medicolegal problem.[1,3-7] A variety of techniques have been developed to obtain initial access into the peritoneal cavity, all of which have been associated with well-described complications. This chapter describes the basic devices and techniques available for peritoneal first entry, reviews the safety record of the common techniques, outlines the management of complications associated with these techniques, and describes the general operative steps in the performance of these techniques. Trocar-related issues that will not be covered in this chapter include port-site hernia, port-site metastasis, injuries related to insertion of secondary trocars, and complications of access for extraperitoneal or retroperitoneal procedures.

DISCLAIMER

It would be difficult to discuss techniques and complications of peritoneal access without referring to specific devices used to gain entry to the peritoneal cavity. So, although specific devices and manufacturers are named in this chapter, such references should be not construed as either endorsement or condemnation, neither explicit nor implicit, of a specific device. I do not have any conflicts of interest to claim; specifically, I do not have any financial interests with the manufacturers of the devices described in this chapter.

LEVEL OF EVIDENCE FOR RECOMMENDATIONS

Unless otherwise stated, recommendations made in this chapter are based on data from uncontrolled clinical series and poorly designed trials. The strength of this type of recommendation, sometimes known as the recommendation's grade or level of evidence, has been described by various authorities as "suggestive" (Agency for Healthcare Research and Quality [AHRQ]),[8] "low" (AHRQ Evidence-Based Practice Center),[9] "level C" (U.S. Preventive Services Task Force),[10] or "grade C" (Oxford Centre for Evidence-Based Medicine).[11]

CURRENT DEVICES IN USE FOR FIRST ENTRY INTO THE PERITONEAL CAVITY

Peritoneal access techniques may be organized into three basic categories: (1) pneumoperitoneum needle insertion; (2) open laparoscopy (Hasson technique); and (3) direct (optical) trocar insertion. Variants of each technique have been described in the surgical literature, and other techniques may exist that have not been published. The profusion of peritoneal access techniques and devices, along with the lack of adequate controlled data, indicates that the best technique or device (in terms of efficacy, safety, ease, and cost) is really not known. In this section, a description of each common device is provided; a review of technique and device safety is given later in the chapter.

Pneumoperitoneum Needle

The pneumoperitoneum needle in general use today originally was described in 1938 by János Veress in Kapuvár, Hungary, as a device to induce pneumothorax.[12] The technique of peritoneoscopy (or celioscopy, or laparoscopy) already had been developed in the early 1900s. The method to gain initial access to the peritoneal cavity back then typically involved (1) direct insertion of a conventional needle to insufflate air into the peritoneal cavity or (2) a surgical cutdown to the peritoneum, with insertion of a needle under direct vision.[13] Subsequent use of laparoscopy with the Veress needle slowly increased during the 20th century, and by the 1970s, the procedure was commonly used by gynecologists (and some gastroenterologists) for diagnosis, tubal ligations, and other minor procedures. At this point, the Veress needle was a common, if not the most common, technique of initial peritoneal access.

The design of the modern Veress needle (Figs. 40-1 and 40-2A) is similar to the original description,[12] consisting of an approximately 2-mm hollow needle containing a spring-loaded

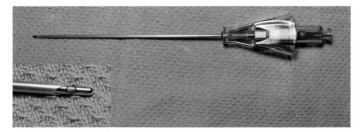

FIGURE 40-1 Pneumoperitoneum (Veress) needle, with tip shown in the inset. Needle is 14 gauge (outer diameter about 2.1 mm).

obturator. The obturator retracts when the needle tip is applied to relatively immobile tissue, permitting the needle to cut a path. After the needle has passed through the immobile tissue and resistance decreases (e.g., the tip enters the peritoneal cavity), the obturator springs back into position, protecting the needle tip. After insertion into the abdomen, gas is insufflated through the needle-obturator assembly, typically through a Luer-Lok connection. In the mid-1990s, there was an effort to produce an "optical" Veress needle,[14] which contained a small-diameter fiberoptic system that could visualize insertion, similar to how current optical trocars function (see later). The optical quality of the Veress "needlescope," however, was limited compared with that of 5- or 10-mm endoscopes. There have only been a few publications with the optical Veress system since its introduction.

A related device that employs the Veress needle is the *radially expanding trocar system* (see Fig. 40-2). Developed in the mid-1990s,[15,16] this multicomponent device consists of a needle-sheath assembly (see Fig. 40-2A and B) and a dilator-cannula assembly (see Fig. 40-2C). The needle-sheath assembly is inserted into the peritoneal cavity as a conventional pneumoperitoneum needle would be (see full description given later), and the abdomen is insufflated. The needle is withdrawn, leaving the sheath in place, and the dilator-cannula assembly then is inserted through the sheath. The sheath is an expandable polymer and accommodates the dilator-cannula as it is inserted (see Fig. 40-2D). After insertion, the dilator component is withdrawn (see Fig. 40-2E), leaving the 12-mm cannula (still within the sheath) for laparoscopic instrumentation. This placement method is somewhat reminiscent of the Seldinger technique used for central venous lines or enterostomy tubes. The purported advantages of a radially expandable system include less abdominal wall trauma (including a smaller fascial incision) compared with nondilating trocar systems, and the lack of need for suture of the fascial defect incurred by the device. Small randomized trials comparing the radially expanding trocar to nonexpanding trocars have shown advantages of the former, but these studies used the Veress needle for initial access in all patients.[17,18]

Open Laparoscopy

Associated with the widespread use of the Veress needle in laparoscopic surgery were rare but potentially devastating bowel and vascular injuries (see Safety Review of Techniques Used to Access the Peritoneal Cavity). These injuries occurred both with the insertion of the pneumoperitoneum needle and with subsequent insertion of the primary trocar—both of these maneuvers, of course, are performed blindly. In an attempt to circumvent this problem, Harrith Hasson, a gynecologist at the Grant Hospital in Chicago, introduced a blunt trocar device in 1971.[19,20] Today, versions of this blunt trocar are generically known as the *Hasson*

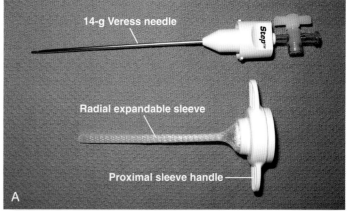

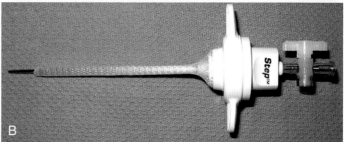

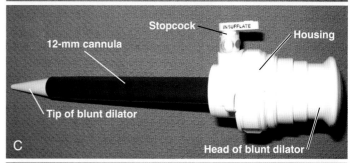

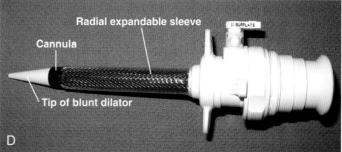

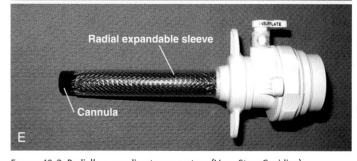

FIGURE 40-2 Radially expanding trocar system (VersaStep, Covidien). **A,** Pneumoperitoneum needle and expandable sleeve, separated. **B,** Needle inserted into sleeve. **C,** Dilator and cannula assembly. **D,** Dilator and cannula inserted into sleeve. **E,** Cannula within sleeve (final in vivo configuration).

cannula (Fig. 40-3), which consists of a blunt obturator sheathed within a cannula. This device typically is inserted into the peritoneal cavity under direct vision with a cutdown at the umbilicus (i.e., a minilaparotomy). The cannula has a cone-shaped plug that helps form a seal against the fascial incision; the cannula is held

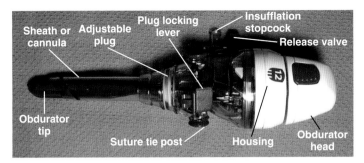

FIGURE 40-3 Blunt trocar (Hasson type) for open laparoscopy. Cannula diameter = 12 mm.

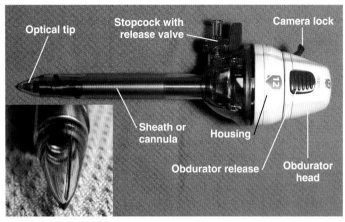

FIGURE 40-4 Optical trocar, with tip shown in the inset (Endopath Xcel, Ethicon Endosurgery). Cannula diameter = 12 mm.

against the abdominal wall with stay sutures that are wrapped around the suture tie posts. The technique of Hasson cannula insertion also is known as *open laparoscopy* (Veress needle access subsequently became known as *closed laparoscopy*). The purported benefits of open laparoscopy include the prevention of vascular injury, gas embolism, and extraperitoneal insufflation and the ability to enter an area with adhesions.

Optical Trocar

Background

In addition to the peritoneal access methods of Veress needle insertion and open laparoscopy, direct trocar insertion without prior pneumoperitoneum was described in 1978 by James Dingfelder, a gynecologist at the University of North Carolina[21]; further descriptions of direct insertion appeared in the gynecologic literature during the 1980s.[22-24] Dingfelder's rationale for direct trocar insertion (as opposed to Veress needle insertion) was to avoid potentially fatal complications of Veress needle misadventures.[21] In addition, he noted that the historical assumption that pneumoperitoneum absolutely had to be established before trocar insertion did not have supporting evidence. As originally described, direct trocar insertion was a blind access procedure; the ports of the 1970s and 1980s did not have optical capabilities. Similar to Veress needle insertion, the success of direct trocar insertion was dependent on a sharp instrument and the skill of the surgeon. Limited controlled data did not find a difference in safety between the Veress needle and direct trocar insertion techniques.[25,26] For all practical purposes, however, nonoptical direct trocar insertion was rendered obsolete by the advent of optical trocar technology in the 1990s.

In 1993, Steven Kaali, a gynecologist in Dobbs Ferry, New York, described an "Opti-Trocar,"[27] which consisted of a conventional trocar with a transparent cutting tip and a pistol-grip handle. With an endoscope housed within the trocar as it was inserted, the surgeon could view the process of abdominal wall penetration in real time. Kaali did not perform direct insertion with this device, but rather established pneumoperitoneum first with a Veress needle. Also in 1993, Andreas Melzer's group in the Department of Surgery at the University of Tübingen, together with the Olympus company, described an "optical scalpel," a trocar with an externally controlled cutting tip that accommodated an endoscope.[28] This device also permitted visual monitoring of transabdominal penetration. Around the same time, a port with a clear conical tip was developed by Riek and colleagues, also at the University of Tübingen[29]; this was the forerunner of Ethicon's Xcel trocar. In addition, U.S. Surgical developed the Visiport device during the early 1990s.[30] Since the late 1990s, a

number of series have been published supporting the safety and efficacy of the optical trocar.[31-36]

Endopath Xcel

The Endopath Xcel Bladeless Trocar (Ethicon Endo-Surgery, Cincinnati, Ohio) (Fig. 40-4) has an obturator with a transparent conical plastic tip, which has an edge that is sharp enough to induce tissue separation during insertion. An endoscope is inserted through the obturator head, allowing the surgeon to monitor insertion progress in real time. This trocar comes in a range of diameters between 5 and 15 mm (and bariatric lengths) and may be used for direct insertion with a 5- or 10-mm laparoscope. The precise definitions of *bladed* and *bladeless* with this trocar are somewhat overlapping because, if enough pressure is used, the plastic conical tip of the Xcel can cut through tissue.

Visiport Plus

The Visiport Plus Optical Trocar (Fig. 40-5) (Covidien, Norwalk, Conn.) consists of a conventional 10-mm cannula through which a pistol-shaped obturator (see Fig. 40-5B) is inserted. The obturator has a clear blunt tip that houses an actuated knife blade (see Fig. 40-5C). With each depression of the device trigger, the knife blade is fired out 1 mm and quickly retracts; the actual motion of the blade cannot be detected with the unaided eye. With the laparoscope inserted through the obturator and the obturator within the tissue of the abdominal wall, the surgeon fires the blade and watches the progress of the tip penetration on the video screen. Of note, the Visiport's product insert strongly recommends that pneumoperitoneum be established before entering the peritoneal cavity with this device; that is, the manufacturer does not recommend that the Visiport be used as a direct insertion device. Of the four optical ports described in this section, the Visiport is the only one that is "bladed."

Kii Fios First Entry

Applied Medical (Rancho Santa Margarita, Calif.) released the Kii Fios First Entry System (Fig. 40-6) in 2008. This is an optical trocar intended for direct insertion without prior pneumoperitoneum. The concept is similar to the Ethicon Xcel trocar, except the Applied Medical device has a port in the distal tip (see Fig. 40-6B and C), which allows relatively rapid insufflation of the peritoneal cavity with just minimal tip penetration (about 3 mm) into the peritoneal cavity. Per the company's website (www.appliedmedical.com), the Kii Fios First Entry device is the

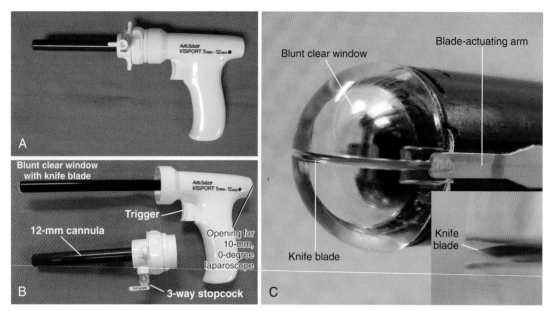

FIGURE 40-5 Optical trocar system with actuated blade (Visiport Plus RPF system, Covidien). **A,** Assembled system. **B,** Blade-containing optical obturator ("gun") and 12-mm cannula, separated. **C,** Close-up of clear window tip, showing recessed blade. *Inset:* lateral view.

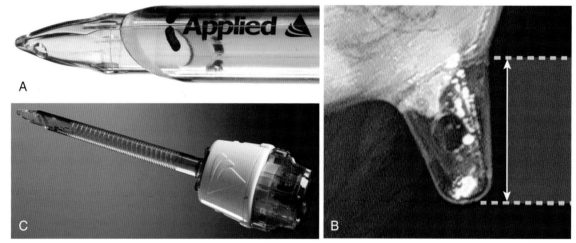

FIGURE 40-6 Optical trocar with insufflation tip (Fios First Entry, Applied Medical). **A,** Close-up of trocar tip. **B,** Intraoperative view of tip entering the peritoneal cavity; distance indicated by *double-headed white arrow* = 3 mm. **C,** Assembled trocar. (Images Courtesy of Applied Medical Resources Corporation. All rights reserved.)

only device with U.S. Food and Drug Administration 510(k) documentation for first entry use. This device comes in 5- to 12-mm diameters, with bariatric lengths.

Genicon Bladeless Tip Trocar

The Genicon (Winter Park, Fla.) Bladeless Visual Tip Trocar and Cannula System (Fig. 40-7) was released in 2005. This system consists of an obturator with a transparent conical tip mounted to a pistol-grip; the obturator assembly is inserted through a cannula (available in 5- to 15-mm diameters, with bariatric lengths). The plastic optical tip permits dissection through tissue under direct endoscope visualization, similar to the Ethicon Xcel and the Applied Medical Fios devices mentioned earlier.

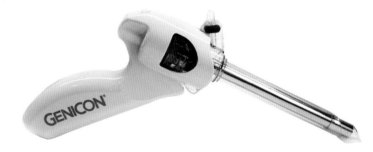

FIGURE 40-7 Genicon Bladeless Tip Trocar System. (Image courtesy of Genicon Corporation.)

Karl Storz EndoTIP

The Karl Storz (Tuttlingen, Germany) Ternamian EndoTIP trocar (*Endo*scopic *T*hreaded *I*maging *P*ort; Fig. 40-8) is an optical device that is designed to be screwed into the abdomen.[37] The purported advantage to this device is that less axial force is needed during insertion compared with nonthreaded ports. This device is not intended for primary insertion before pneumoperitoneum, but rather for insertion after pneumoperitoneum has been established (or for secondary insertion after a laparoscope has been positioned).[38] The description of the EndoTIP is included here for completion.

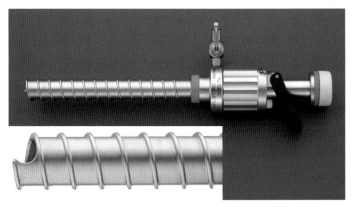

FIGURE 40-8 Ternamian EndoTIP (Endoscopic Threaded Imaging Port, Karl Storz). *Inset:* Close-up of threaded cannula (© 2012 Photo Courtesy of Karl Storz Endoscopy-America, Sugar Land, Tex.).

SAFETY REVIEW OF TECHNIQUES USED TO ACCESS THE PERITONEAL CAVITY

The main complication risks of first entry into the peritoneal cavity during laparoscopy have been injury to (1) major vascular structures (aorta, cava, and iliac vessels) and (2) hollow viscera. Abdominal wall injury and extraperitoneal insufflation also have been of concern, but the consequences of these events generally are less severe than vascular or visceral injury. Gas embolism, although potentially fatal, has been quite rare. The available safety data predominantly derive from pneumoperitoneum needle insertion (closed laparoscopy) and blunt cannula insertion (open laparoscopy); both of these techniques have been in use for decades. In comparison, there are much fewer data available on first entry complications secondary to the more recent technique and devices of optical trocar insertion.

Search Strategy

The following terms were searched using Google Scholar (http://scholar.google.com): *pneumoperitoneum complications, laparoscopy complications, trocar injury, trocar insertion, closed laparoscopy, open laparoscopy, laparoscopic access,* and *laparoscopic entry.* In addition, specific device names (e.g., Xcel, Visiport, optical trocar, VersaStep, Veress, Hasson, radially expanding trocar) were searched. The first 300 results (hits) of each term were reviewed, and the full-text version of each relevant article was retrieved. In addition, bibliographies of major articles were reviewed for further relevant material. Many more articles were identified with the above search strategy than were actually referred to in this chapter. Most of the nonreferenced articles were comparatively small (<500 cases) studies on peritoneal access, either as the primary issue or as component of a general series. For the most part, the data on these smaller studies already have been cataloged and analyzed in one or more systematic reviews; such an exercise was not repeated for this chapter. Instead, the data as collected by these reviews have been summarized here.

Major (Retroperitoneal) Vascular Injury

Vascular injury during insertion of the Veress needle, particularly in the infraumbilical position as is commonly done for gynecologic procedures, has long been known to have a small risk for injury to major vascular structures. Three fourths of these

Table 40-1 Incidence of Major Vascular Injury Associated with First Entry in Laparoscopic Surgery, as Obtained from Systematic Reviews, Large Series, or Surveys

Study	Technique	Injury Rate (%)	No. of Patients
Mintz, 1977[94]	Closed	0.02	99,204
Bergqvist & Bergqvist, 1987[95]	Closed	0.007	75,035
Querleu et al., 1993[96]	Closed	0.02	17,521
Bonjer et al., 1997[58]	Closed	0.075	489,335
Chapron et al., 1998[97]	Closed	0.02	29,966
Harkki-Siren, 1999[98]	Closed	0.01	102,812
Molloy et al., 2002[41]	Closed	0.04	132,851
Jansen et al., 2004[71]	Closed	0.05	52,138
Larobina & Nottle, 2005[99]	Closed	0.044	760,890
Azevedo et al., 2009[72]	Closed	0.014	696,502
Penfield, 1985[100]	Open	0	10,840
Bonjer et al., 1997[58]	Open	0	12,444
Molloy et al., 2002[41]	Open	0	21,292
Larobina & Nottle, 2005[99]	Open	0	22,465
Molloy et al., 2002[41]	Direct	0	16,739

Closed = pneumoperitoneum needle; open = blunt (Hasson) cannula; direct = nonoptical direct insertion of primary trocar without prior pneumoperitoneum.

injuries are arterial, and of these, the aorta is the most common site.[39] In fact, this risk for vascular injury was one of the driving factors for development of the blunt (Hasson) cannula for open laparoscopy.[40] The rates of major vascular injury for various insertion methods, as described in large systematic reviews, are shown in Table 40-1. Essentially, use of the Veress needle can be expected to result in a major vascular injury in one of every 2000 to 10,000 patients. Not surprisingly, the rate of vascular injury secondary to the pneumoperitoneum needle has been higher in controlled studies compared with retrospective studies (1.8 vs. 0.3 per 1000), suggesting that there may be some underreporting of these injuries in retrospective studies.[41]

The Table 40-1 data, as mentioned earlier, largely are derived from the infraumbilical insertion technique. It is suspected, but not yet know with surety, that Veress needle insertion in the left upper abdomen (e.g., at the Palmer point[42]; Fig. 40-9) will reduce the incidence of vascular injury secondary to this instrument.[43,44] In contrast, use of open laparoscopy with the infraumbilical approach all but eliminates the risk for vascular injury. A 2008 Cochrane review calculated a statistically higher incidence of vascular injuries associated with closed laparoscopy compared with open laparoscopy.[41] There have been some case reports of vascular injury with open laparoscopy,[45-47] but these have been secondary to gross technical error (e.g., nicking the aorta with the scalpel during the skin incision) or defective equipment.

In a review of 502 vascular injuries associated with the closed laparoscopy,[2] 46% of the injuries were secondary to the Veress needle itself, and 54% were secondary to the subsequent insertion of the primary trocar (also a blind maneuver). Of course, being confident of which instrument caused an injury when both are inserted blindly may not seem reasonable, but it probably is safe to say that Veress needle injuries actually represent a mix of both needle and primary trocar injuries. With respect to optical trocar insertion, the true incidence of vascular injury[48] is difficult to know because the recorded patient numbers are not as high as

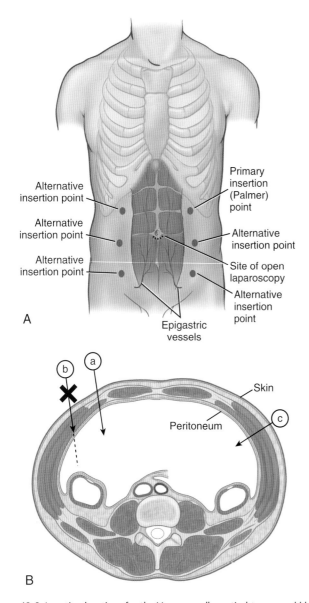

FIGURE 40-9 Insertion locations for the Veress needle, optical trocar, and blunt (Hasson) trocar. Approximate location of epigastric vessels shown. **A** and **B,** Angle of insertion for lateral entry points; transverse plane. *a,* Appropriate angle for device inserted at Palmer point. *b* and *c,* Inappropriate *(b)* and appropriate *(c)* angles, respectively, for a device inserted lateral to Palmer point.

with closed and open laparoscopy. In addition, the optical trocar safety data are somewhat diluted because systematic reviews may include data from studies that used the older technique of direct (nonoptical) insertion.[41,49]

The mortality related to a major vascular injury incurred during first entry into the peritoneal cavity has not been high; in the 2008 Cochrane review on peritoneal access, five deaths were noted, all associated with use of the Veress needle, but none of these was secondary to vascular injury. Major cardiovascular collapse during Veress needle insertion may be secondary to gas embolism and should not be attributed immediately to hemorrhage. In addition, the pattern of delayed mortality from an unrecognized bowel injury does not appear to have an analog in major vascular injury; for instance, delayed rupture of a traumatic pseudoaneurysm is exceedingly rare.[50,51] Most (90%) major vascular injuries incurred during initial access are recognized at the index operation.[41,52,53] The patient who does develop a pseudoaneurysm after laparoscopy usually has a history of Veress needle

access; presentation can occur weeks to months later with pain and gastrointestinal bleeding.[54]

Intestinal Injury

Historically, nearly half of bowel injuries associated with laparoscopic procedures were incurred during peritoneal access.[55] With an increasing number of complex and reoperative abdominal procedures being performed in minimally invasive surgery, the proportion of bowel injuries secondary to access likely will decline. The absolute rates of bowel injury associated with various entry techniques is shown in Table 40-2. Unlike the situation with vascular injury, both closed and open laparoscopy have a defined incidence of bowel injury; some believe that the open (Hasson) technique may have a higher risk for this injury.[41,56] The incidence of bowel injury associated with optical trocar insertion is in the range of 0.05%, although there are fewer data. Essentially, use of any of these techniques can be expected to result in an intestinal injury in 1 of every 1000 to 2000 patients. Importantly, however, intestinal injury associated with Hasson insertion is recognized more frequently than with Veress needle insertion, which can reduce morbidity and mortality secondary to injury from the former device.[57]

Intestinal injury incurred during peritoneal access is more common in general surgical than in gynecologic patients (1.5 vs. 0.4 per 1000)[41]; the reason is not immediately obvious but may be secondary to an increased prevalence of prior abdominal procedures in general surgical patients. In a series of 430 previously published bowel perforations (not all associated with the initial entry),[55] the small intestine was the most common site of injury (56%), followed by the colon (39%). With respect to intestinal injury associated with the pneumoperitoneum needle, most (about 90%) perforations have been presumed to be caused by the blind insertion of the primary trocar, and not the needle per se.[41] Comparing these data to vascular injury, a greater percentage of intestinal injuries has been attributed to insertion of the primary trocar, rather than the Veress needle itself.

The mortality rate of entry-related intestinal injury can range up to 3% to 5%,[55,57] or about 1 mortality for every 20 bowel perforations. Most of these deaths are the result of a missed (i.e., undiagnosed at the index procedure) injury that produces delayed intra-abdominal sepsis.[4] A review by one group found that only one third of intestinal injuries associated with minimally invasive procedures, whether incurred during the access phase or operative phase, were diagnosed during the operation[57]; a review by another group found that bowel injury was diagnosed at operation or within 24 hours in two thirds of the cases.[55] In the 2008 Cochrane review of peritoneal access,[49] two of the five deaths reported were secondary to unrecognized intestinal injury, both from the Veress needle technique.

Gas Embolism

Gas (CO_2) embolism during first entry into the peritoneal cavity has been a complication primarily of the Veress needle, presumably from insertion and insufflation into a major venous structure. There have been no reported cases of gas embolism incurred during access with open laparoscopy.[39] Of course, gas embolism may occur (rarely) during the course of most laparoscopic procedures, possibly through the lumen of a vein that was opened during the course of the dissection. Intravascular insufflation associated with insertion of a Hasson cannula, however, does not appear to be possible. The incidence of gas embolism (also known as *intravascular insufflation*) associated with insertion of the pneumoperitoneum needle in a systemic review of nearly 500,000 closed laparoscopies[58] was 0.0014% (7 cases), or about 1 in every 70,000 cases. The mortality rate in these 7 cases was 100%. In contrast, the mortality rate from gas embolism in a separate case series was only about one third (2 of 7 cases).[59]

Other Injuries

Although vascular and visceral injury remain the most studied and discussed complications associated with first entry into the peritoneal cavity, other less severe injuries can occur, such as abdominal wall hematoma (trocar site bleeding) and extraperitoneal insufflation (not intravascular). The precise incidence of trocar site bleeding is difficult to specify (which may be due in part to underreporting of minor complications) but has been estimated to be 0.2% to 2% of laparoscopic procedures.[60]

Abdominal wall hematoma primarily is incurred at lateral insertion sites (see Fig. 40-9); laceration of the epigastric vessels is a common cause. Computed tomography mapping of the epigastrics demonstrated that they run in a region 4 to 8 cm lateral to the midline.[61] A hematoma generally should not occur with device insertion at the umbilicus, unless the operator veers off the midline. With respect to prevention of abdominal wall hematoma, there may be an advantage with the use of radially

expanding access devices (see Fig. 40-2), which were associated with fewer episodes of trocar bleeding in a Cochrane review compared with nondilating trocars.[49]

Extraperitoneal insufflation can occur during the course of most laparoscopic procedures, but that associated with first entry devices appears to be more common with the use of the Veress needle.[49] The incidence of extraperitoneal insufflation, similar to abdominal wall hematoma, has been difficult to know, presumably because of underreporting.

Failed Entry

Failure to gain access to the peritoneal cavity is another complication of initial entry, but one that usually is not associated with a clinically important injury. The incidence of failed entry also has been difficult to establish. Part of this problem may be secondary to the definition of failure, which in any given patient might be defined as failure at the first attempt to gain access with success on a subsequent attempt, to complete inability to gain access after multiple attempts, with abandonment of the technique and migration to an alternative operative plan. Underreporting also is likely to be an issue in determining the incidence of access failure because this complication in isolation can be perceived as a purely technical failure with minor impact on patient outcome; accordingly, some surgeons may not see any relevance in reporting failed entry. Nevertheless, the 2008 Cochrane review of peritoneal access methods concluded that direct trocar insertion was associated with a decreased rate of access failure compared with the Veress needle insertion.[49]

Overall Mortality Risk

The overall mortality secondary to first entry into the peritoneal cavity was at least 1 in 100,000 laparoscopic procedures in a review of 850,350 previously published cases.[41] For the deaths in which the entry technique was specified ($n = 5$), the Veress needle was used in all cases. Unfortunately, the entry technique was specified in only 20% of the 850,350 cases; there were 5 additional deaths related to initial entry in the nonspecified group (679,847 cases).

Summary of Safety Review: Which Technique Is the Safest?

It has been difficult to demonstrate the safety superiority of one access technique over others because of a lack of adequate controlled data in this area. Although randomized controlled trials have been published on first access methods, these trials have not been sufficiently powered to permit well-grounded conclusions.[49] This lack of controlled data, however, has not deterred some authors from making strong recommendations regarding the use of one peritoneal access method over another. Some authors have advocated the use of open laparoscopy[58,62-64] or optical trocar insertion[35,36] instead of closed laparoscopy because either of the former was safer in their data analysis. Optical trocar insertion initially was thought to be the solution for a lowered-risk entry, but legal databases have revealed numerous injuries from use of these devices (although without the ability to calculate an incidence).[3,5] Most authors have been cautious about issuing any statement about the superiority of any one technique, or have stated that there is no consensus on the best technique for first entry into the peritoneal cavity.[41,49,56,65-71]

One systematic review found that the risk for major injury tended to be higher with open laparoscopy compared with closed laparoscopy; but when the authors removed retrospective data from their analysis, this difference disappeared.[56] The authors suggested that the apparent increase in morbidity with open laparoscopy in the retrospective studies may have been a selection phenomenon, in which a higher-risk patient (e.g., previous operation) would be accessed with open laparoscopy. They then commented that open laparoscopy might be safer than closed laparoscopy in unselected patients.[56]

Similar to other areas of surgery, operator-related factors and patient volume likely play a role in the safety and efficacy of peritoneal access. For example, in Dr. Hasson's own series of 5284 open laparoscopies, there were 21 minor wound infections, 4 minor hematomas, 1 umbilical hernia requiring operation, 1 bowel injury (repaired immediately), no major vascular injuries, and no access failures.[40] This safety record is about as good as can be obtained, but its duplication by other surgeons is not assured. In addition, technical details such as point of device insertion may be seen to play a critical role in the complication rate. In many, if not most, of the data describing open and closed laparoscopy, the point of insertion was at the umbilicus. As implied earlier, the safety profile data of access devices may be different (i.e., better) if the Palmer point[42] (see Fig. 40-9) is routinely used for first entry into the peritoneal cavity.[41]

Management of complications associated with first entry into the peritoneal cavity

Vascular Injury

Management of major retroperitoneal vascular injury incurred during first entry into the peritoneal cavity invariably has been treated with open conversion and conventional vascular repair.[2,53,72] The findings in one of these injuries can vary from a retroperitoneal hematoma to life-threatening free bleeding into the abdomen.[2,53,73-75] Free bleeding from a retroperitoneal vessel into the abdomen may be less likely from a needle injury compared with a trocar injury. Minor bleeding from the omentum or mesentery incurred during first entry may be managed laparoscopically with a sealing device. As mentioned earlier, however, the conservative approach to repair of a major retroperitoneal vascular injury necessitates open conversion and standard vascular repair with proximal and distal control. It also would be prudent to obtain emergency consultation with a vascular surgeon, if one is available. Delayed formation of a pseudoaneurysm also has been described[54]; these cases are managed with vascular surgical consultation.

Intestinal Injury

In the 1990s and 2000s, the management of bowel injury during laparoscopy, whether incurred during first entry or later on, was mostly done with open conversion (about 80% of injuries).[55,72] With better understanding of these injuries and improved instrumentation, however, the management of these injuries can be individualized. For example, a small injury (e.g., Veress needle) to the small intestine that is recognized immediately may be repaired with an imbricating serosal stitch, placed laparoscopically, and the operation may proceed as planned. On the other end of the spectrum, a colon perforation not recognized at the time of injury may require a laparotomy with a possible resection and possible diversion if the patient develops peritonitis and sepsis. Between these two extremes is a spectrum of bowel injury, with varying mechanism (needle vs. trocar), location (small intestine vs. colon; intraperitoneal vs. retroperitoneal), size, associated injury, intestinal spillage, and so forth.

If an intestinal injury is recognized immediately, then repair should be performed immediately. If the injury cannot be sutured with intracorporeal technique, then it may be possible to perform a minilaparotomy directly over the injury, exteriorize the bowel, and repair or resect the involved area. The minilaparotomy then can be closed, and the minimally invasive procedure can be resumed. If the injury is located in a retroperitoneal location (e.g., the posterior right or left colon) or is otherwise difficult to expose laparoscopically, then some sort of conversion (minilaparotomy or otherwise) may be prudent. With promptness and care, a bowel injury that is recognized immediately can be closed before major peritoneal soilage. After repair of an intestinal injury, the surgeon may consider irrigating the abdomen thoroughly with saline, although the utility of such irrigation is difficult to prove.

Mortality from bowel injury incurred during a minimally invasive procedure usually is the result of a missed diagnosis. The patient's symptoms in such a case may include fever, pain, distension, ileus, diarrhea, and leukocytosis; unfortunately, however, the patient's course may be notable for the complete absence of symptoms until right before a rapid and terminal decompensation.[57] The delay in the onset of symptoms after an unrecognized bowel injury can range from several days to several weeks.[55] A typical scenario for missed bowel injury would be a patient who has persistent ileus, persistent pain, or otherwise has a slow recovery after a laparoscopic procedure. The clinicians obtain a computed tomography scan, which shows some nonspecific findings but may show free intraperitoneal air or free fluid. Although either of these findings can be normal after a minimally invasive procedure, they should be viewed as highly suspicious in a patient who is not progressing as expected.

Management of a bowel injury diagnosed in the postoperative period also should be tailored to the patient's clinical status. An intra-abdominal abscess in an otherwise stable patient can be drained by an interventional radiologist. With drainage and appropriate medical care, such an injury should heal with major surgical intervention. Reoperation on a stable patient with an inadequately controlled leak may be attempted laparoscopically in select cases, particularly if the location of the leak is known before the reoperation. If the patient is unstable or otherwise has an injury not amenable to laparoscopic repair, then conventional laparotomy, débridement, repair, and drainage are indicated.

An interesting situation may arise if a bowel injury is incurred during a case in which implantation of a nonresorbable prosthetic mesh is planned, such as during a minimally invasive ventral incisional hernia repair. There typically is an elevated risk for bowel injury during such a case (whether during first entry or the subsequent adhesiolysis) because the typical case involves a previously operated abdomen. The traditional thinking in this situation would dictate that a nonresorbable mesh never should be implanted if the intestinal lumen has been breached because, it is believed, the risk for a disastrous prosthetic infection would be too great. In actual practice, however, there have been poorly documented (unpublished) cases of nonresorbable mesh being implanted during incisional hernia repair in the face of an intestinal injury, with no apparent adverse outcome. The fact that mesh can be placed in the presence of a repaired intestinal injury should not be that surprising because repair (or prophylaxis) of parastomal hernia has been described using nonresorbable mesh with reasonable results.

So what should the surgeon do if, while performing a minimally invasive ventral incisional hernia repair, the colon is entered but quickly controlled and repaired? At present, it probably would be imprudent to advise routine implantation of an intraperitoneal nonresorbable mesh for this scenario. On the other hand, if the mesh is to be placed in the retrorectus space (e.g., during a components separation procedure; see Chapter 28), then there may be less risk for infection, as the data from parastomal hernia surgery have suggested. One empirical alternative in the scenario of bowel injury during ventral herniorrhaphy is to terminate the procedure, give the patient one or two doses of antibiotics, and then reattempt the hernia repair in 72 hours (everyone's schedule permitting). This time period theoretically would allow clearance of the bacterial contamination but avoid re-formation of intraperitoneal adhesions. Another option would be for the surgeon to use a biologic or other resorbable mesh, but this would present different problems (e.g., an elevated recurrence risk).

Gas Embolism

Symptomatic gas embolism during laparoscopic surgery usually is a complication of Veress needle puncture of a large vein with subsequent intravenous insufflation of pneumoperitoneum gas. Asymptomatic gas embolism (as seen with intraoperative transesophageal echocardiography) during laparoscopic procedures actually may be more common than suspected.[76] A symptomatic event, however, is exceedingly rare (about 3 in 100,000 patients[77]) but potentially deadly. The onset of gas embolism may be noted by sudden cardiovascular collapse and "sloshing" heart sounds. Of course, the differential diagnosis of collapse during any laparoscopic procedure is a long list, including tension pneumothorax, cardiac tamponade, hemorrhage, hypovolemia, vasovagal reaction, cardiac dysrhythmia or other dysfunction, acid-base disturbance, drug reaction, and gas embolism. The operating room team quickly needs to consider all of these possibilities if the patient has a sudden cardiovascular collapse. If the decompensation occurs while insufflating with the Veress needle, then gas embolism should be near the top of the differential list.

Extrapolating from animal studies, the lethal intravenous dose of carbon dioxide gas in a human is in the range of 1 liter.[77] If a patient is suspected of having a gas embolism, then gas insufflation immediately is stopped, and the pneumoperitoneum is released. Whether the pneumoperitoneum needle should be withdrawn simultaneously is difficult to know; theoretically, removal of the needle from a large vein could result in bleeding after release of pneumoperitoneum. At this point, however, the patient's presumed problem is venous gas embolism, not venipuncture bleeding, so debating whether to remove the needle probably is not relevant. The patient should be placed into Trendelenburg position with the left side down, in order to trap the gas in the right ventricle. The patient is ventilated with 100% oxygen, and cardiopulmonary resuscitation is performed as necessary.[59] Right heart catheterization with aspiration may be required. If the patient does not stabilize, then an alternative diagnosis needs to be entertained (e.g., arterial injury), which may necessitate an emergency laparotomy.

Abdominal Wall Vessel

A lacerated abdominal wall vessel may be sutured externally under direct vision, or transabdominal stitches may be placed with a suture-passing device. Tamponade of bleeding may be accomplished with an inserted finger or the trocar cannula. Alternatively, a Foley catheter may be inserted through the port site, inflated to 30 cc, and held tight against the parietal peritoneum by clamping the catheter at skin level. Injection of epinephrine can serve as an adjunct for local hemostasis.[25,60]

PERITONEAL ACCESS: OPERATIVE TECHNIQUE

General Considerations

In general, there are three basic techniques to obtain initial access to the peritoneal cavity for a minimally invasive abdominal procedure: (1) insertion of a pneumoperitoneum needle (see Figs. 40-1 and 40-2), commonly known as the Veress needle technique, or closed laparoscopy; (2) insertion of a blunt trocar (see Fig. 40-3) through a minilaparotomy, also known as the Hasson technique or open laparoscopy; and (3) direct insertion of an optical trocar, for which multiple devices are commercially available (see Figs. 40-4 to 40-7). In addition, combinations of these techniques also may be employed, such as (1) Veress needle insertion followed by (2) insertion of an optical trocar.

There are a number of patient- and procedure-specific factors that a surgeon should consider when planning minimally invasive entry into the peritoneal cavity. The suggestions given next regarding this entry are not intended to be absolute recommendations because none is supported with adequate data.

Planned Operation

If the procedure will require access to multiple quadrants or exteriorization of a specimen or segment of bowel (e.g., a colon resection), then open laparoscopy at the umbilicus may be a convenient choice for access because the port position offers a reasonable view to most of the abdomen, and the incision can be enlarged for the exteriorization. If the surgeon only will need ports of 5-mm diameter or less and no extraction incision, then entry with a Veress needle or a 5-mm optical trocar, or both, might be reasonable, if only to avoid a larger incision at the umbilicus. If the surgeon only will need a single large port in a lateral position (e.g., for a stapler), then entry at this site with a 10-mm optical trocar is an option. If the procedure will involve laparoscopic mesh repair of a hernia involving the umbilicus, then lateral first entry might be preferable to periumbilical entry to maintain skin integrity adjacent to the mesh.

Obesity

In the obese subject, the subcutaneous adipose layer generally is thinnest in the upper abdomen toward the midline, but is thicker inferiorly and laterally (particularly if a panniculus is present). The presence of obesity may require the use of "bariatric" ports, which typically have a cannula length of 150 mm, compared with the "regular" length of 100 mm, particularly for ports in the lower and lateral abdomen. If a lateral insertion point (see Fig. 40-9) for a first entry device is elected in the obese subject, then the surgeon should be aware that the curvature of the peritoneal cavity may not be reflected by the curvature of the outer abdominal wall (see Fig. 40-9B). In this case, the device may need to be angled toward the midline so that the peritoneal cavity is not missed (midline angulation of an insertion device should *not* be performed in a thin patient). A reasonably safe first entry location in the obese patient appears to be the Palmer point (see Fig. 40-9),[43] although this has not been demonstrated with controlled data.

Reasonably direct access to the linea alba may be obtained just inferior to the umbilicus (i.e., for open laparoscopy) in nearly all obese subjects, hence the popularity of this location for both open and closed laparoscopy. The relative position of the umbilicus, however, may shift inferiorly with obesity. In such a circumstance, insertion of an infraumbilical Hasson cannula to perform a procedure in the upper abdomen (e.g., a laparoscopic cholecystectomy) may leave the operator with a camera position that is too caudad, compromising the view of procedure. If the surgeon is presented with an umbilicus that has shifted inferiorly in a procedure for which infraumbilical open laparoscopy has been the routine, then alternative first entry higher in the abdomen might be considered to avoid suboptimal camera placement.

Prior Operations

Uncontrolled data have indicated that the risk for injury during initial access is increased in the patient who has a history of prior intra-abdominal surgery.[78-80] Avoidance of a previous laparotomy site during first entry for a laparoscopic procedure is prudent. For example, if a patient is undergoing laparoscopic repair of a ventral incisional hernia, then the safest location for initial peritoneal access will be away from the surgical scar and hernia, which typically means a lateral insertion point. This strategy is particularly important if the surgeon will use a blind entry technique, such as the pneumoperitoneum needle. In fact, it is the opinion of some surgeons that the needle should not be used at all in the presence of previous laparotomy scars. Some authors have recommended that that either open laparoscopy or an optical trocar (instead of the Veress needle) be used in the patient who has a history of abdominal surgery. Data supporting such a view are not definitive, and the Veress needle certainly has been[79,81] and continues to be used by an unknown percentage of surgeons in patients who have undergone previous abdominal procedures.

A related issue is whether it is safe to perform open laparoscopy at the umbilicus if a patient has a periumbilical surgical scar (including previous open laparoscopy). The argument for using the umbilicus in this scenario is that the abdominal entry is performed under direct vision, so the surgeon will be able to diagnose and repair any injury (i.e., bowel perforation) immediately. An equally compelling argument for not using the umbilicus is that an optical trocar may be inserted at a location remote from the umbilicus with a miniscule risk for intra-abdominal injury—so why take the risk at the umbilicus? Again, this is a controversial topic with inadequate controlled data to provide a solid recommendation.

Guidelines for Initial Entry into the Abdomen

The Veress needle technique has the greatest number of published guidelines, recommendations, and instructions,[82-87] most likely because this technique has been in use for peritoneal access for the longest period. The recommendations for use of the Veress needle have been collated in Table 40-3. There are fewer such published guidelines for open laparoscopy[82,83,85,86]; the recommendations for use of the Hasson cannula have been summarized in Table 40-4. Some guidelines for the relatively new technique

Table 40-3 Recommendations for Use of the Pneumoperitoneum (Veress) Needle, Also Known as Closed Laparoscopy, for First Entry into the Peritoneal Cavity during a Laparoscopic Procedure

Avoid previous surgical scars or adhesions
If inserting in periumbilical location in a nonobese patient, aim needle into pelvis
If inserting at lateral location, avoid presumed course of epigastric vessels
If using the Palmer point, consider prior gastric decompression
Level patient positioning (no Trendelenburg)
Thin patients: use extreme caution
Do not lift abdominal wall during insertion
Keep stopcock open during insertion
Mentally visualize location of major vessels during insertion
Avoid wagging the needle side to side as a method to test location
After presumed entry, but before insufflation, perform placement tests (aspiration, saline drop)
Monitor pressure during insufflation (should remain <10 mm Hg)
Fully insufflate abdomen (≥15 mm Hg) before primary trocar insertion (consider temporary high pressure—25 mm Hg—for primary trocar in healthy patients)
After insertion of primary trocar, inspect for injury

Table 40-4 Recommendations for Use of the Blunt (Hasson) Cannula, Also Known as Open Laparoscopy, for First Entry into the Peritoneal Cavity during a Laparoscopic Procedure

Avoid previous surgical scars or adhesions
Stay immediately inferior to the umbilicus, to minimize depth of dissection
Fascial corners are tagged
Confirm intra-abdominal location visually or with palpation before inserting blunt trocar
Withdraw blunt obturator only after abdomen is partially insufflated
After cannula insertion and insufflation, inspect for injury

Table 40-5 Recommendations for Insertion of the Optical Trocar during First Entry into the Peritoneal Cavity for a Laparoscopic Procedure

Avoid previous surgical scars or adhesions
Thin patients: use extreme caution
Level patient positioning (no Trendelenburg)
If inserting at lateral location, avoid presumed course of epigastric vessels
If using the Palmer point, consider prior gastric decompression
Mentally visualize location of major vessels during insertion
Avoid strenuous inward pressure (axial force) and rapid insertion
After trocar insertion and insufflation, inspect for injury

of optical trocar insertion also have been published[83,86]; the available recommendations for this technique are given in Table 40-5.

Technique of Pneumoperitoneum Needle Insertion

With the patient flat, a 2-mm stab incision is made in the skin with a No. 11 scalpel in the left midclavicular line, several fingerbreadths below the costal margin. As discussed earlier, this insertion location sometimes is known as the Palmer point (see Fig. 40-9).[42] This point has been popular for Veress needle insertion because (1) it is in the upper abdomen, where the abdominal wall generally is thinner; (2) it is lateral to the rectus abdominis muscle, thus minimizing the risk for epigastric vessel laceration; (3) there is no underlying solid organ in this location; and (4) in the obese patient, the first intra-abdominal structure to be encountered usually is a fat-laden omentum. The needle is inserted through the stab incision either perpendicular to the skin or slightly angled toward the midline (see Fig. 40-9). As the surgeon advances the needle through the abdominal wall, several yield points ("pops") will be felt through the needle shaft as the needle head breaches successive fascial layers, with a final yield point theoretically occurring when the needle head penetrates the peritoneum.

Of course, the precise moment that the needle head enters the peritoneal cavity cannot be known for certain because Veress needle insertion is a blind maneuver. When the surgeon believes that the needle is within the abdominal cavity, the needle is aspirated with a syringe to ensure that there is no return of blood, gas, or intestinal fluid. The surgeon then may perform a saline drop test, in which saline is injected into the needle, and the needle end is left open to the atmosphere. If the saline flows freely downward, toward the abdomen (flow will be visible because of the clear plastic construction of the head of the Veress needle), then this usually is an indication that the tip of the needle is within the peritoneal cavity. If the needle tip is still within the extraperitoneal space (or some other tissue), then the saline should not flow downward with ease. If the saline does not flow downward, then the needle should be repositioned. The intra-abdominal pressure during subsequent insufflation should remain less than 10 mm Hg; otherwise, the surgeon should be suspicious that the needle is not within the peritoneal cavity.[39]

If the surgeon prefers to insert the Veress needle at the umbilicus, then the patient is placed into slight Trendelenburg position, and the needle is directed into the pelvis (up to 45 degrees from vertical) during insertion in a nonobese subject. In a patient with a normal body mass index, the umbilicus is located just below the level of the aortic bifurcation,[88] hence the recommendation for inferior angulation of the pneumoperitoneum needle. With obesity, however, the location of the umbilicus can shift inferiorly with respect to the bifurcation, and the anterior-posterior patient dimension can increase.[88,89] So in the obese patient, the needle is inserted with less pelvic angulation, staying closer to 0 degrees from vertical. Insertion of the primary trocar, regardless of location, should only be done after complete needle insufflation has been accomplished (i.e., intra-abdominal pressure ≥15 mm Hg). It would be preferable to use the optical insertion technique (see later) for the primary trocar. After the primary trocar has been inserted, inspection for injury is performed.

Although it is my preference not to use the Veress needle on an abdomen with previous surgical scars, this technique has been used by others on previously operated abdomens with reasonable results. Certainly, there are no controlled data that suggest that the Veress needle should not be used if the patient has had a previous abdominal procedure. In the presence of previous abdominal scars, I prefer to use an optical trocar in a site remote from the scars.

Open Laparoscopy

A curvilinear infraumbilical incision is made (see Fig. 40-9); in Hasson's description, a vertical incision is used.[40] In the subcutaneous space, there is a condensation of connective tissue ("midline raphe"), which extends from the periumbilical skin inferiorly and posteriorly, and which correlates with the location of linea alba. This raphe is grasped with a Kocher clamp just inferior to the umbilicus (Fig. 40-10A) and retracted superiorly. The subcutaneous space on either side of the raphe is developed with blunt dissection, staying adjacent to the umbilicus, until the anterior fascia is identified on either side. If the dissection strays from the umbilicus in an overweight patient, then the layer of subcutaneous fat will become thicker, making this access procedure more difficult. Even in obese patients, the distance from the skin to the

anterior fascia should be relatively short, as long as the surgeon stays immediately inferior to the umbilicus.

After the subcutaneous space has been developed on either side of the raphe, this condensation is placed on stretch and then incised down to the linea alba with electrocautery (see Fig. 40-10B). After the raphe has been incised, the infraumbilical linea alba is further cleaned of loose connective tissue. This portion of the procedure is facilitated with lateral retraction provided by Army-Navy or similar retractors (see Fig. 40-10C). If the surgeon has kept the dissection immediately inferior to the umbilicus, then the junction of the umbilical cord remnant with the linea alba should be visible (see Fig. 40-10C). With the wound triangulated between two retractors and the previously placed Kocher clamp, a 1-cm transverse incision is made through the linea alba only, just inferior to its junction with the umbilical cord remnant (see Fig. 40-10D and E).

Stay sutures of 1-0 polyglactin on a short-radius needle are placed in each corner of the fascial incision (see Fig. 40-10D and E), taking bites of both fascial edges (i.e., the suture path is outside-in to inside-out). These stay sutures not only are important for application of traction and anchorage of the Hasson cannula but also function to limit incisional widening from the cannula's plug (see Fig. 40-3) and as part of the incisional closure after the cannula is removed. If each stay suture does not gather up both edges of the fascia at each corner, then the fascia may not seal properly around the plug, pneumoperitoneum may be suboptimal, the fascial defect will progressively enlarge, and so forth. Therefore, stay suture placement in open laparoscopy is an important detail.

Upward traction is placed on the stay sutures, and a blunt-tipped clamp (e.g., a hemostat) is inserted into the fascial incision (see Fig. 40-10F). The fascial anatomy in this location is variable; in some patients, the linea alba, which represents a midline condensation of the anterior and posterior sheaths of the rectus abdominis muscle, may be fused with the underlying transversalis fascia. In this situation, the previously described transverse incision will have crossed all fascial layers, leaving nothing more to traverse but extraperitoneal loose connective tissue and peritoneum. In other subjects, the transversalis fascia forms a discrete layer, also known as *Richet fascia*, posterior to the linea alba in the periumbilical region.[90] With a steady hand on the hemostat and upward traction on the stay sutures, the surgeon delivers a measured yet deliberate "jab" with the clamp. The peritoneum is breached, which should be felt through the clamp as a single "pop." The reach of the jab only should be 1 to 2 cm.

This blunt entry with a clamp should only be done if there has been no previous periumbilical incision and if there is no umbilical hernia. The safety and success of blunt entry with a hemostat tip depends on the lack of intestinal adhesions to the parietal peritoneum directly below the clamp. As long as the bowel is not fixed in this region, then blunt clamp entry as described earlier should not pose a risk for bowel perforation. If the patient does have an umbilical hernia or had a previous periumbilical procedure, then peritoneal incision should be performed under direct vision, as is done during a reoperative laparotomy.

With the hemostat tip in the peritoneal cavity, the jaws are spread to stretch the peritoneal opening. A finger then may be inserted to verify intraperitoneal location, as long as the fascial incision is not widened during the process. The Hasson cannula with blunt obturator then is inserted, the cannula plug is pulled tightly against the fascia by wrapping the stay sutures around the tie posts (see Fig. 40-3), the obturator is removed, and abdominal

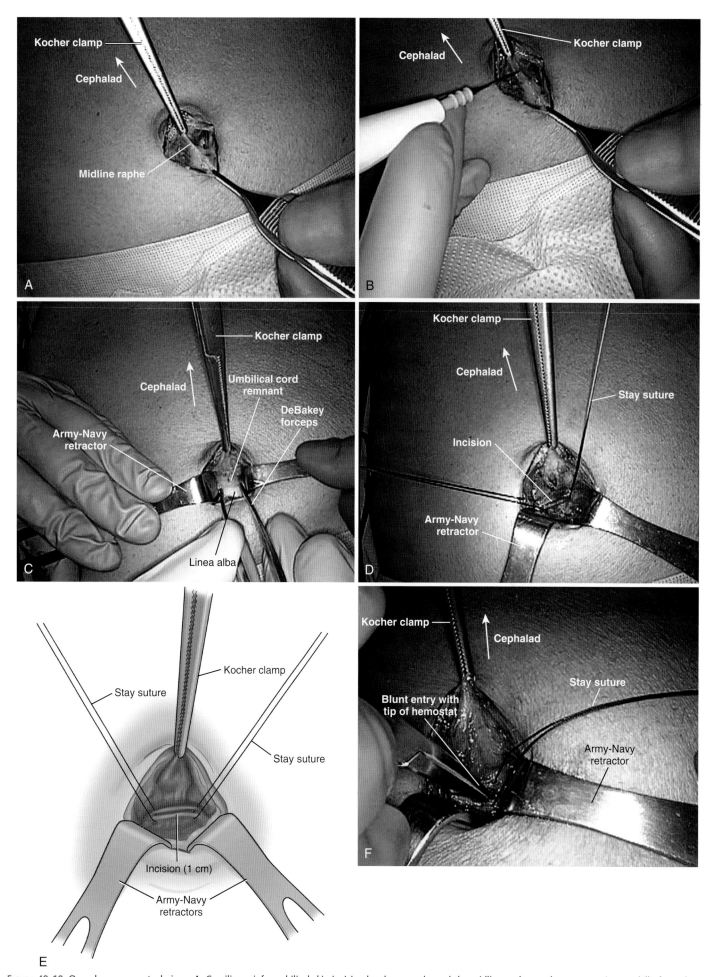

FIGURE 40-10 Open laparoscopy technique. A, Curvilinear infraumbilical skin incision has been made, and the midline raphe can be seen running caudally from the invaginated periumbilical skin; the raphe is placed on stretch between the Kocher clamp and the Adson forceps. B, Exposure of the infraumbilical linea alba by incising the midline raphe with an electrocautery blade. C, Tips of the DeBakey forceps demonstrate the site of the transverse incision through the linea alba for the blunt cannula. D and E, Transverse 1-cm incision has been made through the linea alba, and traction sutures of 1-0 polyglactin have been placed in the incision corners. F, Peritoneal cavity is entered with the closed end of a hemostat.

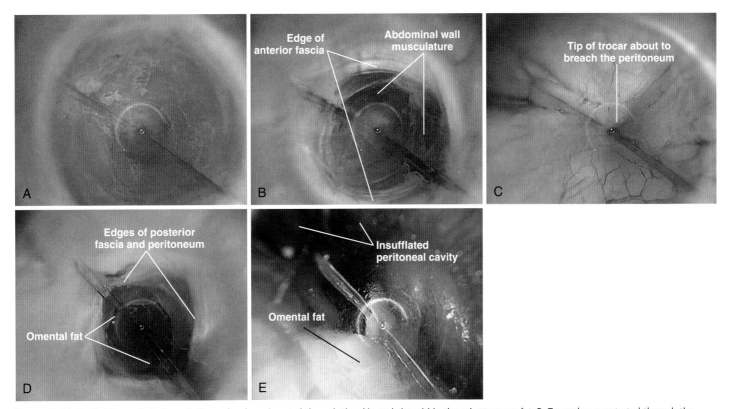

FIGURE 40-11 Optical trocar technique. A, Trocar has been inserted through the skin and sits within the subcutaneous fat. B, Trocar has penetrated through the anterior fascial layer, under which the abdominal wall musculature is visible. C, Trocar has penetrated down to but not through the posterior fascial layer and peritoneum. The center of the trocar is shown just about to breach the peritoneum. D, Tip of trocar has entered the peritoneal cavity; omental fat is present directly beneath. E, CO_2 has been insufflated through the trocar with the camera still inserted, developing an adequate intra-abdominal space into which the trocar may safely be advanced.

insufflation is performed. The laparoscope is inserted during insufflation to confirm positioning and inspect for injury. After completion of the minimally invasive procedure, the fascial incision is closed with interrupted 1-0 polyglactin sutures, using traction on the stay sutures to delineate the corners. The stay sutures then are tied to complete the fascial closure.

Insertion of the Optical Trocar

An optical trocar may be inserted at most locations on the anterior abdominal wall, but similar to the Veress needle, previous transabdominal incisions and known pathology should be avoided. The Palmer point (see Fig. 40-9) often is convenient for optical trocar insertion. A 5- or 10-mm optical trocar (see Figs. 40-4 to 40-7) may be used. A 5- or 10-mm skin incision is made at the Palmer point. A 0-degree laparoscope is inserted into the trocar, and the trocar is inserted through the skin incision and into the subcutaneous fat (Fig. 40-11A). The laparoscope focus is adjusted to bring the fat into clear view.

The skin and abdominal wall is grasped with the nondominant hand inferior to the insertion point, and the abdominal wall is elevated to provide upward counterforce during the insertion. The intent of this counterforce is to prevent excessive depression of the abdominal wall with posterior migration of the trocar tip; otherwise, the tip might get too close to retroperitoneal structures, such as the aorta. If the abdominal wall is not lax enough to permit elevation by hand grasping, then penetrating towel clips may be placed in the skin just superior and inferior to the incision, and the abdominal wall may be elevated with these clips.

With the nondominant hand providing upward traction on the abdominal wall, the dominant hand grasps the trocar-laparoscope assembly and begins the insertion with a combination of downward force and back-and-forth, quarter-turn rotations about the axis of the trocar. If a Visiport device is being used, then less rotation is needed during insertion. The goal of this portion of the procedure is safety, not speed; the downward force on the trocar should be light. Excessive downward force during optical trocar insertion risks a sudden and uncontrolled entry into the peritoneal cavity that, of course, risks injury to the viscera. The surgeon should not burst into the abdomen with one aggressive and unrelenting propulsion of the trocar, but rather should take frequent breaks to assess insertion progress and trocar direction, to regrasp the abdominal wall as needed, and to allow the tissue opportunity to accommodate to the trocar.

The direction of optical trocar insertion should be mostly posterior, with perhaps some medial inclination so that the trocar tip can penetrate the peritoneum with a perpendicular aspect (see Fig. 40-9). It may be helpful for the surgeon to mentally visualize the approximate location of medial structures (e.g., the inferior vena cava) when inserting an optical trocar (or Veress needle) at the Palmer point, particularly if the patient is thin, so that excessive posterior and medial movement is avoided. Such a mental image can help prevent surgeons and surgical trainees from becoming singularly focused on the task of pushing the trocar through the abdominal wall, thereby forgetting about the possible location of the trocar tip.

At the Palmer point, the first fascial layer to be visualized during optical trocar insertion typically will be the anterior sheath of the rectus abdominis (see Fig. 40-11B). This appears as a white layer with the reddish rectus muscle underneath. This is traversed with continuous twisting and downward pressure, as described earlier. If the insertion has been lateral to the rectus sheath, then additional musculofascial layers may need to be traversed before reaching the posterior fascia and parietal peritoneum (see Fig. 40-11C). Arrival at this latter and final layer is signified by a transparent-appearing white layer, through which intra-abdominal structures (typically the omentum, occasionally bowel) may be seen sliding against the inner side. This sliding phenomenon can be enhanced by lateral movement of the trocar-laparoscope assembly against the peritoneum.

With the most posterior layer in view, emphasis is placed on a gradual and controlled intra-abdominal entry, done with the same twisting and downward pressure technique. It is preferable to make a partial entry into the peritoneal cavity first (see Fig. 40-11D) so that about 5 mm of the obturator tip is within the peritoneal cavity. In most cases of Palmer point insertion, the omentum will be the first tissue encountered after the peritoneum is breached; with practice, the surgeon should be able to discern this type of intra-abdominal fat from extraperitoneal fat. With just the obturator tip within the peritoneal cavity, the surgeon should be able to insufflate some gas in order to create enough space (see Fig. 40-11E) so that the cannula can be pushed safely inside the peritoneal cavity. This initial insufflation can be done with the obturator in place; gas should flow (although slowly) around the obturator and into the peritoneal cavity. Of note, the optical trocar in Figure 40-6 has been designed to allow insufflation after the distal 3 mm of the obturator has breached the parietal peritoneum.

After several centimeters of space has been created with insufflation through the partially inserted optical trocar (see Fig. 40-11E), the surgeon can safely push the trocar assembly so that 1 to 2 cm of the cannula is intraperitoneal. The obturator then is removed, and insufflation is completed. The rationale for this technique of partial insertion and partial insufflation before full insertion of the optical trocar is safety; that is, this technique has been presumed to be safer than full insertion before insufflation, although this has not been demonstrated in the literature. After the abdomen has been insufflated, the laparoscope is reinserted into the cannula, inspection for injury is performed, and the intra-abdominal procedure commences. At the end of the procedure, fascial closure of all 10-mm ports is performed.

Insertion Techniques: Who Is Using Which?

In the surgical community, which technique of peritoneal access is the most common? One way to answer this question is with survey data. Most gynecologic surgeons across the world have continued to use closed laparoscopy, according to multiple surveys.[39,71,91-93] The general surgical community also seems to favor the Veress needle,[68] although there are fewer survey data available.

DISCUSSION

As of 2012, there is no definitive evidence demonstrating superiority of one technique of initial peritoneal access over others. The choice of which peritoneal access technique to use largely remains the personal preference of the surgeon. Part of the problem in demonstrating superiority of one technique over another is the relatively large size of a clinical trial that would be needed. Because the complication rates are low, power analyses on this issue have shown that a randomized controlled trial comparing access methods would have to include more than 10,000 patients in each treatment arm. In addition to this difficulty, there would be the issue of standardizing the surgical methods being

tested, and then ensuring that each surgeon participating in the trial was compliant with the surgical protocols that had been standardized. Add to these difficulties the increasingly complex and onerous task of patient recruitment into a clinical trial (particularly one involving surgical techniques), and it would be easy to conclude that a definitive, properly designed trial of initial access methods will not be performed.

So, given the morass of data that are absent of adequate clinical trials, what conclusions can be drawn? The following are some soft conclusions, not to be taken as definitive or final:

- The pneumoperitoneum needle can produce major vascular injuries or gas embolism, at least when used at the umbilicus, but the risk is extremely low.

- Open laparoscopy can result in a similar incidence of bowel injury compared with closed laparoscopy; repair of such an injury usually is not complicated. On the other hand, the risk for major vascular injury with the open technique is lower compared with other entry techniques.

- Optical trocar insertion may be as safe as the other techniques, but more data need to be accrued.

- Use of the Palmer point for needle or trocar insertion may reduce the complication profile, but more data need to be gathered.

- For all access techniques, the risk for injury appears to go up in the presence of previous abdominal surgery.

- The collective published experience in minimally invasive surgery has produced some safety tips and guidelines (reiterated in this chapter) for the safe and effective use of each access technique.

References

1. Fuller J, Ashar BS, Carey-Corrado J: Trocar-associated injuries and fatalities: an analysis of 1399 reports to the FDA, *J Min Invas Gynecol* 12:302–307, 2005.

2. Magrina JF: Complications of laparoscopic surgery, *Clin Obstet Gynecol* 45:469–480, 2002.

3. Bhoyrul S, Vierra MA, Nezhat CR, et al: Trocar injuries in laparoscopic surgery, *J Am Coll Surg* 192:677–683, 2001.

4. Chandler JG, Corson SL, Way LW: Three spectra of laparoscopic entry access injuries, *J Am Coll Surg* 192:478–490, discussion 90-91, 2001.

5. Sharp HT, Dodson MK, Draper ML, et al: Complications associated with optical-access laparoscopic trocars, *Obstet Gynecol* 99:553–555, 2002.

6. Wind J, Cremers JE, van Berge Henegouwen MI, et al: Medical liability insurance claims on entry-related complications in laparoscopy, *Surg Endosc* 21:2094–2099, 2007.

7. Vilos GA: Laparoscopic bowel injuries: Forty litigated gynaecological cases in Canada, *J Obstet Gynaecol Can* 24:224–230, 2002.

8. Agency for Healthcare Research and Quality: Evidence rating. April 13, 2009. Retrieved December 27, 2011, from http://innovations.ahrq.gov/evidencerating.aspx.

9. Owens DK, Lohr KN, Atkins D, et al: AHRQ series paper 5: Grading the strength of a body of evidence when comparing medical interventions—Agency for Healthcare Research and Quality and the effective health-care program, *J Clin Epidemiol* 63:513–523, 2010.

10. Atkins D, Eccles M, Flottorp S, et al: Systems for grading the quality of evidence and the strength of recommendations. I. Critical appraisal of existing approaches. The GRADE Working Group, *BMC Health Serv Res* 4:38, 2004.

11. Oxford Centre for Evidence-Based Medicine: Levels of evidence (March 2009). Retrieved December 27, 2011, from http://www.cebm.net/.

12. Veress J: Neues Instrument zur Ausfuhrung von brust-oder Bauchpunktionen und Pneumothoraxbehandlung, *Dtsch Med Wochenschr* 64:1480–1481, 1938.

13. Anderson ET: Peritoneoscopy, *Am J Surg* 35:136–139, 1937.

14. Schaller G, Kuenkel M, Manegold BC: The optical "Veress-needle"—initial puncture with a minioptic, *Endosc Surg All Technol* 3:55–57, 1995.

15. Turner DJ: A new, radially expanding access system for laparoscopic procedures versus conventional cannulas, *J Am Assoc Gynecol Laparosc* 3:609–615, 1996.

16. Dubrul WR, Tsuji CK: Trocar system having expandable port, *United States Patent* 5,431,676; July 11, 1995.

17. Feste JR, Bojahr B, Turner DJ: Randomized trial comparing a radially expandable needle system with cutting trocars, *JSLS* 4:11–15, 2000.

18. Bhoyrul S, Payne J, Steffes B, et al: A randomized prospective study of radially expanding trocars in laparoscopic surgery, *J Gastrointest Surg* 4:392–397, 2000.

19. Hasson H: A modified instrument and method for laparoscopy, *Am J Obstet Gynecol* 110:886, 1971.

20. Hasson H: Open laparoscopy: A report of 150 cases, *J Reprod Med* 12:234, 1974.

21. Dingfelder JR: Direct laparoscope trocar insertion without prior pneumoperitoneum, *J Reprod Med* 21:45–47, 1978.

22. Saidi M: Direct laparoscopy without prior pneumoperitoneum, *J Reprod Med* 31:684, 1986.

23. Copeland C, Wing R, Hulka JF: Direct trocar insertion at laparoscopy: an evaluation, *Obstet Gynecol* 62:655–659, 1983.

24. Kaali S, Bartfai G: Direct insertion of the laparoscopic trocar after an earlier laparotomy, *J Reprod Med* 33:739, 1988.

25. Philips PA, Amaral JF: Abdominal access complications in laparoscopic surgery, *J Am Coll Surg* 192:525–536, 2001.

26. Yerdel MA, Karayalcin K, Koyuncu A, et al: Direct trocar insertion versus Veress needle insertion in laparoscopic cholecystectomy, *Am J Surg* 177:247–249, 1999.

27. Kaali SG: Introduction of the Opti-trocar, *J Am Assoc Gynecol Laparosc* 1:50–53, 1993.

28. Melzer A, Weiss U, Roth K, et al: Visually controlled trocar insertion by means of the "optical scalpel," *Endosc Surg All Technol* 1:239–242, 1993.

29. Riek S, Bachmann KH, Gaiselmann T, et al: A new insufflation needle with a special optical system for use in laparoscopic procedures, *Obstet Gynecol* 84:476–478, 1994.

30. Sauer JS, Oravecz MG, Greenwald RJ, Kobilansky AI: Optical trocar. US Patent No. 5,441,041; August 15, 1995.

31. String A, Berber E, Foroutani A, et al: Use of the optical access trocar for safe and rapid entry in various laparoscopic procedures, *Surg Endosc* 15:570–573, 2001.

32. Rabl C, Palazzo F, Aoki H, Campos GM: Initial laparoscopic access using an optical trocar without pneumoperitoneum is safe and effective in the morbidly obese, *Surg Innov* 15:126–131, 2008.

33. McKernan JB, Finley CR: Experience with optical trocar in performing laparoscopic procedures, *Surg Laparosc Endosc Percutan Tech* 12:96–99, 2002.

34. Sabeti N, Tarnoff M, Kim J, Shikora S: Primary midline peritoneal access with optical trocar is safe and effective in morbidly obese patients, *Surg Obes Relat Dis* 5:610–614, 2009.

35. Thomas MA, Rha KH, Ong AM, et al: Optical access trocar injuries in urological laparoscopic surgery, *J Urol* 170:61–63, 2003.

36. Mettler L, Schmidt E, Frank V, Semm K: Optical trocar systems: Laparoscopic entry and its complications (a study of cases in Germany), *Gynaecol Endosc* 8:383–390, 1999.

37. Ternamian AM: Laparoscopy without trocars, *Surg Endosc* 11:815–818, 1997.

38. Vilos GA, Vilos AG, Abu-Rafea B, et al: Three simple steps during closed laparoscopic entry may minimize major injuries, *Surg Endosc* 23:758–764, 2009.

39. Pickett SD, Rodewald KJ, Billow MR, et al: Avoiding major vessel injury during laparoscopic instrument insertion, *Obstet Gynecol Clin N Am* 37:387–397, 2010.

40. Hasson HM, Rotman C, Rana N, Kumari NA: Open laparoscopy: 29-year experience, *Obstet Gynecol* 96:763–766, 2000.

41. Molloy D, Kaloo PD, Cooper M, Nguyen TV: Laparoscopic entry: A literature review and analysis of techniques and complications of primary port entry, *Aust N Z J Obstet Gynaecol* 42:246–254, 2002.

42. Palmer R: Safety in laparoscopy, *J Reprod Med* 13:1–5, 1974.

43. Schwartz ML, Drew RL, Andersen JN: Induction of pneumoperitoneum in morbidly obese patients, *Obes Surg* 13:601–604; discussion 4, 2003.

44. Rohatgi A, Widdison AL: Left subcostal closed (Veress needle) approach is a safe method for creating a pneumoperitoneum, *J Laparoendosc Adv Surg Tech* 14:278–280, 2004.

45. Hanney RM, Carmalt HL, Merrett N, Tait N: Vascular injuries during laparoscopy associated with the Hasson technique, *J Am Coll Surg* 188:337–338, 1999.

46. Hanney RM, Carmalt HL, Merrett N, Tait N: Use of the Hasson cannula producing major vascular injury at laparoscopy, *Surg Endosc* 13:1238–1240, 1999.

47. Pring C: Aortic injury using the Hasson trocar: A case report and review of the literature, *Ann Roy Coll Surg Engl* 89:186, 2007.

48. Orvieto M, Breyer B, Sokoloff M, Shalhav AH: Aortic injury during initial blunt trocar laparoscopic access for renal surgery, *J Urol* 171:349–350, 2004.

49. Ahmad G, Duffy JM, Phillips K, Watson A: Laparoscopic entry techniques, *Cochrane Database Syst Rev* 2:CD006583, 2008.

50. Karamoshos K, Mykoniou G, Evagelou J, et al: Sizable pseudoaneurysm of the abdominal aorta after laparoscopic cholecystectomy, *Surg Endosc* 17:661, 2003.

51. Levy MM: Infected aortic pseudoaneurysm following laparoscopic cholecystectomy, *Ann Vasc Surg* 15:477–480, 2001.

52. Guloglu R, Dilege S, Aksoy M, et al: Major retroperitoneal vascular injuries during laparoscopic cholecystectomy and appendectomy, *J Laparoendosc Adv Surg Tech* 14:73–76, 2004.

53. Chapron CM, Pierre F, Lacroix S, et al: Major vascular injuries during gynecologic laparoscopy, *J Am Coll Surg* 185:461–465, 1997.

54. Parthenis DG, Skevis K, Stathopoulos V, et al: Postlaparoscopic iatrogenic pseudoaneurysms of the arteries of the peritoneal and retroperitoneal space: Case report and review of the literature, *Surg Laparosc Endosc Percutan Tech* 19:90, 2009.

55. van der Voort M, Heijnsdijk EA, Gouma DJ: Bowel injury as a complication of laparoscopy, *Br J Surg* 91:1253–1258, 2004.

56. Merlin TL, Hiller JE, Maddern GJ, et al: Systematic review of the safety and effectiveness of methods used to establish pneumoperitoneum in laparoscopic surgery, *Br J Surg* 90:668–679, 2003.

57. Morelli SS, McGovern PG: Laparoscopy in the gynecologic patient: Review of techniques and complications, *Postgrad Obstet Gynecol* 29:1, 2009.

58. Bonjer HJ, Hazebroek EJ, Kazemier G, et al: Open versus closed establishment of pneumoperitoneum in laparoscopic surgery, *Br J Surg* 84:599–602, 1997.

59. Cottin V, Delafosse B, Viale JP: Gas embolism during laparoscopy: A report of seven cases in patients with previous abdominal surgical history, *Surg Endosc* 10:166–169, 1996.

60. Vazquez-Frias JA, Huete-Echandi F, Cueto-Garcia J, Padilla-Paz LA: Prevention and treatment of abdominal wall bleeding complications at trocar sites: Review of the literature, *Surg Laparosc Endosc Percutan Tech* 19:195–197, 2009.

61. Saber AA, Meslemani AM, Davis R, Pimentel R: Safety zones for anterior abdominal wall entry during laparoscopy: A CT scan mapping of epigastric vessels, *Ann Surg* 239:182–185, 2004.

62. Mayol J, Garcia-Aguilar J, Ortiz-Oshiro E, et al: Risks of the minimal access approach for laparoscopic surgery: Multivariate analysis of morbidity related to umbilical trocar insertion, *World J Surg* 21:529–533, 1997.

63. Long JB, Giles DL, Cornella JL, et al: Open laparoscopic access technique: Review of 2010 patients, *JSLS* 12:372–375, 2008.

64. Lal P, Vindal A, Sharma R, et al: Safety of open technique for first-trocar placement in laparoscopic surgery: A series of 6,000 cases, *Surg Endosc* 26:182–188, 2012.

65. Deguara C, Davis C: Laparoscopic entry techniques, *Curr Opin Obstet Gynecol* 23:268–272, 2011.

66. Chapron C, Cravello L, Chopin N, et al: Complications during set-up procedures for laparoscopy in gynecology: Open laparoscopy does not reduce the risk of major complications, *Acta Obstet Gynecol Scand* 82:1125–1129, 2003.

67. Dunne N, Booth MI, Dehn TC: Establishing pneumoperitoneum: Verres or Hasson? The debate continues, *Ann Roy Coll Surg Engl* 93:22–24, 2011.

68. Catarci M, Carlini M, Gentileschi P, Santoro E: Major and minor injuries during the creation of pneumoperitoneum: A multicenter study on 12,919 cases, *Surg Endosc* 15:566–569, 2001.

69. Perunovic RM, Scepanovic RP, Stevanovic PD, Ceranic MS: Complications during the establishment of laparoscopic pneumoperitoneum, *J Laparoendosc Adv Surg Tech* 19:1–6, 2009.

70. Sasmal PK, Tantia O, Jain M, et al: Primary access-related complications in laparoscopic cholecystectomy via the closed technique: experience of a single surgical team over more than 15 years, *Surg Endosc* 23:2407–2415, 2009.

71. Jansen FW, Kolkman W, Bakkum EA, et al: Complications of laparoscopy: An inquiry about closed- versus open-entry technique, *Am J Obstet Gynecol* 190:634–638, 2004.

72. Azevedo JL, Azevedo OC, Miyahira SA, et al: Injuries caused by Veress needle insertion for creation of pneumoperitoneum: a systematic literature review, *Surg Endosc* 23:1428–1432, 2009.

73. Schafer M, Lauper M, Krahenbuhl L: A nation's experience of bleeding complications during laparoscopy, *Am J Surg* 180:73–77, 2000.

74. Saville LE, Woods MS: Laparoscopy and major retroperitoneal vascular injuries (MRVI), *Surg Endosc* 19:1096–1100, 1995.

75. Nordestgaard AG, Bodily KC, Osborne RW Jr, Buttorff JD: Major vascular injuries during laparoscopic procedures, *Am J Surg* 169:543–545, 1995.

76. Fahy BG, Hasnain JU, Flowers JL, et al: Transesophageal echocardiographic detection of gas embolism and cardiac valvular dysfunction during laparoscopic nephrectomy, *Anesth Analg* 88:500–504, 1999.

77. Carlson MA, Frantzides CT: Complications of laparoscopic procedures. In Frantzides CT, editor: *Laparoscopic and Thoracoscopic Surgery*, New York, 1995, Mosby.

78. Marret H, Harchaoui Y, Chapron C, et al: Trocar injuries during laparoscopic gynaecological surgery. Report from the French Society of Gynaecological Laparoscopy, *Gynaecol Endosc* 7:235–241, 1998.

79. Rafii A, Camatte S, Lelievre L, et al: Previous abdominal surgery and closed entry for gynaecological laparoscopy: A prospective study, *Br J Obstet Gynecol* 112:100–102, 2005.

80. Lecuru F, Leonard F, Philippe Jais J, et al: Laparoscopy in patients with prior surgery: Results of the blind approach, *JSLS* 5:13–16, 2001.

81. Dubuisson JB, Chapron C, Decuypere F, De Spirlet M: "Classic" laparoscopic entry in a university hospital: A series of 8324 cases, *Gynaecol Endosc* 8:349–352, 1999.

82. Middlesbrough Consensus Group: A consensus document concerning laparoscopic entry techniques: Middlesbrough, March 19-20, 1999, *Gynaecol Endosc* 8:403–406, 1999.

83. Vilos GA, Ternamian A, Dempster J, et al: Laparoscopic entry: A review of techniques, technologies, and complications, *J Obstet Gynaecol Can* 29:433–465, 2007.

84. Use of the Veress needle to obtain pneumoperitoneum prior to laparoscopy (C-Gyn 7). Consensus statement of the Royal Australian & New Zealand College of Obstetricians & Gynaecologists (RANZCOG) and the Australian Gynaecological Endoscopy Society (AGES), November 2008: Available from http://www.ranzcog.edu.au/.

85. Neudecker J, Sauerland S, Neugebauer E, et al: The European Association for Endoscopic Surgery clinical practice guideline on the pneumoperitoneum for laparoscopic surgery, *Surg Endosc* 16:1121–1143, 2002.

86. Fuller J, Scott W, Ashar B, Corrado J: Laparoscopic trocar injuries: A report from a US Food and Drug Administration Center for Devices and Radiological Health Systematic Technology Assessment of Medical Products Committee (November 2003). Available from http://www.fda.gov/medicaldevices.

87. Semm K, Semm I: Safe insertion of trocars and the Veress needle using standard equipment and the 11 security steps, *Gynaecol Endosc* 8:339–347, 1999.

88. Hurd WW, Bude RO, DeLancey JO, Pearl ML: The relationship of the umbilicus to the aortic bifurcation: Implications for laparoscopic technique, *Obstet Gynecol* 80:48–51, 1992.

89. Hurd WH, Bude RO, DeLancey JO, et al: Abdominal wall characterization with magnetic resonance imaging and computed tomography: The effect of obesity on the laparoscopic approach, *J Reprod Med* 36:473–476, 1991.

90. Moschcowitz AV: Pathogenesis of umbilical hernia, *Ann Surg* 61:570–581, 1915.

91. Lalchandani S, Phillips K: Laparoscopic entry technique—a survey of practices of consultant gynaecologists, *Gynecol Surg* 2:245–249, 2005.

92. Kroft J, Aneja A, Tyrwhitt J, Ternamian A: Laparoscopic peritoneal entry preferences among Canadian gynaecologists, *J Obstet Gynaecol Can* 31:641–648, 2009.

93. Varma R, Gupta JK: Laparoscopic entry techniques: Clinical guideline, national survey, and medicolegal ramifications, *Surg Endosc* 22:2686–2697, 2008.

94. Mintz M: Risks and prophylaxis in laparoscopy: A survey of 100,000 cases, *J Reprod Med* 18:269–272, 1977.

95. Bergqvist D, Bergqvist A: Vascular injuries during gynecologic surgery, *Acta Obstet Gynecol Scand* 66:19–23, 1987.

96. Querleu D, Chapron C, Chevallier L, Bruhat MA: Complications of gynecologic laparoscopic surgery—a French multicenter collaborative study, *N Engl J Med* 328:1355, 1993.

97. Chapron C, Querleu D, Bruhat MA, et al: Surgical complications of diagnostic and operative gynaecological laparoscopy: A series of 29,966 cases, *Hum Reprod* 13:867–872, 1998.

98. Harkki-Siren P: The incidence of entry-related laparoscopic injuries in Finland, *Gynaecol Endosc* 8:335–338, 1999.

99. Larobina M, Nottle P: Complete evidence regarding major vascular injuries during laparoscopic access, *Surg Laparosc Endosc Percutan Tech* 15:119–123, 2005.

100. Penfield AJ: How to prevent complications of open laparoscopy, *J Reprod Med* 30:660–663, 1985.

101. Loffer FD, Pent D: Indications, contraindications and complications of laparoscopy, *Obstet Gynecol Surv* 30:407–427, 1975.

Richard M. Gore, Marc S. Levine, Kiran H. Thakrar, Geraldine M. Newmark, Uday K. Mehta, and Jonathan W. Berlin

Radiology of Minimally Invasive Abdominal Surgery

41

The videos associated with this chapter are listed in the Video Contents and can be found on the accompanying DVDs and on Expertconsult.com.

Over the past two decades, minimally invasive surgery has become the standard of care for a variety of abdominal and pelvic disorders. The increasing popularity of these procedures is related to reduced perioperative and postoperative morbidity, decreased postoperative pain, improved cosmetic results, and faster recovery. Multidetector computed tomography (MDCT), ultrasound, magnetic resonance imaging (MRI), magnetic resonance cholangiopancreatography (MRCP), and positron emission tomography combined with computed tomography (PET-CT) have assumed a primary role in the detection, characterization, and staging of a variety of benign and malignant disorders, many of which are amenable to minimally invasive surgery. These imaging modalities not only are key to the preoperative selection of patients for minimally invasive surgery but are also indispensable in detecting and in many cases treating postoperative complications. This chapter reviews the role of CT, MRI, and ultrasound in managing the patient undergoing the increasingly sophisticated process of minimally invasive abdominal procedures.

IMAGING TECHNIQUES

Multidetector Computed Tomography

Recent improvements in MDCT technology allow thinner collimation and faster scanning that provides multiphasic, high-resolution images of the abdomen and pelvis. These hardware developments, coupled with advances in three-dimensional imaging software and the availability of cheaper data storage capacity, have provided new opportunities for imaging a variety of pathologic processes. Isotropic imaging now is possible, providing two-dimensional multiplanar reformations, CT urography, CT colonography, CT enterography, and three-dimensional imaging formats, with minimal artifacts, and all derived from a single data acquisition. The patient can usually be scanned in less than 15 seconds, allowing for acquisition of thin-section images during multiple phases of the intravenous contrast bolus. This multiphasic evaluation permits high-resolution imaging of not only solid organs and hollow viscera but also the abdominal and pelvic vasculature. The data from these various series then can be reconstructed at thinner intervals and transferred to a workstation, in which multiplanar reformatted images,

maximal-intensity projection images, and three-dimensional volume-rendered images can all be created.

MDCT is ideally suited for imaging the postoperative patient. Opacification of the gastrointestinal (GI) tract with positive contrast material is of critical importance for differentiation among bowel loops, intraperitoneal fluid collections, enlarged lymph nodes, and abscesses. For this purpose, at least 500 mL of dilute (2%) barium sulfate or iodinated compounds should be administered orally or through a nasogastric tube at least 1 hour before the examination. Water-soluble contrast media are preferable if there is any potential risk for intraperitoneal leakage from the GI lumen. Furthermore, water-soluble media tend to stimulate GI peristalsis and more readily opacify the distal small bowel and colon. Intravenous administration of iodinated contrast media is equally important in the detection of abscess and various vascular and parenchymal lesions in the postoperative abdomen. Other modifications, such as rectal contrast enema or scanning the patient in the decubitus or prone position, also are options when attempting to resolve a particular diagnostic dilemma.

The CT examination of the postoperative abdomen should extend from the dome of the diaphragm to the pelvic floor. This approach is warranted because many postoperative complications, particularly abscess and fluid collections, are often located at a site remote from the surgical field because of extension along preexisting anatomic pathways within the abdominal cavity.

Magnetic Resonance Imaging

Significant advances in MRI hardware and software, combined with routine use of phased-array coils and parallel imaging, permit fast and high spatial resolution imaging of the abdomen and pelvis. Short breath-hold scans can produce superb multiphase images without significant peristaltic or respiratory motion artifacts. MRI generally is employed as a secondary imaging test when better characterization of a mass discovered on MDCT or ultrasound is needed.

MRCP is a pivotal tool in the evaluation of pancreaticobiliary disease. This MRI technique exploits the fluid present within the bile ducts, pancreatic duct, and gallbladder, causing the bile and pancreatic juice to have a high signal intensity from which quality endoscopic retrograde cholangiopancreatography (ERCP) images of the ductal system can be created. MRCP can be obtained without the associated complications of ERCP while offering comparable sensitivity, specificity, and accuracy. Thus, bile duct stones and biliary obstruction often are best evaluated with MRCP. When combined with conventional MRI and magnetic resonance angiography, MRCP offers superb preoperative staging of hepatic, biliary tract, and pancreatic primary malignancies.

Ultrasound

Ultrasound is the favored initial imaging test for the evaluation of gallstones, biliary dilation, and cholecystitis and also has a primary role in pediatrics, obstetrics, and gynecology. Ultrasound has several inherent advantages over CT, including lower cost, an ability to perform real-time imaging, portability, a lack of ionizing radiation, and an absence of contraindications. Recent advances in gray-scale and color-flow Doppler techniques, as well as tissue harmonics, have enhanced the ability of ultrasound to identify and characterize abdominal and pelvic masses. In addition, endosonography and transrectal ultrasound are important in the T and N staging of patients with early esophageal, gastric, and rectal cancers.

Combined Positron Emission Tomography and Computed Tomography

Most malignancies exhibit increased metabolic activity that results in increased use of glucose. PET imaging exploits the fact that a glucose analog, ^{18}F-fluorodeoxyglucose (FDG), shows increased intracellular accumulation in malignant tissue. PET-CT is a fixed combination of PET and CT scanners in a combined imaging system. The nearly simultaneous data acquisitions lead to minimization of spatial and temporal mismatches between modalities by eliminating the need to move the patient during the examination. The result is a fused image that provides biologic and anatomic information. Imaging generated from the combination of anatomic and metabolic data often provides more sensitive and specific information concerning the extent of malignancy than anatomic imaging alone. PET-CT is an increasingly popular method for the staging of a number of malignancies (including lung, breast, colorectal, and esophageal cancer), as evident from cancer treatment guidelines, such as those available from the National Comprehensive Cancer Network.

LAPAROSCOPIC CHOLECYSTECTOMY

Since its introduction in the late 1980s, laparoscopic cholecystectomy has become the standard of care for removing the diseased gallbladder. The popularity of this procedure has advanced the popularity of minimally invasive techniques in many other abdominal and pelvic operations.

Preoperative Assessment of Gallstones

Ultrasound is the gold standard for the noninvasive diagnosis of cholelithiasis, with an accuracy of more than 96%. A sonographic diagnosis of cholelithiasis must fulfill three major criteria: (1) an echogenic focus, (2) acoustic shadowing from the focus, and (3) gravitational dependence of the focus. Confidence in the diagnosis is increased if a 5-mm or larger defect meets all three criteria. Stones smaller than 2 to 3 mm may be difficult to visualize. Small stones, however, are usually multiple, which assists in their detection.

The CT appearance of gallstones is variable, depending on their composition, the pattern of calcification, and the presence of lamellation, fissuring, or gas. Stones with high cholesterol content are difficult to visualize because they are isodense with the surrounding bile. Well-calcified stones are readily detected on CT. Stones that are denser than bile may be seen because of a rim or nidus of calcification. The CT attenuation of gallstones correlates more closely with the cholesterol content of the stones than with the calcium content. On CT, gallstones can be simulated by the enhancing mucosa of a contracted gallbladder wall or neck, which often folds upon itself.

On MRI, most gallstones produce little or no signal because of the restricted motion of water and cholesterol molecules in the crystalline lattice of the stone. To optimize gallbladder and ductal stone visualization on MRI, T2-weighted imaging sequences are used that produce bright bile. MRI is superior to CT in detecting small calculi because of the inherent contrast between low-signal-intensity stones and high-signal-intensity bile.

Choledocholithiasis

Choledocholithiasis is found in 7% to 20% of patients undergoing cholecystectomy and in 2% to 4% of patients after cholecystectomy. These stones usually are asymptomatic unless they obstruct the common bile duct (CBD). Small calculi may intermittently cause colicky pain as they obstruct the ampulla of Vater, but they generally pass into the duodenum. Larger stones (between 5 and 10 mm) are difficult to pass and can result in intermittent long-term symptoms and sequelae, such as cholangitis and sepsis.

The detection of bile duct stones is easiest in the setting of biliary dilation. Unfortunately, biliary dilation is present in only 66% to 75% of patients with bile duct stones, so their detection may be difficult. Sonographically, a bile duct stone may appear as an echogenic focus within the fluid-filled duct that may cast an acoustic shadow. A ductal stone also may appear as an echogenic curved line so that only the anterior margin is visualized, with homogeneous echogenicity throughout the stone, or without acoustic shadowing. Adjacent duodenal and colonic gas can make it difficult to image the distal common bile duct. Because of these factors, sonography has a sensitivity of only 18% to 45% in the detection of choledocholithiasis.

As with gallstones, the CT appearance of CBD stones is variable, depending on their composition and pattern of calcification. High-attenuation stones can be seen easily within the duct lumen even in the absence of biliary dilation. Only 20% of CBD stones have a homogeneous high density. Other findings include a rim of high attenuation (which may be difficult to detect when impacted against the duct wall), soft tissue attenuation, and homogeneous near-water attenuation. CBD stones rarely may have sufficient cholesterol to appear lower in attenuation than surrounding bile. MDCT with coronal reformatted images has a sensitivity of 76% to 80% in the detection of bile duct stones.

On MRI, CBD stones appear as foci of low signal intensity surrounded by bright bile on T2-weighted sequences. Stones as small as 2 mm can be detected by this technique, which has a sensitivity of 81% to 100% and a specificity of 85% to 99%. MRCP is superior to CT and ultrasound in selecting which patient may benefit from preoperative ERCP. MRCP has been recommended in the patient with gallstones and a moderate to high suspicion of CBD stones, based on clinical, sonographic, and laboratory data. MRCP can rule out CBD stones in up to 48% of patients with a high preoperative probability of CBD stones.

Acute Cholecystitis

The patient with suspected acute cholecystitis should undergo imaging because 60% to 85% of patients with an unconfirmed diagnosis have other causes of right upper quadrant pain, including peptic ulcer disease, pancreatitis, hepatitis, appendicitis, hepatic congestion from right-sided heart failure, perihepatitis from pelvic inflammatory disease (Fitz-Hugh–Curtis syndrome), right lower lobe pneumonia, right-sided pyelonephritis, nephroureterolithiasis, and so forth. Furthermore, imaging can diagnose severe complications that require immediate surgery, such as emphysematous cholecystitis or perforation.

The patient with suspected acute cholecystitis should have an ultrasound as the initial imaging procedure. If the diagnosis is in doubt after the ultrasound, then hepatobiliary scintigraphy or a CT can be performed. MDCT often is performed initially in many cases because the diagnosis is unclear. CT also may be quite helpful in suspected emphysematous cholecystitis or gallbladder perforation. MRI usually is employed to exclude obstructing and nonobstructing biliary tract stones.

The sonographic findings of acute uncomplicated cholecystitis include gallstones that may be impacted in the cystic duct or gallbladder neck, mural thickening (>3 mm), a three-layered appearance of the gallbladder wall, hazy delineation of the gallbladder, localized pain with maximal tenderness elicited over the gallbladder (sonographic Murphy sign), pericholecystic fluid, and gallbladder distention. Gallstones and the sonographic Murphy sign are the most specific indicators of acute cholecystitis, with a positive predictive value of 92%. The sonographic Murphy sign may be difficult to elicit in obtunded patients and in those who have received pain medication. Of note, Murphy sign may be absent in patients with gangrenous cholecystitis.

The CT findings of acute cholecystitis include gallstones, mural thickening of the gallbladder, mural edema, pericholecystic fluid and inflammation, and transient increased enhancement of the liver parenchyma adjacent to the gallbladder due to hyperemia. As stated before, CT is less sensitive (75%) than ultrasound in the depiction of gallstones. Stones with significant calcification or the presence of gas in a noncalcified stone (the Mercedes Benz sign) are best seen with CT. The CT findings of acute cholecystitis have been divided into major and minor criteria; the former include calculi, mural thickening of the gallbladder, pericholecystic fluid, and subserosal edema, whereas the latter include gallbladder distention and sludge. The overall sensitivity, specificity, and accuracy of CT for the diagnosis of acute cholecystitis are 92%, 99%, and 94%.

MRI rivals ultrasound and CT in the depiction of acute cholecystitis. On postgadolinium T1-weighted images, the findings of acute cholecystitis include increased mural enhancement, mural thickening, and transient increased enhancement of the adjacent liver parenchyma. Findings found on T2-weighted images include gallstones, intramural abscess (appearing as a hyperintense foci in the gallbladder wall), and a thickened gallbladder wall.

Radionuclide cholescintigraphy with technetium-99m–labeled iminodiacetic acid analogs (also known as HIDA scan) was first introduced in the late 1970s. In this examination, hepatic parenchymal uptake of the tracer is observed within 1 minute, with peak activity occurring at 10 to 15 minutes. The bile ducts are usually visualized within 10 minutes, and the gallbladder should fill with isotope within 1 hour, if the cystic duct is patent. If the gallbladder is not identified, then delayed imaging (up to 4 hours after injection) should be performed. Prompt biliary excretion of the isotope without visualization of the gallbladder is the hallmark of acute cholecystitis. False-positive results may occur in patients with abnormal bile flow because of hepatic parenchymal disease or secondary to a prolonged fast with a distended, sludge-filled gallbladder. Delayed gallbladder filling also can be seen in the setting of chronic cholecystitis.

Normal Imaging Findings after Uncomplicated Laparoscopic Cholecystectomy

Occasionally, a patient who has undergone laparoscopic cholecystectomy may present postoperatively with pain, fever, leukocytosis, and jaundice. Such a patient requires additional imaging that may reveal certain and unexpected findings. Normal radiographic findings in this setting are described later.

Pneumoperitoneum

A small amount of pneumoperitoneum commonly is seen following laparoscopic cholecystectomy, as a result of carbon dioxide insufflation. It usually does not require further evaluation in the asymptomatic patient. In the symptomatic patient, however, the presence of pneumoperitoneum does raise the possibility of bowel perforation. This dilemma can be resolved either with a CT scan (with oral contrast) or with an upright chest radiograph that includes the diaphragm. The amount of free air diminishes in the patient without perforation and typically increases in the patient with a bowel perforation. The volume of free air generally is smaller and the window of detection shorter after laparoscopic cholecystectomy compared with open cholecystectomy.

Subcutaneous Emphysema

Subcutaneous emphysema is seen in nearly two thirds of patients, secondary to dissection of carbon dioxide around the trocars into the soft tissue. This finding is not clinically significant and should not be confused with necrotizing fasciitis, which has characteristic regional and systemic signs and symptoms.

Trocar Insertion Trauma

On MDCT, small densities may be seen in the subcutaneous fat of the anterior abdominal wall at the sites of trocar insertion. These densities typically resolve over time; however, there may be a permanent linear scar.

Permanent Surgical Materials

Surgical clips in the gallbladder fossa are identified easily with MDCT. Sonographically, however, clips can mimic CBD stones and also can cause inhomogeneity artifacts on MRI that simulate CBD stones. Absorbable hemostatic sponges may cause diagnostic confusion on CT because they appear as masses with mixed or low attenuation or with central (and occasionally peripheral) gas collections that can be confused with an abscess. Serial CT examinations will show gradual disappearance of this material.

Pulmonic Findings

Lower lobe atelectasis develops in nearly one half of patients, and small pleural effusions may develop in one third. Indeed, pulmonary findings may be more frequent after laparoscopic than open cholecystectomy because of the compressive effects on the lung bases by the pneumoperitoneum in the former procedure.

Postoperative Ileus

Postoperative ileus occurs in nearly one half of patients but usually is not significant because most patients are on a regular diet by the second postoperative day.

Postoperative Fluid Collections

Fluid is seen in the subhepatic space in nearly 20% of patients following both laparoscopic and open cholecystectomy and usually resolves by postoperative day 12. The volume of fluid usually is small and has no clinical consequence. Edema is present in the gallbladder fossa in 22% of patients and probably represents a small collection of bile. Possible causes include interruption of an accessory hepatic duct, which is a persistent embryologic connection between the liver and gallbladder. A CT usually cannot distinguish the source or contents of these fluid collections, but the presence of a large or growing fluid collection is indicative of a complication such as bile duct injury, hemorrhage, or peritonitis. Hepatobiliary scanning and aspiration usually are indicated in this situation. A CT scan should include the pelvis because intra-abdominal fluid may be seen only in the rectouterine pouch (pouch of Douglas) or rectovesical pouch, which are the most dependent portions of the peritoneal cavity in women and men, respectively.

Stone Retention in the Remnant Gallbladder or Cystic Duct

Uncommonly, laparoscopic cholecystectomy may be performed with incomplete excision of the gallbladder secondary to a difficult surgical dissection. This type of case may result in a retained stone within the remnant gallbladder. Because of the limitations in exploring the cystic duct pedicle during a difficult laparoscopic cholecystectomy, a small stone in a particularly long cystic duct remnant may remain. MRCP is superior to both sonography and MDCT in the detection of remnant gallbladder or cystic duct stones.

Common Bile Duct Stones

Retained stones can cause partial or complete biliary obstruction after laparoscopic cholecystectomy. Although intraoperative cholangiography is the gold standard for detecting choledocholithiasis during cholecystectomy, MRCP is valuable in the preoperative and postoperative detection of CBD stones (Fig. 41-1). Small gallstones may migrate into the CBD in the patient with a patulous cystic duct during cephalad retraction of the gallbladder. ERCP is useful in diagnosing and treating these cases.

Bile Leakage

Bile leakage is one of the most common complications of laparoscopic cholecystectomy. Most leaks occur from the cystic duct stump. Other causes include laceration, transection, or thermal injury of the CBD or an unrecognized anomalous duct. CT and ultrasound are the initial imaging studies performed in the postoperative patient with suspected bile leak or biliary sepsis. Although both studies are useful in detecting intra-abdominal fluid collections, neither can differentiate between lymphocele, hematoma, seroma, or biloma (Fig. 41-2). Cross-sectional imaging studies can show a fluid collection in the gallbladder fossa, but such imaging cannot determine whether there is active bile leakage. Hepatobiliary scintigraphy (Fig. 41-3A), ERCP, or

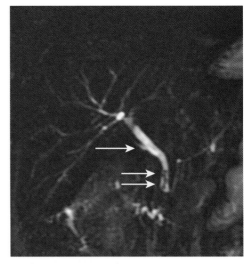

FIGURE 41-1 Retained common bile duct stones shown on magnetic resonance cholangiopancreatography. Multiple low-signal-intensity stones *(short arrows)* are highlighted by high-signal-intensity bile in this patient after laparoscopic cholecystectomy. *Long arrow* indicates cystic duct remnant.

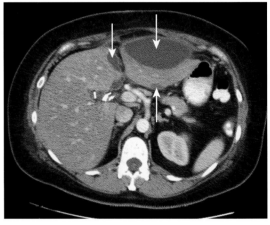

FIGURE 41-2 Postoperative biloma on computed tomography. Several low-density fluid collections *(arrows)* surround the left lobe of the liver 2 weeks after laparoscopic cholecystectomy. Note surgical clips in the gallbladder fossa.

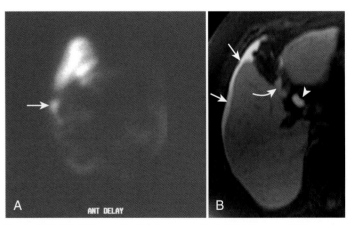

FIGURE 41-3 Bile leak complicating laparoscopic cholecystectomy. **A,** Two-hour delayed image from a hepatobiliary scintigram demonstrating extrabiliary and extraintestinal isotope throughout the peritoneal cavity, but primarily in the Morison pouch *(arrow).* **B,** Magnetic resonance image with Eovist, showing high-signal-intensity contrast material surrounding the liver *(straight arrow),* in the gallbladder fossa *(curved arrow),* and within the common hepatic duct *(arrowhead).*

percutaneous transhepatic cholangiography (PTC) can show an active bile leak and the site of leakage. MRI employing gadoxetate disodium (Eovist), a gadolinium-based agent that is excreted in the bile, also is effective in showing bile leakage (Fig. 41-3B).

Acute Biliary Obstruction and Bile Duct Injury

A bile duct injury typically manifests with biliary dilation (Fig. 41-4) or bile leakage. The site of injury is described according to the Bismuth classification. A Bismuth type 1 injury indicates a remaining (noninjured) common hepatic duct longer than 2 cm; a type 2 injury has a remaining common hepatic duct shorter than 2 cm; a type 3 injury is located at the confluence of the right and left hepatic ducts; a type 4 injury extends into the right and left hepatic ducts. Major ductal injury from laparoscopic cholecystectomy generally is high in the biliary system, and multiple ducts often are involved. Mechanisms of CBD injury include malpositioning of surgical clips, thermal injury from sealing and cauterizing instruments, sharp incision, and en bloc excision.

Late Biliary Obstruction with Stricture

Stricture of the CBD occurring late after laparoscopic cholecystectomy has become a recognized, although uncommon, complication of this procedure. This type of stricture presumably results from mild to moderate thermal injury to the bile duct. Rarely, surgical clips can induce fibrosis or inflammatory changes around the extrahepatic ducts that may lead to a stricture. MRCP is the most effective noninvasive means of diagnosing this type of biliary stricture.

Hemorrhage

Hemorrhage after laparoscopic cholecystectomy (Fig. 41-5) may occur from the cystic artery stump or the right hepatic artery. Bleeding may be secondary to thermal or mechanical injury, as with bile duct injury, or from dislodged hemostatic clips.

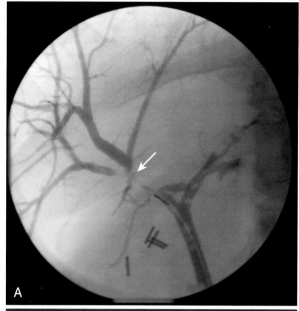

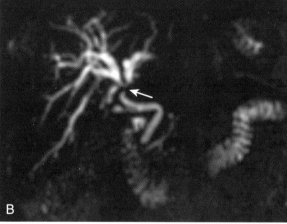

FIGURE 41-4 Bile duct stricture complicating laparoscopic cholecystectomy. A, Endoscopic retrograde cholangiopancreatography image demonstrating a stricture of the right hepatic duct (arrow). There is dilation of the ductal system proximal to this stricture. B, Magnetic resonance cholangiopancreatography image demonstrating a stricture (arrow) at the confluence of the right and left hepatic ducts.

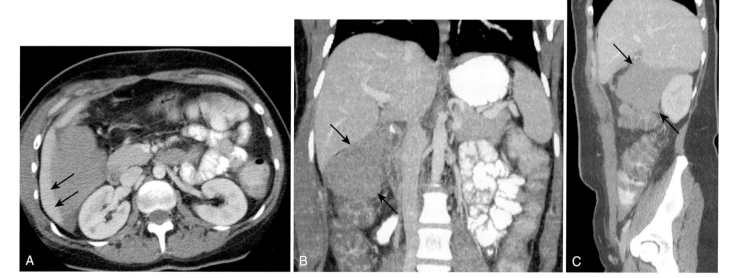

FIGURE 41-5 Hemorrhage following laparoscopic cholecystectomy as seen on multidetector computed tomography. A, Axial slice. B, Coronal reformatted. C, Sagittal reformatted. Arrows indicate a large hematoma originating in the gallbladder fossa.

Bleeding also can occur at a trocar insertion site, from the omentum or abdominal wall. MDCT is the most effective method for detecting bleeding because it will show the hyperdense hemorrhage and may show a focus of active bleeding or a pseudoaneurysm on contrast-enhanced scans. Transcatheter arterial embolization or surgical hemostasis may be considered, particularly if extravasation of the intravenous contrast agent is seen.

Abscess with Retention of Peritoneal Gallstones or Spilled Clips

Gallstone and bile spillage develops in up to one third of patients during laparoscopic cholecystectomy. Dropped stones can lodge in virtually any crevice of the abdominal cavity. The combination of pneumoperitoneum and peritoneal irrigation may disperse the calculi throughout the peritoneal cavity. Stones have been reported in the right pleural space and have eroded into to colon. Abscess formation occurs in about 0.6% of patients in whom bile spillage alone occurs and in 0.6% to 2.9% of cases in whom both bile and stone spillage occurs. An abscess also can be associated with dropped surgical clips. Most abscesses associated with unretrieved peritoneal gallstones or spilled clips are seen in the perihepatic space (Fig. 41-6), but they may occur anywhere in the peritoneal cavity. Visualization of the spilled stone or clip in the abscess is the key to the radiologic diagnosis of this entity. Sonographically, a typical abscess appears as an echogenic focus with posterior acoustic shadowing. On MDCT, a central or eccentric calcified stone or metallic nidus may be identified.

Trocar Site Hernia

An umbilical hernia at the Hasson cannula site is the most common type of trocar hernia, which generally occurs within a few days of surgery and often presents with small bowel obstruction. It can take several months, however, before symptoms of a trocar hernia develop. If the hernia causes small bowel obstruction (Fig. 41-7) and strangulation, operative intervention is needed. A trocar hernia also may be complicated by panniculitis.

Infection

Although intra-abdominal infections are rare following laparoscopic cholecystectomy, trocar site infection is relatively common (Fig. 41-8). A bile leak can produce a localized fluid collection that can become infected or lead to bile peritonitis. The simple presence of postoperative fluid, however, is an unreliable indication of a complication. Postoperative fluid collections may represent bile, blood, serous fluid, lymph, or pus. CT is the most helpful modality for diagnosing intra-abdominal infection. An abscess typically contains gas bubbles; however, pneumoperitoneum is a normal finding in the early postoperative period, and small bubbles of gas do not necessarily mean an abscess. Diagnostic aspiration may be the only means of determining the contents of a fluid collection. If the patient is deteriorating or developing signs of sepsis, a diagnostic aspiration may be indicated.

Complications of Laparoscopy

Abdominal wall bleeding (Fig. 41-9), omental hemorrhage, intra-abdominal vessel injury, retroperitoneal vessel injury, GI perforation, bladder perforation, solid visceral injury, and other injuries can occur with insertion of a trocar. Intra-abdominal injury typically occurs with placement of the first trocar because it is the only one not placed under laparoscopic visualization. For laparoscopic cholecystectomy, this means that most trocar injuries to the viscera will be incurred in the region of the umbilicus. Laceration of a vessel within the abdominal wall (e.g., an epigastric vessel) typically occurs with trocar placement away from the midline.

OBESITY SURGERY

Obesity has become a public health problem of epidemic proportions in the United States. Nearly two thirds of Americans are overweight (body mass index [BMI] >25), and about one third are obese (BMI >30). Bariatric surgery has proved efficacious in achieving sustained weight loss, decreasing the risk for

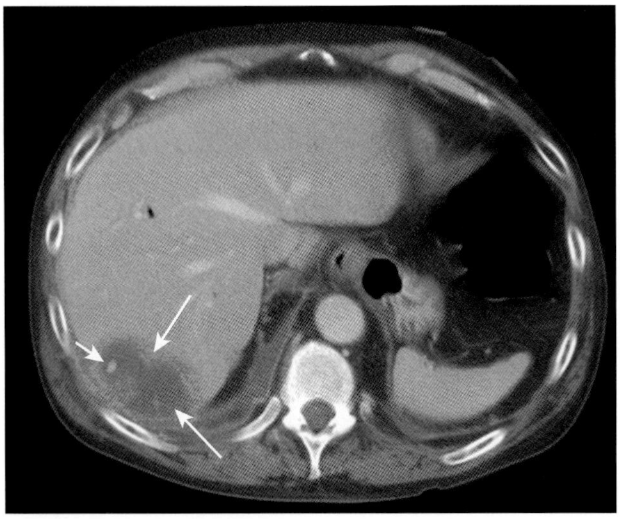

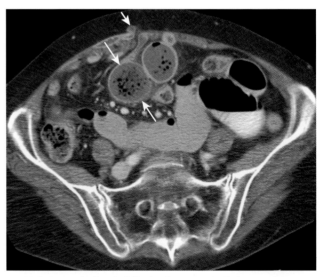

Figure 41-6 Spilled stone during laparoscopic cholecystectomy leading to abscess. Computed tomography scan shows a calcified stone *(short arrow)* within a low-density, thick-walled abscess *(long arrows)* along the posterolateral aspect of the right lobe of the liver.

Figure 41-7 Trocar site hernia following laparoscopic cholecystectomy that resulted in a small bowel obstruction. Computed tomography scan demonstrates a small knuckle of proximal ileum *(short arrow)* incarcerated in the defect. Note the small bowel feces sign *(long arrows)*, with mottled density material within the dilated ileum just proximal to the obstruction.

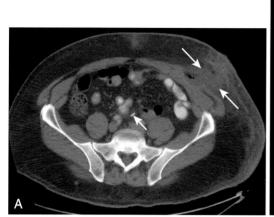
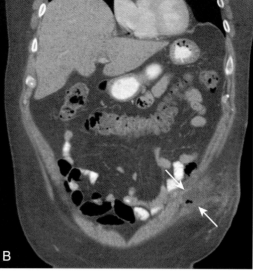
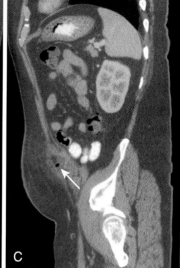

FIGURE 41-8 Trocar site infection visualized with computed tomography, with axial (A), coronal reformatted (B), and sagittal reformatted (C) images. *Long arrows* indicate gas within the abdominal wall; *short arrow* in A shows dropped surgical clip.

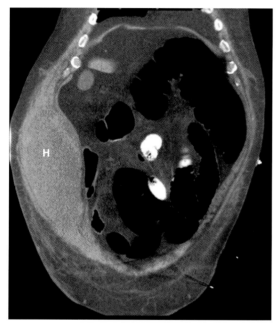

FIGURE 41-9 Abdominal wall hematoma complicating laparoscopic cholecystectomy. Coronal reformatted computed tomography shows a large hematoma (H) involving the right lateral abdominal wall.

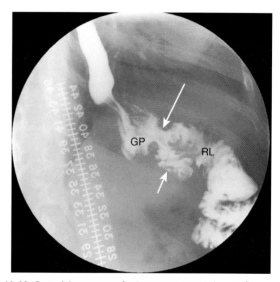

FIGURE 41-10 Gastrojejunostomy of a Roux-en-Y gastric bypass (upper gastrointestinal series). *Short arrow* indicates blind loop of jejunum resulting from the end-to-side anastomosis; *long arrow* shows gastrojejunostomy. GP, gastric pouch; RL, Roux loop of jejunum.

obesity-related morbidity, and improving survival among morbidly obese individuals. Radiographic assessments are important both in the management of weight loss and in the detection of postoperative complications.

Historically, bariatric surgery is categorized into two main types: restrictive and malabsorptive. In restrictive procedures, gastric volume is reduced substantially to decrease caloric intake by promoting early satiety. In malabsorptive procedures, the GI tract is surgically altered to induce malabsorption and diminish caloric intake by the small bowel. In addition, some procedures may be a combination of these two types. Although research into the mechanisms of weight loss after various bariatric procedures has raised questions on these historical definitions, these terms still are in common use. The next sections focus on the imaging involved with two of the more common bariatric procedures, Roux-en-Y gastric bypass (RYGB) and laparoscopic adjustable gastric banding.

ROUX-EN-Y GASTRIC BYPASS

RYGB has become the most commonly performed bariatric procedure in the United States. This technique entails the creation of a 15- to 30-mL gastric pouch that is surgically isolated from the remainder of the stomach (gastric remnant). The pouch can be formed by surgically separating the pouch from the gastric remnant or by simple functional division with the application of staples. The jejunum then is divided approximately 30 to 40 cm distal from the ligament of Treitz, and the distal end is brought up to create an end-to-side gastrojejunostomy with the gastric pouch. The jejunal loop that is connected to the stomach is referred to as the *Roux limb* or *efferent limb*. This limb either is passed through an opening created in the transverse mesocolon (retrocolic) or travels anterior to the transverse colon (antecolic) and is anastomosed to the pouch. Typically, a small afferent limb of jejunum proximal to the gastrojejunostomy ("blind loop") is produced as a result of the end-to-side anastomotic technique (Fig. 41-10). A jejunojejunostomy then is created approximately

100 to 150 cm distal to the gastrojejunostomy, and all mesenteric defects are closed. The RYGB procedure exploits both the restrictive and malabsorptive components to induce weight loss. By varying the length of the Roux limb, the malabsorptive component can be increased or decreased.

Initial imaging is performed on postoperative day 1 with water-soluble contrast material and fluoroscopy to assess for anastomotic leak. In the late postoperative setting, imaging may be performed with either fluoroscopy or CT. CT is employed when fluoroscopic examinations are equivocal or when bowel obstruction or abscess is suspected. Oral contrast material normally can reflux into the afferent limb, and gastric fluid or air can be visualized in the gastric remnant as well.

Anastomotic Leak

Anastomotic leak is one of the most serious complications of RYGB, occurring in 1% to 6% of cases. A postoperative leak can be difficult to diagnose because the patient may present with only tachycardia and abdominal discomfort and have no signs of peritonitis or fever. In addition, the patient's size may lead to a difficult and misleading physical examination. A high index of suspicion is necessary for a clinical diagnosis.

A leak usually occurs within the first 10 days of the procedure. The most common site is the gastrojejunostomy; leak is less common at the distal jejunostomy and bypassed stomach. CT and upper GI series often are complementary in the detection of a leak. The latter study (Fig. 41-11) can detect major and minor leaks with sensitivities of up to 100% and 75%, respectively. A small leak may be difficult to recognize on upper GI series, especially if obtained on the first postoperative day. Sometimes, the only clue to the presence of a leak is opacification of the surgical drain with contrast material. Even a small leak may result in a fluid collection or fistula formation. Gastrogastric and gastrocutaneous fistulas may develop in the rare case. A CT scan can demonstrate a leak or fluid collection that is below the limit of detection for an upper GI series.

A postoperative fluid collection (Fig. 41-12) from an RYGB procedure most commonly develops in the left upper abdomen, particularly in the perisplenic space. Such a collection can evolve into an abscess. An infected collection typically has an enhancing rim, air-fluid levels, and gas bubbles. CT-guided percutaneous abscess drainage often can obviate the need for surgical intervention.

Stomal Stenosis

Stenosis of the gastrojejunostomy (Fig. 41-13) develops in up to 27% of patients who have undergone an RYGB procedure. The typical patient presents with dysphagia, vomiting, dehydration, and excessive weight loss. The diagnosis usually is made with endoscopy or an upper GI series; the latter will show dilation of the gastric pouch and delayed passage of contrast material through the anastomosis. Sometimes, treatment can be performed with endoscopic dilation; if not successful, then surgical revision will be necessary. Stenosis of the jejunojejunostomy is rare and usually requires surgical correction.

Small Bowel Obstruction

Small bowel obstruction develops in 1.3% to 5% of patients after RYGB. Internal hernia and adhesions are the most common causes. Less common causes include incarcerated ventral hernia, gastric pouch bezoar, and intussusception at the enteroenterostomy site. Although the laparoscopic approach is associated with fewer adhesions than the open approach, there is a higher prevalence of internal hernia with the former.

The patient who has undergone RYGB is at risk for three types of internal hernia: (1) through the opening in the transverse mesocolon (Fig. 41-14) through which the Roux limb is brought to the gastric pouch (with the retrocolic technique); (2) through the small bowel mesenteric defect at the gastrojejunostomy site; and (3) through the space posterior to the Roux limb (Peterson type). The herniated bowel may be the Roux limb itself with varying amounts of additional small bowel. Because retrocolic

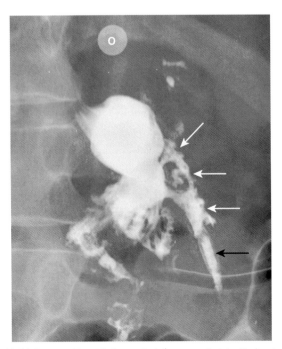

FIGURE 41-11 Roux-en-Y gastric bypass leak (upper gastrointestinal series). There is a leak from the left lateral aspect of gastric pouch into a contained collection (*white arrows*), communicating with an adjacent surgical drain (*black arrow*).

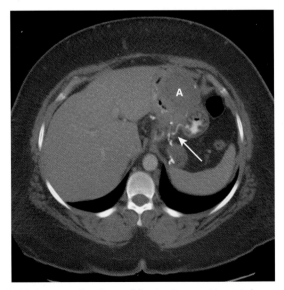

FIGURE 41-12 Postoperative abscess following Roux-en-Y gastric bypass procedure. Computed tomography shows a thick-walled abscess (A) anterior to the anastomotic sutures (*arrow*) in the left upper quadrant.

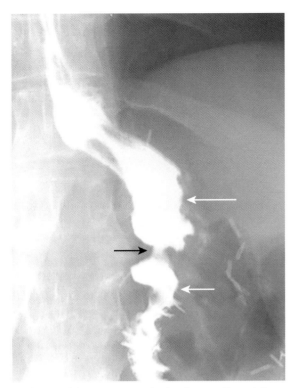

FIGURE 41-13 Gastrojejunostomy stenosis after Roux-en-Y gastric bypass (upper gastrointestinal series). *Long white arrow* indicates gastric pouch; *black arrow* shows gastrojejunostomy stenosis; *short white arrow* indicates proximal Roux loop of jejunum. (From Jha S, Levine MS, Rubesin SE, et al: Detection of strictures on upper gastrointestinal tract radiographic examinations after laparoscopic Roux-en-Y gastric bypass surgery: Importance of projection. *AJR Am J Roentgenol* 186:1090-1093, 2006.)

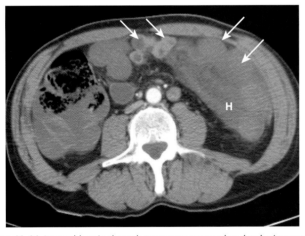

FIGURE 41-14 Internal hernia through transverse mesocolon developing several years after a retrocolic Roux-en-Y gastric bypass procedure, as shown on computed tomography. The *short arrows* indicate clustering of small bowel loops at the mesocolic defect. The *longs arrows* indicate bowel loops that have herniated through the defect; these loops are ischemic (poorly enhancing), and there is hemorrhage (H) in the associated mesentery.

placement of the Roux limb has been shown to be more frequently associated with internal hernia, the antecolic approach has become more popular. Early small bowel obstruction, within 3 days to 3 months of surgery, typically is due to adhesions; an internal hernia generally will develop later.

On upper GI series, an internal hernia may appear as a relatively fixed cluster of small bowel loops seen in the left upper quadrant or midabdomen, with stasis and delayed passage of contrast material. The CT appearance of an internal hernia depends on its location, although abnormal clustering of small

bowel loops and congestion and crowding of the mesenteric vessels are common to all cases. Other signs of internal hernia with CT include swirled appearance of mesenteric fat or vessels, mushroom shape of internal hernia, tubular distal mesenteric fat surrounded by bowel loops, small bowel other than duodenum posterior to the superior mesenteric artery, and right-sided location of the jejunal-jejunal anastomosis.

With an internal hernia of the transverse mesocolon, the cluster of small bowel loops is located posterior to the bypassed stomach and exerts a mass effect on the posterior gastric wall. A hernia through the small bowel mesentery can cause clustering of small bowel loops that are pressed against the anterior abdominal wall, with no overlying omental fat. Peterson-type hernias are very difficult to diagnose and may not be apparent on CT because there is neither a confining border nor a characteristic location. Of note, obstructions resulting from an RYGB operation can result in a closed-loop obstruction with strangulation, which can be lethal. Given the difficulty of diagnosis, it is important to have a high index of suspicion and to closely monitor patients presenting with abdominal pain after RYGB.

Recurrent Weight Gain

Recurrent weight gain can occur for a number of reasons, including disruption of the partitioning staple line of stomach that allows food to flow into the gastric remnant (Fig. 41-15A, B), stretching and volume increase in the gastric pouch (Fig. 41-15C), and widening of the gastrojejunostomy (Fig. 41-15C, D). The causes of these sequelae include patient noncompliance with dietary restrictions, but this is not present in all cases.

Other Complications

As seen in other patients with gastrojejunostomy performed for benign or malignant disease, marginal ulceration can develop on the jejunal side of the anastomosis (Fig. 41-16). Because the collateral mesenteric circulation of the gut is compromised by the formation of the RYGB, vascular compromise of both obstructed and nonobstructed small bowel also may develop (Fig. 41-17).

LAPAROSCOPIC ADJUSTABLE GASTRIC BANDING

Since its approval for use in the United States in 2001, laparoscopic adjustable gastric banding (LAGB) has become an increasingly popular form of bariatric surgery. Under laparoscopic guidance, a band is placed around the proximal portion of the stomach, producing a small gastric pouch. The band is slowly tightened by incremental administration of saline solution through a subcutaneous port into the band, which constricts the band around the stomach and narrows the effective gastric orifice (stoma) through which food may pass. The net effect on the patient is early satiety and weight loss.

Early experience with LAGB in the United States was characterized by frequent complications, including band slippage, esophageal dilation, and stomal stenosis. These complications often necessitated surgical removal of the band and conversion to an RYGB configuration. More recent patient outcomes have since improved substantially, however, as a result of better preoperative screening, improved surgical technique, and more postoperative attention to the individual tailoring of band tightness.

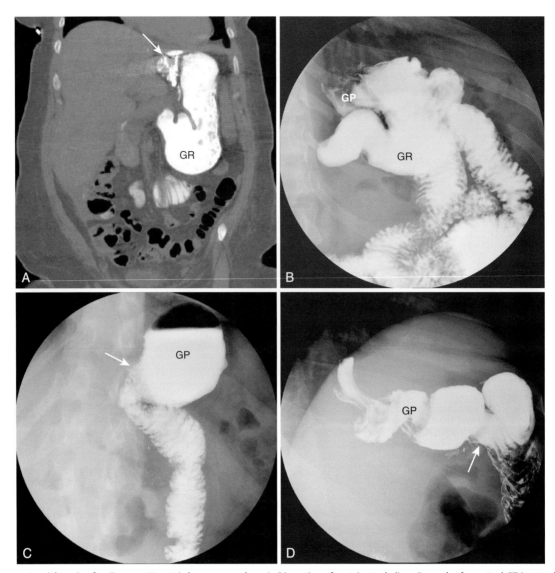

FIGURE 41-15 Recurrent weight gain after Roux-en-Y gastric bypass procedure. **A,** Disruption of gastric staple line. Coronal reformatted CT image showing contrast in both the gastric pouch *(arrow)* and gastric remnant (GR). **B,** Disruption of gastric staple line (upper gastrointestinal [GI] series). Free filling of the GR as well as the proximal jejunum through the gastrojejunostomy. **C,** Stretching and enlargement of both the gastric pouch (GP) and gastrojejunostomy *(arrow)* (upper GI series). **D,** Another example of gastrojejunostomy widening *(arrow)* on an upper GI series.

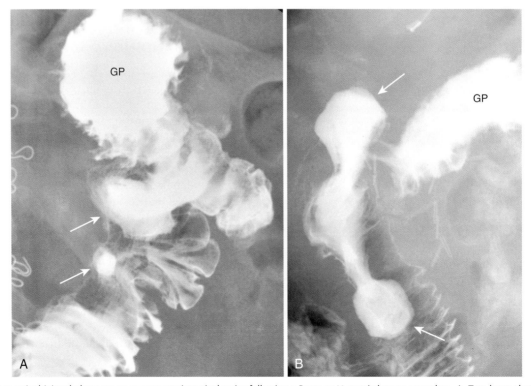

FIGURE 41-16 Giant marginal jejunal ulcers on an upper gastrointestinal series following a Roux-en-Y gastric bypass procedure. **A,** Two large ulcers *(arrows)* are present in the Roux limb just distal to the gastrojejunostomy. **B,** Right posterior oblique image shows two large ulcers *(arrows)* in the Roux limb. Thickened folds also are seen in the proximal jejunum in the region of the more distal ulcer. GP, gastric pouch. (From Ruutiainen AT, Levine MS, Williams NN: Giant jejunal ulcers after Roux-en-Y gastric bypass. *Abdom Imaging* 33:575–578, 2008.)

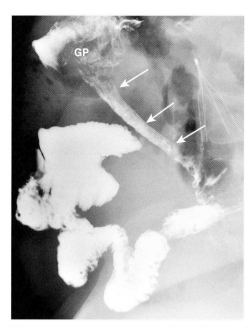

FIGURE 41-17 Ischemic stricture in proximal Roux limb of jejunum (upper gastrointestinal series). *Arrows* indicate a long stricture of the proximal jejunum. A venal caval filter is seen at the upper right. GP, gastric pouch.

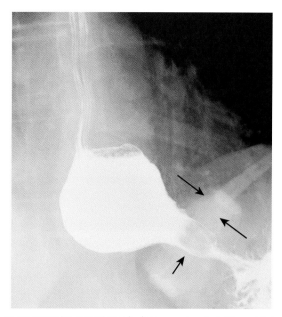

FIGURE 41-18 Excessive constriction by laparoscopic adjustable gastric banding (upper gastrointestinal series). The band *(long arrows)* is causing food impaction *(short arrow)*.

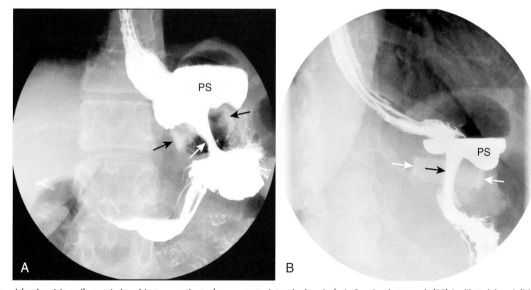

FIGURE 41-19 Slipped (malpositioned) gastric band in two patients (upper gastrointestinal series). **A,** Proximal stomach (PS) is dilated; band *(black arrows)* is positioned transversely, with an overly narrowed stoma *(white arrow)*. **B,** Transversely positioned gastric band *(white arrows)* producing excessive stomal narrowing *(black arrow)* and a dilated PS.

If the LAGB is too loose, then the patient is unlikely to achieve substantial weight loss. Conversely, if the band is too tight (Fig. 41-18), then weight loss may be associated with a variety of obstructive symptoms, including dysphagia, regurgitation, nausea, vomiting, and postprandial substernal and epigastric pain. Some bariatric surgeons perform each band adjustment under fluoroscopic guidance, performing a barium study immediately afterward to assess the tightness of the band. If the band is too tight, then saline can be withdrawn from the band to prevent the development of obstructive symptoms. Other surgeons adjust the band in the office. The decision to add or withdraw saline solution from the band is based on the degree of weight loss and the presence of symptoms suggesting overinflation of the band. In this practice, a follow-up barium study is performed after band adjustment only if obstructive symptoms develop.

In one series, routine fluoroscopic barium studies after LAGB adjustment yielded useful diagnostic information that led to readjustment of the band in 7% of routine adjustments. A stomal diameter less than 6 mm after saline instillation is likely to be associated with obstructive symptoms, so band loosening should be performed. In contrast, a stomal diameter greater than 7 mm is unlikely to be associated with obstructive symptoms, and a diameter of 6 to 7 mm is borderline. A decision to loosen the band in this latter case should be based on the presence or absence of ancillary radiographic findings, such as increased esophageal diameter, pouch dilation, or a prolonged pouch emptying time.

Complications

Early complications of LAGB include malpositioning of the band (Fig. 41-19) and gastric perforation. Regurgitation and pouch esophageal reflux are common early postoperative complications and are exacerbated by dietary noncompliance, but these events persist in patients with insufficient antireflux mechanisms. Radiologic evaluation should determine whether there is (1) obstruction at the site of the band, with an overly narrowed stoma and concentric pouch dilation; (2) eccentric band herniation with concentric pouch dilation; or (3) posterior slippage with eccentric pouch dilation. If none of these complications is identified, then the patient should undergo nutritional counseling to avoid chronic concentric pouch dilation.

Pouch dilation can develop as an early or late complication of LAGB and is classified into three types: (1) acute concentric pouch dilation, (2) chronic concentric pouch dilation, and (3) eccentric pouch dilation. Concentric pouch dilation typically is caused by an overly narrowed stoma and manifests as prestenotic dilation of the proximal fundus. The normal pouch, which should not be larger than 20 mL, can reach dimensions of up to 10 cm in diameter. Rarely, organoaxial volvulus can occur.

Stomal Narrowing

Excessive stomal narrowing most commonly is due to overfilling of the band (Fig. 41-20). Band herniation is a rare cause of acute concentric pouch dilation and manifests as eccentric narrowing of the stoma due to a focal weakness of the band. If the eccentric band herniation occurs superiorly or inferiorly, then the width of the stoma will be underestimated radiographically. If eccentric band herniation occurs anteriorly or posteriorly, however, then the diameter of the stoma will be overestimated. An underestimated stoma probably will lead to a better passage of food with subsequent insufficient weight loss. An overestimated stoma may lead to an overly narrowed stoma with possible concentric pouch dilation. If eccentric band herniation is suspected, then filling of the LAGB system with contrast agent, followed by true en face projections, will be helpful.

If a patient chronically overfills the gastric pouch (i.e., is noncompliant with dietary instructions), then chronic concentric pouch dilation can develop in the presence of a normal stoma. In contrast to an acute concentric pouch dilation, "chronic" concentric pouch dilation is caused by chronic volume overload of the pouch rather than an excessively narrow stoma. The diagnosis of a chronic concentric pouch dilation can be made on the basis of concentric pouch dilation and a normal stomal width.

Eccentric pouch dilation is the third type of pouch abnormality and mostly occurs as a late complication following posterior slippage of the band. Patients present with the same symptoms as with concentric pouch dilation. In cases with severe dislocation of the band (posterior slippage) and extreme eccentric pouch dilation, additional complications, including gastric volvulus (Fig. 41-21), infarction, and penetration, may be observed.

Disconnections

System disconnections are uncommon and can occur at three different locations: (1) at the connection between the port and the catheter; (2) at the connection between the proximal and distal parts of the catheter; and (3) at the connection between the catheter and the band. Disconnection can be caused by manipulation, such as repositioning of the port due to patient discomfort or trauma. Clinically, these patients usually present with insufficient weight loss. Radiographically, this complication is easy to diagnose on a conventional abdominal radiograph. Surgical correction is required.

Transmural Band Penetration

Transmural band penetration (erosion) is a late and rare complication of LAGB surgery. Conditions and events that are associated with band erosion include intraoperative damage of the serosa and outer muscular layers of the gastric wall, nonsteroidal anti-inflammatory drug abuse, and bulimia. A patient with band erosion into the stomach may present with hematemesis that can

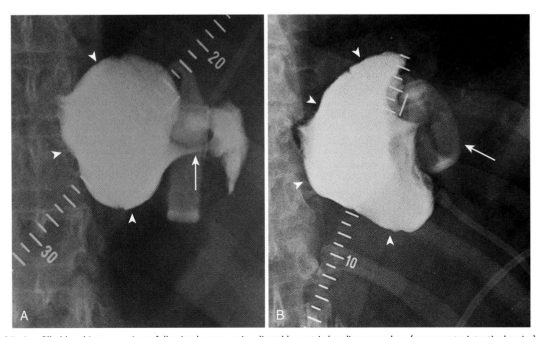

FIGURE 41-20 A and B, Overfilled band in two patients following laparoscopic adjustable gastric banding procedure (upper gastrointestinal series). *Arrowheads* indicate dilated gastric pouch; *arrow* shows luminal narrowing at the level of the band.

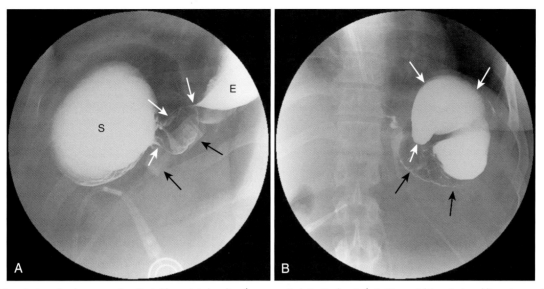

FIGURE 41-21 Gastric volvulus after laparoscopic adjustable gastric banding (upper gastrointestinal series). **A,** Steep right posterior oblique image shows slippage of the band toward the distal stomach (S) with tapered narrowing of the lumen *(small white arrow),* where it traverses the band *(black arrows)* and causes gastric outlet obstruction. A second area of tapered narrowing *(large white arrows)* is present in the distal portion of the esophagus (E) adjacent to the band. **B,** Frontal image from the same examination shows the stomach proximal to the band dilated and rotated so that the gastric body *(large white arrows)* is located above the gastric fundus *(black arrows)* beneath the left hemidiaphragm. Gastric outlet obstruction *(small white arrow)* is present. (From Kicska G, Levine MS, Raper SE, Williams NN: Gastric volvulus after laparoscopic adjustable gastric banding for morbid obesity. *AJR Am J Roentgenol* 189:1469–1472, 2007.)

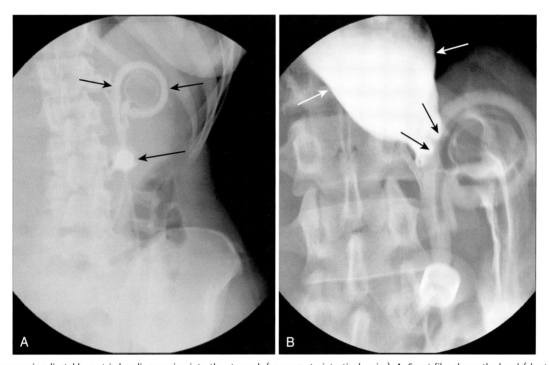

FIGURE 41-22 Laparoscopic adjustable gastric banding erosion into the stomach (upper gastrointestinal series). **A,** Scout film shows the band *(short arrows)* in medial aspect of the left upper quadrant beneath the left hemidiaphragm and connected to the subcutaneous port *(long arrow).* Note vertical orientation of band (instead of the typical transverse-oblique orientation). **B,** Image with contrast demonstrating retrograde migration of the band to the gastroesophageal junction, where it caused high-grade obstruction *(black arrows)* and esophageal dilation *(white arrows).* (From Ruutiainen AT, Levine MS, Dumon K: Intraluminal erosion and retrograde migration of laparoscopic gastric band with high-grade obstruction at gastroesophageal junction. *Surg Obes Relat Dis* April 3, 2010. Epub ahead of print.)

lead to fatal bleeding. On an upper GI series, contrast material outlines the intraluminal portion of the band (Fig. 41-22).

Port Site Infection

As with any implanted foreign body, infection around the port site is another complication of LAGB. Repeated punctures of the port site rarely may lead to a low-grade infection that can be diagnosed at radiographic follow-up. Oral antibiotics usually are sufficient therapy, but occasionally surgical therapy with

local débridement and explantation of the port may be necessary. CT is the preferred means for establishing the diagnosis (Fig. 41-23).

Inadequate Weight Loss

In patients with anatomically optimized bands, unsatisfactory weight loss usually is due to patient noncompliance with dietary instructions, including ingestion of large quantities of calorically dense liquids.

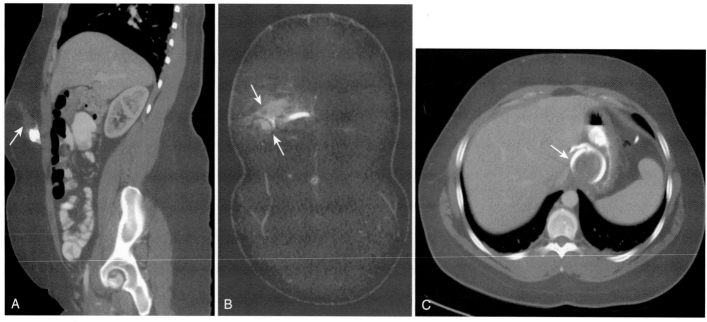

FIGURE 41-23 Infected laparoscopic adjustable gastric banding port. Sagittal **(A)** and coronal **(B)** computed tomography reformatted images show infected fluid *(arrows)* adjacent to the port. **C,** Note the transverse orientation of the band *(arrow)* on the axial image.

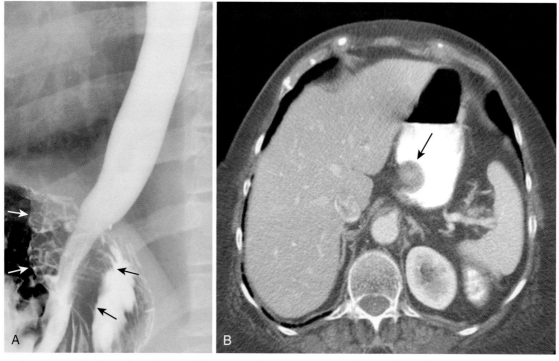

FIGURE 41-24 Normal appearance of a Nissen fundoplication. **A,** Upper gastrointestinal series show the wrap *(arrows)* surrounding the distal esophagus. Note the tapered narrowing of the distal esophagus in the region of the wrap. **B,** Computed tomography scan in a different patient depicts the wrap as a smooth, rounded mass *(arrow)* in the region of the gastroesophageal junction.

FUNDOPLICATION AND HIATAL HERNIA

Laparoscopic procedures with and without mesh commonly are used in the treatment of gastroesophageal reflux and hiatal hernia. The normal appearance of a Nissen wrap on an upper GI series is a large fundal mass with smooth contours and surface. In the steep oblique recumbent position, the distal esophagus smoothly traverses the center of the fundoplication wrap. In contrast to a true fundal mass, the wrap is smooth and symmetrical with a consistent relationship to the distal esophagus (Fig. 41-24). The gastric wrap of a Belsey Mark IV produces a smaller defect than the Nissen fundoplication. The esophagus forms two

distinct angles as it passes through the 270-degree fundoplication. In the Hill procedure, the intra-abdominal esophagus is lengthened, and the angle of His is accentuated. After any successful antireflux procedure, neither a hiatal hernia nor reflux should be seen.

There are a number of well-described temporary and permanent sequelae to these procedures. During the early postoperative period, edema (Fig. 41-25) of the fundoplication wrap may cause transient dysphagia and may be manifested on an upper GI series as a large, smooth fundal mass, along with a smooth, tapered narrowing of the intra-abdominal esophagus and with delayed emptying of contrast material. The edema usually

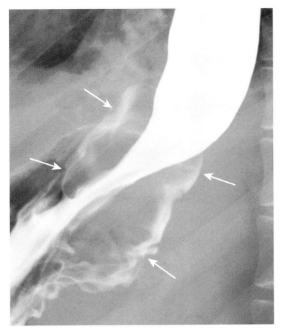

FIGURE 41-25 Edema of the fundoplication wrap in the early postoperative period. Upper gastrointestinal series shows marked enlargement of the wrap *(arrows)*.

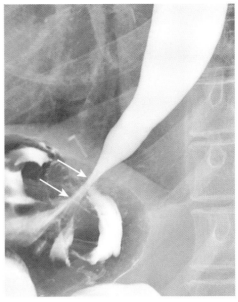

FIGURE 41-26 Esophageal stenosis secondary to an overly tight Nissen wrap (upper gastrointestinal series). *Arrows* indicate narrowed esophageal lumen due to a tight wrap and also to failure of relaxation of the lower esophageal sphincter.

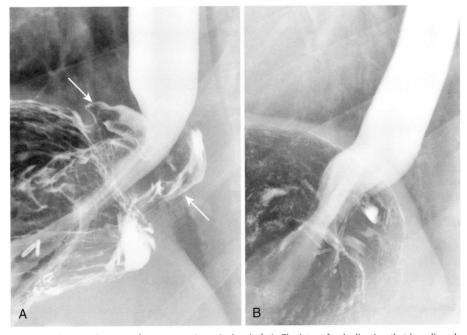

FIGURE 41-27 Various degrees of fundoplication disruption (upper gastrointestinal series). **A,** The intact fundoplication that has slipped so that a portion of the stomach has herniated above the wrap, producing a small hiatal hernia *(arrows)*. **B,** Breakdown of the fundoplication several years after surgery. There is no evidence of a wrap where the esophagus traverses the diaphragm.

subsides after 1 to 2 weeks, and a follow-up esophagram will demonstrate a much smaller defect. Some patients may develop persistent narrowing of the esophagus with dysphagia or the gas-bloat syndrome.

An esophagram also may demonstrate fixed narrowing of the distal esophagus as a result of an overly tight fundoplication wrap or spasm of the lower esophageal sphincter, or both, causing secondary achalasia (Fig. 41-26). Partial disruption of the fundoplication may manifest as a partially intact wrap associated with one or more outpouchings from the gastric fundus or as an hourglass appearance of the stomach as a portion of the fundus slips through the fundoplication (Fig. 41-27A). Disruption of the diaphragmatic sutures (but not the fundoplication sutures) may result in a recurrent hiatal hernia with an intact wrap (Fig. 41-27B). Complete disruption of all sutured tissue presents radiographically as a recurrent hiatal hernia and gastroesophageal reflux without visualization of the fundoplication wrap.

LAPAROSCOPIC SURGERY OF THE HOLLOW VISCERA

Gastrointestinal Tract Malignancies

Accurate tumor localization and preoperative staging are essential in the management of the patient with a gastrointestinal malignancy. Treatment protocols and surgical options are rapidly

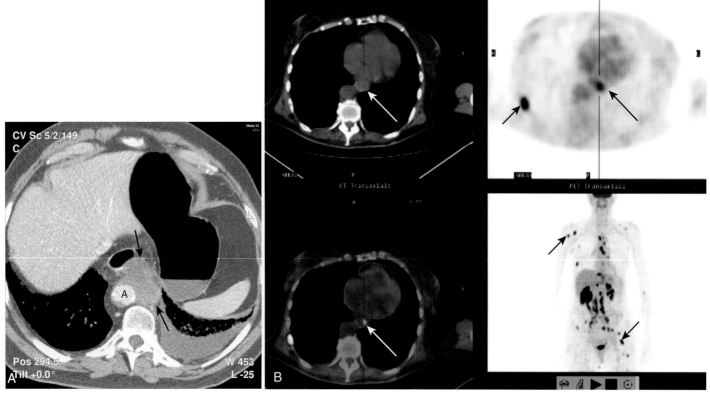

FIGURE 41-28 Adenocarcinoma of the distal esophagus. **A,** Axial computed tomography image demonstrating tumor invasion of the adjacent fat *(arrows)* and distal thoracic aorta (A). **B,** Combined positron emission tomography and computed tomography scan in a different patient shows increased activity in the midesophagus from a squamous cell carcinoma *(long arrows)*. Multiple metastases *(short arrows)* are seen in bone and lymph nodes.

developing for GI oncology patients, and these advances have been matched and partially fueled by the increasing sophistication of the staging capabilities of MDCT, endoscopic ultrasound, transrectal ultrasound, MRI, and PET-CT. These techniques can identify patients with advanced disease who will not benefit from surgery, those with early disease who can be treated by simple mucosal resection, those who will require neoadjuvant therapy, and those who would benefit from a minimally invasive resection.

Esophageal Cancer

When a patient is diagnosed with esophageal cancer (Fig. 41-28), MDCT should be the initial staging tool. It is excellent for the detection of distant metastases and in patients with T3 and T4 lesions. It is less successful, however, in staging N disease and depicting T1 and T2 lesions. Endoscopic ultrasound is superb in diagnosing T1 and T2 disease. PET-CT also is helpful in assessing for the presence or absence of regional and distant lymphadenopathy and metastases. A patient with a T1a N0 esophageal tumor (i.e., confined to the mucosal layer, as opposed to T1b, which invades the submucosa) can undergo mucosal resection, whereas more advanced tumors require more definitive chemotherapy and surgery.

Gastric Cancer

A patient with newly diagnosed gastric cancer (Fig. 41-29) should initially be examined with MDCT. As with esophageal cancer, MDCT is excellent in the detection of distant metastases and in patients with T3 and T4 lesions. It is less successful in staging N disease and depicting T1 and T2 lesions. Endoscopic ultrasound is superb in diagnosing T1 and T2 disease. PET-CT

also is helpful in assessing for the presence or absence of regional and distant lymphadenopathy. A patient with a T1a N0 gastric tumor (confined to the mucosal layer) can undergo mucosal resection, whereas more advanced tumors require more definitive surgery.

Small Bowel Cancer

As with tumors in other portions of the gut, a patient with a small bowel tumor first should undergo MDCT (Fig. 41-30) to locate the tumor, determine the degree of invasion, and assess for the presence of adenopathy or metastases. An octreotide scan also should be performed in the patient with a carcinoid tumor.

Colorectal Cancer

The patient with colon cancer (i.e., not within the rectum) initially should undergo an MDCT of the abdomen and pelvis (Fig. 41-31). This technique is excellent for the detection of metastases, is reasonably good at demonstrating T3 and T4 lesions, and is fair in the depiction of adenopathy. In most cases, no additional preoperative imaging is needed.

The patient with rectal cancer (Fig. 41-32) also should initially undergo MDCT of the chest, abdomen, and pelvis. The chest should be included in this scan because of the higher frequency of pulmonary metastases in patients with rectal cancer. If no regional or distant metastases are identified, transrectal ultrasound is needed to more precisely stage T1 and T2 lesions and to determine N status. In patients with advanced T3 and T4 lesions, MRI is quite accurate in determining the depth of invasion with respect to the mesorectal fascia.

PET-CT also is useful in the detection of metastases to the liver, bone, and lymph nodes that elude detection by

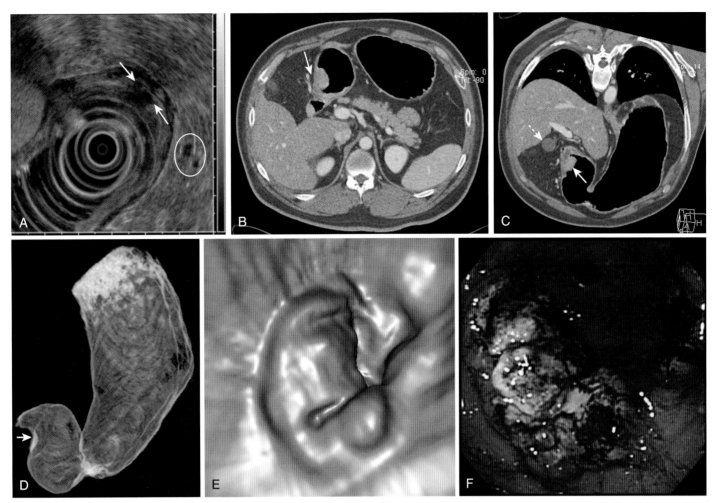

FIGURE 41-29 Gastric cancer. **A,** Endoscopic ultrasound of antral tumor showing tumor invasion of the muscularis propria (hypoechoic layer indicated by *arrows*). Note the spherical, small hypoechoic lymph nodes in the adjacent fat *(oval)*. This tumor likely is T2 N1. **B,** Axial computed tomography (CT) scan shows mural thickening of the distal lesser curvature *(arrow)*. Serosal fat adjacent to the tumor is preserved. **C,** CT image showing an antral mass *(solid arrow)* and enlarged lymph node *(discontinuous arrow)* in the lesser omentum. **D,** Shaded surface display image shows an antral mass deforming the lesser curvature *(arrow)*. Same mass in **D** is shown with virtual endoscopy **(E)** and conventional endoscopy **(F)**. (From Gore RM, Kim JH, Chen C-Y: MDCT, EUS, PET/CT, and MRI in the management of patients with gastric neoplasms. In Gore RM, editor: *Gastric Cancer,* Cambridge, UK, 2010, Cambridge University Press, pp 120–194.)

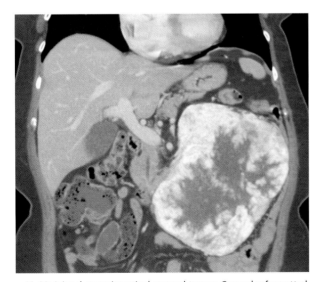

FIGURE 41-30 Jejunal gastrointestinal stromal tumor. Coronal reformatted computed tomography image shows a hypervascular mass in the left upper quadrant.

conventional CT. In addition, PET-CT is superb in detecting recurrent disease in patients with rising carcinoembryonic antigen levels and with normal CT scans. PET-CT also is helpful in patients with limited metastatic disease to the lung and liver, in whom resection (metastectomy) is being considered.

Crohn Disease

Up to 80% of patients with Crohn disease will require operative intervention during the course of their disease. CT and MRI (Fig. 41-33) are the primary noninvasive methods of establishing and staging small bowel disease and guiding medical, surgical, and interventional radiology therapy.

Diverticular Disease

In recent years, laparoscopic resection methods have been applied successfully to diverticulitis of the colon. CT is the primary means of establishing the diagnosis of diverticulitis and associated complications such as intra-abdominal abscess (Fig. 41-34), bowel obstruction, fistula, sinus tracts, pyelophlebitis, and liver abscess. CT also is helpful in the guidance of percutaneous abscess drainage.

Laparoscopic Appendectomy

Although somewhat controversial, laparoscopic appendectomy is believed to have benefits over open appendectomy, including a shorter length of hospital stay, less postoperative pain, earlier postoperative recovery, and a lower complication rate. CT is the gold standard in establishing the diagnosis of appendicitis (Fig. 41-35) and also in the detection of complications such as abscess,

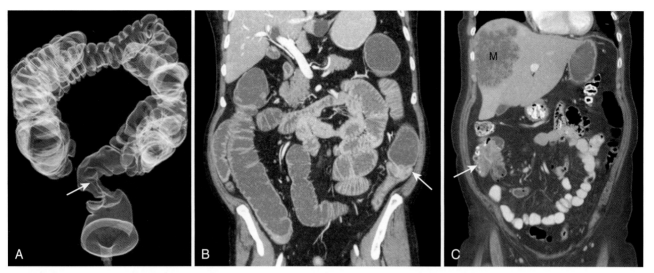

FIGURE 41-31 Colon cancer. **A,** Volume-rendered three-dimensional multidetector computed tomography (CT) image from a CT colonography study, demonstrating an annular constricting lesion of the rectosigmoid junction *(arrow)*. **B,** Obstructing cancer *(arrow)* in the descending colon (coronal reformatted CT image). The obstructed colon and small bowel are fluid filled. **C,** Cecal carcinoma *(arrow)* with a large liver metastasis (M) is shown (coronal reformatted CT image).

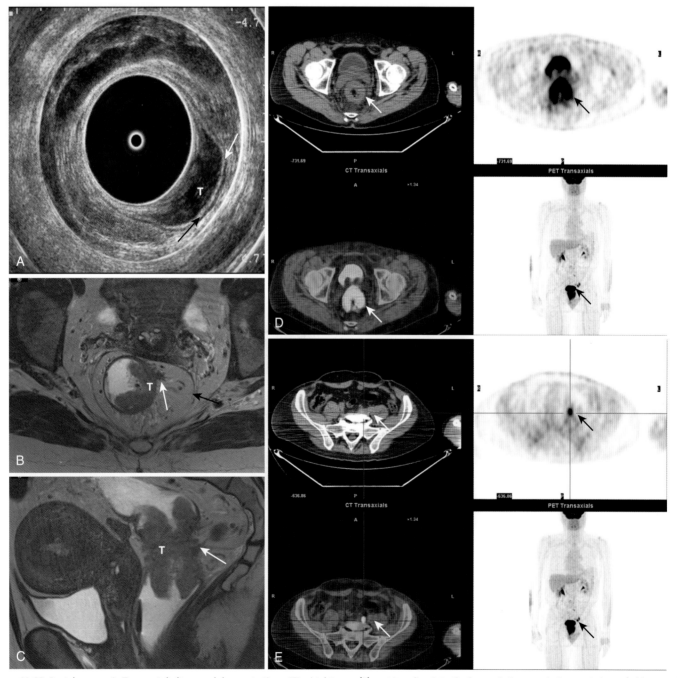

FIGURE 41-32 Rectal cancer. **A,** Transrectal ultrasound demonstrating a T1 rectal tumor (T), not invading into the hypoechoic muscularis propria layer *(white arrow)*. *Black arrow* indicates echogenic submucosa. Axial **(B)** and sagittal **(C)** magnetic resonance images from a different patient demonstrating a T3 rectal cancer (T) invading the mesorectal fat *(white arrows)*. Note that the tumor does not involve the mesorectal fascia *(black arrow)*. **D,** Combined positron emission tomography and computed tomography (PET-CT) scan showing a large PET-avid rectal cancer *(arrows)*. **E,** PET-CT scan in the same patient showing a normal-sized but PET-avid left common iliac lymph node *(arrows),* representing nodal metastasis.

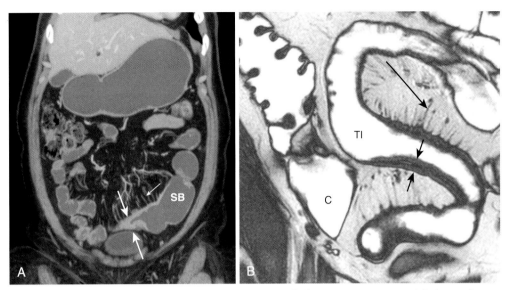

FIGURE 41-33 Crohn disease. **A,** Coronal reformatted image from a computed tomography (CT) enterogram shows mural thickening *(large arrows)* and stenosis of the proximal ileum, associated with engorgement of the vasa rectae *(small arrow)* and dilation of the proximal small bowel (SB). **B,** Coronal image from a magnetic resonance enterography study in a different patient demonstrates mural thickening *(short arrows)* of the terminal ileum (TI) and engorgement of the vasa rectae *(long arrow)*. C, cecum.

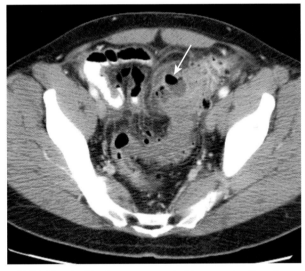

FIGURE 41-34 Diverticulitis shown on computed tomography. There is mural thickening of the sigmoid colon, associated with inflammatory changes in the sigmoid mesocolon and a gas-containing abscess *(arrow)*.

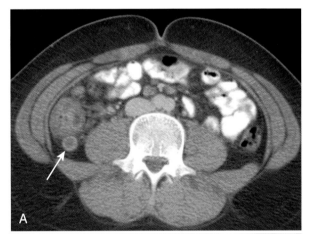

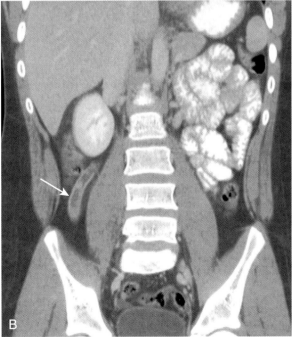

FIGURE 41-35 Uncomplicated appendicitis. Axial **(A)** and coronal reformatted **(B)** multidetector computed tomography images demonstrating a dilated (8.9 mm), retrocecal appendix filled with fluid and debris *(arrows)*.

bowel obstruction, and fistula. If the patient has an appendiceal abscess, then percutaneous drainage (Fig. 41-36) under CT guidance should be considered before appendectomy in order to decrease the risk for postoperative morbidity.

HERNIA

Hernia of the abdominal wall (i.e., ventral and groin regions) is a frequent finding on cross-sectional imaging studies. Complications from surgical repair (both open and laparoscopic), including hernia recurrence, postoperative mesh infection (Fig. 41-37), and various other sequelae of prosthetic materials, may occur in up to 20% of cases. About one half of these complications may require surgical intervention, and MDCT is the primary means of diagnosing these complications.

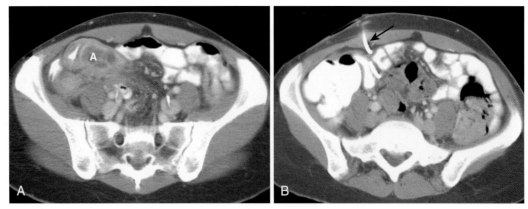

FIGURE 41-36 Appendicitis with abscess. **A,** Computed tomography scan showing a right lower quadrant abscess (A) secondary to appendicitis. **B,** Abscess after percutaneous drainage; *arrow* indicates catheter.

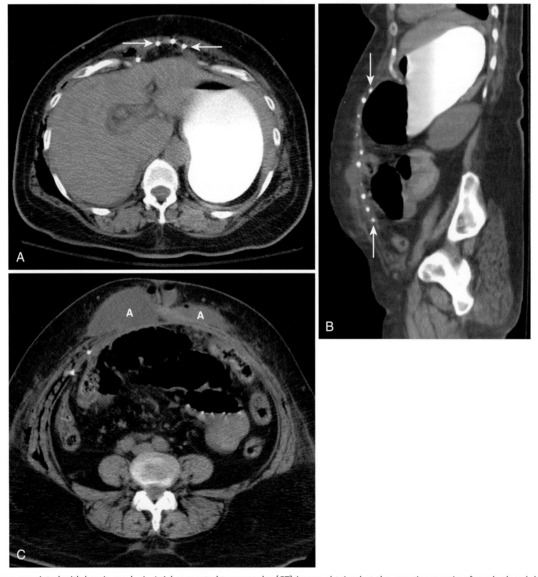

FIGURE 41-37 Abscess associated with hernia mesh. **A,** Axial computed tomography (CT) image obtained at the superior margin of mesh placed during a ventral hernia repair *(arrows)*. **B,** Sagittal reformatted CT image shows the superior/inferior extent of the mesh *(arrows)*. **C,** Axial CT image obtained near a port insertion site shows a complex abscess (A) with air-fluid levels.

Hernia recurrence is the most common complication of hernia repair. Some retrospective studies have suggested that hernia recurrence is less common after laparoscopic repair (up to 7.5% recurrence rate, universal mesh placement) compared with open repair (up to 30% without mesh placement, or up to 10% with mesh placement). MDCT can be the best means of detecting a recurrent hernia because clinical evaluation may be limited owing to the existence of fibrosis or obesity.

A fluid collection (seromas or hematomas) may develop in up to 17% of cases in the immediate postoperative period after hernia repair with mesh. The formation of a collection is related to both the surgical technique and the properties of the particular mesh employed. CT may help identify a fluid collection, differentiate it from a hernia recurrence, and follow it to resolution. A postoperative fluid collection on MDCT studies can have a globular, tubular, or multilobular appearance. Some collections may be loculated with enhancing rims, whereas others may contain air-fluid levels, resemble bowel loops, or even be mistaken for recurrent hernias.

Most seromas resolve spontaneously within 30 days. If the collection persists for more than 6 weeks, steadily grows, produces symptoms, or shows signs of infection, aspiration under imaging guidance should be considered. Image-guided aspiration or drainage may be problematic for large collections located underneath the mesh and may require multiple small-diameter drainage catheters.

Infected postoperative fluid collections develop in 1% to 5% of patients after hernia repair and occur more frequently in older female patients, especially after surgical repair of strangulated and incarcerated hernia. Infected collections tend to present early in the postoperative period (<2 weeks after operation) and constitute an important risk factor for hernia recurrence. The following findings are suspicious for an infected fluid collection: the development of gas or thick septa in a previous "simple" collection; an enhancing rim; fat stranding in surrounding tissues; or the development of a new collection 1 week or more after repair. CT findings alone may not completely characterize the nature of a fluid collection, so imaging-guided aspiration may be needed to establish the diagnosis.

An infected fluid collection may be subcutaneous (superficial) or may involve the mesh (deep). Differentiation in this regard is important because a superficial infection is managed conservatively (e.g., oral antibiotics), whereas a deep infection will require percutaneous drainage or mesh explantation.

An inflammatory reaction to the mesh may lead to fibrosis of the surrounding tissue. This condition may be suspected if the mesh has an asymmetrical or irregular shape on CT. Mesh shrinkage also may occur in this situation. If the mesh is exposed to the peritoneal cavity, then intraperitoneal adhesions may develop, predisposing to small bowel obstruction. Less frequently, the mesh may detach from supporting tissues and migrate within the abdominal wall.

CONCLUSION

State-of-the-art MDCT, MRI, transabdominal ultrasound, endoscopic ultrasound, transrectal ultrasound, and PET-CT are leading to the earlier detection, better characterization, and improved staging of abdominal and pelvic disease. These technical improvements in imaging have been accompanied by equally innovative advances in minimally invasive surgery. Cross-sectional imaging remains the linchpin in individualizing patient treatment by helping to determine which patients will benefit from minimally invasive surgery and by playing a vital role in the diagnosis and treatment of postoperative complications.

Suggested Readings

Aguirre DA, Santosa AC, Casola G, Sirlin CB: Abdominal wall hernias: Imaging features, complications, and diagnostic pitfalls at multi-detector row CT, *Radiographics* 25:1501–1520, 2005.

Ascher SM, Evans SRT, Zeman RK: Laparoscopic cholecystectomy: Intraoperative ultrasound of the extrahepatic biliary tree and the natural history of postoperative transabdominal ultrasound findings, *Semin Ultrasound CT MRI* 14:331–337, 1993.

Blachar A, Blank A, Gavert N, et al: Laparoscopic adjustable gastric banding surgery for morbid obesity: Imaging of normal anatomic features and postoperative gastrointestinal complications, *AJR Am J Roentgenol* 188:472–479, 2007.

Blachar A, Federle MP: Gastrointestinal complications of laparoscopic Roux-en-Y gastric bypass surgery in patients who are morbidly obese: findings on radiography and CT, *AJR Am J Roentgenol* 179:1437–1442, 2002.

Blachar A, Federle MP, Pealer KM, et al: Radiographic manifestations of normal postoperative anatomy and gastrointestinal complications of bariatric surgery, with emphasis on CT imaging findings, *Semin Ultrasound CT MRI* 22:239–251, 2004.

Chandler RC, Srinivas G, Chintapalli KN, et al: Imaging in bariatric surgery: A guide to postsurgical anatomy and common complications, *AJR Am J Roentgenol* 190:122–135, 2008.

Chol JS, Madura JA: The role of minimally invasive treatments in surgical oncology, *Surg Clin North Am* 89:53–57, 2009.

Daly B, Sukumar SA, Krebs TL, et al: Nonbiliary laparoscopic gastrointestinal surgery: Role of CT in diagnosis and management of complications, *AJR Am J Roentgenol* 167:455–459, 1996.

Davidoff AM, Branum GD, Meyers WC: Clinical features and mechanisms of major laparoscopic biliary injury, *Semin Ultrasound CT MRI* 14:338–345, 1993.

Gayer B, Weinstein D, Hertz M, Zissin R: Postsurgical and traumatic lesions of the biliary tract. In Gore RM, Levine MS, editors: *Textbook of Gastrointestinal Radiology*, Philadelphia, 2008, Elsevier-Saunders, 1505–1516.

Gore RM, Berlin JW, Miller FH, et al: Esophageal cancer. In Husband JE, Reznek RH, editors: *Imaging in Oncology*, ed 3, London, 2010, Informa Healthcare, pp 127–158.

Gore RM, Ghahremani GG, Marn CS: Hernias and abdominal wall pathology. In Gore RM, Levine MS, editors: *Textbook of Gastrointestinal Radiology*, ed 3, Philadelphia, 2008, Elsevier-Saunders, pp 2149–2178.

Gore RM, Kim JH, Chen C-Y: MDCT, EUS, PET/CT, and MRI in the management of patients with gastric neoplasms. In Gore RM, editor: *Gastric Cancer*. Cambridge, UK, 2010, Cambridge University Press, pp 120–194.

Gore RM, Masselli G, Caroline DF: Crohn's disease of the small bowel. In Gore RM, Levine MS, editors: *Textbook of Gastrointestinal Radiology*, ed 3, Philadelphia, 2008, Elsevier-Saunders, pp 781–806.

Gore RM, Mehta UK, Berlin JW, et al: Diagnosis and staging of small bowel tumors, *Cancer Imaging* 29:209–212, 2006.

Gore RM, Thakrar KH, Newmark GM, et al: Gallbladder imaging, *Gastroenterol Clin N Am* 39:265–287, 2010.

Gore RM, Yaghmai V, Balthazar E: Diverticular disease of the colon. In Gore RM, Levine MS, editors: *Textbook of Gastrointestinal Radiology*, ed 3, Philadelphia, 2008, Elsevier-Saunders, pp 1019–1038.

Jacobs JE, Balthazar EJ: Diseases of the appendix. In Gore RM, Levine MS, editors: *Textbook of Gastrointestinal Radiology*, ed 3, Philadelphia, 2008, Elsevier-Saunders, pp 1039–1070.

Jha S, Levine MS, Rubesin SE, et al: Detection of strictures on upper gastrointestinal tract radiographic examinations after laparoscopic Roux-en-Y gastric bypass surgery: Importance of projection, *AJR Am J Roentgenol* 186:1090–1093, 2006.

Kicska G, Levine MS, Raper SE, Williams NN: Gastric volvulus after laparoscopic adjustable gastric banding for morbid obesity, *AJR Am J Roentgenol* 189:1469–1472, 2007.

Kim JY, Kim KW, Ahn C-S, et al: Spectrum of biliary and nonbiliary complications of laparoscopic cholecystectomy, *AJR Am J Roentgenol* 191:783–789, 2008.

Martel G, Boushey RP: Laparoscopic colon surgery: Past, present and future, *Surg Clin North Am* 89:867–897, 2006.

McGahan JP, Stein M: Complications of laparoscopic cholecystectomy: Imaging and intervention, *AJR Am J Roentgenol* 165:1089–1097, 1995.

Mehanna MJ, Birjawi G, Moukaddam HA, et al: Complications of adjustable gastric banding, a radiological pictorial review, *AJR Am J Roentgenol* 186:522–534, 2006.

Milsom JW: Laparoscopic surgery in the treatment of Crohn's disease, *Surg Clin North Am* 85:25–34, 2005.

Morrin MM, Kruskal JB, Hochman MG, et al: Radiologic features of complications arising from dropped gallstones in laparoscopic cholecystectomy patients, *AJR Am J Roentgenol* 174:1441–1445, 2000.

Ruutiainen AT, Levine MS, Williams NN: Giant jejunal ulcers after Roux-en-Y gastric bypass, *Abdom Imaging* 33:575–578, 2008.

Sandrasegaran K, Rajesh A, Lall C, et al: Gastrointestinal complications of bariatric Roux-en-Y gastric bypass surgery, *Eur Radiol* 15:254–262, 2005.

Silver R, Levine MS, Williams NN, Rubesin SE: Using radiography to reveal chronic jejunal ischemia as a complication of gastric bypass surgery, *AJR Am J Roentgenol* 181:1365–1367, 2003.

Swenson DW, Levine MS, Rubesin, et al: Utility of routine barium studies after adjustments of laparoscopically inserted gastric bands, *AJR Am J Roentgenol* 194:129–135, 2010.

Thoeni RF, Laufer I: Polyps and colon cancer. In Gore RM, Levine MS, editors: *Textbook of Gastrointestinal Radiology*, ed 3, Philadelphia, 2008, Elsevier-Saunders, pp 1121–1166.

Wehrli NE, Levine MS, Rubesin SE, et al: Secondary achalasia and other esophageal motility disorders after laparoscopic Nissen fundoplication for gastroesophageal reflux disease, *AJR Am J Roentgenol* 189:1464–1468, 2007.

Wiesner W, Schob O, Hauser RS, Hauser M: Adjustable laparoscopic gastric banding in patients with morbid obesity, *AJR Am J Roentgenol* 216:389–394, 2000.

Woodfield CA, Levine MS: The postoperative stomach, *Eur J Radiol* 253:341–352, 2005.

Wright TB, Bertino RB, Bishop AF, et al: Complications of laparoscopic cholecystectomy and their interventional radiologic management, *Radiographics* 13:119–128, 1993.

Yoo C, Levine MS, Redfern RO, et al: Laparoscopic Heller myotomy and fundoplication: Findings and predictive value of early postoperative radiographic studies, *Abdom Imaging* 29:643–647, 2004.

Yu J, Turner MA, Cho SR, et al: Normal anatomy and complications after gastric bypass surgery: Helical CT findings, *Radiology* 231:753–760, 2004.

Surgical Robotics

ELIZABETH M. SCHMIDT, ROBERT E. S. BOWEN, AND DMITRY OLEYNIKOV

The videos associated with this chapter are listed in the Video Contents and can be found on the accompanying DVDs and on Expertconsult.com.

Surgical robotics is a rapidly developing field in which new prototypes are developed on a regular basis by laboratories worldwide. The practical applications have remained relatively few in number. In 2011, surgical robotic devices approved by the U.S. Food and Drug Administration (FDA) and available for hospital use in the United States included the following: (1) the da Vinci Surgical System (approved in 2000); (2) the orthopedic systems ROBODOC and the Mako Rio System (approved in 2008 and 2009, respectively); (3) the CyberKnife radiosurgical system, (approved in 2001); and (4) the cardiac ablation system Sensei (approved in 2009). In addition, a variety of laparoscope holders also have become available. In the near future, however, the array of approved devices should increase. Currently, there are devices under development that expand robotic capabilities for some subspecialties or address the basic limitations of current robotic applications.

Limitations of robotic surgery have included space requirements imposed by the robots, both on the floor of the operating room and in the working space above the operative field. In addition, the generally poor haptic feedback that characterizes contemporary robotic technology has required the surgeon to rely on the interpretation of visual clues when applying force to tissue. Another limitation has been the number of degrees of freedom (DOF), or motion capabilities, that the surgical robot has possessed. As a standard of comparison, the human arm has 7 DOF. Simpler robots with 3 DOF or less are limited to simpler tasks such as camera holding. More complex robots with greater DOF can mimic the human hand and also eliminate the tremor that can accompany hand articulation.

Emerging trends in robotic surgery have included the development of systems with reduced size, improved haptic feedback, expanded operative capability, and greater independence. The last trend may eventually eliminate the need for a surgeon in some cases. Although an exhaustive review of the complex engineering, computer science, and material science required to make these machines is beyond the scope of this chapter, we do discuss some of the newer trends in robotic surgery as they apply to care providers in general and to cardiac, urologic, otolaryngologic, and gynecologic surgery.

GENERAL SURGERY

In the future, the general surgeon may find an operating room robot capable of (1) assisting in procedures that formerly required human assistants, (2) augmenting surgeon capabilities, and (3) performing autonomous procedures. A *surgical assist device* is defined as a tool that aids a surgeon without offering increased capabilities or augmenting surgical skill. Much as a human assistant does, a surgical assist device frees the surgeon to operate at peak skill level by performing tedious tasks ancillary to the primary procedure. Unlike their human counterparts, robots do not suffer from tremor, fatigue, or inconsistency. A *surgeon augmentation device* is defined as a tool that enhances the performance of the surgical procedure. Probably the most well-known example of an augmentation device is the da Vinci Surgical System (Intuitive Surgical, Sunnyvale, Calif.). Augmentation devices are designed to provide improved visualization, increased precision, and reduced invasiveness.

CoBRASurge

The University of Nebraska Medical Center for Advanced Surgical Technology (our laboratory), in association with the University of Nebraska—Lincoln Department of Mechanical Engineering, has created a robot for surgical assistance. The CoBRASurge (Complex Bevel-geared Robot for Advanced Surgery) is a small device for laparoscope tool movement and placement that consists of a compact table-mounted robot with multiple gears and a joystick for movement and control (Fig. 42-1). It uses a bevel-geared mechanism and a spherical mechanism that allow the tools and laparoscope to center on a specific point in space, namely, the trocar. The device mounts to the operating room table, so it does not require floor space. The robot can control a laparoscopic camera and articulated robotic graspers. In its current application, it is controlled from a joystick across the room. Our plans are to engender surgeon control of the robot with a foot joystick. The compact design of this robot allows increased room around the operating table for personnel and instruments.

Laparoscope Soft Tissue Scanner

The laparoscopic soft tissue scanner developed by Vanderbilt University's Medical and Electromechanical Design Laboratory permits preoperative scanning of soft tissue for three-dimensional (3D) image generation that would facilitate instrument placement and needle guidance. This technology could be used for biopsy or tumor excision from deep tissue beds with minimal

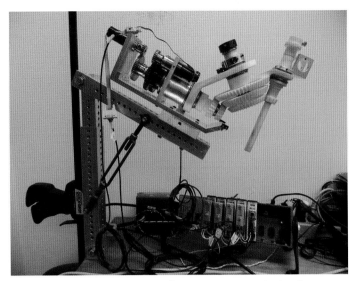

FIGURE 42-1 The CoBRASurge device (Complex Bevel-geared Robot for Advanced Surgery) from the University of Nebraska.

damage to normal tissue. Previous systems with the capability of soft tissue scanning required an open incision to obtain accurate tissue imaging. The small size of the Vanderbilt robot permits surface registration to occur through a single laparoscopic port. The scanner consists of a laser distance device and an optical tracking device and uses conoscopic holography to match scanned tissue point clouds with preoperative 3D computed tomography. This combination allows the surgeon to know organ and tissue placement without requiring substantial soft tissue excavation. It also allows for tissue surface scanning without the need for a large incision or contact with the organ in question, thus eliminating the possibility of contact deformation. Testing with artificial organs (e.g., for liver biopsy) has demonstrated the accuracy of the Vanderbilt robot. This device also may be useful for liver-directed therapy, such as radiofrequency ablation for liver metastasis from colorectal cancer. The Vanderbilt robot furthers the integration of radiologic imaging with virtual operative planning using a minimally invasive approach.

Endoscopy

Current limitations of endoscopy include the need for patient sedation as well as the physical constraints of the endoscope. Capsule endoscopy can be used to examine the whole of the gastrointestinal tract, including the small intestine, which is largely out of the reach of the conventional endoscope. Capsule endoscopes such as the commercially available PillCam (Given Imaging, Duluth, Ga.) are examples of wireless capsule endoscopy (WCE). Currently, WCE relies on the peristaltic action of the gut for anterograde capsule propulsion. There is no capability to guide the camera, revisit a site of interest for photography, or perform a biopsy. Additionally, there currently is no ability to locate the endoscope or identified pathologic process with reasonable precision. There are other WCE devices in development that seek to address these limitations.

VECTOR Capsule Endoscope

The aim of the VECTOR project (Versatile Endoscopic Capsule for gastrointestinal TumOr Recognition and therapy) is to develop a mobile endoscopic robot with future surgical applications. The project currently includes 19 university laboratory participants

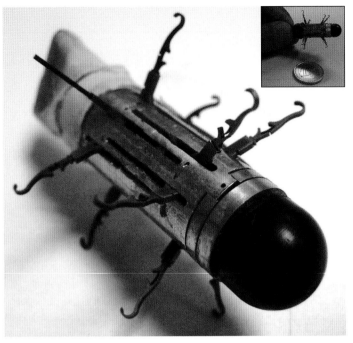

FIGURE 42-2 The original VECTOR capsule. The motorized legs fold out from the main body and allow the capsule to "crawl" along the intestine. (Photo courtesy of P. Valdastri, Center for Research in Microengineering [CRIM], Italy, and R. J. Webster III, Vanderbilt MEDLab.)

in Europe, including the Center for Research in Microengineering (CRIM) in Italy, with input from Vanderbilt University's MED lab. The original VECTOR prototype consisted of a cylindrical body with a camera and two motorized sets of six legs that unfolded from the body of the robot to interact with the intestinal wall (Fig. 42-2). These legs allowed the robot to "walk" insect-like along a small distance in the intestine. The legs are made of heat-treated nitinol, a flexible nickel-titanium alloy with elastic properties designed to reduce the risk for perforation. The robot was engineered to permit passage through a deflated colon in order to reduce one of the main sources of pain from gastrointestinal imaging procedures (i.e., an insufflated colon). This ability is partially facilitated by the robot's unique leg design. The 12 legs are capable of independent motion, which can aid in tight turns, such as the splenic flexure. The robot has been successfully tested in a porcine model. The VECTOR robot may represent an improvement on current swallowable endoscopes because of its movement control and possible future augmentation with accessories, such as for biopsy.

As part of the VECTOR project, the CRIM laboratory has developed other prototype WCEs with the ability to steer and even deploy hemostatic clips. One of their WCEs is equipped with internal permanent magnets that can be steered externally by a magnet on an industrial robotic arm. Although this device also can be controlled manually, the researchers found that robotic control offered greater precision, albeit at the expense of longer procedure times. The WCE has been shown experimentally to be capable of maneuvering in the porcine colon, including against colonic peristalsis. The current prototype measures 14×38 mm (too large to swallow), but the laboratory expects the next generation to be miniaturized sufficiently to allow a patient to ingest. Unlike the VECTOR, the magnet-steered device does require some degree of insufflation, but nevertheless, the latter has shown promise as a practical steered WCE device. A similar device also has been developed that can deploy a nitinol clip to a bleeding site; this has been tested in the porcine intestine.

Other steering mechanisms under development at the CRIM include a swallowable capsule that can navigate the fluid-distended stomach through the use of four propellers. All four propellers are contained at the "rear" of the capsule in order to minimize the risk to the esophagus during swallowing. Simultaneous activation of two ipsilateral propellers is the basis of the steering mechanism. The capsule has been tested successfully in the porcine stomach. The novelty of the propeller-driven "submarine" device relates back to the fact that a typical camera capsule cannot fully investigate gastric disease before the capsule passes through the pylorus. Current capsule cameras cannot be steered to areas of interest in the stomach. The propeller-driven device eventually may provide a workable solution to gastric capsule endoscopy.

Therapeutic Capsule Endoscope

Carnegie Mellon's NanRobotics Laboratory is currently developing a capsule endoscope that can stop and reorient itself during passage through the gastrointestinal system. The robot consists of a cylindrical body with three legs extending from the sides; the legs are covered with a micropatterned elastomer adhesive designed to mimic the feet of a gecko so that the robot can "stick" to the walls of the gut (Fig. 42-3). The legs, when activated, open outward and come in contact with the intestinal lining, causing increased friction and decreasing capsule velocity. Once the area of interest has been examined and biopsied, the legs then peel off, permitting anterograde movement. Further plans for this robot include tools for biopsy and cauterization.

SILS and NOTES Applications

Efforts to accomplish single-incision laparoscopic surgery (SILS), laparoendoscopic single-site surgery (LESS), and natural orifice transluminal endoscopic surgery (NOTES) have presented new challenges to the surgeon. Restricting surgical instruments to one incision, whether in the abdominal or intestinal wall, limits triangulation and visualization. In addition, a NOTES procedure requires flexibility to snake through a natural lumen, but then stiffness to provide an operative platform once the target site is reached. The operating instrument remains bound by the fulcrum effect of one insertion site. Articulating instruments can help, but current iterations allow only modest and relatively stiff articulation; new and improved instrumentation is necessary in this discipline. The robots described later in this chapter attempt to address these needs and to facilitate the performance of single-incision minimally invasive surgical procedures.

ARES (Assembling Reconfigurable Endoluminal Surgical System)

The ARES robot (Fig. 42-4), developed by a consortium of European universities and laboratories, was designed for transgastric surgical applications and represents an attempt to address some of the limitations of endoscopic or natural orifice procedures. The robot consists of multiple modular units molded from an acrylic photopolymer. The current module size is 36.5 mm in length and 15.4 mm in diameter, or about the size of a current "pill cam." These dimensions are designed to allow the patient to swallow the modules. Once in the stomach, the robot undergoes magnetic self-assembly. The researchers have demonstrated a 74% success rate for self-assembly in a model stomach. The robot's placement potentially could be tracked by ultrasonic emissions from one of the modules. Power would be supplied by an onboard battery or with electromagnetic induction. Currently, the design requires a number of modifications to be usable in human surgery.

SPRINT (Single-Port Laparoscopy Bimanual Robot)

Multiple laboratories are working on robots to assist with NOTES and SILS. A consortium of 11 university laboratories and companies in Europe have developed a bimanual robot for single-port laparoscopy, the SPRINT device, which consists of a two separate

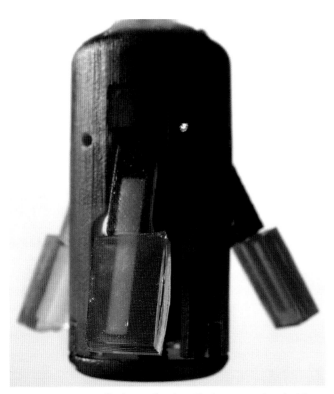

FIGURE 42-3 Carnegie Mellon's capsule robot. The legs are equipped with micropatterned elastomer adhesives to allow adherence to the intestinal wall. (Photo courtesy of M. Sitti, NanoRobotics Laboratory, Carnegie Mellon University.)

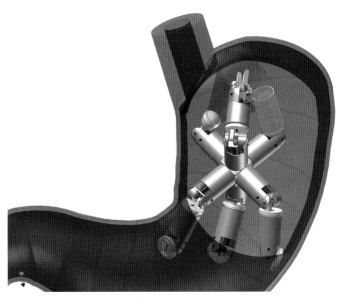

FIGURE 42-4 The ARES device (Assembling Reconfigurable Endoluminal Surgical System) shown assembled within the stomach. (Courtesy of Dr. Kanako Harada.)

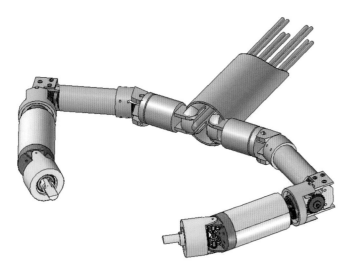

FIGURE 42-5 SPRINT (Single-Port Laparoscopy Bimanual Robot). The arms are capable of 7 degrees of freedom, and the central channel allows for additional equipment passage. (Courtesy of M. Piccigallo, Center for Research in Microengineering, Italy.)

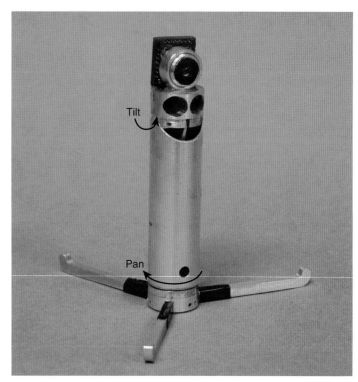

FIGURE 42-6 The pan-and-tilt imaging robot of the University of Nebraska.

camera mechanisms (one panoramic and one stereoscopic) in addition to two articulating arms with 7 DOF each (including tool action) (Fig. 42-5). This system is unique in its ability to insert the robotic arms through the cylindrical access port after the port has been inserted into the abdomen. The robotic arms can be removed and reinserted without removal of the port. This allows for tool changes and repairs, without compromising the position of the remaining arms.

The SPRINT device permits up to four arms to be inserted. Accessory arms in development include a stereoscopic camera holder and a retractor. After the arms have been inserted, there remains a 12-mm central lumen that permits equipment passage (e.g., a sponge for hemostasis) without interrupting the work of the arms. This robot is also being considered for natural orifice surgery. Although this consortium is not the only group that is developing a robot for single-port laparoscopy, the SPRINT device is unique because (1) it permits easy tool transitions, (2) it provides multiple visual components for interpreting the surgical field, and (3) it uses stereoscopic vision with the camera positioned between the two arms.

Mobile Miniature In Vivo Robots

Although most of the robots designed for NOTES focus on access through a single port, we and other researchers at the University of Nebraska—Lincoln and University of Nebraska Medical Center have developed small mobile robots that are deployable within the abdominal cavity. These miniature in vivo robots are capable of providing imaging through onboard cameras as well as tissue manipulation and retraction. Unlike many of their counterparts, they are by definition not restricted by the port size or position because they are not tethered to or in it. Because they can be repositioned, both triangulation and visibility are adjustable. These miniature robots are designed to be either fixed base or mobile. They can be used independently or cooperatively.

One iteration is the pan-and-tilt imaging robot (Fig. 42-6), which has a fixed base. With a diameter of 15 mm, this conical robot can be inserted through a laparoscopic trocar into a strategic position within the peritoneal cavity. Retractable spring-loaded legs then may be abducted to provide stability.

Light-emitting diodes (LEDs) provide illumination for visualization through the onboard adjustable-focus camera. The pan-and-tilt robot can pan 360 degrees with its camera and tilt to 45 degrees. It also can be easily repositioned to accommodate the surgeon's needs.

The pan-and-tilt robot's performance has been tested during porcine laparoscopic cholecystectomy as well as canine prostatectomy. The robot was inserted through a small abdominal incision, and the visualization obtained was used to guide the placement of additional trocars. Secondary views provided by the robot enhanced the visualization provided by the laparoscope. Because visualization and depth perception are some of the limitations of current NOTES technology, the ability to provide enhanced views through this robot may make these procedures safer.

Although the pan-and-tilt robot is stationary, the mobile in vivo imaging robot is designed to navigate the smooth and pliant terrain of the peritoneal cavity using two independently driven helical-profiled wheels. This design provides sufficient traction without creating trauma to the underlying tissue. With dimensions of 15 × 75 mm, the mobile robot can be inserted through a small incision in the abdominal wall or organ. As such, it might provide the sole visualization for a laparoscopic or NOTES procedure. It has been tested successfully as the sole source of visual feedback during porcine cholecystectomy.

In addition, the mobile in vivo robot was fitted for biopsy with a 2.4-mm-wide robotic grasper (Fig. 42-7). With this configuration, the robot has performed liver biopsy in a porcine model by navigating to and visualizing the biopsy site, followed by acquisition of tissue. After the biopsy, the robot is retracted through the entry incision, thus achieving a single-incision biopsy. This robot also has been tested during a NOTES procedure in a porcine model. The robot was introduced into the gastric lumen using a sterile overtube and a standard upper endoscope. The robot successfully explored the gastric cavity and then was introduced into

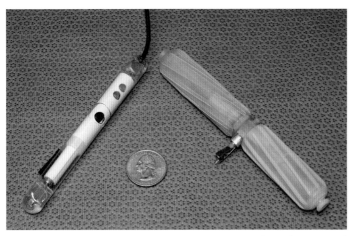

FIGURE 42-7 University of Nebraska's cooperative in vivo robots. The peritoneal imaging robot is on the left, and the mobile in vivo biopsy robot is on the right. (Photo courtesy of S. Farritor, University of Nebraska College of Engineering and Technology.)

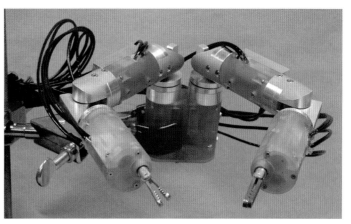

FIGURE 42-8 The dexterous operating robot with two articulating arms, from the University of Nebraska.

the peritoneal cavity through a transgastric incision. The endoscope was advanced through the same gastric incision and used to monitor the robot's activity. The robot and endoscope were then retracted into the stomach, and the gastrotomy was closed.

Our laboratory has produced other miniature in vivo robots that have been used successfully in a cooperative NOTES procedure. The peritoneum-mounted imaging robot (see Fig. 42-7), a device used for lighting and retraction, has been used in conjunction with a standard upper endoscope to explore and manipulate the peritoneal cavity. This robot is composed of an inner housing that contains a lens and focusing mechanism, LEDs for illumination, and a magnetic direct current motor for rotation. These inner components are enclosed within a clear outer housing. A magnetic cap is affixed to each end of the robot. These caps allow manipulation of the robot through movement of an exterior metal handle.

Although the mobile in vivo robots have shown promise in the area of visualization, more complex and dexterous robotic technology will be required for SILS or NOTES procedures. Our laboratory has been developing such a robot for NOTES and SILS use. This dexterous robot (Fig. 42-8) mimics the actions of laparoscopic tools working through separate abdominal wall trocars but uses a robotic platform that is capable of insertion into the peritoneal cavity. The robot consists of two articulating arms independently capable of 4 DOF. Once inserted into the peritoneal cavity, each arm emulates a typical laparoscopic instrument. Unlike a typical laparoscopic instrument inserted through a trocar, however, the robot's arms are not confined by the fulcrum effect of the incision.

The robot is restrained by an external support mounted to the operating room table. The robot is controlled through a remote console located in the operating room. Visual feedback is provided through a standard laparoscope. The current prototype allows the laparoscope to be inserted directly between the robot's arms to allow optimal visualization. The robot's arms currently are fitted with a grasper instrument and cautery arm. It has been used successfully for a porcine cholecystectomy. It can be repositioned from the same incision to reach all four abdominal quadrants. Although the current prototype requires a larger abdominal incision, miniaturization will provide a dexterous robot capable of SILS or NOTES procedures without the current limits of a single incision.

Trauma and Military Applications

One of the emerging applications for robotic surgery is the remote procedure, that is, an operation performed on a patient by a surgeon at a different location using a remote-controlled surgical robot (also known as *telesurgery*). Such technology may someday provide assistance to the military trauma surgeon and perhaps eventually to the general surgeon in remote areas. The idea of master-slave robotic systems is being expanded from the current application of both master and slave in the same room to a separation of many miles. This may allow for the surgeon to be remote from the battlefield or rural area and still provide immediate care via telesurgery.

Raven Robotic Surgical System

The BioRobotics Laboratory at the University of Washington has devised a robotic surgical system for telesurgery. The Raven Robotic Surgical System is a 7-DOF, spherical coordinate cable-actuated system for surgical manipulation. It is designed for both minimally invasive surgery and telesurgery. It has been field-tested in two telesurgery demonstrations, one using an unmanned aerial vehicle to simulate battlefield conditions, and one within the NASA Extreme Environment Mission Operations program (NEEMO). This program uses Aquarius, an underwater laboratory off the coast of Florida, to simulate the harsh environment of space. To test the Raven robot, two nonengineer Aquanauts set up the robot to perform a 2-day telesurgery experiment. Telesurgery has been feasible with the Raven, in part owing to its relatively simple master console (Fig. 42-9). The master console consists of two PHANTOM Omnis, a USB foot pedal, and two computers. One computer runs Skype or iChat for visual data input. The simple but effective design of the master-slave robots is one of the system's greatest attributes. The researchers did note, however, that latency time increased with the remoteness of the telesurgery procedure. Nonetheless, this robotic design suggests that simpler robotic system design may become useful in telesurgery.

UROLOGY

TRUS Robot

One of the main challenges of surgical prostatectomy is to preserve the neurovascular bundle, including cavernous nerve, so that sexual function is not affected. Although the da Vinci robot

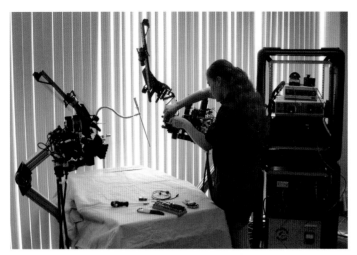

FIGURE 42-9 A researcher adjusts RAVEN before a telesurgery experiment. (Photo courtesy of M. Lum, BioRobotics Laboratory, University of Washington.)

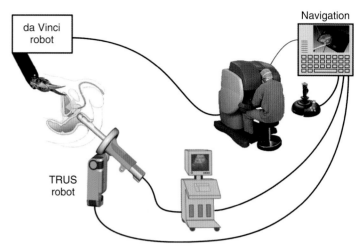

FIGURE 42-10 The setup configuration for the TRUS system. (Diagram courtesy of M. Han, James Buchanan Brady Urological Institute, Johns Hopkins University.)

provides stereoscopic vision and excellent dexterity in a small space, intraoperative bleeding and dense connective tissue can hamper visualization and place vital structures at risk. The James Buchanan Brady Urological Institute at Johns Hopkins University has developed a Trans-Rectal UltraSound (TRUS) probe robot for use in robotic prostatectomy to help overcome these obstacles. The TRUS robot was designed for use in a tandem robotic approach with the da Vinci Surgical System to improve visualization of the prostate, associated blood vessels, and nervous tissue. The robot consists of a rotating ultrasound probe that is placed transrectally, with the robot manipulating the ultrasound probe. The probe can record both ultrasound and Doppler data, allowing a 3D reconstruction of the prostate. The ultrasound also can demonstrate the da Vinci instruments. The surgeon has both a laparoscopic view and appreciation of the ultrasound images from a control console in the operating room (Fig. 42-10). This combination enables the surgeon to recognize the surgical instruments as well as the patient's anatomy during robotic prostatectomy.

MrBot

Image-guided prostate biopsy and needle-based intervention have used ultrasound for imaging. Although ultrasound has the advantage of real-time imaging and ease of use, the sensitivity for prostatic cancer is poor. Moreover, ultrasound is only useful for a transrectal approach. In contrast, magnetic resonance imaging (MRI) has up to 85% sensitivity for prostate tumors larger than 1 cm. MRI is not, however, a technology easily adaptable to robotics. In addition to the obvious preclusion of ferrous metals, the choice of motors is also severely limited; an electric motor can cause significant image artifacts. In response to these issues, the James Buchanan Brady Urological Institute at Johns Hopkins University has developed MrBot, a robot for accessing the prostate. MrBot is a completely nonmagnetic robotic system which is MRI compatible (Fig. 42-11). The control cabinet containing the robot's noncompatible parts stays outside the MRI suite and connects to the robot by hoses. The robot itself is designed to use a number of interchangeable needle drivers, permitting biopsy, thermal ablation, or seed brachytherapy. The robot allows for change of angulation from the same skin incision, a feat not possible through typical template biopsies. The robot has been shown to be accurate to within 1 mm for MRI-guided needle placement in MRI machines up to 7 Tesla. This robot may lead

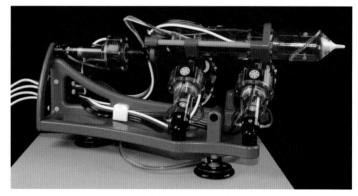

FIGURE 42-11 MrBot prototype. (Photo courtesy of D. Stoianovici, Robotics program, James Buchanan Brady Urological Institute, Johns Hopkins University.)

to image-directed therapy to augment or even replace surgical intervention.

OTOLARYNGOLOGY

Robotic System for Surgery of the Throat and Upper Airways

The surgical field of the throat and upper airways is deep and narrow. Laryngoscopic surgery has experienced little in the way of major advances since the 1980s. The narrow opening of the laryngoscope reduces depth perception and restricts instrumental DOF, which is particularly problematic for suturing. The Advanced Robotics and Mechanism Applications (ARMA) Laboratory at Columbia University, in conjunction with the Department of Otolaryngology at Johns Hopkins University, has designed a robot that uses the existing da Vinci master system coupled to a stereo laparoscope and two robotic slave arms with 20 joint-space DOF (Fig. 42-12). The functional ends of the robotic arms are called *distal dexterity units* (DDUs). Each DDU is capable of rotation about its backbone, enabling precise suturing with a standard curved needle. The researchers have been able to demonstrate the robot's ability to perform bimanual knot tying. The flexible system eventually should be capable of being inserted orally and then maneuvered down the throat. If successful, this system might be one of the first examples of a robotic NOTES device.

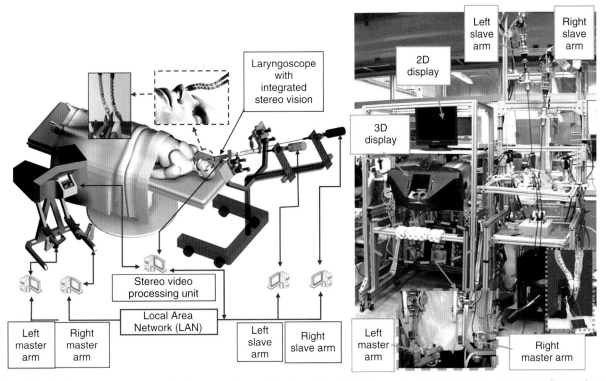

FIGURE 42-12 A minimally invasive surgery system for the upper airways. (Courtesy of Dr. Nabil Simaan, Vanderbilt University, and Dr. Russell H. Taylor, Johns Hopkins University. Modified from Simaan N, Xu K, Kapoor A, et al: Design and integration of a telerobotic system for minimally invasive surgery of the throat. *Int J Robot Res* 28:1134-1153, 2009, Fig. 3.)

CARDIOLOGY

Uniaxial Force Sensor for Minimally Invasive Surgery

The Harvard School of Engineering and Applied Sciences, in conjunction with the University of British Columbia Department of Electrical and Computer Engineering, has developed a uniaxial force sensor for cardiac surgery. This sensor consists of a waterproof 12- × 5.5-mm tube using light transmission and reception to determine force applied (Fig. 42-13). The light-transmitting diodes are separated from phototransistor circuits by an elastic element that is compressed as the force is applied, yielding increased light intensity. The change in light intensity determines the force measurement. The sensor is both waterproof and electrically passive in order to minimize disturbance to normal heart conduction. In addition, the tube is hollow, permitting passage of tools. This device should be useful for cases such as beating-heart mitral valve annuloplasty, in which it is crucial to seat a cardiac valve without causing tissue damage. Porcine experimentation has yielded adequate results. This force sensor advances the concept of operation-specific robotics and should improve haptics for beating-heart surgery.

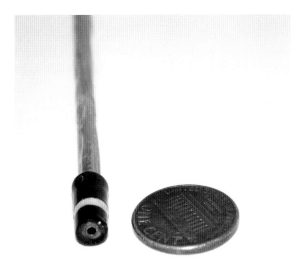

FIGURE 42-13 Uniaxial Force Sensor for cardiac surgery. (Photo courtesy of M. Yip, University of British Columbia Department of Electrical and Computer Engineering.)

Robust Three-Dimensional Motion Tracking for Beating-Heart Surgery

Another obstacle to overcome in beating-heart surgery is the motion of the heart and accompanying respirations. Miniaturized heart stabilizers still are unable to cancel out significant residual motion, leaving the surgeon to manually cancel motion. Researchers at the Montpellier Laboratory of Informatics, Robotics, and Microelectrics (LIRRM) have developed a visual tracking system for robot-assisted beating-heart surgery that allows the surgeon to compensate for the motion of the beating heart. The system uses image markers on the heart in addition to stereoscopic laparoscopy to track tissue motion. A virtually stable workspace synchronizes the motion of the surgical tools with cardiac motion and gives the appearance of a motionless heart to the surgeon.

Visual tracking often is achieved by identifying features of the object to be tracked, particularly for rigid objects. The heart not only is compliant but also has relatively homogenous regions. In addition, the heart's surface is reflective, which can interfere with mapping. The Montpellier researchers overcame these obstacles

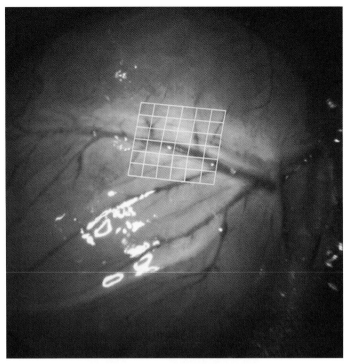

FIGURE 42-14 Robust 3D Motion Tracking for Beating-Heart Surgery. The grid demonstrates tracking results using an image sequence from an in vivo porcine beating heart. (Photo courtesy of R. Richa, Montpellier Laboratory of Informatics, Robotics, and Microelectrics.)

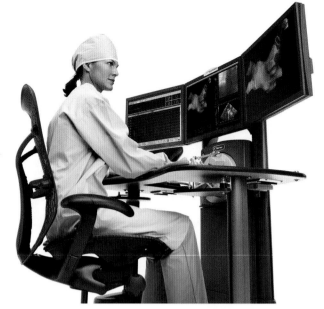

FIGURE 42-15 Sensei X Robotic Catheter System Workstation. (Courtesy of Hansen Medical.)

using a technology called thin-plate spline modeling. They have been able to map an ex vivo porcine heart within 0.19 to 0.24 mm and have demonstrated tracking ability using a video of beating-heart surgery from a da Vinci procedure and also from a beating porcine heart (Fig. 42-14).

Sensei X Robotic Catheter System

The Sensei X Robotic Catheter System (Hansen Medical, Mountain View, Calif.), currently in clinical trials, seeks to improve catheter-based ablation techniques used to treat cardiac arrhythmias. The apparatus consists of a master console with 3D visualization (Fig. 42-15) and an instinctive motion controller, a table-mounted remote catheter manipulator, and an ablation catheter. The catheter's flexibility is provided by 6 DOF. The 3D visualization system facilitates catheter guidance. Catheter guidance also is helped with a haptic sensor on the catheter end that detects changes in pressure, thereby decreasing the risk for tissue damage. It is hypothesized that placing the catheter's movements under robotic control will improve efficacy, decrease procedure time, modify the operator learning curve, and reduce radiation exposure. There are other robots available for catheter ablation, but not with the same degree of haptic feedback and visualization technology. Additionally, other devices rely on magnetic guidance, which makes some patients ineligible for treatment. The Sensei X robot also is able to return with accuracy to sites of treatment. With current catheter ablation technology, both target acquisition and maintenance of stability rely on operator skill. The current technology also requires close proximity of the operator to the radiation source. The Sensei X robot allows the operator to remain meters away from the field, thus reducing the exposure risk.

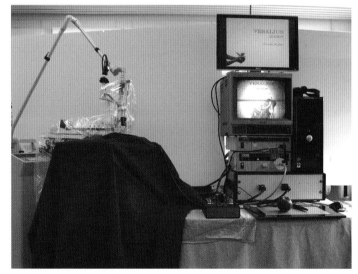

FIGURE 42-16 Setup for Vesalius robot for laser ablation system. (Photo courtesy of H. Tang, Catholic University of Leuven.)

GYNECOLOGY

Laser Ablation System with Intuitive Writing Interface

Researchers at the Catholic University of Leuven have developed a unique system for laser ablation of endometrial implants that uses an intuitive writing interface (Fig. 42-16). Traditionally, ablation of endometrial implants has been accomplished with an operative laparoscope equipped with a carbon dioxide laser. The surgeon would manipulate the laparoscope to direct the laser beam. As with all laparoscopic instruments, only 4 DOF are possible, and gross hand movements of the surgeon are exaggerated at the laser-tissue interface. The Catholic University system includes a laparoscope-positioning robot and a carbon dioxide laser designed for laparoscopic use. The researchers wanted to create a more natural human-computer interface and sought to

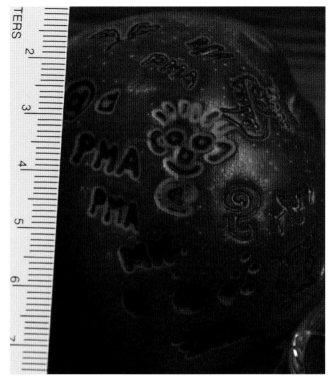

FIGURE 42-17 An example of the precision that can be achieved with the intuitive writing interface of a robotic laser ablation system. (Photo courtesy of H. Tang, Catholic University of Leuven.)

exploit the similarities between drawing or writing and laser ablation. The user interface for this robot uses a stylus on a pad capable of translating human writing into commands for the robot to perform. The surgeon draws with the stylus while watching on a monitor the area to be ablated. This system introduces a novel concept for the user interface, in which "what you draw is what you cut." The intention would be more precise control of the laser. This laser ablation robot may become an alternative to cautery for laparoscopic procedures and may replace the hand-held laser. The researchers have demonstrated the precision of their system using an apple as a tissue surrogate (Fig. 42-17).

CONCLUSION

The use of robotic technology to augment (or even replace) a surgeon is becoming more of a reality. A number of surgical systems already are in use and approved by the FDA. In this chapter we have described some of this technology from a user perspective. The important concepts to the reader include the

ability to understand the current capabilities of surgical robotics, the current challenges with the existing technology, and what may be in the future. Although the da Vinci surgical robot was one of the first units to enjoy practical success, at this point it represents older ways of thinking about robotic manipulation. The da Vinci system mimics the surgeon's capabilities but does not transcend the surgeon's limitations. Surgical robots of the future may need to present a paradigm shift to surgical practice in order to be successful. Machines will need to be purpose-built for specific procedures, allowing the surgeon to accomplish tasks that could not be accomplished without that robot. Our own work in miniature robotics has taught us that a problem-based approach to surgical robotics can facilitate the development and testing of new technologic improvements by concentrating on the necessary tasks. A small robot that can be inserted through a natural orifice and enables the surgeon to perform laparoscopic manipulation should decrease the difficulty and increase the feasibility of natural orifice procedures compared with that possible with current instrument technology. In the future, these and other technologies undoubtedly will be smarter, faster, and less expensive, similar to the way that minimally invasive surgical instrumentation progressed from the 1990s to the present. Similar to the advent of minimally invasive surgery, it is foreseeable that robotic technology will change surgical paradigms in the decades to come.

Suggested Readings

Glass P, Cheung E, Sitti M: A legged anchoring mechanism for capsule endoscopes using micropatterned adhesives, *IEEE Trans Biomed Eng* 55:2759–2767, 2008.

Hillel AT, Kapoor A, Simaan N, et al: Applications of robotics for laryngeal surgery, *Otolaryngol Clin North Am* 41:781–791, vii, 2008.

Kanagaratnam P, Koa-Wing M, Wallace DT, et al: Experience of robotic catheter ablation in humans using a novel remotely steerable catheter sheath, *J Interv Card Electrophysiol* 21:19–26, 2008.

Lathrop RA, Hackworth DM, Webster RJ 3rd: Minimally invasive holographic surface scanning for soft-tissue image registration, *IEEE Trans Biomed Eng* 57:1497–1506, 2010.

Lehman A, Tiwari M, Shah B, et al: Recent advances in the CoBRASurge robotic manipulator and dexterous miniature in vivo robotics for minimally invasive surgery, *Proc IMechE Part C: J Mech Eng Sci* 224:1–8, 2010.

Mozer PC, Partin AW, Stoianovici D: Robotic image-guided needle interventions of the prostate, *Rev Urol* 11:7–15, 2009.

Macura KJ, Stoianovici D: Advancements in magnetic resonance-guided robotic interventions in the prostate, *Top Magn Reson Imaging* 19:297–304, 2008.

Rentschler ME, Dumpert J, Platt SR, et al: Natural orifice surgery with an endoluminal mobile robot, *Surg Endosc* 21:1212–1215, 2007.

Toenies J, Tortora G, Simf M, et al: Swallowable medical devices for diagnosis and surgery: The state of the art, *Proc ImechE PartC: J Mech Eng Sci* 224:1397–1414, 2009.

Yip MC, Yuen SG, Howe RD: A robust uniaxial force sensor for minimally invasive surgery, *IEEE Trans Biomed Eng* 57:1008–1011, 2010.

TIMOTHY M. RUFF, CONSTANTINE T. FRANTZIDES, AND ALEXANDER T. FRANTZIDES

New Minimally Invasive Surgery Technologies

The videos associated with this chapter are listed in the Video Contents and can be found on the accompanying DVDs and
on Expertconsult.com.

In the chapter titled "The Future of Laparoscopy" in the 1995 textbook, *Laparoscopic and Thoracoscopic Surgery*, we predicted that "we will see drastic changes both in techniques and instrumentation" for laparoscopy. At that time, laparoscopy had become the preferred method for cholecystectomy, and fundoplication and herniorrhaphy were "on their way to being accepted." Indeed, the advantages of laparoscopic surgery over open surgery are becoming more and more accepted. These include better visualization, decreased postoperative pain, decreased length of stay, and a faster recovery. In oncologic surgery, it is often possible to begin adjuvant therapy much sooner because the much smaller wounds heal much quicker, and there is in general a faster recovery from the surgery. In the early stages of laparoscopy, visionaries and innovators recognized that optics and imaging systems needed to be refined for more advanced procedures to be performed, and they have. Additionally, robotics were predicted to invade the operating suite, and they have found an increasing number of uses. Laparoscopic staplers were expected to be developed; they are now in widespread use and are continuing to be improved. Indeed, during the past two decades, many new technologies have been developed in laparoscopy, and several others are in an evolutionary state.

As can be seen from the preceding chapters, there has been a tremendous advancement in the scope of laparoscopic surgery during the past two decades. For a new technology to become successful, it needs to improve on the currently available technology—whether it is safer, smaller, cheaper, more user-friendly, or in some other way better. Indeed, appropriate coverage for all new technologies in minimally invasive surgery would be far beyond the scope of this chapter. The intent is simply to mention the highlights of new technologies. This advancement in technology has not been possible without the assistance of the medical industry to produce better, more technologically advanced devices to perform more complicated surgeries using smaller and smaller incisions. All these technologic advancements need to be accomplished without compromising patient safety, yet also at a reasonable cost, so that the payers will continue to reimburse for the surgical procedures. This chapter introduces some of the newer technologies in the field of laparoscopic surgery in general, as provided by certain manufacturers. Surgical robotics are well covered in Chapter 42. It should be noted that similar technologies have been produced by different companies, and this chapter seeks to demonstrate an example of each.

MINIMALLY INVASIVE SURGERY STAPLERS

Surgical staplers are used in a variety of laparoscopic and thoracoscopic surgical procedures. Characteristics of an effective stapler include the ability to manage tissue variability, the ability to staple thick tissues effectively, the ability to staple with staggered compression, the ability to optimize hemostasis and burst pressure strength, and the ability to improve tissue retention during manipulation and transaction. The stapler must be ergonomically easy to grasp as well as being usable by a variety of hand sizes and strengths. An example of such a stapler that satisfies all of these characteristics is the recently released Endo GIA Ultra Universal Stapler (Covidien, Norwalk, Conn.) (Fig. 43-1). In addition, this stapler can be used as a grasper alone before firing the staples. Other companies produce similar products.

There are also a variety of staple heights available for each type of reload for the surgical stapler. Usually, the stapler reloads are color coded according to the staple height, to allow for better recognition in the operating room. The larger staple height is better for thicker tissue, whereas the smaller height is more applicable to thinner tissue, or even vascular tissue. It is important to match staple height to the tissue to be stapled. Too tall of a staple may result in an inadequate seal as well as a potential for hemorrhage, whereas too short of a staple may not penetrate the tissue fully, potentially resulting in an anastomotic leak. Covidien has recently improved on the staple reloads with the Tri-Staple Technology (Fig. 43-2). This technology varies the staple height in a given reload to facilitate use over a broader range of tissue thickness and also includes a stronger fixed anvil for easier maneuverability. The cartridge face is stepped, as opposed to being flat in previous versions of the reload. This encourages lateral diffusion of tissue fluids during clamping and firing, which decreases the force required to compress the tissue. A stronger knife blade assists with cutting of thicker tissues, and larger anvil buckets are used to ensure good staple formation. The Extra Thick (black) reloads with the Tri-Staple Technology allow the reload to staple tissue up to 3-mm thick using 5-mm staples. This is especially useful for challenging cases such as bariatric revisions as well as pulmonary lobectomies in radiated tissue. The Endo GIA Curved Tip Reloads with Tri-Staple Technology include a gold-colored curved tip at the distal end of the reload, providing enhanced visualization of the anvil tip (Fig. 43-3). This curved tip can be used for blunt dissection and tissue manipulation before firing

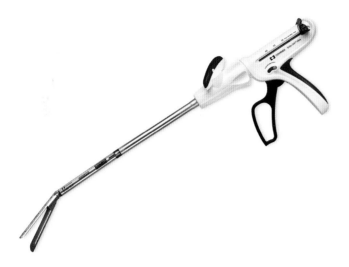

FIGURE 43-1 Endo GIA Ultra Universal Stapler (Covidien, Norwalk, Conn.).

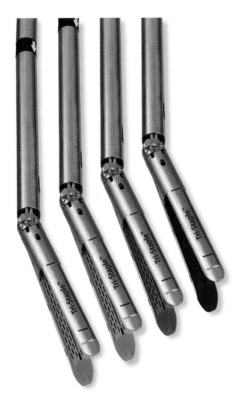

FIGURE 43-2 Endo GIA Tri-Staple Reloads (Covidien, Norwalk, Conn.) with a variety of staple heights.

the stapler. A radiopaque flexible introducer can be mounted onto the curved tip, assisting with placement of the stapler onto a target structure.

LAPAROSCOPIC INSTRUMENTS

The technology behind minimally invasive surgical instruments continues to evolve. Although several companies produce various types of laparoscopic instruments, Snowden-Pencer (San Diego, Calif.) has developed instruments that are able to be disassembled, thus allowing visual inspection of surfaces during the cleaning process (Fig. 43-4). In addition, hand fatigue has been reduced with a newly stylized handle to more evenly distribute pressure, as well as thumb actuation ridges for easier operation and

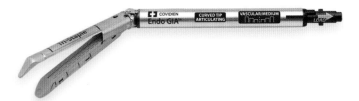

FIGURE 43-3 Endo GIA Tri-Staple Reload with Gold Tip (Covidien, Norwalk, Conn.) used for blunt dissection and tissue manipulation prior to firing the stapler.

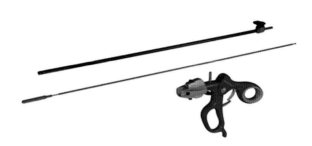

FIGURE 43-4 Laparoscopic ergonomic take-apart instrument (Snowden-Pencer, San Diego, Calif.).

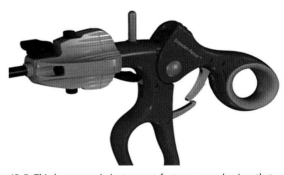

FIGURE 43-5 This laparoscopic instrument features a mechanism that can be used with or without the ratchet function (Snowden-Pencer, San Diego, Calif.).

cushioned inserts to reduce thumb pressure. There is also an integrated ratchet mechanism that allows the same instrument to be used either with or without the ratchet, thus greatly improving versatility (Fig. 43-5).

Laparoscopy inherently prevents surgeons from using their hands directly on the tissue. Several types of metal have been used to grasp tissue, but these can cause traumatic injury to the tissue if grasped too strongly or dropping of the tissue if grasped too loosely. Secure atraumatic graspers are an essential part of any advanced laparoscopic procedure. An example is the atraumatic minimally invasive surgery grasper, in which the jaws have a disposable membrane made of a hydrophobic porous proprietary mesh that allows a gentle yet secure grip on the tissue, thus avoiding tissue trauma (Trigonon Inc., Milwaukee, Wis.) (Fig. 43-6).

LAPAROSCOPES

Minimally invasive surgery has historically been performed with laparoscopes using either a 0-, 30-, or 45-degree viewing direction. Although the variety of angles in the laparoscope is

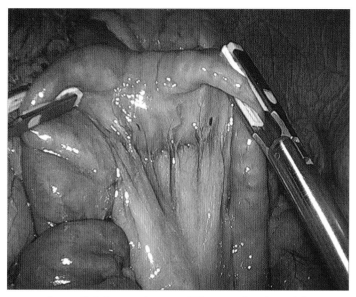

FIGURE 43-6 Atraumatic grasper (Trigonon, Milwaukee, Wis.).

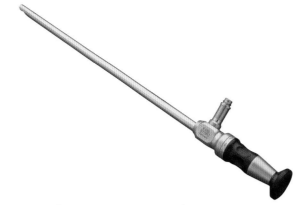

FIGURE 43-7 EndoCAMeleon rigid endoscope (Karl Storz, Tuttlingen, Germany).

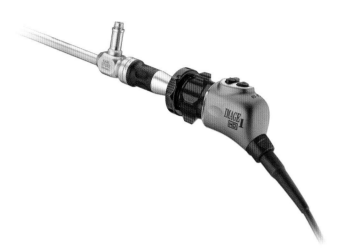

FIGURE 43-8 Image 1 HD video platform and autoclavable H3-ZA camera head (Karl Storz, Tuttlingen, Germany).

advantageous for seeing around various structures, changing from one angle to another involves removing the laparoscope, disconnecting the camera and light source and reconnecting them to the new laparoscope, cleaning the lens, and reinserting the laparoscope to the correct position. In the past, attempts were made to view a variety of angles using a device similar to the flexible endoscope. Unfortunately, this resulted in the surgeon frequently becoming disoriented because of the frequent changes in the camera angle as well as the creation of blind spots. Karl Storz (Tuttlingen, Germany) has developed the EndoCAMeleon rigid endoscope, which gives a variable viewing direction (Fig. 43-7). The rotation is accomplished with a knob that rotates the viewing direction anywhere between 0 and 120 degrees, but all in a single plane. This variable rotation greatly decreases disorientation, makes intraoperative laparoscope changes obsolete, and therefore reduces operative time.

VIDEO EQUIPMENT

The human eye can recognize only 780 horizontal lines of image resolution on a monitor screen. The camera and video equipment are already up to this standard with the commonly available high-definition (HD) video. The video platform can also improve visualization of the surgical field. By use of the full HD technology with 16:9 aspect, the surgeon is provided with improved depth perception and color contrast for optimal surgical performance, decreasing eye fatigue during long procedures. An example of such technology is the Image 1 HD video platform and autoclavable H3-ZA camera head (Karl Storz) (Fig. 43-8). Additional detail can be provided using a second camera to create a three-dimensional image, such as is done with the commercially available robot.

BIOLOGIC MESH

There are several indications for prosthesis placement, such as for repair of any of a wide variety of hernias, urinary incontinence, reconstruction of the pelvic floor, abdominal and thoracic wall repair, and muscle flap reinforcement. Biologic mesh is produced from a variety of sources, depending on the manufacturer. Synthetic mesh, although much less expensive, can be prone to

infection, erosion, and adhesions. Its long-term durability, however, is much better than that of the biologic products. Biologic mesh is less likely to become infected by bacteria, and therefore its main indication is in the presence of an infected, or potentially infected, field. It is also much less likely to erode into a vital structure. If there is a need for mesh in the presence of any type of potentially infected field, such as during the construction of any type of bowel anastomosis, the biologic mesh would be more appropriate than the synthetic mesh. An example of a biologic mesh is the Veritas Collagen Matrix made by Synovis (St. Paul, Minn.). It minimizes tissue attachment to the matrix in the case of direct contact with viscera. Its thin and pliable character allows for easy laparoscopic use; can be introduced through a trocar, fixated with sutures, staples, or tacks; and readily adapts to the anatomic structure.

Veritas is a bovine pericardium whose processing reduces the potential immunogenicity without interfering with host cell infiltration, revascularization, or gradual replacement with host tissue. This results in a non-cross-linked biologic implant that is acellular, highly biocompatible, and nonantigenic. This allows the mesh to remodel, making the repair histologically indistinguishable from the adjacent host tissue. Bovine pericardium is predominantly type I collagen with very little elastin that allows for a high resistance to stretch and remains pliable and strong, despite being thin. Its resistance to wear and tear as well as the ease of use is why bovine pericardium has been used for many decades in neurologic, vascular, and cardiac procedures as well as in soft tissue repair of abdominal and thoracic defects.

In two recently published trials studying Veritas as well as other biologic meshes, several important characteristics were studied. When looked at collectively, the composite score showed that Veritas Collagen Matrix scored the highest at all time points studied (1, 6, and 12 months).

Synovis has also applied the technology behind Veritas Collagen Matrix into a staple line reinforcement, called Peri-Strips Dry. The use of Peri-Strips Dry has been shown to allow for a stronger staple line with significantly fewer anastomotic leaks and surgical complications as well as a decrease in bleeding. It is available for both linear and circular staplers and can be used in essentially any soft tissue anastomosis. However, there is concern about using any staple line reinforcement in any kind of anastomosis in which staple lines cross each other, such as with gastrojejunostomy when using a circular stapler.

NATURAL ORIFICE TRANSLUMINAL ENDOSCOPIC SURGERY

The application of natural orifice transluminal endoscopic surgery (NOTES) is still years away from its routine use. It is covered in detail in Chapter 14. It involves using a natural body orifice to obtain access to the peritoneal cavity, most commonly either the mouth or vagina, but also access through the rectum and even urethra has been reported. NOTES can be applied with the assistance of laparoscopy—usually an additional trocar for retraction assistance, or "pure-NOTES," in which no other incisions are made. There have been several instances of NOTES being used, most commonly cholecystectomy. Other surgeries reportedly performed include Heller myotomy, sentinel lymph node biopsy with sigmoid colon resection, sleeve gastrectomy, nephrectomy, tubal sterilization, and splenectomy. The advantages include many of those of traditional laparoscopic surgery, although with pure-NOTES, there is no skin incision. Several issues with NOTES are currently being investigated. Studies are ongoing in regard to the best method of closure of the gastrotomy as well as the best method of beginning the initial pneumoperitoneum. Ongoing improvements in technology will be necessary to allow NOTES to advance further, including the development of flexible instruments such as graspers, clip appliers, and even staplers. As intriguing as NOTES is from a technologic standpoint, it remains to be seen how far it will advance into everyday use.

PREDICTION OF THE FUTURE OF MINIMALLY INVASIVE SURGERY

There are many frontiers to which laparoscopic surgery may advance, for the betterment of patients. These depend on technologic improvements and on surgeons working together with industry.

Image Converter

It is well known that the ideal placement for the camera is in the same view as the operating surgeon. In advanced laparoscopic procedures such as gastric bypass and incisional hernia repair, the camera is often located 180 degrees from the surgeon, producing a mirror image to the surgeon. Even experienced laparoscopic surgeons often have difficulty when the camera is located on the opposite side of the patient from the surgeon. An image converter will take the digital image and reverse it left to right, and possibly upside-down as well. Studies have shown that when an image converter is applied, thus eliminating the mirror image, both novice and experienced surgeons are able to complete various tasks in a trainer much quicker and more accurately. Further development of this rather straightforward device would significantly improve surgeon performance in situations of mirror-image visualization.

Levitation

Prognosticators have hypothesized about the use of magnetic levitation in minimally invasive surgery. Pneumoperitoneum would be introduced by the method of the surgeon's choice through a single standard trocar. Small, possibly even microscopic, "bullets" could then be inserted through the trocar. A magnetic field would then be created in three dimensions, which could be controlled, to "levitate" the bullet-like devices or even small transformers. The transformers could have specific abilities, such as cutting, grasping, or coagulating. They could also be multifunctional, like a Swiss Army Knife. For example, one could be equipped with a surveillance camera and controlled remotely by levitation, providing images from a variety of angles and thus improving visualization. Obviously, realization of this idea is still several years away.

Data Glove

Commercially available data gloves on the market today are used in virtual reality simulations. The data glove is worn on the operator's hand and contains many sensors that convert the motion of the fingers to a digital signal that can be transmitted to a remote location. It is theorized that this could find several applications in surgery (Fig. 43-9). This may be used to operate remotely, thus expanding the outreach of advanced surgical care to underserved rural areas. There has always been a concern about the astronaut in deep space who needs urgent surgery. The data glove may be applicable to allow an Earth-based surgeon to perform the operation on the astronaut in space. In addition, the data glove may find application in the training and evaluation of surgeons, in the terms of an advanced simulator.

Nanotechnology

Nanotechnology is the science of systems in which the key component or the whole system itself measures 1 to 100 nanometers, or about 1000 times thinner than a common sheet of paper. There are an amazing, and ever-increasing, number of potential uses of nanotechnology (Fig. 43-10). Disease detection and drug delivery directly to a specific location in the human body could someday be accomplished with nanotechnology. Also, nanocrystals can be attached to cells and then imaged to track the cellular processes at the level of a single cell. Antimicrobial coatings, such as the commonly used silver, but also gold or even diamonds, can be applied with the use of nanotechnology. Conceivably, biomedical sensors could be developed to alert a patient or doctor about changes in commonly measured values, such as heart rate and blood glucose levels. Artificial organs and tissue can be engineered with the use of nanotechnology to assist in hernia surgery and transplantation surgery. The smart scalpel is a gold-based device that can give the surgeon the touch sensitivity of the

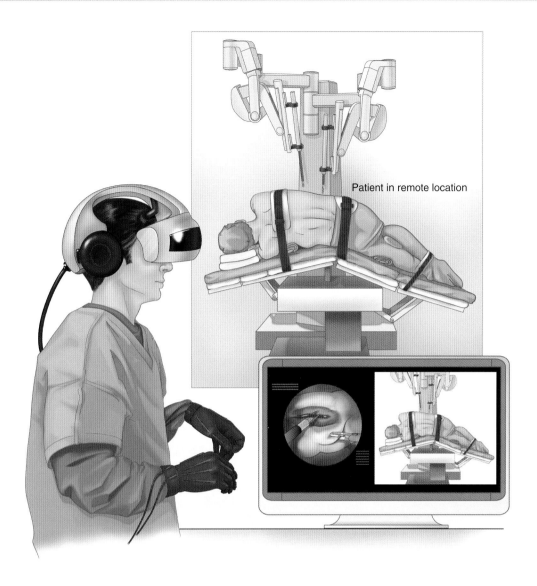

FIGURE 43-9 Remotely controlled operation with a data glove. (Redrawn from Frantzides CT, editor: *Laparoscopic and Thoracoscopic Surgery*, St. Louis, 1995, Mosby.)

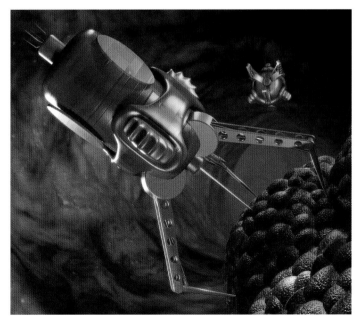

FIGURE 43-10 Medical nanorobot injecting a drug into a tumor. (Courtesy of Roger Harris/Photo Researchers Inc.)

human finger. A new Harmonic scalpel is being developed that distinguishes between soft tissue, blood vessel, and bone. Nano-tweezers use the energy of laser light to manipulate tiny nanoscale objects with the goal of removing or replacing sections of genes or cells. Nanobots are being developed to be introduced through a major artery, enter the aorta, measure the valve pressure gradients, and possibly even repair the valve.

Bioglue

Biologic glue has been used in various types of surgeries, including vascular and transplantation surgery. However, its use has been recently expanded to include mesh fixation for inguinal hernia mesh, crural reinforcement for a large intrathoracic stomach, and even ventral hernias. This may reduce the need for tacking devices, possibly helping to decrease postoperative pain. Applications of enteric anastomosis using biologic glue, either alone or as reinforcement for sutures or staples, have been studied and may someday be used routinely. There has been a report of a bioglue used successfully on an inferior venal caval anastomosis in an animal.

CONCLUSION

This is an exciting time in minimally invasive surgery. Not that long ago, surgeons were limited to the scalpel and a small selection of suture material. There is now an ever-expanding selection of tools and devices to help perform increasingly complex procedures easier, faster, and with better results and to help patients recover more quickly and resume their normal activities sooner. There are also several intriguing technologies on the horizon that will continue to be developed and refined, such as NOTES, the data glove, levitation, and the image converter. Nanotechnology will continue to find further applications as well.

ACKNOWLEDGMENTS

Pictures and videos of products have been provided by Covidien, V. Mueller/Snowden Pencer, Trigonon Inc., Karl Storz, and Synovis.

DISCLOSURE

Dr. Constantine T. Frantzides is the inventor of the atraumatic graspers.

Suggested Readings

Angrisani L, Cutolo PP, Buchwald JN, et al: Laparoscopic reinforced sleeve gastrectomy: Early results and complications, *Obes Surg* 21:783–793, 2011.

Arnold W, Shikora SA: A comparison of burst pressure between buttressed versus non-buttressed staple-lines in an animal model, *Obes Surg* 15:164–171, 2005.

Deeken CR, Melman L, Jenkins ED, et al: Histologic and biomechanical evaluation of crosslinked and non-crosslinked biologic meshes in a porcine model of ventral incisional hernia repair, *J Am Coll Surg* 212:880–888, 2011.

Frangou C: Is nanotechnology the next revolution in surgery? *Gen Surg News* 36:1, 6, 8–9, 2009.

Frantzides, CT, Carlson, MA: The future of laparoscopic surgery. In Frantzides CT, editor: *Laparoscopic and Thoracoscopic Surgery*, St. Louis, 1995, Mosby, pp 285–288.

Gill RS, Al-Adra DP, Mangat H, et al: Image inversion and digital mirror-image technology aid laparoscopic surgery task performance in the paradoxical view: A randomized controlled trial, *Surg Endosc* 25:3535–3539, 2011.

Johnston WK 3rd, Low RK, Das S: Image converter eliminates mirror imaging during laparoscopy, *J Endourol* 17:327–331, 2003.

Melman L, Jenkins ED, Hamilton NA, et al: Early biocompatibility of crosslinked and non-crosslinked biologic meshes in a porcine model of ventral hernia repair, *Hernia* 15:157–164, 2011.

Mintz Y, Horgan S, Cullen J, et al: NOTES: A review of the technical problems encountered and their solutions, *J Laparoendosc Adv Surg Tech* 18:583–587, 2008.

Nau P, Ellsion E, Muscarella P, et al: A review of 130 humans enrolled in transgastric NOTES protocols at a single institution, *Surg Endosc* 25:1004–1011, 2011.

Ramirez MC, Rodriguez J, Varghese F, et al: Reinforced circular stapler in bariatric surgery, *JSLS* 14:358–363, 2010.

Sajid MS, Khatri K, Singh K, Sayegh M: Use of staple-line reinforcement in laparoscopic gastric bypass surgery: A meta-analysis, *Surg Endosc* 25:2884–2891, 2011.

Shikora SA, Kim JJ, Tarnoff ME: Comparison of permanent and nonpermanent staple line buttressing materials for linear gastric staple lines during laparoscopic Roux-en-Y gastric bypass, *Surg Obes Relat Dis* 4:729–734, 2008.

Sodergren M, Clark J, Athanasiou T, et al: Natural orifice transluminal endoscopic surgery: Critical appraisal of applications in clinical practice, *Surg Endosc* 23:680–687, 2009.

Spector D, Perry Z, Konobeck T, et al: Comparison of hemostatic properties between collagen and synthetic buttress materials used in staple line reinforcement in a swine splenic hemorrhage model, *Surg Endosc* 25:1148–1152, 2011.

Tomikawa M, Xu H, Hashizume M: Current status and prerequisites for natural orifice transluminal endoscopic surgery (NOTES), *Surg Today* 40:909–916, 2010.

Index

Page numbers followed by "f" indicate figures, "t" indicate tables.